RN Adult Medical Surgical Nursing
Review Module Edition 8.0

Contributors

Audrey Knippa, MS, MPH, RN, CNE
Nursing Education Coordinator and
  Content Project Leader

Sheryl Sommer, PhD, MSN, RN
Director, Nursing Curriculum and
  Education Services

Brenda Ball, MEd, BSN, RN
Nursing Education Specialist

Lois Churchill, MN, RN
Nursing Education Specialist

Carrie B. Elkins, DHSc, MSN, PHCNS, BC
Nursing Education Specialist

Mary Jane Janowski, MA, BSN, RN
Nursing Resource Specialist

Karin Roberts, PhD, MSN, RN, CNE
Nursing Education Coordinator

Mendy G. Wright, DNP, MSN, RN
Nursing Education Specialist

Derek Prater, MS Journalism
Lead Product Developer and Editorial Project Leader

Erika A. Archer, BS Education, Foreign Language
Product Developer

Johanna Barnes, BA Journalism
Product Developer

Chris Crawford, BS Journalism
Product Developer

Hilary E. Groninger, BS Journalism
Product Developer

Megan E. Herre, BS Journalism
Product Developer

Amanda Lehman, BA English
Product Developer

Joanna Shindler, BA Journalism
Product Developer

Brant L. Stacy, BS Journalism, BA English
Product Developer

Consultants

Christi Blair, MSN, RN

Tracey Bousquet, BSN, RN

Joyce Campbell, MSN, CCRN, FNP-BC

Fleurdeliza T. Cuyco, BSN

Deb Johnson-Schuh, MSN, RN

Terri Lemon, MSN, RN

Veronica Njie-Carr, PhD, APRN-BC

INTELLECTUAL PROPERTY NOTICE

IMPORTANT NOTICE TO THE READER

USER'S GUIDE

Welcome to the Assessment Technologies Institute® RN Adult Medical Surgical Nursing Review Module Edition 8.0. The mission of ATI's Content Mastery Series® review modules is to provide user-friendly compendiums of nursing knowledge that will:

- Help you locate important information quickly.

- Assist in your remediation efforts.

- Provide exercises for applying your nursing knowledge.

- Facilitate your entry into the nursing profession as a newly licensed RN.

Organization

This review module is organized into units covering the foundations of nursing care (Unit 1), body systems and physiological processes (Units 2 to 13), and perioperative nursing care (Unit 14). Chapters within these units conform to one of three organizing principles for presenting the content:

- Nursing concepts

- Procedures (diagnostic and therapeutic)

- Systems disorders

Nursing concepts chapters begin with an overview describing the central concept and its relevance to nursing. Subordinate themes are covered in outline form to demonstrate relationships and present the information in a clear, succinct manner.

Procedures chapters include an overview describing the procedure(s) covered in the chapter. These chapters will provide you with nursing knowledge relevant to each procedure, including indications, interpretations of findings, client outcomes, nursing actions, and complications.

Systems disorders chapters include an overview describing the disorder(s) and/or disease process. These chapters may provide information on health promotion and disease prevention before addressing assessments, including risk factors, subjective data, and objective data. Next, you will focus on collaborative care, including nursing care, medications, interdisciplinary care, therapeutic procedures, surgical interventions, care after discharge, and client outcomes. Finally, you will find complications related to the disorder, along with nursing actions in response to those complications.

Application Exercises

Questions are provided at the end of each chapter so you can practice applying your knowledge. The Application Exercises include both NCLEX-style questions, such as multiple-choice and multiple-select items, and questions that ask you to apply your knowledge in other formats, such as short-answer and matching items. After the Application Exercises, an answer key is provided, along with rationales for the answers.

NCLEX® Connections

To prepare for the NCLEX-RN, it is important for you to understand how the content in this review module is connected to the NCLEX-RN test plan. You can find information on the detailed test plan at the National Council of State Boards of Nursing's Web site: https://www.ncsbn.org/. When reviewing content in this review module, regularly ask yourself, "How does this content fit into the test plan, and what types of questions related to this content should I expect?"

To help you in this process, we've included NCLEX Connections at the beginning of each unit and with each question in the Application Exercises Answer Keys. The NCLEX Connections at the beginning of each unit will point out areas of the detailed test plan that relate to the content within that unit. The NCLEX Connections attached to the Application Exercises Answer Keys will demonstrate how each exercise fits within the detailed content outline.

These NCLEX Connections will help you understand how the detailed content outline is organized, starting with major client needs categories and subcategories and followed by related content areas and tasks. The major client needs categories are:

- Safe and Effective Care Environment
  - Management of Care
  - Safety and Infection Control
- Health Promotion and Maintenance
- Psychosocial Integrity
- Physiological Integrity
  - Basic Care and Comfort
  - Pharmacological and Parenteral Therapies
  - Reduction of Risk Potential
  - Physiological Adaptation

An NCLEX Connection might, for example, alert you that content within a unit is related to:

- Reduction of Risk Potential
  - Diagnostic Tests
    - Evaluate the results of diagnostic testing and intervene as needed.

Icons

Icons are used throughout the review module to draw your attention to particular areas. Keep an eye out for these icons:

 This icon indicates an Overview, or introduction, to a particular subject matter. Descriptions and categories will typically be found in an Overview.

 This icon is used for the Application Exercises and the Application Exercises Answer Keys.

 This icon is used for NCLEX connections.

This icon is used for gerontological content. When you see this icon, take note of information that is specific to aging or the care of older adult clients.

This icon is used for content related to safety. When you see this icon, take note of safety concerns or steps that nurses can take to ensure client safety and a safe environment.

 This icon indicates that a media supplement, such as a graphic, an animation, or a video, is available. If you have an electronic copy of the review module, this icon will appear alongside clickable links to media supplements. If you have a hardcopy version of the review module, visit www.atitesting.com for details on how to access these features.

Feedback

ATI welcomes feedback regarding this review module. Please provide comments to: comments@ atitesting.com.

Table of Contents

Unit 5 Nursing Care of Clients With Hematologic Disorders

Unit 6 Nursing Care of Clients With Fluid/Electrolyte/Acid-Base Imbalances

Unit 9 Nursing Care of Clients With Reproductive Disorders

Unit 10 Nursing Care of Clients With Musculoskeletal Disorders

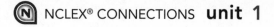

UNIT 1: FOUNDATIONS OF NURSING CARE FOR ADULT CLIENTS

- Health, Wellness, and Illness

- Emergency Nursing Principles and Management

NCLEX® CONNECTIONS

When reviewing the chapters in this unit, keep in mind the relevant sections of the NCLEX® outline, in particular:

CLIENT NEEDS: HEALTH PROMOTION AND MAINTENANCE

Relevant topics/tasks include:
- Health and Wellness
  - ○ Encourage client participation in appropriate behavior modification programs related to health and wellness.
- Health Promotion/Disease Prevention
  - ○ Educate the client on actions to promote/maintain health and prevent disease.

CLIENT NEEDS: PHYSIOLOGICAL ADAPTATION

Relevant topics/tasks include:
- Hemodynamics
  - ○ Intervene to improve the client's cardiovascular status.
- Illness Management
  - ○ Educate the client about managing illness.
- Medical Emergencies
  - ○ Apply knowledge of pathophysiology when caring for a client experiencing a medical emergency.

UNIT 1	FOUNDATIONS OF NURSING CARE FOR ADULT CLIENTS
Chapter 1	Health, Wellness, and Illness

Overview

- Health and wellness combine in a state of optimal physical functioning along with a feeling of emotional and social contentment. Wellness involves the ability to adapt emotionally and physically to a changing state of health and environment.

- Illness is an altered level of functioning in response to a disease process. Disease is a condition that results in the physiological alteration in the composition of the body.

- Nurses must understand the variables affecting health/wellness/illness and how they relate to a client's health needs.

Health and Wellness

- Aspects of health and wellness

  ○ Physical – able to perform activities of daily living

  ○ Emotional – adapts to stress; expresses and identifies emotions

  ○ Social – interacts successfully with others

- A client's state of health and wellness is constantly changing and adapting to a continually fluctuating external and internal environment.

  ○ The external environment

    ▪ Social – crime versus safety, poverty versus prosperity, and peace versus social unrest

    ▪ Physical – access to health care, sanitation, availability of clean water, and geographic isolation

  ○ The internal environment includes cumulative life experiences, cultural and spiritual beliefs, age, gender, and other support systems.

- The level of health and wellness is unique to each individual and relative to the individual's usual state of functioning.

  ○ For example: A person with rheumatoid arthritis who has a strong support system and positive outlook may consider himself healthy while functioning at an optimal level with minimal pain.

- Variables

  - Modifiable – may be changed such as smoking, nutrition, health education and awareness, and exercise

  - Nonmodifiable – cannot be changed, such as gender, age, developmental level, and genetic traits

- Desired outcomes are to obtain and maintain optimal state of wellness and function.

  - Can be achieved through health education and positive action (smoking cessation, weight loss, seeking health care)

- The health/wellness/illness continuum is an assessment tool that is used to measure the level of wellness.

  - It is used as a model to compare the present state of health of a client to that of his previous state of health. It may be useful as an assessment guide and also as a tool to set goals and find ways to improve the client's state of health. The health care professional can assist the client to see at what point he is at on the continuum and seek ways to move toward optimal wellness.

  - The degree of wellness is relative to the usual state of wellness for a client.

  - The range of health to illness runs from optimal wellness to severe illness.

  - At the center of the continuum is the client's normal state of health.

  - Level of health/illness is assessed in comparison to the norm for a client.

Illness

- Response to disease may be influenced by:

  - Degree of physical changes as a result of the disease process.

  - Perceptions by self and others of the disease, which may be influenced by various reliable and unreliable sources of information, such as friends, magazines, TV and the Internet.

  - Cultural values and beliefs.

  - Denial or fear of illness.

  - Social demands and time constraints.

Nursing Care

- Evaluate the health needs of a client and create strategies to meet those needs.

- Health/wellness assessment

  - Physical assessment

  - Evaluating health perceptions

  - Identifying risks to health/wellness

  - Identifying access to health care

- Identifying obstacles to compliance and adherence

  o Perceptions of illness – awareness of the severity of the illness

  o Confidence in the provider

  o Belief in the prescribed therapy

    ■ For example: A person who has had a negative experience with the health care system, may not trust the health care provider and may not follow the advice and comply with the treatment prescribed.

  o Availability of support systems

  o Family role and function (One member of the family may be the family caregiver and may neglect caring for him/herself.)

  o Financial restrictions that may lead to prioritized health care (A parent may seek medical care for children, but not for him/herself.)

- Health promotion and disease prevention – Use health education and awareness to reduce risk factors and promote health care.

- Interventions:

  o Provide resources to strengthen coping abilities.

  o Encourage use of support systems during times of illness and stress.

  o Identify obstacles to health and wellness and create strategies to reduce these obstacles.

  o Identify ways to reduce health risks and improve compliance.

  o Develop health education methods to improve health awareness and reduce health risks.

CHAPTER 1: HEALTH, WELLNESS, AND ILLNESS

 Application Exercises

1. An older adult client is newly diagnosed with type 2 diabetes mellitus. He is prescribed glipizide (Glucotrol XL) PO once a day. He comes to the clinic for a follow-up appointment 2 weeks later. He tells the nurse that he lives alone and it is hard to follow his diet and remember to take his pills. Which of the following obstacles to health care compliance should the nurse recognize in this client? (Select all that apply.)

_____ Lack of belief in the prescribed therapy

_____ Age

_____ Gender

_____ Availability of support systems

_____ Awareness of the severity of the illness

2. A health care clinic is using the health-wellness-illness continuum tool to evaluate the level of wellness for clients. Which of the following clients should be placed at the center of the continuum?

A College student who has influenza-like symptoms.

B. An older adult client who is newly diagnosed with diabetes mellitus.

C. A new mother who has a urinary tract infection.

D. An older adult client who has a long history of well-controlled rheumatoid arthritis.

3. The role of the health care professional in health, wellness, and illness includes which of the following? (Select all that apply.)

_____ Enlist strategies to alter nonmodifiable variables to health and wellness.

_____ Evaluate health perceptions.

_____ Identify risks to health and wellness.

_____ Identify obstacles to compliance and adherence.

_____ Encourage use of support systems.

CHAPTER 1: HEALTH, WELLNESS, AND ILLNESS

 Application Exercises Answer Key

1. An older adult client is newly diagnosed with type 2 diabetes mellitus. He is prescribed glipizide (Glucotrol XL) PO once a day. He comes to the clinic for a follow-up appointment 2 weeks later. He tells the nurse that he lives alone and it is hard to follow his diet and remember to take his pills. Which of the following obstacles to health care compliance should the nurse recognize in this client? (Select all that apply.)

__X__	**Lack of belief in the prescribed therapy**
_____	Age
_____	Gender
__X__	**Availability of support systems**
__X__	**Awareness of the severity of the illness**

Age and gender are not considered obstacles to health care compliance. Some other obstacles include client perception of the illness, financial restrictions, lack of transportation, and fear and distrust of the health care system.

 NCLEX® Connection: Physiological Adaptation: Illness Management

2. A health care clinic is using the health-wellness-illness continuum tool to evaluate the level of wellness for clients. Which of the following clients should be placed at the center of the continuum?

A College student with influenza-like symptoms.

B. An older adult client who is newly diagnosed with diabetes mellitus.

C. A new mother with a urinary tract infection.

D. An older adult client with a long history of well-controlled rheumatoid arthritis.

The college student, older adult newly diagnosed with diabetes mellitus, and mother who has a urinary tract infection are experiencing alterations in health, placing them on the illness side of the continuum.

 NCLEX® Connection: Physiological Adaptation: Illness Management

3. The role of the health care professional in health, wellness, and illness includes which of the following? (Select all that apply.)

	Enlist strategies to alter nonmodifiable variables to health and wellness.
X	**Evaluate health perceptions.**
X	**Identify risks to health and wellness.**
X	**Identify obstacles to compliance and adherence.**
X	**Encourage use of support systems.**

Nonmodifiable variables are variables that cannot be changed, such as gender, age, and genetic traits. The health care professional can evaluate health perceptions, identify risk to health and wellness, identify obstacles to compliance and adherence, and encourage the use of support systems.

Ⓝ NCLEX® Connection: Physiological Adaptation: Illness Management

UNIT 1	FOUNDATIONS OF NURSING CARE FOR ADULT CLIENTS
Chapter 2	Emergency Nursing Principles and Management

Overview

- Emergency nursing principles are the guidelines that nurses follow to assess and manage emergency situations for both a client and multiple clients.

- Nurses must have the ability to identify emergent situations and rapidly assess and intervene when life-threatening conditions exist. Emergent conditions are common to all nursing environments.

- Emergency nursing principles

  - Primary survey

  - Airway/cervical spine, breathing, circulation, disability, and exposure (ABCDE) principle

  - Triage guidelines

  - Basic First-Aid

  - Cardiac arrest and CPR

Primary Survey

- A primary survey is a rapid assessment of life-threatening conditions. It should take no longer than 60 seconds to perform.

- The primary survey should be completed systematically so conditions are not missed.

- Standard precautions attire – gloves, gowns, eye protection, face masks, and shoe covers – must be worn to prevent contamination with bodily fluids.

- The ABCDE principle guides the primary survey.

ABCDE Principle

- Emergency care is guided by the principle of ABCDE.

- Airway/Cervical Spine

  - This is the most important step in performing the primary survey. If a patent airway is not established, subsequent steps of the primary survey are futile.

  - If a client is awake and responsive, the airway is open.

- o   If a client's ability to maintain an airway is lost, it is important to inspect for blood, broken teeth, vomitus, or other foreign materials in the airway that may cause an obstruction.

- o   If the client is unresponsive without suspicion of trauma, the airway should be opened with a head-tilt-chin-lift maneuver.

  - ▪   This is the most effective manual technique for opening a client's airway.

  - ▪   Do NOT perform this technique on clients who have a potential cervical spine injury.

  - ▪   The nurse should assume a position at the head of the client, place one hand on his forehead, and the other on his chin. His head should be tilted while his chin is lifted superiorly. This lifts the tongue out of the laryngopharynx and provides for a patent airway.

- o   If the client is unresponsive with suspicion of trauma, the airway should be opened with a modified jaw thrust maneuver.

  - ▪   The nurse should assume a position at the head of the client, and place both hands on either side of the client's head. Locate the connection between the maxilla and the mandible. Lift the jaw superiorly while maintaining alignment of the cervical spine.

- o   Once the airway is opened, it should be inspected for blood, broken teeth, vomitus, and secretions. If present, obstructions should be cleared with suction or a finger-sweep method.

- o   The open airway can be maintained with airway adjuncts, such as an oropharyngeal or nasopharyngeal airway.

- o   A bag-valve-mask with a 100% oxygen source is indicated for clients who need additional support during resuscitation.

- •   Breathing

  - o   Once a patent airway is achieved, the presence and effectiveness of breathing should be assessed.

  - o   Breathing assessment

    - ▪   Auscultation of breath sounds

    - ▪   Observation of chest expansion and respiratory effort

    - ▪   Notation of rate and depth of respirations

    - ▪   Identification of chest trauma

  - o   If a client is not breathing or is breathing inadequately, manual ventilation should be performed by a bag-valve-mask with supplemental oxygen or mouth-to-mask ventilation until a bag-valve-mask can be obtained.

- •   Circulation

  - o   Once adequate ventilation is accomplished, circulation is assessed.

  - o   Nurses should assess heart rate, blood pressure, and perfusion.

- o Interventions geared toward restoring effective circulation

  - CPR

  - Hemorrhage control (direct pressure should be applied to visible, significant external bleeding)

  - Obtaining IV access

  - Infusion of fluids and/or blood

- o An IV should be inserted using a large-bore catheter into the antecubital fossa (bend of the elbow). Lactated Ringer's and 0.9% normal saline are typical resuscitation fluids.

- o Shock may develop if circulation is compromised. Shock is the body's response to inadequate tissue perfusion and oxygenation. It manifests with an increased heart rate and hypotension and may result in tissue ischemia and necrosis.

- o Interventions to alleviate shock include:

  - Administer oxygen.

  - Apply pressure to bleeding that is obvious.

  - Elevate the client's feet to shunt blood to vital organs.

  - Administer fluids and blood products as ordered.

  - Monitor vital signs.

  - Remain with the client and provide reassurance and support for anxiety.

- Disability

  - o Disability is a quick assessment to determine the client's level of consciousness.

  - o The AVPU mnemonic is useful.

    - A – Alert

    - V – Responsive to voice

    - P – Responsive to pain

    - U – Unresponsive

  - o The Glasgow Coma Scale is another widely used method.

    - Components include eye opening, verbal response, and motor response.

  - o Neurologic assessment must be repeated at frequent intervals to assure immediate response to any change.

- Exposure

  - o The nurse should remove all of the client's clothing for a complete physical assessment.

  - o Clothing should be cut away during a resuscitation situation.

  - o Evidence such as bullets, drugs, or weapons may need to be preserved.

- o Hypothermia is a primary concern for clients. Hypothermia leads to vasoconstriction and impaired oxygenation.
- o To prevent hypothermia
  - Remove wet clothing from the client.
  - Cover the client with blankets.
  - Increase the temperature of the room.
  - Infuse warmed fluids as prescribed.

Triage Guidelines

- Triage Under Usual Conditions
  - o Triage guidelines ensure that clients with the highest acuity needs receive the quickest treatment.
  - o Clients are categorized based upon their acuity. One example of a triage framework is the Emergent, Urgent, Nonurgent model.
    - Emergent triage indicates a life- or limb-threatening situation.
    - Urgent triage indicates that the client should be treated soon, but that the risk posed is not life-threatening.
    - Nonurgent cases can generally wait for an extended length of time without serious deterioration.
- Triage Under Mass Casualty Conditions
  - o This is a military form of triage that is implemented with a focus of achieving the greatest good for the greatest number of people.
  - o Classifications
    - Emergent or Class I – identified with a red tag indicating an immediate threat to life
    - Urgent or Class II – identified with a yellow tag indicating major injuries that require immediate treatment
    - Nonurgent or Class III – identified with a green tag indicating minor injuries that do not require immediate treatment
    - Expectant or Class IV – identified with a black tag indicating one who is expected and allowed to die

Basic First-Aid

- Complete the primary survey before performing First-Aid.
- Bleeding
  - o Identify any sources of external bleeding and apply direct pressure to the wound site.
  - o DO NOT remove impaled objects.

- o Internal bleeding may require intravascular volume replacement with fluids and/or blood products or surgical intervention.

- Fractures and Splinting

  - o Assess the site for swelling, deformity, and skin integrity.

  - o Assess temperature, distal pulses, and mobility.

  - o Apply a splint to immobilize the fracture. Cover any open areas with a sterile cloth if available.

  - o Reassess neurovascular status after splinting.

- Sprains

  - o Refrain from weight-bearing.

  - o Apply ice to decrease inflammation.

  - o Apply a compression dressing to minimize swelling.

  - o Elevate the affected limb.

- Heat Stroke

  - o Heat stroke must be identified quickly and be treated aggressively.

  - o Signs and symptoms of a heat stroke include hypotension, tachypnea, tachycardia, anxiety, confusion, unusual behavior, seizures, and coma.

  - o Rapid cooling must be achieved

    - ▪ Remove the client's clothing.

    - ▪ Place ice packs over the major arteries (axillae, chest, groin, neck).

    - ▪ Immerse the client in a cold water bath.

    - ▪ Wet the client's body, then fan with rapid movement of air.

- Frostnip and Frost Bite

  - o Frostnip does not lead to tissue injury and may be treated by warming.

  - o Frostbite presents as white, waxy areas on exposed skin, and tissue injury occurs.

  - o Frostbite may be full- or partial-thickness.

  - o The affected area should be warmed in a water bath 38° to 41° C (100.4° to 105.8° F).

  - o Pain medication should be provided.

  - o A tetanus vaccination should be provided.

- Burns

  - o Burns may result from an electrical current, chemicals, radiation, and/or flames.

    - ▪ Remove the agent (electrical current, radiation source, chemical).

    - ▪ Smother any flames that are present.

- Perform a primary survey.
- Cover the client and maintain NPO status.
- Elevate the client's extremities if not contraindicated (presence of a fracture).
- Perform a head-to-toe assessment and estimate the surface area and thickness of burns.
- Administer fluids and a tetanus toxoid.

- Altitude-Related Illnesses

  - Clients may become hypoxic in high altitudes.
  - Signs and symptoms
    - Throbbing headache
    - Nausea
    - Vomiting
    - Dyspnea
    - Anorexia
  - Nursing interventions
    - Administer oxygen
    - Descend to a lower altitude
    - Provide pharmacological therapy, such as steroids and diuretics, if indicated
  - Altitude sickness can progress to cerebral and pulmonary edema and should be treated immediately.

Cardiac Arrest and CPR

- Cardiac Arrest

  - Cardiac arrest, the sudden cessation of cardiac function, is characterized by the absence of a carotid pulse in the adult and child 1 year to adolescent. In infant's up to 1 year, cardiac arrest is the absence of a brachial pulse. If no brachial pulse, check the infant's carotid pulse. The brachial pulse is checked first because the carotid pulse may be difficult to palpate due to the fatty tissue of the infant's neck.

  - Assessment
    - The client's skin has an ashy appearance.
    - The client has no respirations.
    - The client's pupils are dilated.
  - Findings
    - Ventricular fibrillation (VF) is the cause of sudden, nontraumatic cardiac arrest in 80 to 90% of victims.

- Cardiac arrest may also occur following respiratory arrest. Sometimes, electrical activity is present, but is not sufficient enough to stimulate effective cardiac contractions. This condition is called pulse-less electrical activity.

- In children and infants, cardiac arrest is often secondary to hypoxemia or shock.

- Without sufficient cardiac output, the brain will suffer cell anoxia (cell death) within 4 to 6 min, with death following shortly thereafter.

- An interdisciplinary team will provide care during in-facility cardiac arrests. This team should include nurses, physicians, respiratory therapists, laboratory personnel, and chaplain services.

- Management of cardiac arrest depends on prompt recognition of signs and symptoms and the introduction of therapeutic interventions directed at artificially sustaining circulation and ventilation.

- Goals for management of cardiac arrest

  - Rapid identification of the signs and symptoms of cardiac arrest

  - Quick initiation of both circulatory and respiratory support

  - Activation of the emergency medical system

  - Utilization of emergency equipment and cardiac monitoring

  - Stabilization of the client following the arrest

  - Diagnosis and treatment of the cause of the cardiac arrest

- CPR is the process of externally supporting the circulation and respirations of an individual who has experienced a cardiac arrest. Defibrillation is used in the presence of ventricular fibrillation and ventricular tachycardia. Neither of these rhythms provide sufficient cardiac output to support life. CPR and defibrillation significantly increases the client's chances of survival when initiated immediately.

- Prefacility care greatly improves the chance of survival for client's who have experienced cardiac arrest.

- **CPR**

  - CPR is a combination of basic interventions designed to sustain oxygen and circulation to vital organs until more advanced interventions can be initiated to correct the cause of the cardiac arrest.

  - Basic interventions can be delivered by trained citizens, but advanced interventions require more sophisticated training and certification and the use of emergency equipment.

  - CPR is a series of emergency procedures directed at artificially providing a client with circulation (chest compressions) and oxygenation (ventilations) in the absence of cardiac output.

  - CPR is a component of basic life support (BLS) and advanced cardiac life support (ACLS).

- ○ The goal of BLS is to provide oxygen to the vital organs until appropriate advanced resuscitation measures can be initiated or until resuscitative efforts are ordered to be stopped. BLS involves Airway, Breathing and Circulation (ABCs) of CPR:
  - Airway
    - □ Confirm the absence of spontaneous respirations.
    - □ Establish a patent airway.
    - □ Provide the Heimlich maneuver if the airway is obstructed with a foreign object.
    - □ Use abdominal thrusts for clients who are unconscious.
  - Breathing
    - □ Provide artificial respirations (ventilations) to deliver oxygen into the blood in an attempt to prevent cell anoxia.
  - Circulation
    - □ Confirm the absence or presence of a pulse.
    - □ Provide external support of circulation (chest compressions) to transport oxygenated blood to the brain.
- ○ The goal of ACLS is the return of spontaneous breathing and circulation. In addition to the ABCs of BLS, ACLS involves:
  - Diagnosis of underlying cardiac dysrhythmias. Pharmacological interventions are dependent upon the rhythm identified. Defibrillation may be required. This involves delivering a premeasured shock to the heart to interrupt the aberrant rhythm and allow the natural pacemaker of the heart to initiate beats.
  - Insert an oropharyngeal or endotracheal airway with bag ventilation and supplemental oxygen.
  - Administer of IV fluids.
  - Administer IV antidysrhythmic medications.
- ○ The chain of survival is a series of interventions directed at the resuscitation of the cardiac arrest victim. It involves:
  - Early activation of the emergency medical services.
  - Early CPR/early defibrillation.
  - Early ACLS care.
- • Nursing Responsibilities During a Cardiac Arrest
  - ○ The nurse assisting during a cardiac arrest must:
    - Be knowledgeable about the facility's procedure for alerting members of the code team to the presence of an emergency.
    - Use the current BLS and ACLS guidelines from the American Heart Association (AHA).

- Be knowledgeable about facility policies/procedures and the location and operation of emergency equipment (crash cart).

- Have current certification for basic life support and/or advanced cardiac life support skills.

o Nursing responsibilities

- Know the client's status regarding resuscitation (The nurse must know whether or not the client has a current Do-Not-Resuscitate order.).

- Maintain airway patency.

- Assess the depth and rate of respirations.

- Provide chest compressions at the proper rate and depth for age (See the chart on the following page.).

- Assess vital signs for effectiveness of chest compressions and ventilations.

- Defibrillate the client when indicated.

- Obtain and maintain IV access.

- Provide medications as prescribed.

- Monitor laboratory values (ABGs, CBC, electrolytes).

- Document all interventions and medications.

- AHA guidelines – BLS for Infants, Children, and Adults*

MANEUVER	ADULT (ADOLESCENT AND OLDER)	CHILD (1 YEAR TO ADOLESCENT)	INFANT (UNDER 1 YEAR)
Activate emergency response number.	Activate this when a victim is found unresponsive. If asphyxial arrest is likely, call the number after 5 cycles (2 min) of CPR.	Activate this after performing 5 cycles of CPR. For sudden, witnessed collapse, activate its after verifying that the victim is unresponsive.	
Airway	Head tilt, chin lift (for suspected trauma, use jaw thrust)		
Initial breaths	2 breaths at 1 second/breath	2 effective breaths at 1 second/breath	
Perform rescue breaths without chest compressions.	10 to 12 breaths/ min (approx. 1 breath every 5 to 6 seconds)	12 to 20 breaths/min (approximately 1 breath every 3 to 5 seconds)	

MANEUVER	ADULT (ADOLESCENT AND OLDER)	CHILD (1 YEAR TO ADOLESCENT)	INFANT (UNDER 1 YEAR)
Perform rescue breaths for CPR with advanced airway.	8 to 10 breaths/min (approximately 1 breath every 6 to 8 seconds)		
Foreign-body airway obstruction	Abdominal thrusts		Back slaps and chest thrusts
Circulation	Carotid	Carotid or femoral	Brachial or femoral
Compression landmarks	Center of chest, between nipples		Just below nipple line
Compression method	2 hands: heel of one hand, other hand on top	2 hands: heel of one hand, other hand on top 1 hand: heel of one hand only	1 rescuer: 2 fingers 2 rescuers: 2 thumb-encircling hands
Compression depth	1 ½ to 2 inches	Approximately ⅓ to ½ the depth of the chest	
Compression rate	Approximately 100/min		
Compression-ventilation ratio	30:2 (1 or 2 rescuers)	30:2 (1 rescuer) 15:2 (2 rescuers)	

Table based on AHA guidelines for healthcare providers.
Source: American Heart Association. American Heart Association 2005 Guidelines for CPR and ECC. Retrieved December 30, 2009, from: http://www.americanheart.org/presenter.jhtml?identifier=3035517.

- The AHA guidelines for basic life support and advanced life support are updated on a regular basis.

- These updates are based on research and aggregate client outcomes.

- Since most cases of adult cardiac arrest are caused by ventricular fibrillation or ventricular tachycardia, early defibrillation is essential. When a defibrillator is immediately available (and ventricular fibrillation or ventricular tachycardia is confirmed) the client is defibrillated prior to the initiation of CPR. A standard defibrillator or an automated external defibrillator (AED) may be used. Although the occurrence of cardiac arrest is rare in the pediatric population, the nurse must also be prepared to use a defibrillator when indicated.

- AHA ACLS Protocols

  ○ VF or pulseless ventricular tachycardia (VT)

    ■ Perform CPR (stop when the defibrillator is ready).

    ■ Provide oxygen.

- Defibrillate: 200 joules.
- Defibrillate: 300 joules.
- Defibrillate: 360 joules.
  - □ If using a preprogrammed AED, 360 joules will automatically be delivered.
- Establish IV access.
- Administer epinephrine 1 mg IV push every 3 to 5 min or vasopressin 40 units IV x 1 only (switch to epinephrine if no response).
- Defibrillate: 360 joules within 30 to 60 seconds.
- Consider the following medications.
  - □ Amiodarone hydrochloride (Cordarone)
  - □ Lidocaine hydrochloride (Xylocaine)
  - □ Magnesium sulfate
  - □ Procainamide (Procan SR)
  - □ Sodium bicarbonate
- o Pulseless electrical activity (PEA)
  - Perform CPR.
  - Provide oxygen.
  - Defibrillate for VF or pulseless VT.
  - Establish IV access.
  - Consider the most common causes.
    - □ 5 H's
      - ‣ Hypovolemia
      - ‣ Hypoxia
      - ‣ Hydrogen ion accumulation, resulting in acidosis
      - ‣ Hyperkalemia or hypokalemia
      - ‣ Hypothermia
    - □ 5 T's
      - ‣ Tables (accidental or deliberate drug overdose)
      - ‣ Tamponade (cardiac)
      - ‣ Tension pneumothorax
      - ‣ Thrombosis (coronary)
      - ‣ Thrombosis (pulmonary)
  - Administer epinephrine 1 mg IV push every 3 to 5 min.
  - If PEA rate is slow (bradycardic), administer atropine 1 mg IV every 3 to 5 min (maximum total dose 0.04 mg/kg).

- ○ Asystole
  - ▪ Perform CPR.
  - ▪ Provide oxygen.
  - ▪ Defibrillate for VF or pulseless VT.
  - ▪ Confirm true asystolic rhythm.
  - ▪ Establish IV access.
  - ▪ Begin immediate transcutaneous pacing, if possible.
  - ▪ Give epinephrine 1 mg push every 3 to 5 min.
  - ▪ Administer atropine 1 mg IV every 3 to 5 min (maximum total dose 0.04 mg/kg).
  - ▪ Consider ceasing resuscitation if asystole persists.
- • Using Conventional Defibrillators
  - ○ The following steps represent the safe and effective method for delivering shocks to a client who has VF.
    - ▪ Turn on the defibrillator.
    - ▪ Set the energy level at 200 joules for monophasic defibrillators (or clinically equivalent for biphasic energy level).
    - ▪ Turn on the "lead select" switch on the paddles or, if monitor leads are used, Lead I, II, or III.
    - ▪ Place gel on the paddles or apply conductor pads on the client's chest.
    - ▪ Position the paddles or remote defibrillation pads on the client's sternum apex.
    - ▪ Look at the monitor display and evaluate the rhythm (succeeding steps presume that VF/VT is present).
    - ▪ State to the team members, "Charging defibrillator. Stand clear!"
    - ▪ Press the "Charge" button on the apex paddle (right hand) or on the defibrillator controls.
    - ▪ Once the defibrillator is fully charged, clearly state the following chant (or some suitable equivalent) before each shock:
      - ☐ "I'm going to shock on three. One, I'm clear." (Check to be sure there is no contact with the client, the stretcher, or the equipment.)
      - ☐ "Two, you're clear." (Visually check to ensure that no one is touching the client, the stretcher, or the ventilatory adjuncts, including the tracheal tube.
      - ☐ "Three, everybody's clear." (Check to be sure all is clear before pressing the "shock" buttons.)
    - ▪ Put 25 lb of pressure on both paddles.
    - ▪ Press both of the paddle "discharge" buttons at the same time.

- Look at the monitor. If VF/VT is still displaying, recharge the defibrillator immediately. If there is any question about the client's rhythm display (a lead is dislodged or the paddles are not showing the correct signal), check for a pulse.

- Shock at 200 to 300 joules, then at 360 joules for monophasic defibrillators (or a clinically equivalent biphasic energy level), repeating the aforementioned statements.

Expected Pharmacological Action

- Catecholamine adrenergic agonists cannot be taken by the oral route, do not cross the blood-brain barrier, and their duration of action is short.

RECEPTORS	SITE/RESPONSE
Alpha$_1$	• Activation of receptors in arterioles of skin, viscera and mucous membranes, and veins lead to vasoconstriction.
Beta$_1$	• Heart stimulation leads to increased heart rate, increased myocardial contractility, and increased rate of conduction through the atrioventricular (AV) node. • Activation of receptors in the kidney leads to the release of renin.
Beta$_2$	• Activation of receptors in the arterioles of the heart, lungs, and skeletal muscles lead to vasodilation. • Bronchial stimulation leads to bronchodilation. • Activation of receptors in uterine smooth muscle causes relaxation. • Activation of receptors in the liver cause glycogenolysis. • Skeletal muscle receptor activation leads to muscle contraction.
Dopamine	• Activation of receptors in the kidney cause the renal blood vessels to dilate.

Emergency Medications

RECEPTORS	PHARMACOLOGICAL ACTION	THERAPEUTIC USE
epinephrine (Adrenaline)		
Alpha$_1$	• Vasoconstriction	• Slows absorption of local anesthetics • Manages superficial bleeding • Reduces congestion of nasal mucosa • Increases blood pressure
Beta$_1$	• Increases heart rate • Strengthens myocardial contractility • Increases rate of conduction through the AV node	• Treatment of AV block and cardiac arrest
Beta$_2$	• Bronchodilation	• Asthma

RECEPTORS	PHARMACOLOGICAL ACTION	THERAPEUTIC USE
dopamine (Intropin)		
Low dose – dopamine (2 to 5 mcg/kg/min)	• Renal blood vessel dilation	• Shock • Heart failure

Moderate dose – dopamine (5 to 10 mcg/kg/min)
Beta$_1$
	• Renal blood vessel dilation
	• Increases:
	  ○ Heart rate
	  ○ Myocardial contractility
	  ○ Rate of conduction through the AV node
	  ○ Blood pressure	

High dose – dopamine (>10 mcg/kg/min)
Beta$_1$
Alpha$_1$
	• Renal blood vessel vasoconstriction
	• Increases:
	  ○ Heart rate
	  ○ Myocardial contractility
	  ○ Rate of conduction through the AV node
	  ○ Blood pressure
	  ○ Vasoconstriction	

dobutamine (Dobutrex)		

Beta$_1$	• Increases:
	  ○ Heart rate
	  ○ Myocardial contractility
	  ○ Rate of conduction through the AV node
		• Heart failure

Side/Adverse Effects: Nursing Interventions and Client Education

SIDE/ADVERSE EFFECTS	NURSING INTERVENTIONS/CLIENT EDUCATION
epinephrine (Adrenaline)	
Vasoconstriction from activation of alpha$_1$ receptors in the heart can lead to hypertensive crisis.	• Provide the client with continuous cardiac monitoring. • Report changes in the client's vital signs to the primary care provider.
Beta$_1$ receptor activation in the heart can cause dysrhythmias. Beta$_1$ receptor activation also increases the workload of the heart and oxygen demand, leading to the development of angina.	• Provide the client with continuous cardiac monitoring. • Monitor the client closely for dysrhythmias, change in heart rate, and chest pain. • Notify the primary care provider if the client experiences dysrhythmias, an elevated heart rate, or chest pain, and treat per protocol.
dopamine (Intropin)	
Beta$_1$ receptor activation in the heart can cause dysrhythmias. Beta$_1$ receptor activation also increases the workload of the heart and oxygen demand, leading to the development of angina.	• Provide the client with continuous cardiac monitoring. • Monitor the client closely for dysrhythmias, change in heart rate, and chest pain. • Notify the primary care provider of signs of dysrhythmias, elevated heart rate, and chest pain, and treat per protocol.
Necrosis can occur from extravasation of high doses of dopamine.	• Infuse dopamine into the central line. Monitor the IV site carefully. • Discontinue the infusion at first sign of irritation.
dobutamine (Dobutrex)	
Increased HR	• Provide the client with continuous cardiac monitoring. • Report changes in the client's vital signs to the primary care provider.

Contraindications/Precautions

- Pregnancy Risk Category C – epinephrine, dopamine

- Pregnancy Risk Category B – dobutamine

  o These medications are contraindicated in clients with tachydysrhythmias and ventricular fibrillation.

  o Use cautiously in clients with hyperthyroidism, angina, history of MI, hypertension, and diabetes mellitus.

Medication/Food Interactions: Nursing Interventions and Client Education

MEDICATION/FOOD INTERACTIONS	NURSING INTERVENTIONS/CLIENT EDUCATION
MAOIs – inactivates epinephrine; therefore, MAOIs will prevent this inactivation and thereby, prolong and intensify the effects of epinephrine.	• Avoid the use of MAOIs in clients who are receiving epinephrine.
Tricyclic antidepressants – block the uptake of epinephrine, which will prolong and intensify the effects of epinephrine.	• Clients taking these medications concurrently may need a lower dose of epinephrine.
General anesthetics – can cause the heart to become hypersensitive to the effects of epinephrine, which leads to dysrhythmias.	• Perform continuous ECG monitoring of the client. • Notify the primary care provider if the client experiences chest pain, dysrhythmias, or an elevated heart rate.
Alpha-adrenergic blocking agents, such as phentolamine, block action at alpha receptors. They do not interact with dobutamine.	• Phentolamine may be used to treat epinephrine toxicity.
Beta-adrenergic blocking agents, such as propranolol, block the action at beta receptors.	• Propranolol may be used to treat chest pain and dysrhythmias.
Diuretics promote the beneficial effect of dopamine.	• Monitor the client for therapeutic effects.

Nursing Interventions and Client Education

- Medications must be administered by continuous IV infusion.
- Use IV pump to control infusion.
- Titrate dosage based on the client's blood pressure response.
- Stop the infusion at the first sign of infiltration. Extravasation can be treated with a local injection of an alpha-adrenergic blocking agent, such as phentolamine.
- Assess/monitor the client for chest pain. Notify the primary care provider if the client experiences chest pain.
- Provide continuous ECG monitoring. Notify the primary care provider if the client experiences tachycardia or dysrhythmias.

Client Outcomes

- The client will have improved tissue perfusion.

- The client will maintain adequate gas exchange.

- The client will have a patent airway.

- The client will have an improved mental status.

- The client will have an improved adequate cardiac function.

CHAPTER 2: EMERGENCY NURSING PRINCIPLES AND MANAGEMENT

Ⓐ Application Exercises

Scenario: A client arrives in the emergency department after falling off his mountain bike. He is alert, oriented, and able to move all of his extremities. He has a compound fracture to his left tibia, as well as several scrapes and bruises. He was not wearing a helmet. His vital signs are blood pressure 98/60 mm Hg, heart rate 104/min, respiratory rate 24/min, and temperature 37.2° C (99° F).

1. Which of the following actions should the nurse first take?

    A. Obtain IV access.

    B. Assess the client's airway.

    C. Check the client's pulse.

    D. Assess the client's neurological status.

2. How should the nurse prioritize the interventions?

3. Several minutes later, the client's vital signs have changed. They now read blood pressure 78/45 mm Hg, heart rate 131/min, respiratory rate 34/min, and temperature 37° C (99° F). The client is unable to answer questions and is mumbling incoherently. What is the likely explanation for the change in his status? What should the nurse do next?

4. A client who is unresponsive is brought to the emergency department by his spouse. She states, "He was working in the yard and dropped to the ground." Which of the following techniques should the nurse use to open the client's airway?

    A. Head tilt, chin lift

    B. Modified jaw thrust

    C. Hyperextension of the head

    D. Flexion of the head

5. Which of the following are appropriate interventions for a client who had heat stroke? (Select all that apply.)

    _____ Immerse the client in cold water.

    _____ Encourage the client to walk it off.

    _____ Apply ice packs to the client's groin and axillae.

    _____ Keep the client's clothing on to avoid sun exposure.

    _____ Administer a tetanus vaccination to the client.

6. Number the following steps in the correct order to reflect the proper performance of CPR for the adult client.

_____ Position the client.

_____ Perform ventilation.

_____ Open the airway.

_____ Start compressions.

_____ Check for breathing.

_____ Check for a spontaneous pulse.

_____ Check for unresponsiveness.

_____ Call for help.

_____ Check for circulation (carotid pulse/signs of circulation).

7. A client is brought to the emergency department after she fell through the ice on a pond while ice skating. She is unresponsive but is breathing slowly. Which of the following findings should the nurse expect to find?

A. Hyperglycemia

B. Hypoglycemia

C. Hyperthermia

D. Hypothermia

CHAPTER 2: EMERGENCY NURSING PRINCIPLES AND MANAGEMENT

 Application Exercises Answer Key

Scenario: A client arrives in the emergency department after falling off his mountain bike. He is alert, oriented, and able to move all of his extremities. He has a compound fracture to his left tibia, as well as several scrapes and bruises. He was not wearing a helmet. His vital signs are blood pressure 98/60 mm Hg, heart rate 104/min, respiratory rate 24/min, and temperature 37.2° C (99° F).

1. Which of the following actions should the nurse first take?

    A. Obtain IV access.

    B. Assess the client's airway.

    C. Check the client's pulse.

    D. Assess the client's neurological status.

    By following the ABCDE framework, the nurse should know that assessing the client's airway is the first action to take. Checking the client's pulse, obtaining IV access and assessing the client's neurological status are all parts of the assessment; however, they are not the first actions the nurse should take.

 NCLEX® Connection: Physiological Adaptation: Medical Emergencies

2. How should the nurse prioritize the interventions?

    The nurse should start with a primary survey using the ABCDE mnemonic. The client has a patent airway and is breathing, evidenced by the fact that he is talking. Since the client was not wearing a helmet and did fall, his head and neck should be immobilized until a cervical spine injury can be ruled out. The nurse should next assess circulation. IV access should be obtained, and perfusion should be assessed with blood pressure and pulse. The AVPU mnemonic can be used to assess the client's disability or neurological status. Lastly, the client's clothing should be removed to allow for a complete physical assessment. However, the room should be kept warm to prevent hypothermia.

 NCLEX® Connection: Physiological Adaptation: Medical Emergencies

3. Several minutes later, the client's vital signs have changed. They now read blood pressure 78/45 mm Hg, heart rate 131/min, respiratory rate 34/min, and temperature 37° C (99° F). The client is unable to answer questions and is mumbling incoherently. What is the likely explanation for the change in his status? What should the nurse do next?

It is possible that internal bleeding is occurring from hidden injuries. The nurse should expect to administer warmed fluids and/or blood products to replenish his intravascular volume and administer oxygen to prevent hypoxia. The client may also require a surgical intervention to stop the bleeding.

Ⓝ **NCLEX® Connection: Physiological Adaptation: Hemodynamics**

4. A client who is unresponsive is brought to the emergency department by his spouse. She states, "He was working in the yard and dropped to the ground." Which of the following techniques should the nurse use to open the client's airway?

A. Head tilt, chin lift

B. Modified jaw thrust

C. Hyperextension of the head

D. Flexion of the head

The head tilt, chin lift is used for a client who is unresponsive without suspicion of trauma. The modified jaw thrust is used with a client who is unresponsive following a motor vehicle crash. Hyperextension and flexion of the head can cause further injury.

Ⓝ **NCLEX® Connection: Physiological Adaptation: Medical Emergencies**

5. Which of the following are appropriate interventions for a client who had heat stroke? (Select all that apply.)

__X__	**Immerse the client in cold water.**
_____	Encourage the client to walk it off.
__X__	**Apply ice packs to the client's groin and axillae.**
_____	Keep the client's clothing on to avoid sun exposure.
_____	Administer a tetanus vaccination to the client.

Immersing the client in cold water and applying ice packs to the groin and axillae are appropriate interventions for heat stroke. The client should stop all activity to conserve energy. All clothing should be removed prior to immersing the client in cold water. A tetanus vaccination is not indicated for a heatstroke; however, it is indicated for frostnip and frostbite.

Ⓝ **NCLEX® Connection: Physiological Adaptation: Medical Emergencies**

6. Number the following steps in the correct order to reflect the proper performance of CPR for the adult client.

3	Position the client.
6	Perform ventilation.
4	Open the airway.
8	Start compressions.
5	Check for breathing.
9	Check for a spontaneous pulse.
1	Check for unresponsiveness.
2	Call for help.
7	Check for circulation (carotid pulse/signs of circulation).

According to the ABC priority framework, the following order is indicated to perform CPR for an adult client.

 NCLEX® Connection: Physiological Adaptation: Medical Emergencies

7. A client is brought to the emergency department after she fell through the ice on a pond while ice skating. She is unresponsive but is breathing slowly. Which of the following findings should the nurse expect to find?

   A. Hyperglycemia

   B. Hypoglycemia

   C. Hyperthermia

   D. Hypothermia

Hypothermia would be the expected finding for this client. Hyperglycemia, hypoglycemia, and hyperthermia would not be expected.

 NCLEX® Connection: Physiological Adaptation: Pathophysiology

UNIT 2: NURSING CARE OF CLIENTS WITH NEUROSENSORY DISORDERS

- Diagnostic and Therapeutic Procedures
- Central Nervous System Disorders
- Peripheral Nervous System Disorders
- Sensory Disorders
- Neurologic Emergencies

NCLEX® CONNECTIONS

When reviewing the chapters in this unit, keep in mind the relevant sections of the NCLEX® outline, in particular:

CLIENT NEEDS: BASIC CARE AND COMFORT	CLIENT NEEDS: PHARMACOLOGICAL AND PARENTERAL THERAPIES	CLIENT NEEDS: REDUCTION OF RISK POTENTIAL
Relevant topics/tasks include:	Relevant topics/tasks include:	Relevant topics/tasks include:
• Nonpharmacological Comfort Interventions	• Adverse Effects/ Contraindications/Side Effects/Interactions	• Diagnostic Tests
○ Assess the client's need for pain management and intervene as needed using non-pharmacological comfort measures.	○ Provide information to the client on common side effects/ adverse effects/ potential interactions of medications and when to notify the provider.	○ Compare the client's diagnostic findings with pretest results.
• Mobility/Immobility	• Expected Actions/Outcomes	• Potential for Complications of Diagnostic Tests/ Treatments/Procedures
○ Assess the client for mobility, gait, strength, and motor skills.	○ Evaluate the client's use of medications over time.	○ Intervene to prevent potential neurological complications.
• Nutrition and Oral Hydration	• Pharmacological Pain Management	• Therapeutic Procedures
○ Assess the client's ability to eat.	○ Use pharmacological measures for pain management, as needed.	○ Apply knowledge of related nursing procedures and psychomotor skills when caring for clients undergoing therapeutic procedures.

UNIT 2	NURSING CARE OF CLIENTS WITH NEUROSENSORY DISORDERS
Section	Diagnostic and Therapeutic Procedures
Chapter 3	Neurologic Diagnostic Procedures

Overview

- Neurologic assessment and diagnostic procedures are used to evaluate neurologic function by testing indicators such as mental status, motor functioning, electrical activity, and intracranial pressure.

- Neurologic assessment and diagnostic procedures that nurses should be knowledgeable about include:

  - Cerebral angiogram

  - Cerebral computed tomography (CT) scan

  - Electroencephalography (EEG)

  - Glasgow Coma Scale (GCS)

  - Intracranial pressure (ICP) monitoring

  - Lumbar puncture (spinal tap)

  - Magnetic resonance imaging (MRI) scan

  - Positron emission tomography (PET) and single-photon emission computed tomography (SPECT) scans

  - Radiography (x-ray)

Cerebral Angiogram

- A cerebral angiogram provides visualization of the cerebral blood vessels.

  - Digital subtraction angiography "subtracts" the bones and tissues from the images, providing x-rays with only the vessels apparent.

  - The procedure is performed within the radiology department, because x-ray images provide documentation of blood vessel integrity.

- Indications

  - A cerebral angiogram is used to assess the blood flow to and within the brain, identify aneurysms, and define the vascularity of tumors (useful for surgical planning). It may also be used therapeutically to inject medications that treat blood clots or to administer chemotherapy.

- Preprocedure

  - If the client is pregnant, a determination of the risks to the fetus versus the benefits of the information obtained by this procedure should be made.

  - Nursing Actions

    - Instruct the client to refrain from consuming food or fluids for 4 to 8 hours prior to the procedure.

    - Assess for allergy to shellfish or iodine, which would require the use of a different contrast media. Any history of bleeding requires additional monitoring to assure clotting after the procedure

    - Ensure that the client is not wearing any jewelry.

    - A mild sedative is usually administered prior to the procedure and vital signs are continuously monitored during the procedure.

  - Client Education

    - Instruct the client about the importance of not moving during the procedure and about the need to keep the head immobilized.

- Intraprocedure

  - The client is placed on a radiography table, where the client's head is secured.

  - A catheter is placed into an artery (usually in the groin or the neck), dye is injected, and x-ray pictures are taken.

  - The catheter is removed once all pictures are taken.

  - Additional sedation may be provided during the procedure, if required.

- Postprocedure

  - Nursing Actions

    - The area is closely monitored to assure that clotting occurs.

    - Movements are restricted for 8 to 12 hours to prevent rebleeding at the catheter site.

- Complications

  - Bleeding

    - There is a risk for bleeding at the entry site.

    - Nursing Actions

      - Check the insertion site frequently.

      - If bleeding does occur, dressings should be reinforced and not removed. Pressure should also be applied.

Cerebral Computed Tomography (CT) Scan

- A CT scan provides cross-sectional images of the cranial cavity. A contrast media may be used to enhance the images.

- Indications

  o A CT scan can be used to identify tumors and infarctions, detect abnormalities, monitor response to treatment, and guide needles used for biopsies.

- Preprocedure

  o If the client is pregnant, a determination of the risks to the fetus versus the benefits of the information obtained by this procedure should be made.

  o Nursing Actions

    ▪ If contrast media and/or sedation is expected:

      □ Instruct the client to refrain from consuming food or fluids for 4 to 8 hr prior to the procedure.

      □ Assess for allergy to shellfish or iodine, which would require the use of a different contrast media.

      □ Assess renal function (BUN), because contrast media is excreted by the kidneys.

    ▪ Because this procedure is performed with the client in a supine position, placing pillows in the small of the client's back may assist in preventing back pain. The head must be secured to prevent unnecessary movement during the procedure

    ▪ Ensure that the client's jewelry is removed prior to this procedure. In general, clients wear a hospital gown to prevent any metals from interfering with the x-rays.

- Intraprocedure

  o The client must lie supine with the head stabilized during the procedure.

  o Although CT scanning is painless, sedation may be provided.

- Postprocedure

  o Nursing Actions

    ▪ There is no follow-up care associated with a CT scan.

    ▪ If contrast media is injected, monitor the site to assure clotting has occurred.

    ▪ If sedation is administered, monitor the client until stable.

Electroencephalography (EEG)

- This noninvasive procedure assesses the electrical activity of the brain and is used to determine if there are abnormalities in brain wave patterns.

- Indications

  o EEGs are most commonly performed to identify and determine seizure activity, but they are also useful for detecting sleep disorders and behavioral changes.

- Preprocedure

  o Nursing Actions

    ▪ Review medications with the provider to determine if they should be continued prior to this procedure.

  o Client Education

    ▪ Instruct the client to wash his hair prior to the procedure and eliminate all oils, gels, and sprays.

    ▪ If indicated, instruct the client, to be sleep-deprived, because this provides cranial stress, increasing the possibility of seizure activity occurring during the procedure.

- Intraprocedure

  o The procedure generally takes 1 hr.

  o There are no risks associated with this procedure.

  o With the client resting in a chair or lying in bed, small electrodes are placed on the scalp and connected to a brain wave machine or computer.

  o Electrical signals produced by the brain are recorded by the machine or computer in the form of wavy lines. This documents brain activity.

  o Notations are made when stimuli are presented or when sleep occurs. (Flashes of light or pictures may be used during the procedure to assess the client's response to stimuli.)

  o An EEG provides information about the ability of the brain to function and highlights areas of abnormality.

- Postprocedure

  o Client Education

    ▪ Instruct the client that normal activities may be resumed.

Glasgow Coma Scale (GCS)

- This assessment concentrates on neurologic function and is useful to determine the level of consciousness and monitor response to treatment. The GCS is reported as a number, which allows health care providers to immediately determine if neurologic changes have occurred.

- Indications

  o GCS scores are helpful in determining changes in the level of consciousness for clients with head injuries, space occupying lesions or cerebral infarctions, and encephalitis. This is important because complications related to neurologic injuries may occur rapidly and require immediate treatment.

- Interpretation of Findings

  ○ The best possible GCS score is 15. In general, total scores of the GCS correlate with the degree or level of coma.

  ○ Less than 8 – Associated with severe head injury and coma

  ○ 9 to 12 – Indicate a moderate head injury

  ○ Greater than 13 – Reflect minor head trauma

- Procedure

  ○ The GCS is calculated by using appropriate stimuli (a painful stimulus may be necessary) and then assessing the client's response in three areas.

    ■ Eye opening (E) – The best eye response, with responses ranging from 4 to 1

      □ 4 = Eye opening occurs spontaneously.

      □ 3 = Eye opening occurs secondary to voice.

      □ 2 = Eye opening occurs secondary to pain.

      □ 1 = Eye opening does not occur.

    ■ Verbal (V) – The best verbal response, with responses ranging from 5 to 1

      □ 5 = Conversation is coherent and oriented.

      □ 4 = Conversation is incoherent and disoriented.

      □ 3 = Words are spoken, but inappropriately.

      □ 2 = Sounds are made, but no words.

      □ 1 = Vocalization does not occur.

    ■ Motor (M) – The best motor response, with responses ranging from 6 to 1

      □ 6 = Commands are followed.

      □ 5 = Local reaction to pain occurs.

      □ 4 = There is a general withdrawal to pain.

      □ 3 = Decorticate posture (adduction of arms, flexion of elbows and wrists) is present.

      □ 2 = Decerebrate posture (abduction of arms, extension of elbows and wrists) is present.

      □ 1 = Motor response does not occur.

- o Responses within each subscale are added, with the total score quantitatively describing the client's level of consciousness. E + V + M = Total GCS
  - ■ In critical situations, where head injury is present and close monitoring is required, subscale results may also be documented. Thus, a GCS may be reported as either a single number, indicating the sum of the subscales (3 to 15), or as 3 numbers, one from each subscale result, and the total (E3 V3 M4 = GCS 13). This allows providers to determine specific neurologic function.
  - ■ Intubation limits the ability to use GCS summed scores. If intubation is present, the GCS may be reported as two scores, with modification noted. This is generally reported as "GCS 5t" (with the t representing the intubation tube).

Intracranial Pressure (ICP) Monitoring

- An ICP monitor is a device inserted into the cranial cavity that records pressure and is connected to a monitor that shows a picture of the pressure waveforms.

  - o Monitoring ICP facilitates continual assessment and is more precise than vague clinical manifestations.

  - o The insertion procedure is always performed by a neurosurgeon in the operating room, emergency department, or critical care unit. This procedure is rarely used unless the client is comatose, so there is minimal need for pain medication and preprocedural teaching.

- Three Basic Types of ICP Monitoring Systems

  - o Intraventricular catheter (also called a ventriculostomy)
    - ■ A fluid-filled catheter is inserted into the anterior horn of the lateral ventricles (most often on the right side) through a burr hole. The catheter is connected to a sterile drainage system with a three-way stopcock that allows simultaneous monitoring of pressures by a transducer connected to a bedside monitor and drainage of CSF.

  - o Subarachnoid screw or bolt
    - ■ A special hollow, threaded screw or bolt is placed into the subarachnoid space through a twist-drill burr hole in the front of the skull, behind the hairline. The bolt is connected by fluid-filled tubing to a transducer leveled at the approximate location of the lateral ventricles.

  - o Epidural or subdural sensor
    - ■ A fiber-optic sensor is inserted into the epidural space through a burr hole. The fiber-optic device measures changes in the amount of light reflected from a pressure-sensitive diaphragm in the catheter tip. The cable is connected to a precalibrated monitor that displays the numerical value of ICP. This method of monitoring is noninvasive because the device does not penetrate the dura.

- Indications

  ○ ICP monitoring is useful for early identification and treatment of increased intracranial pressure. Clients who are comatose and/or have GCS scores of 8 are candidates for ICP monitoring.

  ○ Client Presentation

    ▪ Symptoms of increased ICP include severe headache, deteriorating level of consciousness, restlessness, irritability, dilated or pinpoint pupils, slowness to react, alteration in breathing pattern (Cheyne Stokes respirations, central neurologic hyperventilation, apnea), deterioration in motor function, and abnormal posturing (decerebrate, decorticate, flaccidity).

- Interpretation of Findings

  ○ Normal ICP is 10 to 15 mm Hg. Persistent elevation of ICP extinguishes cerebral circulation, which will result in brain death if not treated urgently.

- Preprocedure

  ○ The head is shaved around the insertion location. The site is then cleansed with an antibacterial solution.

- Intraprocedure

  ○ Local anesthetic can be used to numb the area if the client's GCS indicates some level of consciousness (GCS 8 to 11).

  ○ Insertion and care of any ICP monitoring device requires surgical aseptic technique to reduce the risk for CNS infection.

- Postprocedure

  ○ Nursing Actions

    ▪ Maintain system integrity at all times. There is a risk of serious, life-threatening infection.

    ▪ Inspect the insertion site at least every 24 hr for redness, swelling, and drainage. Change the sterile dressing covering the access site per facility protocol.

    ▪ ICP monitoring equipment must be balanced and recalibrated per facility protocols.

    ▪ After the insertion procedure, observe ICP waveforms, noting the pattern of waveforms and monitoring for increased ICP (a sustained elevation of pressure above 15 mm Hg).

    ▪ Assess the client's clinical status and monitor routine and neurologic vital signs every hour as needed.

- Calculate cerebral perfusion pressure (CPP) hourly. To calculate CPP, subtract ICP from mean arterial pressure (MAP).

    □ CPP = MAP – ICP

    □ MAP = [(2 x diastolic) + systolic]/3

- CPP should be maintained above 70 to 80 mm Hg.

- Complications

  ○ Infection and bleeding

    - The insertion and maintenance of an ICP monitoring system can cause infection and bleeding.

    - Nursing Actions

      □ Follow strict surgical aseptic technique.

      □ Perform sterile dressing changes per facility protocol.

      □ Keep drainage systems closed.

      □ Limit monitoring to 3 to 5 days.

      □ Irrigate the system only as needed to maintain patency.

Lumbar Puncture (Spinal Tap)

- A lumbar puncture is a procedure during which a small amount of cerebrospinal fluid (CSF) is withdrawn from the spinal canal and then analyzed to determine its constituents.

- Indications

  ○ This procedure is used to detect the presence of certain diseases (multiple sclerosis, syphilis), infection, and malignancies. A lumbar puncture may also be used to administer medication or chemotherapy directly to spinal fluid.

- Preprocedure

  ○ The risks versus the benefits of a lumbar puncture should be discussed with the client prior to undertaking this procedure.

    - A lumbar puncture is associated with severe complications, especially when performed in the presence of increased ICP (brain herniation).

    - Lumbar punctures for clients with bleeding disorders or taking anticoagulants may result in bleeding that compresses the spinal cord.

  ○ Nursing Actions

    - Ensure that all the client's jewelry has been removed and that the client is wearing only a hospital gown.

    - Instruct the client to void prior to the procedure.

    - Clients should be positioned to stretch the spinal canal. This may be done by having the client assume a "cannonball" position while on one side or by having the client stretch over an overbed table if sitting is preferred.

- Intraprocedure

  - The area of the needle insertion is cleansed, and a local anesthesia is injected.

  - This is not a painful procedure; there should be little need for pain or relaxing medication other than the local anesthesia.

  - The needle is inserted and the CSF is withdrawn, after which the needle is removed.

  - A manometer may be used to determine the opening pressure of the spinal cord, which is useful if increased pressure is a consideration.

- Postprocedure

  - CSF is sent to the pathology department for analysis.

  - Nursing Actions

    - Monitor the puncture site. The client should remain lying for several hours to ensure that the site clots.

  - Client Education

    - Once stable, advise the client that normal activities may be resumed.

- Complications

  - CSF leakage

    - If clotting does not occur, CSF may leak, resulting in a headache and increasing the potential for infection.

Magnetic Resonance Imaging (MRI) Scan

- An MRI scan provides cross-sectional images of the cranial cavity. A contrast media may be used to enhance the images.

  - Unlike CT scans, MRI images are obtained using magnets, thus the consequences associated with radiation are avoided. This makes this procedure safer for women who are pregnant.

  - The use of magnets precludes the ability to scan a client who has an artificial device, (pacemakers, surgical clips, intravenous access port). If these are present, shielding may be done to prevent injury.

  - MRI-approved equipment must be used to monitor vital signs and provide ventilator/oxygen assistance to clients undergoing MRI scans.

- Indications

  - MRI scans may be used to detect abnormalities, monitor response to treatment, and guide needles used for biopsies.

  - MRIs are capable of discriminating soft tissue from tumor or bone. This makes the MRI scan more effective at determining tumor size and blood vessel location.

- Preprocedure
  - Nursing Actions
    - Ensure that the client's jewelry is removed prior to this procedure. The client should wear a hospital gown to prevent any metals from interfering with the magnet.
    - If sedation is expected, the client should refrain from food or fluids for 4 to 8 hr prior to the procedure.
    - Determine if the client has a history of claustrophobia and explain the tight space and noise.
    - Health care providers (and family members) who are in the scanning area while the magnet is on must remove all jewelry, pagers, and phones to prevent damage to themselves or the magnet.
    - Because this procedure is performed with the client in a supine position, placing pillows in the small of the client's back may assist in preventing back pain. The head must be secured to prevent unnecessary movement during the procedure.
- Intraprocedure
  - The client must lie supine with the head stabilized.
  - MRI scanning is noisy, and earplugs or sedation may be provided.
- Postprocedure
  - Nursing Actions
    - No follow-up care is required after an MRI scan.
    - If contrast media is injected, monitor the site to assure clotting has occurred.
    - If sedation is administered, monitor the client until stable.

PET and SPECT Scans

- PET and SPECT scans are nuclear medicine procedures that produce three-dimensional images of the head. These images can be static (depicting vessels) or functional (depicting brain activity).
  - A glucose-based tracer is injected into the blood stream prior to the PET/SPECT scan. This initiates regional metabolic activity, which is then documented by the PET/SPECT scanner.
  - A CT scan may be performed after a PET/SPECT scan, as this provides information regarding brain activity and pathological location.
- Indications
  - A PET/SPECT scan capture of regional metabolic is most useful in determining tumor activity and/or response to treatment. PET/SPECT scans are also able to determine the presence of dementia, indicated by the inability of the brain to respond to the tracer.

- Preprocedure

  ○ PET/SPECT scans use radiation, thus the risk/benefit consequences to any client who may be pregnant must be discussed.

  ○ Nursing Actions

    ▪ Assess for a history of diabetes mellitus. While this condition does not preclude a PET/SPECT scan, alterations in the client's medications may be necessary to avoid hyperglycemia or hypoglycemia before and after this procedure.

- Intraprocedure

  ○ While the pictures are being obtained, the client must lie flat with the head restrained.

  ○ This procedure is not painful and sedation is rarely necessary.

- Postprocedure

  ○ Nursing Actions

    ▪ There is no follow-up care after a PET/SPECT scans.

    ▪ Because the tracer is glucose based and short acting (less than 2 hr), it is broken down within the body as a sugar, not excreted.

Radiography (X-Ray)

- An x-ray uses electromagnetic radiation to capture images of the internal structures of an individual.

  ○ A structure's image is light or dark relative to the amount of radiation the tissue absorbs. The image is recorded on a radiograph, which is a black and white image that is held up to light for visualization. Some are recorded digitally and are available immediately.

  ○ X-rays must be interpreted by a radiologist, who documents the findings.

- Indications

  ○ X-ray examinations of the skull and spine can reveal fractures, curvatures, bone erosion and dislocation, and possible soft tissue calcification, all of which can damage the nervous system.

- Preprocedure

  ○ Nursing Actions

    ▪ There is no special preprocedure protocol for x-rays that do not use contrast. X-rays are often the first diagnostic tool used after an injury (rule out cervical fracture in head trauma), and they can be done without any preparation.

    ▪ Determine if female clients are pregnant.

    ▪ Ensure that the client's jewelry is removed and that no clothes cover the area.

- o Client Education
  - ■ Explain that the amount of radiation used in contemporary x-ray machines is very small.
- Intraprocedure
  - o Client Education
    - ■ Instruct the client to remain still during the procedure.
- Postprocedure
  - o Nursing Actions
    - ■ No postprocedure care is required.
  - o Client Education
    - ■ Inform the client when results will be available.

CHAPTER 3: NEUROLOGIC DIAGNOSTIC PROCEDURES

(A) Application Exercises

Scenario: A nurse is caring for a client who was admitted following a motor vehicle crash. The client is exhibiting symptoms of increasing intracranial pressure (ICP) from a suspected closed head injury. He is admitted to the ICU for a ventriculostomy.

1. The client's wife asks the nurse what the procedure entails. Which of the following responses is appropriate?

    A. "An incision will be made in the skin, and the ventriculostomy tube will be inserted just under the skin."

    B. "Moderate discomfort will be felt as a small hole is drilled in his skull."

    C. "Your husband will have a large dressing that will cover the operative site and ventriculostomy."

    D. "A catheter will be attached to a bedside monitor that will continuously measure intracranial pressure."

2. Which of the following should be the nurse's highest priority concern for the client after the ventriculostomy is placed?

    A. Headache

    B. Infection

    C. Hemorrhage

    D. Hypoxia

3. The nurse should recognize that which of the following client behaviors suggest an increase in ICP? (Select all that apply.)

    _____ Severe headache

    _____ Motor, verbal, and eye-opening responses to deep pain only

    _____ Pupils equal at 5 mm

    _____ Arms flexed with internal rotation and plantar flexion of legs

    _____ Glasgow Coma Scale score of 3

    _____ Deep tendon reflexes of 2+ in the lower extremities

    _____ Blood pressure of 168/58 mm Hg and heart rate of 48/min

    _____ Shallow breaths followed by period of apnea, then deep breaths

4. A nurse is caring for a client who is scheduled for a cerebral angiogram with contrast dye. Which of the following client statements should the nurse communicate to the health care provider? (Select all that apply.)

_____ "I may be pregnant."

_____ "I take Coumadin."

_____ "I am on an antihypertensive."

_____ "I am allergic to shellfish."

_____ "I am allergic to latex."

5. A nurse is providing education to a client who is to undergo an electroencephalogram (EEG) the next day. Which of the following information should the nurse include in the teaching?

A. "Do not wash your hair the morning of the procedure."

B. "Try to stay awake most of the night prior to the procedure."

C. "The procedure will take approximately 15 minutes."

D. "You will need to lie flat for 4 hours after the procedure."

CHAPTER 3: NEUROLOGIC DIAGNOSTIC PROCEDURES

Ⓐ Application Exercises Answer Key

Scenario: A nurse is caring for a client who was admitted following a motor vehicle crash. The client is exhibiting symptoms of increasing intracranial pressure (ICP) from a suspected closed head injury. He is admitted to the ICU for a ventriculostomy.

1. The client's wife asks the nurse what the procedure entails. Which of the following responses is appropriate?

    A. "An incision will be made in the skin, and the ventriculostomy tube will be inserted just under the skin."

    B. "Moderate discomfort will be felt as a small hole is drilled in his skull."

    C. "Your husband will have a large dressing that will cover the operative site and ventriculostomy."

    D. "A catheter will be attached to a bedside monitor that will continuously measure the intracranial pressure."

    The purpose of a ventriculostomy is to measure and drain cerebral spinal fluid. The ventriculostomy will be connected to a monitor that will provide ICP readings. The ventriculostomy will be inserted into a ventricle of the brain through a small burr hole that is drilled in the skull. This is not usually a painful procedure because there are no pain receptors in the brain or skull. Only a small, sterile dressing will be necessary over the wound after the procedure.

Ⓝ NCLEX® Connection: Reduction of Risk Potential, Potential for Complications of Diagnostic Tests/Treatments/Procedures

2. Which of the following should be the nurse's highest priority concern for the client after the ventriculostomy is placed?

    A. Headache

    B. Infection

    C. Hemorrhage

    D. Hypoxia

    If the ventriculostomy is not maintained using sterile technique, an infection may result in meningitis, which could be life threatening. Although a client with increased ICP may experience headaches, hemorrhage, and hypoxia, these findings are not complications directly related to the ventriculostomy.

Ⓝ NCLEX® Connection: Reduction of Risk Potential, Potential for Complications of Diagnostic Tests Treatments Procedures

3. The nurse should recognize that which of the following client behaviors suggest an increase in ICP? (Select all that apply.)

__X__ **Severe headache**

__X__ **Motor, verbal, and eye-opening responses to deep pain only**

_____ Pupils equal at 5 mm

__X__ **Arms flexed with internal rotation and plantar flexion of legs**

__X__ **Glasgow Coma Scale score of 3**

_____ Deep tendon reflexes of 2+ in the lower extremities

__X__ **Blood pressure of 168/58 mm Hg and heart rate of 48/min**

__X__ **Shallow breaths followed by a period of apnea, then deep breaths**

A severe headache; deteriorating level of consciousness; abnormal posturing (decorticate in this case); Cushing's reflex/triad of hypertension, bradycardia, and widened pulse pressure (110 mm Hg in this case); and alterations in respiratory pattern (Cheyne-Stokes respirations in this case) are signs of increased ICP. Normal pupil findings include 3 to 5 mm size with reactivity to light. Deep tendon reflexes of 2+ in the lower extremities is a normal neurological finding.

 NCLEX® Connection: Physiological Adaptation, Alterations in Body Systems

4. A nurse is caring for a client who is scheduled for a cerebral angiogram with contrast dye. Which of the following client statements should the nurse communicate to the health care provider? (Select all that apply.)

__X__ **"I may be pregnant."**

__X__ **"I take Coumadin."**

_____ "I am on an antihypertensive."

__X__ **"I am allergic to shellfish."**

_____ "I am allergic to latex."

The health care provider should be notified if a client is or could be pregnant due to the risks to the fetus secondary to injection of contrast material. Allergies to shellfish or iodine are also contraindications to contrast dye if client is taking warfarin (Coumadin) this should also be reported to the health care provider due to the potential for bleeding post procedure. There are no contraindications to contrast dye for clients who are taking antihypertensives or are allergic to latex.

NCLEX® Connection: Reduction of Risk Potential, Potential for Complications of Diagnostic Tests/Treatments/Procedures

5. A nurse is providing education to a client who is to undergo an electroencephalogram (EEG) the next day. Which of the following information should the nurse include in the teaching?

    A. "Do not wash your hair the morning of the procedure."

    B. "Try to stay awake most of the night prior to the procedure."

    C. "The procedure will take approximately 15 minutes."

    D. "You will need to lie flat for 4 hours after the procedure."

The client should be instructed to wash his hair prior to the procedure and to stay awake the night before the procedure if possible. An EEG usually takes approximately 1 hr and there are no activity restrictions post procedure.

Ⓝ **NCLEX® Connection: Reduction of Risk Potential, Diagnostic Tests**

UNIT 2	NURSING CARE OF CLIENTS WITH NEUROSENSORY DISORDERS
Section	Diagnostic and Therapeutic Procedures
Chapter 4	Pain Management

Overview

- Effective pain management includes the use of pharmacological and nonpharmacological pain management therapies. Invasive therapies such as nerve ablation may be appropriate for intractable cancer-related pain.

- Clients have a right to adequate assessment and management of pain. Nurses are accountable for the assessment of pain. A nurse's role is that of an advocate and educator for effective pain management.

- Nurses have a priority responsibility for the continual assessment of a client's pain level and to provide individualized interventions. They should assess the effectiveness of the interventions 30 to 60 min after implementation.

- Assessment challenges may occur with clients who are cognitively impaired or on a ventilator.

- Undertreatment of pain is a serious health care problem. Consequences of undertreatment of pain include physiological and psychological components.

  o Acute/chronic pain can cause anxiety, fear, and depression.

  o Poorly managed acute pain may lead to chronic pain syndrome.

Physiology of Pain

- Transduction is the conversion of painful stimuli to an electrical impulse through peripheral nerve fibers (nociceptors).

- Transmission occurs as the electrical impulse travels along the nerve fibers and is regulated by neurotransmitters.

- The point at which one feels pain is known as the pain threshold.

- The amount of pain one is willing to bear is known as pain tolerance.

SUBSTANCES THAT INCREASE PAIN TRANSMISSION AND CAUSE AN INFLAMMATORY RESPONSE	SUBSTANCES THAT DECREASE PAIN TRANSMISSION AND PRODUCE ANALGESIA
• Substance P • Prostaglandins • Bradykinin • Histamine	• Serotonin • Endorphins

- Perception or awareness of pain occurs in the brain and is influenced by thought and emotional processes.

- Modulation occurs in the spinal cord, causing muscles to contract reflexively, moving the body away from painful stimuli.

Pain Categories

ACUTE PAIN	CHRONIC PAIN
• Acute pain is protective, temporary, usually self-limiting, and resolves with tissue healing. • Physiological responses (sympathetic nervous system) are fight-or-flight responses (tachycardia, hypertension, anxiety, diaphoresis, muscle tension). • Behavioral responses include grimacing, moaning, flinching, and guarding. • Interventions include treatment of the underlying problem.	• Chronic pain is not protective; it is ongoing or recurs frequently, lasting longer than 6 months and persisting beyond tissue healing. • Physiological responses do not usually alter vital signs, but the client may experience depression, fatigue, and a decreased level of functioning. • Psychosocial implications may lead to disability. • Chronic pain may not have a known cause, and it may not respond to interventions. • Management of pain is aimed at symptomatic relief. • Chronic pain can be malignant or nonmalignant.

NOCICEPTIVE PAIN	NEUROPATHIC PAIN
<ul><li>Nociceptive pain arises from damage to or inflammation of tissue other than that of the peripheral and central nervous systems.</li><li>It is usually throbbing, aching, and localized.</li><li>This pain typically responds to opioids and nonopioid medications.</li><li>Types of nociceptive pain<ul><li>Somatic – in bones, joints, muscles, skin, or connective tissues</li><li>Visceral – in internal organs such as the stomach or intestines. It can cause referred pain in other body locations not associated with the stimulus</li><li>Cutaneous – in the skin or subcutaneous tissue</li></ul></li></ul>	<ul><li>Neuropathic pain arises from abnormal or damaged pain nerves.</li><li>It includes phantom limb pain, pain below the level of a spinal cord injury, and diabetic neuropathy.</li><li>Neuropathic pain is usually intense, shooting, burning, or described as "pins and needles."</li><li>This pain typically responds to adjuvant medications (antidepressants, antispasmodic agents, skeletal muscle relaxants).</li></ul>

- Risk Factors for Undertreatment of Pain

  o Cultural and societal attitudes

  o Lack of knowledge

  o Fear of addiction

  o Exaggerated fear of respiratory depression

  o Anxiety about making errors in administration of pain medication

- Populations at Risk for Undertreatment of Pain

  o Infants

  o Children

  o Older adults

  o Clients with substance abuse problems

- Causes of Acute and Chronic Pain

  o Trauma

  o Surgery

  o Cancer (tumor invasion, nerve compression, bone metastases, associated infections, immobility)

  o Arthritis

  o Fibromyalgia

- o Neuropathy

- o Diagnostic or treatment procedures (injection, intubation, radiation)

- The Pain Experience is Affected by:

  - o Age.

    - Infants cannot verbalize or understand their pain.

    - Older adult clients may have multiple pathologies that cause pain and limit function.

  - o Fatigue, which can increase sensitivity to pain.

  - o Genetic sensitivity, which can increase or decrease the amount of pain an individual can tolerate.

  - o Cognitive function.

    - Clients who are cognitively impaired may not be able to report pain or report it accurately.

  - o Prior experiences, which can increase or decrease sensitivity depending on whether or not adequate relief was obtained.

  - o Anxiety and fear, which can increase sensitivity to pain.

  - o Support systems that are present and can decrease sensitivity to pain.

  - o Culture, which may influence how a client expresses pain or the meaning given to it.

Assessment

- According to noted pain experts Margo McCaffery and Chris Pasero, pain is whatever the person experiencing it says it is, and it exists whenever the person says it does. The client's report of pain is the most reliable diagnostic measure of pain. Self-report using standardized pain scales is useful for clients who are older than 7 years. Specialized pain scales are available for use with younger children.

- Pain should be assessed and recorded frequently, and may be considered the fifth vital sign.

- Subjective data can be obtained using a symptom analysis.

PARAMETERS	ASSESSMENT
The location is described using anatomical terminology and landmarks.	Ask, "Where is your pain? Does it radiate anywhere else?" Ask the client to point to the location.
Quality refers to how the pain feels. Feelings of pain include: sharp, dull, aching, burning, stabbing, pounding, throbbing, shooting, gnawing, tender, heavy, tight, tiring, exhausting, sickening, terrifying, torturing, nagging, annoying, intense, and/or unbearable.	Ask the client, "What does the pain feel like?" Give the client more than two choices ("Is the pain throbbing, burning, or stabbing?").

PARAMETERS	ASSESSMENT
Intensity, strength, and severity are "measures" of the pain. Visual analog scales (e.g., description scale, number rating scale) can be used to: • Measure pain. • Monitor pain. • Evaluate the effectiveness of interventions.	Ask the client the following questions: • "How much pain do you have now?" • "What is the worst/best the pain has been?" • "How would you rate your pain on a scale of 0 to 10?"
Timing – onset, duration, frequency	Ask the following questions: • "When did it start?" • "How long does it last?" • "How often does it occur?" • "Is it constant or intermittent?"
Setting – how the pain affects daily life or how ADLs affect the pain	Ask the following questions: • "Where are you when the symptoms occur?" • "What are you doing when the symptoms occur?" • "How does the pain affect your sleep?" • "How does the pain affect your ability to work and do your job?"
Associated symptoms that should be noted include fatigue, depression, nausea, and anxiety.	Ask, "What other symptoms do you experience when you are feeling pain?"
Aggravating/relieving factors	Ask the following questions: • "What makes the pain better?" • "What makes the pain worse?" • "Are you currently taking any prescription, herbal, or over-the-counter medications?"

- Objective Data
  - Behaviors complement self-report and assist in pain assessment of clients who are nonverbal.
    - Facial expressions (grimacing, wrinkled forehead), and body movements (restlessness, pacing, guarding)
    - Moaning, crying
    - Decreased attention span
- Acute pain temporarily increases blood pressure, pulse, and respiratory rate. Eventually, increases in vital signs will stabilize despite the persistence of pain. Therefore, physiologic indicators may not be an accurate measure of pain over time.

Nonpharmacological Pain Management

- Cutaneous (skin) stimulation – transcutaneous electrical nerve stimulation (TENS), heat, cold, therapeutic touch, and massage

 View Media Supplement: TENS unit (Video)

- - Interruption of pain pathways
  - Cold for inflammation
  - Heat to increase blood flow and to reduce stiffness
- Distraction
  - Includes ambulation, deep breathing, visitors, TV, and/or music
- Relaxation
  - Includes meditation, yoga, and/or progressive muscle relaxation
- Imagery
  - Focuses on a pleasant thought to divert focus
  - Requires an ability to concentrate
- Acupuncture – vibration or electrical stimulation via tiny needles inserted into the skin and subcutaneous tissues at specific points
- Reduction of pain stimuli in the environment
- Elevation of extremities that are edematous help to promote venous return and decrease swelling

Pharmacological Interventions

- Analgesics are the mainstay for relieving pain. The three classes of analgesics are nonopioids, opioids, and adjuvants.
- Nonopioid analgesics, such as acetaminophen, ibuprofen, and aspirin, are appropriate for treating mild to moderate pain.
  - Acetaminophen has analgesic and antipyretic effects. NSAIDs have analgesic, anti-inflammatory, antiplatelet, and antipyretic effects.
  - Be aware of the hepatotoxic effects of acetaminophen. A client who has a healthy liver should take no more than 4 g/day. Be aware of opioids that contain acetaminophen, such as hydrocodone bitartrate 5 mg and acetaminophen 500 mg (Vicodin).
  - Monitor the client for salicylism (tinnitus, vertigo, decreased hearing acuity).
  - Prevent gastric upset in the client by administering the medication with food or antacids.
  - Monitor the client for bleeding with long-term NSAID use.

- Opioid analgesics (morphine sulfate, fentanyl [Sublimaze], codeine) are appropriate for treating moderate to severe pain (postoperative pain, MI pain, cancer pain).

  o Following a PRN schedule, manage a client's acute severe pain with short-term, (24 to 48 hr) around-the-clock opioids.

  o The parenteral route is preferred for immediate, short-term relief of acute pain. The oral route is the preferred route for chronic, nonfluctuating pain.

  o Consistent timing and dosing of opioid administration will provide consistent pain control.

  o It is essential to monitor and intervene for adverse effects of opioid use.

    ▪ Constipation – Use a preventative approach (monitoring of bowel movements, fluids, fiber intake, exercise, stool softeners, stimulant laxatives, enemas).

    ▪ Orthostatic hypotension – Advise the client to sit or lie down if symptoms of lightheadedness or dizziness occur. Instruct the client to avoid sudden changes in position by slowly moving from a lying to a sitting or standing position. Provide assistance with ambulation as needed.

    ▪ Urinary retention – Monitor the client's I&O, assess for distention, administer bethanechol (Urecholine), and catheterize as prescribed.

    ▪ Nausea/vomiting – Administer antiemetics, advise the client to lie still and/or move slowly, and eliminate odors.

    ▪ Sedation – Monitor the client's level of consciousness and take safety precautions. Sedation usually precedes respiratory depression.

    ▪ Respiratory depression – Monitor the client's respiratory rate prior to and following administration of opioids (especially in clients who are opioid-naïve). Initial treatment of respiratory depression and sedation is generally a reduction in opioid dose. If necessary, slowly administer diluted naloxone (Narcan) as prescribed to reverse opioid effects.

- Adjuvant analgesics enhance the effects of nonopioids, help alleviate other symptoms that aggravate pain (depression, seizures, inflammation), and are useful for treatment of neuropathic pain.

  o Adjuvant medications

    ▪ Anticonvulsants – carbamazepine (Tegretol)

    ▪ Antianxiety agents – diazepam (Valium)

    ▪ Tricyclic antidepressants – amitriptyline (Elavil)

    ▪ Antihistamine – hydroxyzine (Vistaril)

    ▪ Glucocorticoids – dexamethasone (Decadron)

    ▪ Antiemetics – ondansetron hydrochloride (Zofran)

- PCA is a medication delivery system that allows the client to self-administer safe doses of opioid narcotics.

  o Constant plasma levels are maintained by small, frequent doses.

- o The client experiences less lag time between identified need and delivery of medication, which increases the client's sense of control and may decrease the amount of medication needed.

- o Commonly used opioids are morphine sulfate and hydromorphone (Dilaudid).

- o Client teaching is an important aspect of successful PCA therapy.

- o The client is the only person who should push the PCA button to prevent inadvertent overdosing.

- Other strategies for effective pain management

  - o Take a proactive approach by giving the client analgesics before pain becomes too severe. It takes less medication to prevent pain than to treat pain.

  - o Instruct the client to report developing or recurrent pain and to not wait until pain is severe (for PRN orders of pain medication).

  - o Educate the client regarding misconceptions about pain.

  - o Assist the client to reduce fear and anxiety.

  - o Create a treatment plan that includes both nonpharmacological and pharmacological pain relief measures.

Complications and Nursing Implications

- Undertreatment of pain is a serious complication and may lead to increased anxiety with acute pain and depression with chronic pain. Assess/monitor the client for pain frequently, and intervene as appropriate.

- Sedation, respiratory depression, and coma can occur as a result of overdosing. Sedation always precedes respiratory depression.

  - o Identify clients who are high-risk (older adult clients, clients who are opioid-naïve).

  - o Carefully titrate doses while closely monitoring respiratory status.

  - o Stop the opioid and give the antagonist naloxone (Narcan) if the client's respirations are less than 8/min and shallow, or if the client is difficult to arouse.

  - o Identify the cause of sedation.

  - o Use a sedation scale in addition to a pain rating scale to assess a client's pain, especially when administering opioids.

CHAPTER 4: PAIN MANAGEMENT

 Application Exercises

1. When caring for clients experiencing pain, a nurse should recognize that which of the following substances decrease pain transmission. (Select all that apply.)

_____ Substance P

_____ Serotonin

_____ Bradykinin

_____ Endorphins

_____ Histamine

2. A nurse is performing a pain assessment on a client. Which of the following subjective data describes the quality of the client's pain?

A. "My pain is so bad that I cannot sleep at night."

B. "My pain feels like a tight feeling in my chest."

C. "My pain started last week after I went for a hike."

D. "My pain feels better if I rest in an upright position."

3. Which of the following statements describes nociceptive pain? (Select all that apply.)

_____ Arises from nerves damaged by pain

_____ Well localized

_____ Responds well to opioid analgesics

_____ May result in referred pain

_____ Associated with phantom limb pain

4. A nurse is caring for a postoperative client. Which of the following assessment findings is the most reliable indicator that the client is experiencing pain?

A. Blood pressure of 166/90 mm Hg

B. Pain rating of 9 on a scale of 0 to 10

C. Client grimaces when bed is moved

D. Client refuses to eat breakfast

CHAPTER 4: PAIN MANAGEMENT

 Application Exercises Answer Key

1. When caring for clients experiencing pain, a nurse should recognize that which of the following substances decrease pain transmission. (Select all that apply.)

_____	Substance P
__X__	**Serotonin**
_____	Bradykinin
__X__	**Endorphins**
_____	Histamine

Serotonin and endorphins are natural substances within the body that decrease pain transmission. Substance P, bradykinin, and histamine all increase pain transmission.

 NCLEX® Connection: Physiological Adaptation: Pathophysiology

2. A nurse is performing a pain assessment on a client. Which of the following subjective data describes the quality of the client's pain?

A. "My pain is so bad that I cannot sleep at night."

B. "My pain feels like a tight feeling in my chest."

C. "My pain started last week after I went for a hike."

D. "My pain feels better if I rest in an upright position."

Option B describes the quality of the pain, referring to how the pain feels to the client. This is typically a description such as throbbing, sharp, dull, or tight feeling. Option A describes associated symptoms such as difficulty sleeping, nausea, and anxiety. Option C describes the timing of the pain. Option D describes a relieving factor.

 NCLEX® Connection: Reduction of Risk Potential: System-Specific Assessment

3. Which of the following statements describes nociceptive pain? (Select all that apply.)

_____	Arises from nerves by damaged pain
__X__	**Usually well localized**
__X__	**Responds well to opioid analgesics**
__X__	**May result in referred pain**
_____	Associated with phantom limb pain

Nociceptive pain is usually localized, responds well to opioid analgesics, and may result in referred pain. Neuropathic pain arises from damaged pain nerves and is associated with phantom limb pain.

 NCLEX® Connection: Physiological Adaptation: Pathophysiology

4. A nurse is caring for a postoperative client. Which of the following assessment findings is the most reliable indicator that the client is experiencing pain?

    A. Blood pressure of 166/90 mm Hg

    B. Pain rating of 9 on a scale of 0 to 10

    C. Client grimaces when bed is moved

    D. Client refuses to eat breakfast

The client's self-report of pain using a standardized pain scale is the most reliable indicator of pain. Vital signs, nonverbal communication, and other actions may be indicators of pain, but are not the most reliable.

(N) NCLEX® Connection: Reduction of Risk Potential: System-Specific Assessment

UNIT 2	NURSING CARE OF CLIENTS WITH NEUROSENSORY DISORDERS
Section	Central Nervous System Disorders
Chapter 5	Meningitis

Overview

- Meningitis is an inflammation of the meninges, which are the membranes that protect the brain and spinal cord.

- Viral, or aseptic, meningitis is the most common form of meningitis and commonly resolves without treatment.

- Bacterial, or septic, meningitis is a contagious infection with a high mortality rate. The prognosis depends on how quickly care is initiated.

- A meningitis vaccine is available for high-risk populations, such as residential college students.

Health Promotion and Disease Prevention

- Ensure infants receive *Haemophilus influenzae* type b (Hib) vaccine on schedule.

- Pneumococcal polysaccharide vaccine (PPSV) – Vaccinate adults who are immunocompromised, who have a chronic disease, who smoke cigarettes, or who live in a long-term care facility. CDC guidelines should be followed for revaccination. Give one dose to adults older than 65 years of age who have not previously been vaccinated nor have history of disease.

- Ensure that adolescents receive the meningococcal vaccine (MCV4) (*Neisseria meningitidis*) on schedule and prior to living in a residential setting in college. Individuals in other communal living conditions (military) should also be immunized.

  - Client Education

    - Use an insect repellant when risk of being bitten by a mosquito exists.

Assessment

- Risk Factors

  - Viral meningitis

    - Viral illnesses such as the mumps, measles, herpes, and arboviruses (West Nile)

  - Bacterial meningitis

- Bacterial-based infections, such as otitis media, pneumonia, or sinusitis, in which the infectious micro-organism is *Neisseria meningitidis, Streptococcus pneumoniae, or Haemophilus influenzae*
- Immunosuppression
- Invasive procedures, skull fracture, or penetrating head wound (direct access to cerebrospinal fluid)
- Overcrowded or communal living conditions

- Subjective Data

  ○ Excruciating, constant headache

  ○ Nuchal rigidity (stiff neck)

  ○ Photophobia (sensitivity to light)

- Objective Data

  ○ Physical Assessment Findings

    - Fever and chills
    - Nausea and vomiting
    - Altered level of consciousness
    - Positive Kernig's sign (resistance and pain with extension of the client's leg from a flexed position)
    - Positive Brudzinski's sign (flexion of extremities occurring with deliberate flexion of the client's neck)

View Media Supplement:
- Positive Kernig's Sign (Video)   • Positive Brudzinski's Sign (Video)

    - Hyperactive deep tendon reflexes
    - Tachycardia
    - Seizures
    - Red macular rash (meningococcal meningitis)
    - Restlessness, irritability

  ○ Laboratory Tests

    - Urine, throat, nose, and blood culture and sensitivity

      □ Perform culture and sensitivity of various body fluids to identify possible infectious bacteria and an appropriate broad-spectrum antibiotic. Not definitive for meningitis but can guide initial selection of antimicrobial.

    - CBC

      □ Elevated WBC count

- o Diagnostic Procedures
  - ■ Cerebrospinal fluid (CSF) analysis
    - □ CSF analysis is the most definitive diagnostic procedure. CSF is collected during a lumbar puncture performed by the provider.
    - □ Results indicative of meningitis
      - ▶ Appearance of CSF – cloudy (bacterial) or clear (viral)
      - ▶ Elevated WBC
      - ▶ Elevated protein
      - ▶ Decreased glucose (bacterial)
      - ▶ Elevated CSF pressure
    - □ New enteroviral diagnostic test can be done on CSF to determine if infectious agent is viral or bacterial in 2.5 hr.
  - ■ CT scan and MRI
    - □ A CT scan or an MRI may be performed to identify increased intracranial pressure (ICP) and/or an abscess.

Collaborative Care

- • Nursing Care
  - o Isolate the client as soon as meningitis is suspected.
  - o Maintain isolation precautions per hospital policy.
  - o This should be droplet precautions which requires a private room or a room with cohorts, wearing of a surgical mask when within 3 feet of the client, appropriate hand hygiene, and the use of designated equipment, such as blood pressure cuff and thermometer. Continue until antibiotics have been administered for 24 hr.
  - o Implement fever-reduction measures, such as a cooling blanket, if necessary.
  - o Report meningococcal infections to the public health department.
  - o Decrease environmental stimuli.
    - ■ Provide a quiet environment.
    - ■ Minimize exposure to bright light (natural and electric).
  - o Maintain bed rest with the head of the bed elevated to 30°.
  - o Maintain client safety, such as seizure precautions.
  - o Replace fluid and electrolytes as indicated by laboratory values.
  - o Older adult clients are at an increased risk for secondary complications, such as pneumonia.

- Medications
  - Ceftriaxone (Rocephin) or cefotaxime (Claforan)
    - Antibiotics given until culture and sensitivity results are available. Effective for bacterial infections.
  - Phenytoin (Dilantin)
    - Anticonvulsants given if ICP increases or client experiences a seizure.
  - Acetaminophen (Tylenol), ibuprofen (Motrin)
    - Analgesics for headache and/or fever – nonopioid to avoid masking changes in the level of consciousness.
  - Ciprofloxacin (Cipro), rifampin (Rifadin)
    - Prophylactic antibiotics given to individuals in close contact with the client.
- Client Outcomes
  - The client's ICP and neurological status will return to their premeningitis parameters.
  - The client's headache, photophobia, and nuchal rigidity will resolve.

Complications

- Increased ICP (possibly to the point of brain herniation)
  - Meningitis can cause ICP to increase.
  - Nursing Actions
    - Monitor for signs of increasing ICP (decreased level of consciousness, pupillary changes, and widening pulse pressure).
    - Provide interventions to reduce ICP (positioning and avoidance of coughing and straining).
    - Mannitol can be administered via IV.
- Syndrome of inappropriate antidiuretic hormone (SIADH)
  - SIADH can be a complication of meningitis.
  - Nursing Actions
    - Monitor for signs and symptoms (dilute blood, concentrated urine).
    - Provide interventions, such as the administration of demeclocycline (Declomycin) and restriction of fluid.

- Septic emboli (leading to disseminated intravascular coagulation or cardiovascular accident)

  ○ Septic emboli can form during meningitis and travel to other parts of the body, particularly the hands.

  ○ Development of gangrene will necessitate an amputation.

 View Media Supplement: Gangrenous Toe (Image)

  ○ Nursing Actions

    ▪ Monitor circulatory status of extremities and coagulation studies.

    ▪ Report any alterations immediately to the provider.

CHAPTER 5: MENINGITIS

 Application Exercises

Scenario: A college student presents to the emergency department after her roommate found her lying with her left thigh flexed toward her abdomen. The client reports a severe headache and a stiff neck. Initial assessment by the nurse reveals a positive Kernig's sign and a positive Brudzinski's sign. Bacterial meningitis is suspected.

1. What is the significance of the positive Kernig's and Brudzinski's signs?

2. Which of the following additional findings should the nurse expect to find upon assessment? (Select all that apply.)

    _____ Pain and stiffness when flexing the neck

    _____ Report of severe headache

    _____ Hypoactive deep tendon reflexes

    _____ Flexion of knees when head is raised

    _____ History of multiple mosquito bites while camping

3. A nurse is reviewing the health record of students newly admitted to a university. The nurse should ensure that the students living in dormitories are appropriately immunized because they are at risk for developing meningitis secondary to what organism?

    A. *Streptococcus pneumoniae*

    B. *Neisseria meningitidis*

    C. *Bartonella henselae*

    D. *Rickettsia rickettsii*

4. Which of the following nursing interventions are appropriate for a client who has meningitis at risk for increased ICP? (Select all that apply.)

    _____ Implement seizure precautions.

    _____ Perform neurological checks once each day.

    _____ Administer morphine for the report of neck and generalized pain.

    _____ Turn off room lights and television.

    _____ Administer prescribed broad-spectrum antibiotics after blood cultures are obtained.

    _____ Encourage the client to cough and deep breathe frequently.

CHAPTER 5: MENINGITIS

 Application Exercises Answer Key

Scenario: A college student presents to the emergency department after her roommate found her lying with her left thigh flexed toward her abdomen. The client reports a severe headache and a stiff neck. Initial assessment by the nurse reveals a positive Kernig's sign and a positive Brudzinski's sign. Bacterial meningitis is suspected.

1. What is the significance of the positive Kernig's and Brudzinski's signs?

Both signs are indications of the meningeal irritation that may occur as a result of septic or bacterial meningitis.

 NCLEX® Connection: Physiological Adaptation: Infectious Disease

2. Which of the following additional findings should the nurse expect to find upon assessment? (Select all that apply.)

   X   **Pain and stiffness when flexing the neck**

   X   **Report of severe headache**

   _____   Hypoactive deep tendon reflexes

   X   **Flexion of knees when head is raised**

   _____   History of multiple mosquito bites while camping

A client who has bacterial meningitis will exhibit pain and stiffness of the neck, positive Kernig's sign, flexion of the knees when the head is raised (positive Brudzinski's sign), and a severe headache. Hyperactive deep tendon reflexes is expected with meningitis and mosquito bites cause viral meningitis, not bacterial.

 NCLEX® Connection: Physiological Adaptation: Infectious Disease

3. A nurse is reviewing the health record of students newly admitted to a university. The nurse should ensure that the students living in dormitories are appropriately immunized because they are at risk for developing meningitis secondary to what organism?

A. *Streptococcus pneumoniae*

B. *Neisseria meningitidis*

C. *Bartonella henselae*

D. *Rickettsia rickettsii*

All students entering college, particularly those living in a dormitory, should be immunized against *Neisseria meningitidis*. While *Streptococcus pneumoniae* can cause meningitis, it is not recommended as an immunization in this population. *Bartonella henselae* and *Rickettsia rickettsii* are organisms that can also cause meningitis, but an immunization against them is not available.

 NCLEX® Connection: Physiological Adaptation: Infectious Disease

4. Which of the following nursing interventions are appropriate for a client who has meningitis at risk for increased ICP? (Select all that apply.)

   X   **Implement seizure precautions.**

          Perform neurological checks once each day.

          Administer morphine for the report of neck and generalized pain.

   X   **Turn off room lights and television.**

   X   **Administer prescribed broad-spectrum antibiotics after blood cultures are obtained.**

          Encourage the client to cough and deep breathe frequently.

Clients who have meningitis who are at risk for increased ICP should be under seizure precautions, the lights and television should be turned off, and once blood cultures are obtained, broad spectrum antibiotics should be administered. Neurological checks need to be performed more frequently than once a day (usually every 1 to 2 hr), opioids are avoided because they can mask changes in the client's level of consciousness, and coughing increases ICP so it should only be done as necessary, not on a frequent, routine basis.

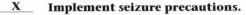 NCLEX® Connection: Physiological Adaptation: Medical Emergencies

UNIT 2	NURSING CARE OF CLIENTS WITH NEUROSENSORY DISORDERS
Section	Central Nervous System Disorders
Chapter 6	Seizures and Epilepsy

Overview

- Seizures are abrupt, abnormal, excessive and uncontrolled electrical discharge of neurons within the brain that may cause alterations in the level of consciousness and/or changes in motor and sensory ability and/or behavior.

- Epilepsy is the term used to define the medical disorder characterized by chronic recurring abnormal brain electrical activity.

- The International Classification of Epileptic Seizures uses three broad categories to describe seizures: generalized, partial or focal/local, and unclassified or idiopathic.

Assessment

- Risk Factors

    o Genetic predisposition – absence seizures tend to occur in families

    o Acute febrile state – particularly among infants and children under the age of 2 years

    o Head trauma – may be early or late onset (up to 9 months) and incidence is increased when the head trauma includes a skull fracture

    o Cerebral edema – especially when it occurs acutely and seizure activity tends to disappear when the edema is successfully treated

    o Abrupt cessation of antiepileptic drugs (AEDs) – as a rebound activity

    o Infection – if intracranial, a result of increased intracranial pressure; if systemic, a result of the persistent febrile state

    o Metabolic disorder – a result of insufficient or excessive chemicals within the brain such as occurs with hypoglycemia or hyponatremia

    o Exposure to toxins – especially those associated with rubber and tanning industries (leather tanning, not sun tanning)

    o Brain tumor – if benign, seizures are caused by the increased bulk associated with the tumor; if malignant, associated with the ability of the brain tissue to function

    o Hypoxia – results in a decreased oxygen level of the brain; necessary for neuronal activity

- o Acute drug and alcohol withdrawal – dehydration that accompanies withdrawal creating a toxic level of the drug in the body

- o Fluid and electrolyte imbalances – results in abnormal levels of nutrients required for neuronal function

- o With older adult clients, increased seizure incidence is associated with cerebrovascular diseases.

- o Triggering Factors

  - ▪ Increased physical activity

  - ▪ Excessive stress

  - ▪ Overwhelming fatigue

  - ▪ Acute alcohol ingestion

  - ▪ Excessive caffeine intake

  - ▪ Exposure to flashing lights

  - ▪ Specific chemicals, such as cocaine, aerosols and inhaling glue products

- • Subjective and Objective Data

  - o Generalized seizure

    - ▪ A generalized seizure is also called a tonic-clonic seizure (previously referred to as a grand mal seizure).

    - ▪ It may begin with an aura (alteration in vision, smell, or emotional feeling).

    - ▪ A generalized seizure begins with a 15- to 20-second tonic episode (stiffening of muscles) and loss of consciousness.

    - ▪ A 1- to 2-min clonic episode (rhythmic jerking of the extremities) follows the tonic episode.

    - ▪ Breathing may stop during the tonic phase and become irregular during the clonic phase.

    - ▪ Cyanosis can accompany breathing irregularities.

    - ▪ Biting of the cheek or tongue can occur during clonic phase.

    - ▪ Incontinence can also accompany a seizure.

    - ▪ During the postictal phase, a period of confusion and sleepiness follows the seizure.

    - ▪ Tonic seizure

      - □ During a seizure, only the tonic phase is experienced.

      - □ The seizure usually lasts only a few seconds.

      - □ A loss of consciousness does not occur.

      - □ This type of seizure is much less common than a tonic-clonic seizure.

- Clonic seizure
  - Only the clonic phase is experienced.
  - Fatigue does not usually follow the seizure.
  - This type of seizure is much less common than a tonic-clonic seizure.
- Absence seizure
  - Absence seizures are most common in children.
  - The seizure consists of a loss of consciousness lasting a few seconds.
  - This type of seizure is associated with blank staring.
  - Baseline neurological function is resumed after seizures, with no apparent sequela.
- Myoclonic seizure
  - Myoclonic seizures consist of brief jerking or stiffening of the extremities, which may be symmetrical or asymmetrical.
  - This type of seizure lasts for seconds.
- Atonic or akinetic seizure
  - Atonic or akinetic seizures are characterized by a few seconds in which muscle tone is lost.
  - The seizure is followed by a period of confusion.
  - The loss of muscle tone frequently results in falling.

- Partial or focal/local seizure
  - Complex partial seizure
    - Complex partial seizures have associated automatisms (behaviors that the client is unaware of, such as lip smacking or picking at clothes).
    - The seizure can cause a loss of consciousness for several minutes.
    - Amnesia may occur immediately prior to and after the seizure.
  - Simple partial seizures
    - Consciousness is maintained throughout simple partial seizures.
    - Seizure activity may consist of unusual sensations, a sense of déjà vu, autonomic abnormalities, such as changes in heart rate and abnormal flushing, unilateral abnormal extremity movements, pain or offensive smell.
- Unclassified or idiopathic seizures do not fit into other categories. These types of seizures account for half of all seizures activities and occur for no known reason.
- Laboratory Tests
  - Should include alcohol and illicit drug levels, HIV testing, and, if suspected, screen for the presence of excessive toxins.

○ Diagnostic Procedures

- Electroencephalogram (EEG)

  □ An EEG records electrical activity and may identify the origin of seizure activity.

  □ Client Education

  ‣ No caffeine for 6 to 9 hr prior to the procedure.

  ‣ Wash hair before the procedure (no oils, sprays) and after the procedure to remove electrode glue.

  ‣ May be asked to take deep breaths and/or be exposed to flashes of a strobe light during the procedure.

  ‣ Sleep may be withheld prior to test and possibly induced during test.

- Magnetic resonance imaging (MRI), computed tomography imaging (CT)/ computed axial tomography (CAT) scan, positron emission tomography (PET) scan, cerebrospinal fluid (CSF) analysis, skull x-ray, can all be used to identify or rule out potential causes of seizures.

Collaborative Care

- Nursing Care

View Media Supplement: Seizure Precautions (Video)

○ During a seizure:

- Protect the client from injury (move furniture away, hold head in lap if on the floor).

- Position client to provide a patent airway.

- Be prepared to suction oral secretions.

- Turn the client to the side to decrease the risk of aspiration.

- Loosen restrictive clothing.

- Do not attempt to restrain the client.

- Do not attempt to open jaw or insert airway during seizure activity (may damage teeth, lips, and tongue). Do not use padded tongue blades.

- Document onset and duration of seizure and client findings/observations prior to, during, and following the seizure (level of consciousness, apnea, cyanosis, motor activity, incontinence).

○ Post seizure:

- Maintain the client in a side-lying position to prevent aspiration and to facilitate drainage of oral secretions.

- Check vital signs.

- Assess for injuries.
- Perform neurological checks.
- Allow the client to rest if necessary.
- Reorient and calm the client (may be agitated or confused).

- Institute seizure precautions including placing the bed in the lowest position and padding the side rails to prevent future injury.
- Determine if client experienced an aura, which can possibly indicate the origin of seizure in the brain.
- Try to determine possible trigger (fatigue).

- Medications
  - Administer prescribed antiepileptic drugs (AED), such as phenytoin (Dilantin).
    - Nursing Considerations
      - Initial goal is to control seizure activity using only one medication. If the chosen medication is not effective either the dose is increased, or another medication is added or substituted.
      - Therapeutic levels are determined by blood tests. These are performed on a routine schedule to assure compliance and effectiveness of the medication.
      - Medications should be taken at the same time every day to enhance effectiveness.
      - Be aware of drug-drug adverse effects and drug-food adverse effects. These are specific to the medication.
      - Allergic reactions to these medications are rare, yet may occur immediately or late in therapy. If allergic, another medication may be substituted.
      - Some antiepileptic medications cause oral gum overgrowth. Routine oral hygiene and dental visits can minimize this side effect.
      - When using phenytoin, specific instructions should include avoidance of oral contraceptives, as this medication decreases their effectiveness. Warfarin (Coumadin) should also not be given with this medication.

- Interdisciplinary Care
  - Refer client to a social service to aid in obtaining medications if cost will affect the client's ability to adhere to the medication routine.
  - If employment is affected by seizure activity, referral to social agencies for financial support and vocational evaluation.
  - If seizure activity affects a school-age child's performance in the classroom, this condition should be reported to the disability office, which can develop specialized interventions or facilitate an Individualized Education Program (IEP).
  - Discrimination on the basis of epilepsy is illegal in all states.

- Surgical Interventions

  ○ Surgical interventions include placement of a vagal nerve stimulator and excision of the portion of the brain causing the seizures for intractable seizures.

  ○ Vagal nerve stimulator

  > **(M) View Media Supplement:** Vagal Nerve Stimulator (Image)

    ▪ The vagal nerve stimulator is a device implanted into the left chest wall and connected to an electrode placed on the left vagus nerve.

    ▪ This procedure is performed under general anesthesia.

    ▪ The device is then programmed to administer intermittent stimulation of the brain via stimulation of the vagal nerve, at a rate specific to the client's needs.

    ▪ Client Education

      □ In addition to routine stimulation, the client may initiate vagal nerve stimulation by holding a magnet over the implantable device, at the onset of seizure activity. This either aborts the seizure, or lessens its severity.

  ○ Surgical removal or interruption of brain tissue causing seizure activity

    ▪ Requires an open craniotomy that may be performed with the client awake, in an effort to assure that only abnormal brain tissue is destroyed.

    ▪ EEG monitoring or brain stimulation activities are done during this lengthy procedure to identify the abnormal brain tissue.

    ▪ Anterior temporal lobe resection may also be undertaken to treat refractory complex partial seizures.

    ▪ These procedures have associated morbidities, including infection, loss of cerebral function, and a lack of success in preventing seizures.

    ▪ Nursing Actions

      □ Provide client education regarding seizure management.

        ▸ The importance of monitoring AED levels and maintaining therapeutic medication levels.

        ▸ Possible medication interactions (decreased effectiveness of oral contraceptives).

      □ Encourage the client to wear a medical identification tag at all times.

      □ Instruct the client to research the driving laws for individuals with a history of seizures in his state. Some states restrict or limit the driving of an individual with a recent history of seizures.

- Client Outcomes

  ○ The client will experience a decreased incidence of seizures.

  ○ The client will be compliant with the medication regimen.

Complications

- Status epilepticus

  - This is prolonged seizure activity occurring over a 30-min time frame. The complications associated with this condition are related to decreased oxygen levels, inability of the brain to return to normal functioning, and continued assault on neuronal tissue. This acute condition requires immediate treatment to prevent loss of brain function, which may become permanent.

  - Nursing Actions

    - Maintain an airway, provide oxygen, establish IV access, perform EKG monitoring, and monitor pulse oximetry and ABG results.

    - As prescribed, administer a loading dose of diazepam (Valium) or lorazepam (Ativan) followed by a continuous infusion of phenytoin (Dilantin).

CHAPTER 6: SEIZURES AND EPILEPSY

 Application Exercises

1. A client is admitted for surgical repair of an inguinal hernia. The client has a seizure disorder and states that he thinks he is about to have a seizure. Which of the following nursing interventions should be implemented? (Select all that apply.)

_____ Provide privacy.

_____ Ease the client to the floor if standing.

_____ Move furniture away from the client.

_____ Loosen the client's clothing.

_____ Insert airway or a padded tongue blade.

_____ Protect the client's head with padding.

_____ Restrain the client to protect from injury.

2. Which of the following is a priority intervention for a nurse caring for a client who has just experienced a generalized seizure?

A. Keep the client in a side-lying position.

B. Take the client's vital signs.

C. Reorient the client to the environment.

D. Check the client for injuries.

3. A client calls a clinic and tells the nurse that her morning dose of phenytoin (Dilantin) was accidentally skipped and it is now 3 hr before the next dose is due. The client typically takes phenytoin 3 times a day. Which of the following actions should the nurse tell the client to take?

A. Take a double dose of the medication at the next scheduled time.

B. Wait until the next scheduled time and take a regular dose.

C. Take the skipped dose now and take another dose at the next scheduled time.

D. Wait until the next day to take additional doses and then resume the regular schedule.

4. A nurse is providing education for a client who is scheduled to have an EEG the following day. Which of the following instructions is appropriate to provide?

A. Decaffeinated coffee can be consumed the morning of the procedure.

B. Hair should not be washed prior to the procedure.

C. Food may not be consumed the morning of the procedure.

D. Get plenty of sleep prior to the test.

CHAPTER 6: SEIZURES AND EPILEPSY

 Application Exercises Answer Key

1. A client is admitted for surgical repair of an inguinal hernia. The client has a seizure disorder and states that he thinks he is about to have a seizure. Which of the following nursing interventions should be implemented? (Select all that apply.)

__X__	**Provide privacy.**
__X__	**Ease the client to the floor if standing.**
__X__	**Move furniture away from the client.**
__X__	**Loosen the client's clothing.**
_____	Insert airway or a padded tongue blade.
__X__	**Protect the client's head with padding.**
_____	Restrain the client to protect from injury.

   Privacy should be provided to the client if possible. The nurse should ease the client to the floor to prevent falling. If there is any furniture close by, it should be moved away from the client to prevent injury. The client's clothing should be loosened and the head protected with padding or using the nurse's lap. Current evidence shows that insertion of an airway or a padded tongue blade is dangerous and can injure the client, so neither should be done. Restraint of the client can also cause injury and should be avoided.

   NCLEX® Connection: Physiological Adaptation: Alterations in Body Systems

2. Which of the following is a priority intervention for a nurse caring for a client who has just experienced a generalized seizure?

   A. Keep the client in a side-lying position.

   B. Take the client's vital signs.

   C. Reorient the client to the environment.

   D. Check the client for injuries.

   The greatest risk to the client is aspiration during the postictal phase. Therefore, the priority intervention is to keep the client in a side-lying position so secretions can drain from the mouth. Taking the client's vital signs, reorienting the client to the environment, and checking the client for injuries are important, but not the priority at this time.

   NCLEX® Connection: Physiological Adaptation: Alterations in Body Systems

3. A client calls a clinic and tells the nurse that her morning dose of phenytoin (Dilantin) was accidentally skipped and it is now 3 hr before the next dose is due. The client typically takes phenytoin 3 times a day. Which of the following actions should the nurse tell the client to take?

    A. Take a double dose of the medication at the next scheduled time.

    B. Wait until the next scheduled time and take a regular dose.

    C. Take the skipped dose now and take another dose at the next scheduled time.

    D. Wait until the next day to take additional doses and then resume the regular schedule.

The client should not take an extra dose of phenytoin or miss any remaining doses for the day. It is important that anticonvulsant medication be taken on a regular basis to maintain a consistent blood level. Taking a double dose increases the risk for toxicity. If it is within 4 hr of the next dose, the client should wait and take the next regularly scheduled dose.

Ⓝ NCLEX® Connection: Pharmacological and Parenteral Therapies: Expected Actions/ Outcomes

4. A nurse is providing education for a client who is scheduled to have an EEG the following day. Which of the following instructions is appropriate to provide?

    A. Decaffeinated coffee can be consumed the morning of the procedure.

    B. Hair should not be washed prior to the procedure.

    C. Food may not be consumed the morning of the procedure.

    D. Get plenty of sleep prior to the test.

Caffeine-containing products should be avoided 6 to 9 hr prior to an EEG, but decaffeinated products and food can be consumed. Hair should be washed prior to the EEG and, if possible, the client should not sleep the night prior to the procedure.

Ⓝ NCLEX® Connection: Reduction of Risk Potential: System Specific Assessment

UNIT 2	NURSING CARE OF CLIENTS WITH NEUROSENSORY DISORDERS
Section	Central Nervous System Disorders
Chapter 7	Parkinson's Disease

Overview

- Parkinson's disease (PD) is a progressively debilitating disease that grossly affects motor function. It is characterized by four primary symptoms: tremor, muscle rigidity, bradykinesia (slow movement), and postural instability. These symptoms occur due to overstimulation of the basal ganglia by acetylcholine.

- The secretion of dopamine and acetylcholine in the body produce inhibitory and excitatory effects on the muscles respectively.

- Overstimulation of the basal ganglia by acetylcholine occurs because degeneration of the substantia nigra results in decreased dopamine production. This allows acetylcholine to dominate making smooth, controlled movements difficult.

- Treatment of PD focuses on increasing the amount of dopamine or decreasing the amount of acetylcholine in a client's brain.

- As PD is a progressive disease, there are 5 stages of involvement.

  ○ Stage 1 – Unilateral shaking or tremor of one limb.

  ○ Stage 2 – Bilateral limb involvement occurs making walking and balance difficult.

  ○ Stage 3 – Physical movements slow down significantly, affecting walking more.

  ○ Stage 4 – Tremors may decrease but akinesia and rigidity make day-to-day tasks difficult.

  ○ Stage 5 – Client unable to stand or walk, is dependent for all care, and may exhibit dementia.

Assessment

- Risk Factors

  ○ Onset of symptoms between age 40 to 70

  ○ More common in men

  ○ Genetic predisposition

  ○ Exposure to environmental toxins

- Subjective Data

  o Report of fatigue

  o Report of decreased manual dexterity over time

- Objective Data

> **(M) View Media Supplement:** Assessment Findings with Parkinson's Disease (Video)

  o Physical Assessment Findings

  ▪ Stooped posture

  ▪ Slow, shuffling, and propulsive gait

  ▪ Slow, monotonous speech

  ▪ Tremors/pill-rolling tremor of the fingers

  ▪ Muscle rigidity

  ▪ Bradykinesia/akinesia

  ▪ Mask-like expression

  ▪ Autonomic symptoms (orthostatic hypotension, flushing, diaphoresis)

  ▪ Difficulty chewing and swallowing

  ▪ Drooling

  ▪ Dysarthria

  ▪ Progressive difficulty with ADLs

  ▪ Mood swings

  ▪ Cognitive impairment (dementia)

  o Laboratory Tests

  ▪ There are no definitive diagnostic procedures.

  ▪ Diagnosis is made based on symptoms, their progression, and by ruling out other diseases.

Collaborative Care

- Nursing Care

  o Administer the client's medications at prescribed times.

  ▪ Monitor medication effectiveness and make recommendations for changes in dosage and time of administration to provide best coverage.

- o Monitor swallowing and maintain adequate nutrition. Consult speech and language therapist to assess swallowing if the client demonstrates a risk for choking.

  - Consult the client's dietician for appropriate diet.

  - Document the client's weight at least weekly.

  - Keep a diet intake log.

  - Encourage fluids and document intake.

  - Provide smaller, more frequent meals.

  - Add commercial thickener to thicken food.

  - Provide supplements as prescribed.

- o Maintain client mobility for as long as possible.

  - Encourage exercise, such as yoga (may improve mental status as well).

  - Encourage use of assistive devices as disease progresses.

  - Encourage range-of-motion (ROM) exercises.

  - Teach the client to stop occasionally when walking to slow down speed and reduce risk for injury.

  - Pace activities by providing rest periods.

  - Assist the client with ADLs as needed (hygiene, dressing).

- o Promote client communication for as long as possible.

  - Teach the client facial muscle strengthening exercises.

  - Encourage the client to speak slowly and to pause frequently.

  - Use alternate forms of communication as appropriate.

  - Refer client to a speech-language pathologist.

- o Monitor client's mental and cognitive status

  - Observe for signs of depression and dementia.

  - Provide a safe environment (no throw rugs, encourage the use of an electric razor).

  - Assess personal and family coping with the client's chronic, degenerative disease.

  - Provide a list of community resources (support groups) to the client and the client's family.

  - Refer the client to a social worker or case manager as condition advances (financial issues, long-term home care, and respite care).

- Medications

  - o May take several weeks of use before improvement of symptoms is seen.

  - o While the client is taking a combination of medications, maintenance of therapeutic medication levels is necessary for adequate control.

- o Dopaminergics
    - When given orally, medications, such as levodopa (Dopar), are converted to dopamine in the brain, increasing dopamine levels in the basal ganglia.
    - Dopaminergics may be combined with carbidopa (Sinemet) to decrease peripheral metabolism of levodopa requiring a smaller dose to make the same amount available to the brain. Side effects are subsequently less.
    - Due to medication tolerance and metabolism, the client's dosage and administration times must be adjusted to avoid periods of poor mobility.
    - Nursing Considerations
        - □ Monitor for the "wearing-off" phenomenon and dyskinesias (problems with movement), which can indicate the need to adjust the dosage or time of administration or the need for a medication holiday.
- o Dopamine agonists
    - Dopamine agonists such as bromocriptine (Parlodel) and pramipexole (Mirapex) activate release of dopamine. May be used in conjunction with a dopaminergic for better results.
    - Nursing Considerations
        - □ Monitor for orthostatic hypotension, dyskinesias, and hallucinations.
- o Anticholinergics
    - Anticholinergics such as benztropine (Cogentin) and trihexyphenidyl (Artane) help control tremors and rigidity
    - Nursing Considerations
        - □ Monitor for anticholinergic effects (dry mouth, constipation, urinary retention).
- o Catechol O-methyltransferase (COMT) inhibitors
    - COMT inhibitors such as entacapone (Comtan) decrease the breakdown of levodopa making more available to the brain as dopamine. Can be used in conjunction with a dopaminergic and dopamine agonist for better results.
    - Nursing Considerations
        - □ Monitor for dyskinesia/hyperkinesia when used with levodopa.
        - □ Assess for diarrhea.
        - □ Dark urine is a normal finding.
- o Antivirals
    - Antivirals such as amantadine (Symmetrel) stimulate release of dopamine and prevent its reuptake.
    - Nursing Considerations
        - □ Monitor for swollen ankles and discoloration of the skin.
        - □ Client may also experience atropine-like effects.

- Interdisciplinary Care

  - Since PD is a degenerative, neurological disorder, long-term treatment and care must be accommodated.

  - During the later stages of the disorder, the client will need referrals to and support from such disciplines as speech therapists, occupational therapists, physical therapists, social service, culminating with placement in a long-term care facility.

- Surgical Interventions

  - Stereotactic pallidotomy

    - Stereotactic pallidotomy is the destruction of a small portion of the brain within the globus pallidus through the use of brain imaging and electrical stimulation.

    - Target area is identified with a CT scan or an MRI.

    - Mild electrical stimulation is provided through a burr hole to a target area.

    - Client is assessed for a decrease in tremors and muscle rigidity.

    - When a decrease is elicited, a temporary lesion is formed and the client is reassessed.

    - If symptomatic relief is demonstrated, a permanent lesion is made.

    - Nursing Actions

      - Assess for a neurological impairment and brain hemorrhage postoperatively.

  - Deep brain stimulation

    - An electrode is implanted in the thalamus.

    - A current is delivered through an implanted pacemaker generator.

    - The goal of the current is to interfere with electrical conduction in tremor cells decreasing tremors.

    - Nursing Actions

      - Monitor for infection, brain hemorrhage, or stroke-like symptoms.

    - Client Education

      - The client will need to be instructed on how to use a magnet to adjust the current.

      - The battery to the magnet will need to be replaced every few years.

- Client Outcomes

  - The client's medication will be scheduled so the "wearing-off" phenomenon does not occur.

  - The client will ambulate safely through the use of assistive devices.

  - The client will maintain adequate hydration and nutrition via appropriate diet and thickened liquids.

Complications

- Aspiration pneumonia

    o As PD advances in severity, alterations in chewing and swallowing will worsen, increasing the risk for aspiration.

    o Nursing Actions

    - Use swallowing precautions to decrease the risk for aspiration.

    - Develop individual dietary plan based on the speech therapist's recommendations.

    - Have a nurse in attendance when the client is eating.

    - Encourage the client to eat slowly and chew thoroughly before swallowing.

    - Feed the client in an upright position and have suction equipment on standby.

- Altered cognition (dementia, memory deficits)

    o Clients in advanced stages of PD may exhibit altered cognition in the form of dementia and memory loss.

    o Nursing Actions

    - Acknowledge the client's feelings.

    - Provide for a safe environment.

    - Develop a comprehensive plan of care with the family, client, and interdisciplinary team.

CHAPTER 7: PARKINSON'S DISEASE

 Application Exercises

Scenario: An older adult male was diagnosed with PD 2 years ago. In spite of his condition, he is able to live independently with his partner of 59 years. He takes levodopa (Dopar) with carbidopa (Sinemet) to control his disease. The couple have two adult children who live nearby and offer assistance when needed. Due to a recent episode of pneumonia, the client is receiving home health visits.

1. Which of the following questions should the home health nurse ask to determine if the medications are being given in appropriate dosages and times?

    A. "Is your weight remaining the same?"

    B. "Can you see the television from a comfortable distance?"

    C. "Are you having periods when walking is more difficult?"

    D. "Do you experience any night sweats?"

2. What is the advantage, if any, of administering the medications levodopa and carbidopa at the same time?

    A. Carbidopa prevents the peripheral metabolism of levodopa making a smaller dose of levodopa necessary.

    B. Carbidopa stimulates the release of dopamine while levodopa provides a synthetic supplement.

    C. There is no advantage. One medication treats the tremors, while the other medication prevents cognitive deterioration.

    D. There is no advantage. The medications can be given at separate times with the same results.

3. A client has a new prescription for bromocriptine (Parlodel) for the management of PD. Which of the following instructions should the nurse provide to the client to manage common side effects?

    A. Rise slowly when standing up.

    B. Increase dietary fiber and fluid intake.

    C. Chew sugarless gum.

    D. Wear sunscreen when outdoors.

4. Which of the following findings should be expected by a nurse caring for a client who has PD? (Select all that apply.)

    _____ Decreased vision

    _____ Pill-rolling tremor of the fingers

    _____ Shuffling gait

    _____ Drooling

    _____ Bilateral ankle edema

    _____ Lack of facial expressions

    _____ Emotional lability

    _____ Frequent periods of sleep

CHAPTER 7: PARKINSON'S DISEASE

 Application Exercises Answer Key

Scenario: An older adult male was diagnosed with PD 2 years ago. In spite of his condition, he is able to live independently with his partner of 59 years. He takes levodopa (Dopar) with carbidopa (Sinemet) to control his disease. The couple have two adult children who live nearby and offer assistance when needed. Due to a recent episode of pneumonia, the client is receiving home health visits.

1. Which of the following questions should the home health nurse ask to determine if the medications are being given in appropriate dosages and times?

 A. "Is your weight remaining the same?"

 B. "Can you see the television from a comfortable distance?"

 C. "Are you having periods when walking is more difficult?"

 D. "Do you experience any night sweats?"

 Periods of increased difficulty walking may indicate that the client is having periods when the medication is "wearing off" and an adjustment of dosage is indicated. The client's weight, vision, and occurrence of night sweats are not related to the medication dosage for PD.

  NCLEX® Connection: Pharmacological and Parenteral Therapies, Expected Actions/ Outcomes

2. What is the advantage, if any, of administering the medications levodopa and carbidopa at the same time?

 A. Carbidopa prevents the peripheral metabolism of levodopa making a smaller dose of levodopa necessary.

 B. Carbidopa stimulates the release of dopamine while levodopa provides a synthetic supplement.

 C. There is no advantage. One medication treats the tremors, while the other medication prevents cognitive deterioration.

 D. There is no advantage. The medications can be given at separate times with the same results.

 Carbidopa is given concurrently with levodopa because it prevents the peripheral metabolism of levodopa causing a smaller dose of levodopa to be necessary. Levodopa is not a synthetic supplement, it is converted to dopamine in the brain. Both carbidopa and levodopa are usually given together because of their synergistic action, which include a decrease in tremors and prevention of cognitive deterioration.

  NCLEX® Connection: Pharmacological and Parenteral Therapies, Expected Actions/ Outcomes

3. A client has a new prescription for bromocriptine (Parlodel) for the management of PD. Which of the following instructions should the nurse provide to the client to manage common side effects?

    A. Rise slowly when standing up.

    B. Increase dietary fiber and fluid intake.

    C. Chew sugarless gum.

    D. Wear sunscreen when outdoors.

    Orthostatic hypotension is a common side effect of bromocriptine. Rising slowly when standing up will decrease the risk of dizziness and lightheadedness. Bromocriptine does not have anticholinergic effects, so it is not necessary to instruct the client to increase dietary fiber and fluid intake and chew sugarless gum. Wearing sunscreen when outdoors is good health promotion but does not relate to the side effects of bromocriptine.

 NCLEX® Connection: Pharmacological and Parenteral Therapies, Adverse Effects/Contraindications/Side Effects/Interactions

4. Which of the following findings should be expected by a nurse caring for a client who has PD? (Select all that apply.)

    _____ Decreased vision

    __**X**__ **Pill-rolling tremor of the fingers**

    __**X**__ **Shuffling gait**

    __**X**__ **Drooling**

    _____ Bilateral ankle edema

    __**X**__ **Lack of facial expressions**

    __**X**__ **Emotional lability**

    _____ Frequent periods of sleep

    A client who has PD will experience pill-rolling tremors of the fingers, a shuffling gait, drooling, a lack of facial expressions, and emotional lability. Ankle edema and decreased vision are not direct effects of PD. Sleep disturbances are experienced rather than frequent periods of sleep.

 NCLEX® Connection: Reduction of Risk Potential, System Specific Assessment

UNIT 2	NURSING CARE OF CLIENTS WITH NEUROSENSORY DISORDERS
Section	Central Nervous System Disorders
Chapter 8	Alzheimer's Disease

⊚ Overview

- Alzheimer's disease (AD) is a nonreversible type of dementia that progressively develops through seven stages over many years. A special framework made up of seven stages has been designed to categorize the disease and its signs and symptoms. The framework is based on three general stages: early stage, mid stage, and late stage.

- AD is a type of dementia. Dementia is defined as multiple cognitive deficits that impair memory and can affect language, motor skills, and/or abstract thinking.

- Some people die 4 to 6 years after diagnosis, but others can live with the disease for up to 20 years.

- AD is responsible for 60% of dementia cases in clients over 65 years of age.

- ⓖ Age is the number one known risk factor for AD, which usually occurs after the age of 65.

- AD is characterized by memory loss, problems with judgment, and changes in personality.

- Severe physical decline occurs along with deteriorating cognitive functions.

Assessment

- Risk Factors

  ⓖ
  - ○ Advanced age

  - ○ Genetic predisposition

  - ○ Environmental agents (herpes virus, metal, or toxic waste)

  - ○ Previous head injury

  ⓖ
  - ○ Apolipoprotein E

- Subjective and Objective Data

STAGE	SIGNS AND SYMPTOMS
Stage 1: No impairment (Normal function)	• No memory problems
Stage 2: Very mild cognitive decline (May be normal age-related changes or very early signs of AD)	• Forgetfulness, especially of everyday objects (eyeglasses or wallet) • No memory problems evident to provider, friends, or coworkers
Stage 3: Mild cognitive decline (Problems with memory or concentration may be measurable in clinical testing or during a detailed medical interview)	• Mild cognitive deficits, including losing or misplacing important objects • Decreased ability to plan • Short-term memory loss noticeable to close relatives • Decreased attention span • Difficulty remembering words or names • Difficulty in social or work situations
Stage 4: Moderate cognitive decline (Mild or early-stage AD; medical interview will detect clear-cut deficiencies)	• Personality changes – appearing withdrawn or subdued, especially in social or mentally challenging situations • Obvious memory loss • Limited knowledge and memory of recent occasions, current events, or personal history • Difficulty performing tasks that require planning and organizing (paying bills or managing money) • Difficulty with complex mental arithmetic
Stage 5: Moderately severe cognitive decline (Moderate or mid-stage AD)	• Increasing cognitive deficits emerge • Inability to recall important details such as address, telephone number, or schools attended, but memory of information about self and family remains intact • Disorientation and confusion as to time and place
Stage 6: Severe cognitive decline (Moderately severe or mid-stage AD)	• Memory difficulties continue to worsen • Loss of awareness of recent events and surroundings • May recall own name, but unable to recall personal history • Significant personality changes are evident (delusions, hallucinations, and compulsive behaviors) • Wandering behavior • Requires assistance with usual daily activities such as dressing, toileting, and other grooming • Normal sleep/wake cycle is disrupted • Increased episodes of urinary and fecal incontinence

STAGE	SIGNS AND SYMPTOMS
Stage 7: Very severe cognitive decline (Severe or late-stage AD)	• Ability to respond to environment, speak, and control movement is lost • Unrecognizable speech • General urinary incontinence • Inability to eat without assistance and impaired swallowing • Gradual loss of all ability to move extremities (ataxia)

Alzheimer's Association National Office (2009), Stages of Alzheimer's, Retrieved April 27, 2009, From: http://www.alz.org/alzheimers_disease_stages_of_alzheimers.asp.

- ○ Laboratory Tests

  - ■ Genetic testing for the presence of apolipoprotein E. can determine if late onset dementia is due to AD.

- ○ Diagnostic Procedures

  - ■ There is no definitive diagnostic procedure, except brain tissue examination upon death.

  - ■ Magnetic resonance imaging (MRI), computed tomography (CT) imaging/computed axial tomography (CAT) scan, positron emission tomography (PET) scan, and electroencephalogram (EEG) may be performed to rule out other possible causes of symptoms.

Collaborative Care

- • Nursing Care

  - ○ Assess cognitive status, memory, judgment, and personality changes.

  - ○ Initiate bowel and bladder program with the client based on a set schedule.

  - ○ Encourage the client and family to participate in an AD support group.

  - ○ Provide a safe environment.

  - ○ Keep the client on a sleeping schedule and monitor for irregular sleeping patterns.

  - ○ Provide verbal and nonverbal ways to communicate with the client.

  - ○ Offer snacks or finger foods if the client is unable to sit for long periods of time.

  - ○ Check the client's skin weekly for breakdown.

  - ○ Provide cognitive stimulation:

    - ■ Offer varied environmental stimulations such as walks, music, or craft activities.

    - ■ Keep a structured environment and introduce change gradually (client's daily routine or a room change).

    - ■ Use a calendar to assist with orientation.

    - ■ Use short directions when explaining an activity or care the client needs, such as a bath.

- Be consistent and repetitive.
- Use therapeutic touch.
  - Provide memory training:
    - Reminisce with the client about the past.
    - Use memory techniques such as making lists and rehearsing.
    - Stimulate the client's memory by repeating the client's last statement.
  - Avoid overstimulation (keep noise and clutter to a minimum and avoid crowds).
  - Promote consistency by placing commonly used objects in the same location and using a routine schedule.
    - Reality orientation (early stages)
    - Easily viewed clock and single day calendar
    - Pictures of family and pets
    - Frequent reorientation to time, place, and person
  - Validation therapy (later stages)
    - Acknowledge the client's feelings.
    - Don't argue with the client; this will lead to the client becoming upset.
    - Reinforce and use repetitive actions or ideas cautiously.
  - Promote self-care as long as possible. Assist the client with activities of daily living as appropriate.
  - Speak directly to the client in short, concise sentences.
  - Reduce agitation (use calm, redirecting statements; provide a diversion).
  - Provide a routine toileting schedule.
- Medications
  - Most medications for clients who have dementia attempt to target behavioral and emotional problems, such as anxiety, agitation, combativeness, and depression.
  - These medications include antipsychotics, antidepressants, and anxiolytics. Clients receiving these medications should be closely monitored for adverse effects.
  - AD medications temporarily slow the course of the disease and do not work for all clients.
  - Pharmacotherapeutics is based on the theory that AD is a result of depleted levels of the enzyme acetyltransferase, which is necessary to produce the neurotransmitter acetylcholine.
  - Benefits for those clients who do respond to medication include improvements in cognition, behavior, and function.
  - If a client fails to improve with one medication, a trial of one of the other medications is warranted.

- o Donepezil hydrochloride (Aricept)

  - Prevents the breakdown of acetylcholine (ACh), which increases the amount of ACh available. This results in increased nerve impulses at the nerve sites.

  - Cholinesterase inhibitors help slow this process down.

  - Nursing Considerations

    - □ Observe the client for frequent stools and or upset stomach when taking donepezil hydrochloride.

    - □ Monitor the client for dizziness and or headache. The client may feel lightheaded or have an unsteady gait.

    - □ Use caution when administering this medication to clients who have asthma or COPD.

- Interdisciplinary Care

  - o Refer the client to social services and case managers for possible adult day care facilities or long-term care facilities.

  - o Refer the client to the Alzheimer's Association and community outreach programs. This can include in-home care or respite care.

- Therapeutic Procedures

  - o Alternative therapy

    - Estrogen therapy for women may prevent Alzheimer's disease, but it is not useful in decreasing the effects of pre-existing dementia.

    - Ginkgo biloba, an herbal product taken to increase memory and blood circulation, can cause a variety of side effects and medication interactions. If a client is using ginkgo biloba or other nutritional supplements, that information should be shared with health care providers.

- Care after Discharge

  - o Refer to social services and case managers for long-term/home management.

  - o Alzheimer's Association, community outreach programs and support groups

  - o Client Education

    - Educate family/caregivers about illness, methods of care, and adaptation of the home environment.

    - Home safety measures to be implemented may include:

      - □ Removing scatter rugs.

      - □ Installing door locks that cannot be easily opened, and place alarms on doors.

      - □ Keeping a lock on the water heater and thermostat; keeping the water temperature tuned down to a safe level.

      - □ Providing good lighting, especially on stairs.

- □ Installing handrails on stairs and marking step edges with colored tape.

- □ Placing the mattress on the floor.

- □ Removing clutter and clearing hallways for walking.

- □ Securing electrical cords to baseboards.

- □ Keeping cleaning supplies in locked cupboards.

- □ Installing handrails in the bathroom, at bedside, and in the tub; placing a shower chair in the tub.

- □ Having the client wear a medical identification bracelet if living at home with caregiver.

- □ Monitoring for improvement in memory and the client's quality of life.

- ■ Support for caregivers

  - □ Determine teaching needs for the client, especially for family members, when the client's cognitive ability is progressively declining.

  - □ Review the resources available to the family as the client's health declines. Include long-term care options. A wide variety of home care and community resources, such as respite care, may be available to the family in many areas of the country, and these resources may allow the client to remain at home rather than in an institution.

- Client Outcomes

  - ○ The client will remain free from injury.

  - ○ The client will sleep 5 to 6 hr every night.

  - ○ The client will be able to perform self-care independently with verbal assistance.

CHAPTER 8: ALZHEIMER'S DISEASE

 Application Exercises

1. A nurse is providing teaching to an older adult client who has AD and his wife, who cares for him full time at home. The client is unable to care for himself and needs assistance with taking his medications. The client has been prescribed donepezil hydrochloride (Aricept). Which of the following statements made by the wife indicates the teaching has been effective regarding donepezil hydrochloride?

    A. "This medication should increase my husband's appetite."

    B. "This medication should help my husband sleep better."

    C. "This medication should help my husband's daily function."

    D. "This medication should increase my husband's energy level."

2. A nurse is making a home visit to a client who has AD. The client is often disoriented to time and place, is unsteady on his feet, and has a history of wandering. His wife is fearful that he will wander outside or injure himself in the home. Which of the following safety measures should the nurse instruct the wife to implement? (Select all that apply.)

    _____ Remove floor rugs.

    _____ Have door locks that can be easily opened.

    _____ Provide good lighting, especially along the stairs.

    _____ Install handrails along the stairs, and in the bathroom.

    _____ Keep the mattress on the floor.

    _____ Secure electrical cords to baseboards.

3. A nurse is caring for a client who has AD and keeps falling. Which of the following actions should the nurse take first to keep the client safe?

    A. Keep the call-light close to the client.

    B. Place the client in a room close to the nurses' station.

    C. Encourage the client to ask for help when he needs assistance.

    D. Remind the client to wait for assistance when he gets up unattended.

CHAPTER 8: ALZHEIMER'S DISEASE

 Application Exercises Answer Key

1. A nurse is providing teaching to an older adult client who has AD and his wife, who cares for him full time at home. The client is unable to care for himself and needs assistance with taking his medications. The client has been prescribed donepezil hydrochloride (Aricept). Which of the following statements made by the wife indicates the teaching has been effective regarding donepezil hydrochloride?

    A. "This medication should increase my husband's appetite."

    B. "This medication should help my husband sleep better."

    C. "This medication should help my husband's daily function."

    D. "This medication should increase my husband's energy level."

Donepezil hydrochloride helps slow the progression of AD. It can also help improve behavior and daily function. It does not help with the client's appetite, sleep, or energy level.

NCLEX® Connection: Pharmacological and Parenteral Therapies: Expected Actions/ Outcomes

2. A nurse is making a home visit to a client who has AD. The client is often disoriented to time and place, is unsteady on his feet, and has a history of wandering. His wife is fearful that he will wander outside or injure himself in the home. Which of the following safety measures should the nurse instruct the wife to implement? (Select all that apply.)

__X__	**Remove floor rugs.**
_____	Have door locks that can be easily opened.
__X__	**Provide good lighting, especially along the stairs.**
__X__	**Install handrails along the stairs, and in the bathroom.**
__X__	**Keep the mattress on the floor.**
__X__	**Secure electrical cords to baseboards.**

Removing floor rugs can decrease the client's risk of falling. Good lighting can also decrease the risk for falling in dark areas, such as stairways. Installing handrails on the stairs and in the bathroom can be useful for the client to hold on to when his gait is unsteady. By securing electrical cords to baseboards and placing the client's mattress on the floor, the client's risk of falling or tripping is decreased. Easy-to-open door locks increase the risk for a client who wanders to get out of his home and get lost.

NCLEX® Connection: Reduction of Risk Potential: Potential for Alterations in Body Systems

3. A nurse is caring for a client who has AD and keeps falling. Which of the following actions should the nurse take first to keep the client safe?

    A. Keep the call-light close to the client.

    B. Place the client in a room close to the nurses' station.

    C. Encourage the client to ask for help when he needs assistance.

    D. Remind the client to wait for assistance when he gets up unattended.

Moving the client's room close to the nurses' station provides constant supervision by the nurse and staff to keep the client safe. Keeping the call-light close to the client, encouraging the client to ask for help, and reminding the client to wait for assistance when he gets up are all part of the nursing process, but not first priorities. The client may not always remember to use the call-light and ask for help when needed.

Ⓝ NCLEX® Connection: Reduction of Risk Potential: Potential for Alterations in Body Systems

UNIT 2	NURSING CARE OF CLIENTS WITH NEUROSENSORY DISORDERS
Section	Central Nervous System Disorders
Chapter 9	Brain Tumors

 Overview

- Brain tumors occur in any part of the brain and are classified according to the cell or tissue of origin. Types of brain tumors include: malignant gliomas (neuroglial cells), benign meningiomas (meninges), pituitary tumors, acoustic neuromas (acoustic cranial nerve).

- Primary malignant brain tumors originate from neuroglia tissue and rarely metastasize outside of the brain. Secondary malignant brain tumors are lesions that are metastases from a primary cancer located elsewhere in the body. Cranial metastatic lesions are most common from breast, kidney, and gastrointestinal tract cancers.

- Benign brain tumors develop from the meninges or cranial nerves and do not metastasize. These tumors have distinct boundaries and cause damage either by the pressure they exert within the cranial cavity and/or by impairing the function of the cranial nerve.

- Brain tumors that occur in the cerebral hemispheres above the tentorium cerebelli are classified as supratentorial tumors. Those below the tentorium cerebelli, such as tumors of the brainstem and cerebellum, are classified as infratentorial tumors.

- Brain tumors apply pressure to surrounding brain tissue, resulting in decreased outflow of cerebrospinal fluid, increased intracranial pressure, cerebral edema, and neurological deficits. Tumors that involve the pituitary gland may cause endocrine dysfunction.

- Malignant brain tumors are associated with a high overall mortality rate.

Health Promotion/Disease Prevention

- There are no routine screening procedures to detect brain tumors.

Assessment

- Risk Factors

  ○ The cause is unknown, but several risk factors have been identified including:

    ▪ Genetics

    ▪ Environmental agents

    ▪ Exposure to ionizing radiation

    ▪ Exposure to electromagnetic fields

    ▪ Previous head injury

- Subjective and Objective Data
  - ○ Physical Assessment Findings
    - Dysarthria
    - Dysphagia
    - Positive Romberg sign
    - Positive Babinski's sign
    - Vertigo
    - Hemiparesis
    - Cranial nerve dysfunction (inability to discriminate sounds, loss of gag reflex, loss of blink response)
  - ○ Signs/symptoms specific to supratentorial brain tumors
    - Severe headache – worse upon awakening but gets better over time
    - Visual symptoms (blurring, visual field deficit)
    - Seizures
    - Loss of voluntary movement or the inability to control movement
    - Change in cognitive function (memory loss, language impairment)
    - Change in personality, inability to control emotions
    - Nausea with or without vomiting
  - ○ Signs/symptoms specific to infratentorial brain tumors
    - Hearing loss or ringing in the ear
    - Facial drooping
    - Difficulty swallowing
    - Nystagmus, crossed eyes, or decreased vision
    - Autonomic nervous system (ANS) dysfunction
    - Ataxia or clumsy movements
    - Hemiparesis
    - Cranial nerve dysfunction (e.g., inability to discriminate sounds, loss of gag reflex, loss of blink response)

View Media Supplement:

- Nystagmus (Animation)
- Babinski's Reflex (Video)
- Testing for Romberg Sign (Video)

- ○ Laboratory Tests
    - ■ CBC and differential to rule out anemia or malnutrition
    - ■ Alcohol and illicit drug screen to rule out these as causes of abnormal physical examination
    - ■ TB and HIV screening if social conditions warrant
- ○ Diagnostic Procedures
    - ■ X-ray, computed tomography (CT) imaging scan, magnetic resonance imaging (MRI), brain scan, position emission tomography (PET) scan, and cerebral angiography are all used to determine the size, location, and extent of the tumor.
    - ■ Cerebral biopsy – performed to identify cellular pathology
        - □ This procedure may be performed in the surgical suite or in a radiology specialty suite.
        - □ Diagnostic procedure may be used to guide the biopsy, such as a CT or MRI scan. Image guiding systems, which utilize CT or MRI scan information, may be used in the surgical suite.
        - □ A piece of cerebral tissue that appears abnormal on the CT/MRI scan is obtained. This tissue is then sent to pathology, where diagnostic tests are performed.
        - □ Benefit – Biopsy is minimally disruptive to the rest of the brain, provides a decreased recovery time and is not associated with the risks of an open craniotomy.
        - □ Negative – Biopsy does not remove or debulk the tumor, the diagnostic determination by pathology may be inconclusive (related to insufficient tissue), and a misdiagnosis can occur if the tumor contains many types of tissue or the specimen is taken from one site.
        - □ Client Education
            - ‣ Include specific instruction regarding medications.
                - ▷ If the client is on antiepileptic medications, these must be continued to prevent seizure activity.
                - ▷ If the client is on aspirin products, these should be discontinued at least 72 hr prior to the procedure to minimize the risk of intracerebral bleeding.
                - ▷ Other medications may be held prior to the procedure.
                - ▷ Normally, preprocedure activities may be resumed after the client recovers from the general anesthetic. Care of the incision should include keeping the area clean and dry. If sutures are in place, they need to be removed 1 to 7 days later. Driving or other dangerous activities should be avoided until follow-up appointment occurs and diagnosis is known.

Collaborative Care

- Nursing Care

  o Maintain airway (monitor oxygen levels, administer oxygen as needed, monitor lung sounds).

  o Monitor neurological status, in particular, assessing for changes in level of consciousness, neurological deficits, and occurrence of seizures.

  o Maintain client safety (assist with transfers and ambulation, provide assistive devices as needed).

  o Implement seizure precautions.

  o Administer medications as prescribed.

- Medications

  o Nonopioid analgesics are used to treat headaches.

    ▪ Opioid medications are avoided as they tend to decrease the client's level of consciousness.

  o Corticosteroids are used to reduce cerebral edema.

    ▪ Corticosteroid medications quickly reduce cerebral edema and may be rapidly administered to maximize their effectiveness.

    ▪ Chronic administration is used to control cerebral edema associated with the presence or treatment of benign or malignant brain tumors.

  o Anticonvulsant medications are used to control or prevent seizure activity.

    ▪ Anticonvulsant medications suppress the neuronal activity within the brain, which prevents seizure activity.

    ▪ There are several classifications of antiepileptic medications, each specifically designed to treat specific seizure behavior.

  o H2-antagonists are used to decrease the acid content of the stomach, reducing the risk of stress ulcers.

    ▪ H2-antagonist medications are administered during acute or stressful periods, such as after surgery, at the initiation of chemotherapy or during the first several radiation therapy treatments.

    ▪ The impact of these treatments, together with the necessity of corticosteroids, place the client at risk for stress ulcers. This is primarily preventative treatment.

  o Antiemetics are used if nausea with or without vomiting is present.

    ▪ Nausea and vomiting may be present as a result of the increased intracranial pressure, the site of the tumor, or the treatment required.

    ▪ These medications are administered as prescribed, and may be provided as a preventative intervention, especially when the treatment is associated with nausea and/or vomiting.

- Interdisciplinary Care

  - Initiate appropriate referrals (social services, support groups, medical equipment, and physical, speech, and occupational therapy).

  - Treatments include steroids, surgery, chemotherapy, conventional radiation therapy, stereotactic radiosurgery, and clinical trials. Chemotherapy and/or conventional radiation therapy may be administered prior to surgery to reduce the bulk of the tumor.

  - In most cases when the tumor is benign, surgery is a curative treatment. However, these tumors can regrow, thus radiation and/or chemotherapy may be provided to prevent recurrence.

  - Some tumors may be "malignant by location" meaning that while the pathology is benign, the location makes the mortality rate associated with them high.

  - In cases where the tumor is a metastatic lesion from a primary lesion elsewhere in the body, treatments are palliative in nature. These treatments may consist of surgery, radiation, and chemotherapy, in any combination, and are aimed at controlling intracerebral lesions.

- Surgical Interventions

  - Craniotomy – complete or partial resection of brain tumor through surgical opening in the skull

    - Nursing Actions

      - Preoperatively

        ▸ Explain the procedure to the client, answering all appropriate questions and providing emotional support.

        ▸ Questions regarding the surgery and its outcomes should be written, in an effort to ensure all questions are answered.

        ▸ The client's significant other should be present to hear the responses and avoid miscommunication/misunderstanding.

        ▸ If the client is on aspirin, these medications need to be stopped at least 72 hr prior to the procedure.

        ▸ If the client is taking alternative/complementary medications or receiving treatments, these should be made known to the provider.

        ▸ A living will and durable power for health care decisions should be completed.

        ▸ Medications should be administered as prescribed. An antianxiety or muscle relaxant medication can be administered, if requested, and provided by the provider.

      - Postoperatively

        ▸ Client's vital signs and neurological status should be closely monitored, including using the Glasgow Scale.

> ► The head of the client should be elevated 30° and placed in a neutral position.

> ► Pain should be adequately treated.

> ► Straining activities (moving up in bed and attempting to have a bowel movement) should be avoided to prevent increased intracranial pressure. Postoperative bleeding and seizure activity are the greatest risks.

Complications

- Syndrome of inappropriate antidiuretic hormone (SIADH)

  ○ This is a condition where fluid is retained as a result of an overproduction of vasopressin or antidiuretic hormone (ADH) from the posterior pituitary gland.

  ○ The condition occurs when the hypothalamus has been damaged and can no longer regulate the release of ADH.

  ○ Treatment of SIADH consists of fluid restriction, desmopressin acetate tablets (DDAVP), and treatment of hyponatremia.

  ○ If SIADH is present, the client may be disorientated, report of a headache, and/or vomit.

  ○ If severe or untreated, this condition may cause seizures and/or a coma.

- Diabetes insipidus (DI)

  ○ This is a condition where large amounts of urine are excreted as a result of a deficiency of ADH from the posterior pituitary gland.

  ○ The condition occurs when the hypothalamus has been damaged and can no longer regulate the release of ADH.

  ○ Treatment of DI consists of massive fluid replacement, careful attention to laboratory values, and replacement of essential nutrients as indicated.

CHAPTER 9: BRAIN TUMORS

 Application Exercises

1. A nurse is caring for a client who is having surgery for the removal of an encapsulated acoustic tumor. Which of the following potential complications should the nurse monitor for postoperatively? (Select all that apply.)

_____ Increased intracranial pressure (ICP)

_____ Hemorrhagic shock

_____ Hydrocephalus

_____ Hypoglycemia

_____ Meningitis

_____ Seizures

2. A nurse is caring for a client who has just undergone a craniotomy for a supratentorial tumor. Which of the following postoperative prescriptions should the nurse clarify with the provider?

A. Dexamethasone (Decadron) 30 mg IV bolus BID

B. Morphine sulfate 2 mg IV bolus PRN every 2 hr for pain

C. Ondansetron (Zofran) 4 mg IV bolus PRN every 4 to 6 hr for nausea

D. Phenytoin (Dilantin) 100 mg IV bolus TID

3. Which of the following assessment findings indicates increased ICP? (Select all that apply.)

_____ Disoriented to time and place

_____ Restlessness and irritability

_____ Unequal pupils

_____ ICP 15 mm/Hg

_____ Headache

4. A client who has an expanding brain tumor is prescribed dexamethasone (Decadron). Which of the following are true regarding steroid therapy? (Select all that apply.)

_____ It is prescribed to reduce cerebral swelling.

_____ Hypoglycemia is an expected adverse effect.

_____ It can result in weight gain.

_____ It has a diuretic effect.

_____ It can cause fluid retention.

CHAPTER 9: BRAIN TUMORS

 Application Exercises Answer Key

1. A nurse is caring for a client who is having surgery for the removal of an encapsulated acoustic tumor. Which of the following potential complications should the nurse monitor for postoperatively? (Select all that apply.)

   X   **Increased intracranial pressure (ICP)**

   _____   Hemorrhagic shock

   X   **Hydrocephalus**

   _____   Hypoglycemia

   X   **Meningitis**

   X   **Seizures**

A client who has had a craniotomy should be monitored postoperatively for increased ICP and the development of hydrocephalus. Secondary to infection, meningitis can also develop, as well as seizures. While hypovolemic shock can occur secondary to SIADH, hemorrhagic shock is not a concern. An alteration in glucose metabolism is not usually a postoperative concern after this surgery.

 NCLEX® Connection: Reduction of Risk Potential: Potential for Complications of Diagnostic Tests/Treatments/Procedures

2. A nurse is caring for a client who has just undergone a craniotomy for a supratentorial tumor. Which of the following postoperative prescriptions should the nurse clarify with the provider?

   A. Dexamethasone (Decadron) 30 mg IV bolus BID

   B. Morphine sulfate 2 mg IV bolus PRN every 2 hr for pain

   C. Ondansetron (Zofran) 4 mg IV bolus PRN every 4 to 6 hr for nausea

   D. Phenytoin (Dilantin) 100 mg IV bolus TID

Narcotic analgesics should be avoided postoperatively due to the CNS depressant effects the medication has that can make an assessment of the client's level of consciousness difficult. Dexamethasone, ondansetron, and phenytoin do not have CNS depressant effects.

 NCLEX® Connection: Pharmacological and Parenteral Therapies: Adverse Effects/ Contraindications/Side Effects/Interactions

3. Which of the following assessment findings indicates increased ICP? (Select all that apply.)

__X__ **Disoriented to time and place**

__X__ **Restlessness and irritability**

__X__ **Unequal pupils**

_____ ICP 15 mm/Hg

__X__ **Headache**

Normal ICP is less than or equal to 10 to 15 mm/Hg, so an ICP of 15 mm/Hg is within the expected reference range. Changes in level of consciousness are an early indicator of increased ICP. Increased ICP can cause behavior changes, such as restlessness and irritability. Unequal pupils indicates pressure on the oculomotor nerve secondary to increased ICP. A headache is a symptom of increased ICP.

Ⓝ NCLEX® Connection: Reduction of Risk Potential: System Specific Assessment

4. A client who has an expanding brain tumor is prescribed dexamethasone (Decadron). Which of the following are true regarding steroid therapy? (Select all that apply.)

__X__ **It is prescribed to reduce cerebral swelling.**

_____ Hypoglycemia is an expected adverse effect.

__X__ **It can result in weight gain.**

_____ It has a diuretic effect.

__X__ **It can cause fluid retention.**

Dexamethasone is a common steroid prescribed to reduce cerebral edema. Hyperglycemia, fluid retention, and weight gain are adverse effects of dexamethasone.

Ⓝ NCLEX® Connection: Pharmacological and Parenteral Therapies: Expected Actions/ Outcomes

UNIT 2	NURSING CARE OF CLIENTS WITH NEUROSENSORY DISORDERS
Section	Central Nervous System Disorders
Chapter 10	Multiple Sclerosis and Amyotrophic Lateral Sclerosis

Overview

- Multiple sclerosis (MS) and amyotrophic lateral sclerosis (ALS) are both neurologic diseases that affect the spinal cord typically resulting in difficulties with gait, strength, and motor function.

- MS is an autoimmune disorder characterized by development of plaque in the white matter of the central nervous system (CNS). This plaque damages the myelin sheath and interferes with impulse transmission between the CNS and the body.

- ALS is a disease of the upper and lower motor neurons characterized by muscle weakness progressing to muscle atrophy and eventually paralysis and death. ALS does not involve autonomic changes, sensory alterations, or cognitive changes.

MULTIPLE SCLEROSIS

Overview

- MS follows several possible courses. The most common is:

  - Relapsing and remitting – the disease is marked by relapses and remissions that may or may not return the client to their previous baseline level of function. Overtime, the client may eventually progress to the point of quadriplegia.

- MS is a chronic and progressive disease with no known cure and symptoms progress in severity over time. Initial symptoms may be so vague that diagnosis is not made for several years.

- Life expectancy is not adversely affected by this disease.

Assessment

- Risk Factors

  - The onset of MS is typically between 20 and 40 years of age and occurs twice as often in women. The etiology of MS is unknown. There is a family history (first-degree relative) of MS in many cases.

  - Since MS is an autoimmune disease, there are factors that trigger relapses.

- ■ Viruses and infectious agents
- ■ Living in a cold climate
- ■ Physical injury
- ■ Emotional stress
- ■ Pregnancy
- ■ Fatigue
- ■ Overexertion
- ■ Temperature extremes
- ■ Hot shower/bath
- Subjective and Objective Data
    - ○ Fatigue – especially of the lower extremities
    - ○ Pain or paresthesia
    - ○ Diplopia, changes in peripheral vision, decreased visual acuity
    - ○ Uhthoff's sign (a temporary worsening of vision and other neurological functions commonly seen in clients with MS, or clients predisposed to MS, just after exertion or in situations where they are exposed to heat)
    - ○ Tinnitus, vertigo, decreased hearing acuity
    - ○ Dysphagia – swallowing difficulties
    - ○ Dysarthria (speech difficulties – slurred and nasal speech)
    - ○ Muscle spasticity
    - ○ Ataxia and/or muscle weakness
    - ○ Nystagmus
    - ○ Bowel dysfunction (constipation, fecal incontinence)
    - ○ Bladder dysfunction (areflexia, urgency, nocturia)
    - ○ Cognitive changes (memory loss, impaired judgment)
    - ○ Sexual dysfunction
    - ○ Laboratory Tests
        - ■ Cerebrospinal fluid analysis – elevated protein level and a slight increase in WBCs
    - ○ Diagnostic Procedures
        - ■ Magnetic resonance imaging (MRI)
            - □ An MRI of the brain and spine is used to reveal plaques which is most diagnostic.

Collaborative Care

- Nursing Care

  - Nurses caring for clients who have MS should monitor:

    - Visual acuity

    - Speech patterns – fatigue with talking

    - Swallowing

    - Activity tolerance

    - Skin integrity

  - Encourage fluid intake and other measures to decrease the risk of developing a urinary tract infection. Assist the client with bladder elimination (intermittent self-catheterization, bladder pacemaker, Credé [placing manual pressure on abdomen over the bladder to expel urine]).

  - Monitor cognitive changes and take interventions to maintain function (reorient the client, place objects used daily in routine places).

  - Facilitate effective communication (dysarthria) through the use of a communication board.

  - Apply alternating eye patches to treat diplopia. Teach scanning techniques.

  - Exercise and stretch involved muscles (avoid fatigue and overheating).

  - Utilize energy conservation measures.

  - Promote and maintain safe home and hospital environment to reduce the risk of injury (walk with wide base of support, assistive devices, skin precautions).

- Medications

  - Azathioprine (Imuran) and cyclosporine (Sandimmune)

    - Immunosuppressive agents are used to reduce the frequency of relapses.

    - Nursing Considerations

      - Monitor for long-term effects.

      - Be alert for signs and symptoms of infection.

      - Assess for hypertension.

      - Assess for kidney dysfunction.

  - Prednisone (Deltasone)

    - Corticosteroids are used to reduce inflammation in acute exacerbations.

    - Nursing Considerations

      - Monitor for increased risk of infection, hypervolemia, hypernatremia, hypokalemia, hyperglycemia, gastrointestinal bleeding, and personality changes.

- ○ Dantrolene (Dantrium), tizanidine (Zanaflex), baclofen (Lioresal), and diazepam (Valium)
  - ▪ Antispasmodics are used to treat muscle spasticity.
  - ▪ Intrathecal baclofen can be used for severe cases of MS.
  - ▪ Nursing Considerations
    - ▫ Observe for increased weakness.
    - ▫ Monitor for liver damage if on tizanidine or dantrolene.
  - ▪ Client Education
    - ▫ Report increased weakness to provider.
    - ▫ Report jaundice to provider.
    - ▫ Avoid stopping baclofen abruptly.
- ○ Interferon beta (Betaseron)
  - ▪ Immunomodulators are used to prevent or treat relapses.
- ○ Carbamazepine (Tegretol)
  - ▪ Anticonvulsants are used for paresthesia.
- ○ Docusate sodium (Colace)
  - ▪ Stool softeners are used for constipation.
- ○ Propantheline (Pro-Banthine)
  - ▪ Anticholinergics are used for bladder dysfunction.
- ○ Primidone (Mysoline) and clonazepam (Klonopin)
  - ▪ Beta-blockers are used for tremors.
- Interdisciplinary Care
  - ○ Plan for disease progression. Provide community resources and respite services for the client and family.
  - ○ Consider referral to occupational and physical therapy for home environment assessment to determine safety and ease of mobility. Use adaptive devices to assist with activities of daily living.
  - ○ Refer to speech language therapist for dysarthria and dysphagia.
- Client Outcomes
  - ○ The client will be able to ambulate without assistance and independently perform ADLs.
  - ○ The client will avoid triggers and exhibit fewer relapses.

AMYOTROPHIC LATERAL SCLEROSIS

Overview

- Amyotrophic lateral sclerosis (ALS) is a degenerative neurological disorder of the upper and lower motor neurons that result in deterioration and death of the motor neurons. This results in a progressive paralysis and muscle wasting that eventually causes respiratory paralysis and death. Cognitive function is not usually affected.

- ALS is also known as Lou Gehrig's disease, after the professional baseball player who died of this disease in 1941.

- Death usually occurs within 3 to 5 years of the initial symptoms due to respiratory failure. The cause of ALS is unknown and there is no cure.

- Health Promotion and Disease Prevention

  o Client Education

    ▪ Genetic counseling is suggested for family members of clients who have ALS.

Assessment

- Risk Factors

  o ALS affects more men than women, often developing between the ages of 40 to 70.

- Subjective Data

  o Fatigue

  o Twitching and cramping of muscles

- Objective Data

  o Physical Assessment Findings

    ▪ Muscle weakness – usually begins in one part of the body

    ▪ Muscle atrophy

    ▪ Dysphagia

    ▪ Dysarthria

    ▪ Hyperreflexia of deep tendon reflexes

  o Laboratory Tests

    ▪ Creatine kinase (CK-BB) level – Increased

  o Diagnostic Procedures

    ▪ Electromyogram (EMG)

      ▫ Reduction in number of functioning motor units of peripheral nerves

- Muscle biopsy
  - □ Reduction in number of motor units of peripheral nerves and atrophic muscle fibers

Collaborative Care

- Nursing Care
  - o Maintain a patent airway and suction and/or intubate as needed.
  - o Monitor ABGs and administer oxygen, intermittent positive pressure ventilation, bilevel positive airway pressure, or mechanical ventilation as needed.
  - o Keep the head of the bed at 45°; turn, cough, and deep breathe every 2 hr; conduct incentive spirometry/chest physiotherapy.
  - o Facilitate effective communication (dysarthria) with the use of a communication board or a speech language therapist referral.
  - o Assess coping and depression.
  - o Assess swallow reflex and ensure safety with oral intake. Thicken fluids as needed.
  - o Meet nutritional needs for calories, fiber, and fluids. When no longer able to swallow, provide enteral nutrition as prescribed.
  - o Utilize energy conservation measures.
  - o Address the client's interest in the establishment of advance directives/living wills.
- Medications
  - o Riluzole (Rilutek)
    - Glutamate antagonist that can slow the deterioration of motor neurons by decreasing the release of glutamic acid. Must be taken early in disease process. Will add approximately 2 to 3 months of life to the client's overall lifespan.
    - Nursing Considerations
      - □ Monitor liver function tests – hepatotoxic risk.
      - □ Assess for dizziness, vertigo, and somnolence.
    - Client Education
      - □ Avoid drinking alcohol.
      - □ Take medication at evenly spaced regular intervals (e.g., every 12 hr).
      - □ Store medication away from bright light.
  - o Baclofen (Lioresal), dantrolene sodium (Dantrium), diazepam (Valium)
    - Antispasmodics are used to decrease spasticity.

- Interdisciplinary Care

  o Initiate appropriate referrals (dietician, social service, physical therapy, occupational therapy, clinical psychologist) for extended care in the home or a long-term care facility as client's condition deteriorates.

  o Consider referral to a speech pathologist for speech and swallowing issues.

  o Consider hospice referral to provide support to the client and family coping with the terminal phase of the illness.

- Client Outcomes

  o The client will remain independent in ADLs until severe weakness and paralysis develops.

  o The client will be able to remain in the home with support services available to meet his needs.

  o The client will be free of infections (respiratory, urinary, integument).

Complications

- Pneumonia

  o Pneumonia can be caused by respiratory muscle weakness and paralysis contributing to ineffective airway exchange.

  o Nursing Actions

    ▪ Assess respiratory status routinely and provide antimicrobial therapy as indicated.

- Respiratory failure

  o Respiratory failure may necessitate mechanical ventilation.

  o Nursing Actions

    ▪ Assess respiratory status and be prepared to provide ventilatory support as needed per the client's advance directives.

CHAPTER 10: MULTIPLE SCLEROSIS AND AMYOTROPHIC LATERAL SCLEROSIS

(A) Application Exercises

Scenario: A home health care nurse is interviewing a client who is newly diagnosed with multiple sclerosis (MS). The client is upset over her increasing loss of mobility, decreased visual acuity, and the severe fatigue that worsens as the day progresses. In addition, the client states she is experiencing mood swings that she cannot control. As the client has a decreased libido, she is also worried about her relationship with her husband. The client tells the nurse she and her husband had planned a pregnancy, but now they have been forced to put their lives on hold.

1. Which of the following is appropriate for the nurse to assess to determine the extent of the client's MS? (Select all that apply.)

    _____ Motor dysfunction

    _____ Cognitive dysfunction

    _____ Emotional lability

    _____ Skin lesions

    _____ Cerebellar dysfunction

    _____ Bowel and bladder dysfunction

    _____ Alopecia

    _____ Fatigue

2. Which of the following actions should the nurse take to help the client increase mobility and lessen fatigue?

3. Which of the following findings might have exacerbated the client's MS? (Select all that apply.)

    _____ Influenza

    _____ Long-term use of NSAIDs

    _____ Large meal intake

    _____ Recent insomnia

    _____ Stress

    _____ Snow skiing

4. A nurse is caring for a client admitted to the hospital with respiratory difficulty after being diagnosed with ALS approximately 1 year ago. Which of the following client findings should the nurse anticipate? (Select all that apply.)

_____ Muscle weakness

_____ Loss of sensation

_____ Fluctuations in blood pressure

_____ Muscle atrophy

_____ Incontinence

_____ Ineffective cough

_____ Loss of cognitive function

5. A client recently diagnosed with ALS is being placed on riluzole (Rilutek). Which of the following instructions should the nurse give the client?

A. "Take riluzole at bedtime."

B. "Do not take riluzole with dairy products."

C. "Avoid consuming alcoholic beverages while taking riluzole."

D. "Monitor your blood pressure daily while taking riluzole."

CHAPTER 10: MULTIPLE SCLEROSIS AND AMYOTROPHIC LATERAL SCLEROSIS

Ⓐ Application Exercises Answer Key

Scenario: A home health care nurse is interviewing a client who is newly diagnosed with multiple sclerosis (MS). The client is upset over her increasing loss of mobility, decreased visual acuity, and the severe fatigue that worsens as the day progresses. In addition, the client states she is experiencing mood swings that she cannot control. As the client has a decreased libido, she is also worried about her relationship with her husband. The client tells the nurse she and her husband had planned a pregnancy, but now they have been forced to put their lives on hold.

1. Which of the following is appropriate for the nurse to assess to determine the extent of the client's MS? (Select all that apply.)

__X__	**Motor dysfunction**
__X__	**Cognitive dysfunction**
__X__	**Emotional lability**
_____	Skin lesions
__X__	**Cerebellar dysfunction**
__X__	**Bowel and bladder dysfunction**
_____	Alopecia
__X__	**Fatigue**

The nurse should assess for motor and cognitive dysfunction, emotional lability, cerebellar dysfunction, bowel and bladder dysfunction, and fatigue in relation to the involvement of the CNS. Skin lesions and alopecia do not typically occur in relation to MS.

Ⓝ **NCLEX® Connection: Reduction of Risk Potential: System Specific Assessment**

2. Which of the following actions should the nurse take to help the client increase mobility and lessen fatigue?

It is important to encourage the client to conserve her energy and increase mobility by using assistive devices such as canes, walkers, and wheelchairs. In addition, for safety, the client should wear nonslip, flat, shoes that tie. The nurse should check the client's home environment to make certain that lighting is adequate, and that cords and throw rugs are removed to prevent the client from falling. The client should schedule major activities in the morning and then plan rest periods during the afternoon. The nurse should arrange with the physical and occupational therapy departments to make periodic home visits if able and if the client's insurance company allows for it.

 NCLEX® Connection: Physiological Adaptation: Illness Management

3. Which of the following findings might have exacerbated the client's MS? (Select all that apply.)

   X   **Influenza**

          Long-term use of NSAIDs

          Large meal intake

   X   **Recent insomnia**

   X   **Stress**

   X   **Snow skiing**

Emotional and physical stress, such as insomnia, marital stress, and snow skiing, as well as an illness, such as influenza, can cause an exacerbation of MS. There is no relationship between the use of NSAIDs and eating habits and MS.

 NCLEX® Connection: Physiological Adaptation: Pathophysiology

---

4. A nurse is caring for a client admitted to the hospital with respiratory difficulty after being diagnosed with ALS approximately 1 year ago. Which of the following client findings should the nurse anticipate? (Select all that apply.)

   X   **Muscle weakness**

          Loss of sensation

          Fluctuations in blood pressure

   X   **Muscle atrophy**

   X   **Incontinence**

   X   **Ineffective cough**

          Loss of cognitive function

ALS is a deteriorating disease of the motor system characterized by muscle weakness progressing to muscle atrophy and eventually paralysis and death. ALS does not involve autonomic changes, sensory alterations, or cognitive changes.

 NCLEX® Connection: Reduction of Risk Potential: System Specific Assessment

5. A client recently diagnosed with ALS is being placed on riluzole (Rilutek). Which of the following instructions should the nurse give the client?

A. "Take riluzole at bedtime."

B. "Do not take riluzole with dairy products."

C. "Avoid consuming alcoholic beverages while taking riluzole."

D. "Monitor your blood pressure daily while taking riluzole."

Riluzole is hepatotoxic so alcoholic beverages should be avoided to decrease the risk of liver damage. It should be taken on an empty stomach every 12 hr, either 1 hr before or 2 hr after meals. The medication does not affect blood pressure.

 NCLEX® Connection: Pharmacological and Parenteral Therapies: Adverse Effects/ Contraindications/Side Effects/Interactions

UNIT 2	NURSING CARE OF CLIENTS WITH NEUROSENSORY DISORDERS
Section	Peripheral Nervous System Disorders

Chapter 11   Guillain-Barré Syndrome

 Overview

- Guillain-Barré syndrome (GBS) develops in relation to acute destruction of the myelin sheath of peripheral nerves due to an autoimmune disorder that results in varying degrees of muscle weakness and paralysis.

> **Ⓜ** **View Media Supplement:**   Nerve with Myelin Sheath (Image)

- After the acute phase, remyelination occurs, re-establishing nerve functions. However, aggregates of lymphocytes can cause secondary damage, which can delay recovery or result in permanent deficits.

- Chronic inflammatory demyelinating polyneuropathy (CIDP) is a different type of GBS that progresses over a very long period, and recovery is rare.

- Three stages characterize the course of GBS:

  o Initial period – 1 to 4 weeks; onset of symptoms until neurological deterioration stops.

  o Plateau period – several days to 2 weeks; no deterioration, and no improvement occurs.

  o Recovery period – 4 to 6 months and up to 2 years; remyelination and return of muscle strength.

- Etiology is unknown – evidence indicates a cell-mediated immunologic reaction. A history of a recent viral event is reported by many clients.

Assessment

- Risk Factors

  o Recent (within 1 to 3 weeks) history of:

    ▪ Acute illness (upper respiratory infection, gastrointestinal illness)

    ▪ Viruses such as Epstein-Barr virus (EBV) or cytomegalovirus (CMV)

    ▪ Vaccination (swine flu vaccination)

    ▪ Surgery

- Subjective Data

  o Client report of increasing weakness with no recollection of injury.

  o Client report of a virus within the previous 1 to 3 weeks.

- Objective Data

  o Acute progressive muscle weakness and paralysis

    ▪ Ascending (initially, bilateral lower extremity muscles are affected then progresses upward through arms and thorax).

    ▪ Recovery is in descending order (initially, facial muscles recover, then improvement progresses downward).

  o Muscle flaccidity without muscle atrophy

  o Paresthesias – creeping/crawling sensations across skin

  o Cranial nerve symptoms (diplopia, facial weakness, dysarthria, dysphagia)

  o Decreased/absent deep tendon reflexes

  o Signs of respiratory compromise when muscle weakness reaches thorax

  o Autonomic dysfunction (fluctuating blood pressure, dysrhythmias)

  o Diagnostic Procedures

    ▪ Electromyography (EMG) and nerve conduction velocity (NCV)

      □ Shows evidence of denervation after 4+ weeks

    ▪ WBC count

      □ Leukocytosis can develop.

    ▪ Lumbar puncture (LP)

      □ Shows the distinguishing characteristic GBS finding of an increase in protein within the cerebrospinal fluid without an increase in cell count.

Collaborative Care

- Nursing Care

  o Monitor respiratory status (rate and depth of respirations, pulse oximetry, ABGs). Have oxygen, suction equipment, and intubation tray readily available.

  o Keep the head of the bed at 45°; have the client turn and cough, deep breathe, and use an incentive spirometer every 2 hr; institute chest physiotherapy if indicated.

  o Monitor heart rhythms for irregularities and bradycardia.

  o Monitor blood pressure and respond to fluctuations as needed (beta-blocker administration for hypertension, IV fluids for hypotension).

  o Assess for difficulty articulating words (dysarthria). Provide an alphabet board if the client can still use his hands.

- ○ Assess for difficulty swallowing and choking. Request swallowing study be completed if the client is having difficulty swallowing food or liquids. Keep the client NPO until results are available.

- ○ Assess pain level if client is experiencing paresthesia. Change position at least every 2 hr and apply ice or heat for discomfort.

- ○ Take measures to prevent skin breakdown. The client may not be able to change position or feel pain when skin breakdown is occurring.

- ○ Provide comfort measures (frequent repositioning, ice, heat, massage, distraction).

  - ▪ Monitor cranial nerve function and intervene to maintain safety accordingly (risk of aspiration, risk for injury).

- ○ Assess coping strategies and depression. Provide reassurance to the client because cognitive functions are not affected.

- ○ Administer medications as prescribed.

- Medications

  - ○ Morphine

    - ▪ An analgesic given for pain and paresthesias

    - ▪ Nursing Considerations

      - □ Monitor for respiratory depression and constipation.

  - ○ IV Immunoglobulin (IVIg)

    - ▪ Given to suppress attack on immune system

    - ▪ Nursing Considerations

      - □ Monitor for side effects, such as chills, fever, myalgia, and for possible complications including anaphylaxis or renal failure.

  - ○ Neurontin (Gabapentin)

    - ▪ Given for neuropathic pain

    - ▪ Nursing Considerations

      - □ Assess for confusion, depression, drowsiness, and ataxia.

- Interdisciplinary Care

  - ○ Initiate appropriate referrals (social services, physical therapy, occupational therapy).

- Therapeutic Procedures

  - Plasmapheresis – A treatment where blood is removed from the body, ran through a separator, and the circulating antibodies are removed from the plasma. This procedure decreases the attack against the myelin sheath. This may be done several times over a period of several weeks.

    - Nursing Actions

      - Preprocedure

        - Assess vital signs, laboratory values, and weight.

      - Intraprocedure

        - Assess for dizziness and hypotension.

        - Maintain patency of shunts during the procedure (one is usually placed in each upper extremity).

      - Postprocedure

        - Apply pressure dressing.

        - Monitor for infection.

        - Assess laboratory values.

          - Monitor for the possible complications of hypovolemia, hypokalemia, and hypocalcemia.

    - Client Education

      - Instruct the client that the procedure will typically last 2 to 5 hr.

- Care after Discharge

  - Client Education

    - Clients with significant paralysis will be discharged to a rehabilitation facility. The duration of the stay will depend on how quickly the myelin sheath damage heals and if residual disabilities remain. Once discharged from rehabilitation, therapies will continue on an outpatient or in-home basis for several months.

    - Clients will need varying levels of support upon discharge in relation to the severity of paralysis.

    - Referrals will need to be made, with the assistance of social services, for a home health nurse, home health aide, and in-home physical and occupational therapists.

    - If the client is not mobile, many adaptations may also need to be made to the home to make it wheelchair accessible.

- Client Outcomes
  - The client will be free of complications of immobility.
  - The client will be able to resume ADLs.
  - The client's muscle strength and functioning will return to baseline.

Complications

- Respiratory compromise
  - Recognize progressing paralysis and be prepared to intervene promptly.
  - Nursing Actions
    - Monitor respiratory status (rate and depth of respirations, pulse oximetry, ABGs).
    - Have oxygen, suction equipment, and intubation tray readily available.
    - Provide assistance in mobilization and removal of secretions.

CHAPTER 11: GUILLAIN-BARRÉ SYNDROME

 Application Exercises

1. A nurse is admitting a client who is tentatively diagnosed with GBS due to progressive paralysis of the lower extremities. Which of the following client reports is relevant in regard to the diagnosis of GBS?

    A. Recent head trauma

    B. History of systemic lupus erythematosus

    C. History of upper respiratory infection

    D. Recent tick bite

2. A nurse is caring for a client admitted with GBS 1 week ago. The nurse notes that the client's pulse oximetry reading is 88%, respirations are 32/min and shallow, and decreased lung sounds are found in the base of each lung. Which of the following equipment should the nurse plan to place at the client's bedside?

    A. An incentive spirometer

    B. An intubation tray

    C. A nasogastric tube

    D. A can of thickener

3. A nurse is assessing a client who is on a rehabilitation unit and was diagnosed with GBS 1 month ago. Which of the following client findings should the nurse anticipate? (Select all that apply.)

    _____   Muscle weakness

    _____   Muscle atrophy

    _____   Incontinence

    _____   Ineffective cough

    _____   Hyperreflexia

4. A client who has GBS and is on a rehabilitation unit asks the nurse if he will ever walk again. His symptoms began 1 month ago. Which of the following responses by the nurse is appropriate?

    A. "It is doubtful, since you have not shown any improvement."

    B. "Your physical therapist is better able to answer that question."

    C. "Most individuals do walk again, but it may take up to two years."

    D. "Your ability to walk will depend on how hard you work in therapy."

CHAPTER 11: GUILLAIN-BARRÉ SYNDROME

 Application Exercises Answer Key

1. A nurse is admitting a client who is tentatively diagnosed with GBS due to progressive paralysis of the lower extremities. Which of the following client reports is relevant in regard to the diagnosis of GBS?

    A. Recent head trauma

    B. History of systemic lupus erythematosus

    C. History of upper respiratory infection

    D. Recent tick bite

    A history of an upper respiratory or gastrointestinal infection, stress, such as surgery/trauma, or a recent vaccination within the last 1 to 3 weeks is a common finding in clients who have GBS. There is no relationship between head trauma, systemic lupus erythematosus, or tick bites to GBS.

     NCLEX® Connection: Physiological Adaptation: Pathophysiology

2. A nurse is caring for a client admitted with GBS 1 week ago. The nurse notes that the client's pulse oximetry reading is 88%, respirations are 32/min and shallow, and decreased lung sounds are found in the base of each lung. Which of the following equipment should the nurse plan to place at the client's bedside?

    A. An incentive spirometer

    B. An intubation tray

    C. A nasogastric tube

    D. A can of thickener

    An endotracheal intubation tray, as well as a bag valve mask, and suctioning equipment should be placed at the client's bedside in case he needs respiratory support. Involvement of the respiratory muscles is a potential complication of GBS. An incentive spirometer will be of limited use if the client's respiratory muscles are affected. The client findings also do not indicate difficulty swallowing, so an NG tube and thickener are not indicated.

     NCLEX® Connection: Physiological Adaptation: Medical Emergencies

3. A nurse is assessing a client who is on a rehabilitation unit and was diagnosed with GBS 1 month ago. Which of the following client findings should the nurse anticipate? (Select all that apply.)

___X___ **Muscle weakness**

_____ Muscle atrophy

___X___ **Incontinence**

___X___ **Ineffective cough**

_____ Hyperreflexia

A characteristic of GBS is muscle weakness without atrophy. An ineffective cough and incontinence are likely due to muscle weakness. The client's reflexes are decreased or absent.

NCLEX® Connection: Reduction of Risk Potential: System Specific Assessment

4. A client who has GBS and is on a rehabilitation unit asks the nurse if he will ever walk again. His symptoms began 1 month ago. Which of the following responses by the nurse is appropriate?

A. "It is doubtful, since you have not shown any improvement."

B. "Your physical therapist is better able to answer that question."

C. **"Most individuals do walk again, but it may take up to two years."**

D. "Your ability to walk will depend on how hard you work in therapy."

Clients who have GBS usually begin to show significant improvement within 4 to 6 months. However, in severe cases, recovery can take up to 2 years. A client's rate of recovery is based on the rate and amount of remyelination necessary for normal nerve conduction to resume. Even if the client works hard in therapy, remyelination must occur for improvement in muscle innervations.

NCLEX® Connection: Physiological Adaptation: Alterations in Body Systems

UNIT 2	NURSING CARE OF CLIENTS WITH NEUROSENSORY DISORDERS
Section	Peripheral Nervous System Disorders
Chapter 12	Myasthenia Gravis

Overview

- Myasthenia gravis (MG) is a progressive autoimmune disease that produces severe muscular weakness. It is characterized by periods of exacerbation and remission. Muscle weakness improves with rest.

- It is caused by antibodies that interfere with the transmission of acetylcholine at the neuromuscular junction.

Assessment

- Risk Factors

  - Associated with rheumatoid arthritis, scleroderma, and systemic lupus erythematosus

  - Causes

    - Co-existing autoimmune disorder

    - Frequently associated with hyperplasia of the thymus gland

  - Factors that trigger exacerbations

    - Infection

    - Stress, emotional upset, and fatigue

    - Pregnancy

    - Increases in body temperature (fever, sunbathing, hot tubs)

- Subjective Data

  - Progressive muscle weakness

  - Diplopia (double vision)

  - Difficulty chewing and swallowing

  - Respiratory dysfunction

  - Bowel and bladder dysfunction

  - Poor posture

  - Fatigue after exertion

- Objective Data

  ○ Physical Assessment Findings

    ▪ Impaired respiratory status (difficulty managing secretions, poor respiratory effort)

    ▪ Decreased swallowing ability

    ▪ Poor muscle strength, especially of the face, eyes, and proximal portion of major muscle groups

    ▪ Incontinence

    ▪ Drooping eyelids – unilateral or bilateral

  ○ Diagnostic Procedures

    ▪ Tensilon testing

      □ Baseline assessment of the cranial muscle strength is done.

      □ Edrophonium chloride (Tensilon) is administered.

        ‣ Medication inhibits the breakdown of acetylcholine, making it available for use at the neuromuscular junction. A positive test results in marked improvement in muscle strength that lasts approximately 5 min.

      □ Nursing Actions

        ‣ Assist provider in administering this test.

        ‣ Observe for complications such as fasciculations around the eyes and face as well as cardiac arrhythmias.

        ‣ Have atropine available, which is the antidote for edrophonium chloride (bradycardia, sweating, and abdominal cramps).

      □ Client Education

        ‣ Explain purpose of the test to the client.

        ‣ Encourage the client to follow the providers directions in moving previously affected muscles.

        ‣ Discourage the client from demonstrating improvement by increasing effort, which could skew the test results.

    ▪ Electromyography

      □ Shows the neuromuscular transmission characteristics of MG.

      □ Decrease in amplitude of the muscle is demonstrated over a series of consecutive muscle contractions.

Collaborative Care

- Nursing Care

  - Assess and intervene as needed to maintain a patent airway (muscle weakness of diaphragm, respiratory, and intercostal muscles).

  - Assess swallowing to prevent aspiration. Keep oxygen, endotracheal intubation, and suctioning equipment, and a bag valve mask available at the client's bedside.

  - Use energy conservation measures. Allow for periods of rest.

  - Provide small, frequent high-calorie meals and schedule at times when medication is peaking.

  - Have the client sit upright when eating and use thickener in liquids as necessary.

  - Apply a lubricating eye drop during the day and ointment at night if the client is unable to completely close his eyes. The client may also need to patch or tape his eye shut at night to prevent damage to the cornea.

    - Encourage the client to wear a medical identification wristband or necklace at all times.

  - Administer medications as prescribed and at specified times.

- Medications

  - Anticholinesterase agents

    - Cholinesterase inhibitor medications are the first line in therapy.

    - Nursing Considerations

      □ Ensure that the medication is given at the specified time – usually 4 times a day.

      □ If periods of weakness are observed, discuss change in administration times with the provider.

      □ Use cautiously in clients who have a history of asthma or cardiac dysrhythmias.

    - Client Education

      □ Take with food to address gastrointestinal side effects.

      □ Eat within 45 min of taking the medication to strengthen chewing and reduce the risk for aspiration.

      □ Stress the importance of maintaining therapeutic levels and taking the medication at the same time each day.

  - Pyridostigmine (Mestinon) and neostigmine (Prostigmin)

    - Used to increase muscle strength in the symptomatic treatment of MG. It inhibits the breakdown of acetylcholine and prolongs its effects.

- Nursing Considerations
  - Assess the client for a history of seizures.
  - Use cautiously in clients who have a history of asthma and cardiovascular disease.
  - Immunosuppressants such as azathioprine (Imuran) and prednisone (Deltasone)
    - Immunosuppressants are given during exacerbations when pyridostigmine is not adequately effective.
    - Since MG is an autoimmune disease, immunosuppressants decrease the production of antibodies.
    - A corticosteroid, such as prednisone, is the first medication of choice. Cytotoxic medications, such as azathioprine (Imuran), are given if corticosteroids are ineffective.
    - Nursing Considerations
      - Monitor for infection.
      - Taper use gradually.
    - Client Education
      - Explain to the client the importance of slowly tapering off of a corticosteroid.
      - Tell the client to observe for signs of infection and take precautions against exposure to viruses and contaminants.
  - IV immunoglobulins (IVIg) – acute management
    - IVIg, an immunoglobulin, may be prescribed for MG that does not respond to the above treatments.

- Interdisciplinary Care
  - Consult physical therapy for durable medical equipment needs.
  - Consult occupational therapy for assistive devices to facilitate ADLs.
  - Consult with a speech and language therapist if weakening of facial muscles impacts communication or swallowing.

- Therapeutic Procedures
  - Plasmapheresis – removes circulating antibodies from the plasma. This is usually done several times over a period of days and may continue on a regular basis for some clients.
    - Nursing Actions
      - Preprocedure
        - Assess vital signs, laboratory values, and weight.

□ Intraprocedure

▸ Assess for dizziness and hypotension.

▸ Maintain the patency of shunts during the procedure (one is usually placed in each upper extremity).

□ Postprocedure

▸ Apply a pressure dressing.

▸ Monitor for infection.

▸ Assess laboratory values.

▸ Monitor for the possible complications of hypovolemia, hypokalemia, and hypocalcemia.

■ Client Education

□ Instruct the client that the procedure will typically last 2 to 5 hr.

- Surgical Interventions

  ○ Thymectomy – removal of the thymus gland is done to attain better control or complete remission.

    ■ May take months to years to see results due to the life of the circulating T cells.

  ○ Nursing Actions

    ■ Postoperatively, monitor the client's respiratory status closely. Depending on the type of surgical procedure (transcervical using a video-assisted thoracoscope versus the open sternal split), the client may be intubated and have a chest tube.

    ■ Make sure the client is turned, coughs, and deep breathes every 2 hr.

    ■ Observe the client for signs of a pneumo- or hemothorax.

- Client Outcomes

  ○ Client will not experience periods of fatigue that interfere with the ability to perform ADLs.

  ○ Client will verbalize the importance of taking medication regularly and at the prescribed time.

Complications

- Myasthenic crisis and cholinergic crisis

  ○ Myasthenic crisis occurs when the client is experiencing a stressor that causes an exacerbation of MG, such as infection, or is taking inadequate amounts of cholinesterase inhibitor.

  ○ Cholinergic crisis occurs when the client has taken too much cholinesterase inhibitor.

  ○ The symptoms of both can be very similar (muscle weakness, respiratory failure).

  ○ The client's highest risk for injury is due to respiratory compromise and failure.

Complications and Nursing Implications

MYASTHENIC CRISIS UNDERMEDICATION	CHOLINERGIC CRISIS OVERMEDICATION
Respiratory muscle weakness – mechanical ventilation	Muscle twitching to the point of respiratory muscle weakness – mechanical ventilation
Myasthenic symptoms (weakness, incontinence, fatigue)	Cholinergic symptoms – hypersecretions (nausea, diarrhea, respiratory secretions) and hypermotility (abdominal cramps)
Hypertension	Hypotension
Temporary improvement of symptoms with administration of Tensilon	• Tensilon has no positive effect on symptoms, it can actually worsen symptoms (more anticholinesterase – more cholinergic symptoms). • Symptoms improve with the administration of an anticholinergic medication, such as atropine.

CHAPTER 12: MYASTHENIA GRAVIS

(A) Application Exercises

Scenario: A client is recovering from a myasthenic crisis during which time he suffered respiratory distress requiring mechanical ventilation for several days. The provider believes an earlier episode of gastroenteritis triggered the crisis.

1. What is myasthenic crisis and what symptoms most likely prompted the client to seek medical attention?

2. Why is the client's earlier episode of gastroenteritis suspected to be the trigger for the myasthenic crisis?

3. Why is it necessary to teach the client to recognize a cholinergic crisis?

4. A nurse is preparing to assist the provider in testing a client for MG. Which of the following medications should the nurse have available for the provider to administer?

     A. Pyridostigmine (Mestinon)

     B. Edrophonium chloride (Tensilon)

     C. Atropine sulfate (Atropair)

     D. Azathioprine (Imuran)

5. Which of the following should the nurse do for a client who has ptosis? (Select all that apply.)

     _____ Apply lubricating eye drops during the day.

     _____ Add a thickener to liquids.

     _____ Support the neck with pillows.

     _____ Tape eyes shut at night.

     _____ Provide for periods of rest during the day.

6. A nurse instructs a client who has MG about home care and the risk factors that can exacerbate the disease. Which of the following client statements indicates a need for further teaching?

     A. "I should take my medication 45 minutes before breakfast, lunch, and dinner."

     B. "I have suction equipment at home in case I start to choke."

     C. "I will soak in the hot tub every day."

     D. "I ordered a medical identification bracelet and will wear it every day."

CHAPTER 12: MYASTHENIA GRAVIS

 Application Exercises Answer Key

Scenario: A client is recovering from a myasthenic crisis during which time he suffered respiratory distress requiring mechanical ventilation for several days. The provider believes an earlier episode of gastroenteritis triggered the crisis.

1. What is myasthenic crisis and what symptoms most likely prompted the client to seek medical attention?

> **A myasthenic crisis is the sudden onset of muscular weakness that may be related to a stressful event, undermedication, systemic infection, surgery, or trauma. Symptoms are the same as with the primary disease, only more severe (weakness, fatigue, dysphagia, dysarthria, choking, respiratory distress).**

 NCLEX® Connection: Physiological Adaptation: Medical Emergencies

2. Why is the client's earlier episode of gastroenteritis suspected to be the trigger for the myasthenic crisis?

> **Gastroenteritis is an infectious disease. It places stress on the body and causes vomiting and diarrhea, which may have resulted in the client insufficiently medicating himself.**

 NCLEX® Connection: Physiological Adaptation: Pathophysiology

3. Why is it necessary to teach the client to recognize a cholinergic crisis?

> **A cholinergic crisis is caused by too much medication. It must be differentiated from a myasthenic crisis in order to select the correct treatment. A cholinergic crisis produces gastrointestinal symptoms, which differ from those of a myasthenic crisis but may be confused with acute gastroenteritis.**

 NCLEX® Connection: Physiological Adaptation: Illness Management

4. A nurse is preparing to assist the provider in testing a client for MG. Which of the following medications should the nurse have available for the provider to administer?

    A. Pyridostigmine (Mestinon)

    B. Edrophonium chloride (Tensilon)

    C. Atropine sulfate (Atropair)

    D. Azathioprine (Imuran)

Edrophonium chloride is a short-acting anticholinesterase medication used to diagnose MG. A positive test is demonstrated by increased muscle strength in affected muscles shortly after IV administration. Pyridostigmine, atropine sulfate, and azathioprine are not medications used to diagnose MG. They may, however, be used in the treatment of the disease.

 NCLEX® Connection: Pharmacological and Parenteral Therapies: Expected Actions/ Outcomes

5. Which of the following should the nurse do for a client who has ptosis? (Select all that apply.)

    __X__   **Apply lubricating eye drops during the day.**

    _____   Add a thickener to liquids.

    _____   Support the neck with pillows.

    __X__   **Tape eyes shut at night.**

    _____   Provide for periods of rest during the day.

Ptosis is the drooping of an eyelid caused by weakness of the muscles of the eyelids. This weakness can cause the eyelids to not close completely making them at risk for corneal dryness and deterioration. Application of lubricating drops and taping the eyes shut at night will help protect the corneas from dryness. Since ptosis relates to an eye complication, adding thickener to liquids, supporting the neck with pillows, and providing for rest periods during the day are not relevant to the issue.

 NCLEX® Connection: Physiological Adaptation: Illness Management

6. A nurse instructs a client who has MG about home care and the risk factors that can exacerbate the disease. Which of the following client statements indicates a need for further teaching?

    A. "I should take my medication 45 minutes before breakfast, lunch, and dinner."

    B. "I have suction equipment at home in case I start to choke."

    C. "I will soak in the hot tub every day."

    D. "I ordered a medical identification bracelet and will wear it every day."

Hot temperatures and hot water can cause a client with MG to have an exacerbation of symptoms. Hot baths and hot tubs should be avoided. The other statements indicate an understanding of the risk factors for exacerbations of MG.

 NCLEX® Connection: Physiological Adaptation: Illness Management

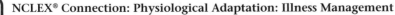

UNIT 2	NURSING CARE OF CLIENTS WITH NEUROSENSORY DISORDERS
Section	Sensory Disorders
Chapter 13	Disorders of the Eye

Overview

- Disorders of the eye can be caused by injury, disease process, and the aging process.

- Disorders of the eye that nurses should be knowledgeable about include:

  - Reduced vision

  - Macular degeneration

  - Retinal detachment

  - Cataracts

  - Glaucoma

- Macular degeneration (often called age-related macular degeneration – AMD) is the central loss of vision which affects the macula of the eye.

- There is no cure for macular degeneration.

- The number one cause for vision loss in people over the age of 60 is AMD.

REDUCED VISION

Overview

- Visual acuity of 20/200 or less with corrective lenses constitutes legal blindness.

- Reduced visual acuity can be unilateral (one eye) or bilateral (both eyes).

Health Promotion and Disease Prevention

- Teach clients to wear sunglasses while outside.

- Educate clients to wear protective eye wear while working in areas, such as welding or yard work.

- Teach clients to avoid rubbing their eyes.

- Encourage annual eye examinations and good eye health, especially for adults over the age of 40.

Assessment

- Risk Factors

  (G)

  - Age is the most significant risk factor for visual sensory alterations.
  - Presbyopia – age-related loss of the eye's ability to focus on close objects
  - Cataracts – opacity of lens
  - Glaucoma – loss of peripheral vision
  - Diabetic retinopathy – microaneurysms
  - Macular degeneration – loss of central vision
  - Eye infection, inflammation, or injury
  - Brain tumor

- Subjective Data

  - Frequent headaches
  - Frequent eye strain
  - Blurred vision
  - Poor judgment of depth
  - Diplopia – double vision

- Objective Data

  - Tendency to close or favor one eye
  - Poor hand-eye coordination
  - Diagnostic Procedures
    - Ophthalmoscopy
      - An ophthalmoscope is used to examine the back part of the eyeball (fundus), including the retina, optic disc, macula, and blood vessels.
    - Visual acuity tests
      - Visual acuity tests include the Snellen and Rosenbaum eye charts.
    - Tonometry
      - Tonometry is used to measure intraocular pressure (IOP). IOP (normal is 10 to 21 mm Hg) is elevated with glaucoma, especially angle-closure glaucoma.

(M) **View Media Supplement:** Intraocular Pressure (Image)

- ▪ Gonioscopy
  - □ Gonioscopy is used to examine the iridocorneal angle or anterior chamber of the eyes.
    - ▸ Slit lamp
      - ▹ The slit lamp is used to exam the anterior portion of the eye, such as the cornea, anterior chamber, and the lens.

Collaborative Care

- ● Nursing Care
  - ○ Nurses should monitor:
    - ▪ Visual acuity using the Snellen and Rosenbaum eye charts – both measure distance vision.
      - □ The Snellen method has the client stand 20 feet away.
      - □ The Rosenbaum method has the client hold the chart 14 inches away from his eyes.
    - ▪ External and internal eye structures (ophthalmoscope)
    - ▪ Functional ability
  - ○ Assess how the client is adapting to her environment to maintain safety.
    - ▪ Increase the amount of light in a room.
    - ▪ Arrange the home to remove hazards, such as eliminating throw rugs.
    - ▪ Provide phones with large numbers and/or auto dial.
  - ○ Provide the client with adaptive devices that accommodate for reduced vision.
    - ▪ Magnifying lens and large print books/newspapers
    - ▪ Talking devices, such as clocks and watches
- ● Medications
  - ○ Anticholinergics, such as atropine (Isopto Atropine ophthalmic solution)
    - ▪ Anticholinergics are used for intraocular exams/surgery. They provide mydriasis (dilation of the pupil) and cycloplegia (ciliary paralysis).
    - ▪ Client Education
      - □ Adverse effects include reduced accommodation, blurred vision, and photophobia. With systemic absorption, there could be anticholinergic effects (tachycardia, decreased secretions).
- ● Care after Discharge
  - ○ Initiate referrals as appropriate to social services, support groups, and reduced-vision resources.

○ Client Education

■ Wear sunglasses to protect eyes.

■ Wear eye protection to prevent injury to the eye.

■ Wash hands before and after treating the eye with medication.

■ Promote smoking cessation if the client is a smoker.

■ Limit alcohol intake.

■ Keep blood pressure and cholesterol under control.

■ Clients who have diabetes mellitus should keep blood glucose under control.

■ Eat foods rich in antioxidants, such as green, leafy vegetables.

■ Encourage adults 40 or older to have an annual examination including a measurement of IOP.

● Client Outcomes

○ The client will be free of injury to the eye.

○ The client will maintain level of vision and report any changes.

○ The client will be free of pain and report any changes to his provider.

○ The client will be free of infection and report any changes to his provider.

Complications

● Risk for Injury

○ Reduced vision places clients at a higher risk for injury. In particular, disturbed visual sensory perception is a well-known risk factor for injury and mortality in older adults.

○ Nursing Actions

■ Monitor for safety risks, such as the ability to drive safely, and intervene to reduce risks.

○ Client Education

■ Encourage annual eye examinations and good eye health.

RETINAL DETACHMENT

Overview

● Retinal detachment is a painless separation of the retina from the epithelium, resulting in the loss of vision in fields corresponding to the separation.

● Retinal detachment is a medical emergency, and the assistance of a provider should be sought immediately.

Health Promotion and Disease Prevention

- Take precautions when engaging in sports that can cause a blow to the head or the eye.

Assessment

- Risk Factors

  o Nearsightedness

  o Family history

  o Previous cataract surgery

  o Eye injury

  o Retinal tear – trauma

  o Fibrous vitreous tissue – pulls retina

  o Exudate – forms under retina

- Subjective and Objective Data

  o The onset is abrupt.

  o Bright flashes of light can occur.

  o Floating dark spots, commonly referred to as floaters, can be seen.

  o "Curtain drawing over visual field" sensation can occur.

  o An examination reveals a sudden loss of vision without pain.

  o Diagnostic Procedures

    ▪ A detached retina can be determined with an ophthalmoscope examination. Depending on the type of retinal tear, laser and/or surgery can be used as an intervention.

Collaborative Care

- Nursing Care

  o Restrict activity to prevent additional detachment.

  o Cover the affected eye with an eye patch.

- Medications

  o Terramycin with dexamethasone (TobraDex-ophthalmic solution)

    ▪ Antibiotic-steroid combination

    ▪ Prevents infection and decreases inflammation of the eye

    ▪ Client Education

      □ Remind the client to instill the drops as prescribed to prevent infection and inflammation.

- Interdisciplinary Care
  - A retinal specialist should be consulted for surgery.
- Surgical Interventions
  - Scleral buckling
    - Scleral buckling involves local or general anesthesia for the application of a silicone sponge held in place with stitches or an encircling band to promote attachment. An infiltration of a gas bubble can be done at the same time to push the retina back against the wall of the eye.
  - Retinal rebinding
    - The application of diathermy (high-frequency current), cryotherapy (freezing probes), or photocoagulation (laser beams) are used to create an inflammatory response for the purpose of rebinding the retina.
    - Nursing Actions
      - Provide information about the procedure for the client.
      - Rest the eye prior to the procedure.
      - An eye patch and shield are applied, and the client will lie with the affected eye up, or as prescribed, if a gas bubble is injected during the procedure.
      - Administer analgesics, antiemetics, antibiotics, and anti-inflammatory medications as prescribed.
    - Client Education
      - Avoid activities that cause rapid eye movement (reading, writing) for a specified period of time.
      - Wear sunglasses while outside or in brightly lit areas.
      - Rest the eye.
      - Contact the surgeon immediately if there is acute pain of the affected eye.
      - Contact the surgeon immediately if the eye has discharge or bleeds.
- Care after Discharge
  - Set up services, such as community outreach programs, meals on wheels, and services for the blind.
    - Client Education
      - Instruct the client to avoid activities that increase IOP, such as:
        - Bending over at the waist
        - Sneezing
        - Coughing
        - Straining
        - Vomiting

- ▸ Head hyperflexion

- ▸ Restrictive clothing, such as tight shirt collars

- ☐ The client should report if any changes occur, such as lid swelling, decreased vision, bleeding or discharge, a sharp, sudden pain in the eye, and/or flashes of light or floating shapes.

- • Client Outcomes

  - ○ The client will remain free from injury to the affected eye.

  - ○ The client will remain free from infection.

  - ○ The client will be pain free.

  - ○ The client will have improved vision as result of retinal surgery.

Complications

- • Loss of vision

  - ○ The final visual result is not always known for several months postoperatively. More than one attempt at repair of the eye may be required.

  - ○ Client Education

    - ■ The greatest risk for permanent progressive loss of vision is when the detachment is not treated prior to extension to the macula. Therefore, it is important for clients to know and recognize signs of detachment and to seek professional help immediately.

CATARACTS

Overview

- • A cataract is an opacity in the lens of an eye that impairs vision.

- • There are three types of cataracts:

  - ○ A subcapsular cataract begins at the back of the lens.

  - ○ A nuclear cataract forms in the center (nucleus) of the lens.

  - ○ A cortical cataract forms in the lens cortex and extends from the outside of the lens to the center.

 View Media Supplement: Cataracts (Image)

Health Promotion and Disease Prevention

- • Teach clients to wear sunglasses while outside.

- • Educate clients to wear protective eye wear while performing hazardous activities, such as welding and yard work.

- • Encourage annual eye examinations and good eye health, especially in adults over the age of 40.

Assessment

- Risk Factors

  - Advanced age
  - Diabetes
  - Heredity
  - Smoking
  - Trauma
  - Excessive exposure to the sun
  - Chronic corticosteroid use

- Subjective Data

  - Decreased visual acuity (prescription changes, reduced night vision)
  - Blurred vision
  - Diplopia – double vision
  - Glare and light sensitivity – photo sensitivity
  - History of visual problems

- Objective Data

  - Physical Assessment Findings
    - Progressive and painless loss of vision
    - Visible opacity
    - Absent red reflex
  - Diagnostic Procedures
    - Cataracts can be determined upon examination of the lens with an ophthalmoscope.

Collaborative Care

- Nursing Care

  - Check the client's visual acuity using the Snellen and Rosenbaum charts.
  - Examine the external and internal eye structures using an ophthalmoscope.
  - Determine the client's functional capacity due to decreased vision.
  - Increase the amount of light in a room.

- o Provide the client with adaptive devices that accommodate for reduced vision.

    - Magnifying lens and large print books/newspapers

    - Talking devices, such as clocks

- Medications

    - o Cholinesterase inhibitor (Atropine 1% ophthalmic solution)

        - This medication prevents pupil constriction for prolonged periods of time and relaxes muscles in the eye. It is used to dilate the eye preoperatively and for visualization of the eye's internal structures.

        - Nursing Considerations

            □ The medication has a long duration, but a slow onset.

        - Client Education

            □ Remind the client that the medication takes more than 24 hr to begin working.

    - o Acetazolamide (Diamox – oral medication)

        - Acetazolamide is administered preoperatively to reduce IOP, to dilate pupils, and to create eye paralysis to prevent lens movement.

        - Nursing Considerations

            □ Always ask the client if he is allergic to sulfa. Acetazolamide is a sulfa-based medication.

- Interdisciplinary Care

    - o An ophthalmologist should be consulted for cataract surgery.

- Surgical Interventions

    - o Surgical removal of the lens

        - A small incision is made and the lens is either removed in one piece, or in several pieces, after being broken up using sound waves. The posterior capsule is retained. A replacement or intraocular lens is inserted. Replacement lenses can correct refractive errors, resulting in improved distant vision.

        - Nursing Actions

            □ Postoperative care should focus on:

                ▸ Preventing infection.

                ▸ Administering ophthalmic medications.

                ▸ Providing pain relief.

                ▸ Teaching the client about self-care at home.

        - Client Education

            □ Wear sunglasses while outside or in brightly lit areas.

            □ Report signs of infection, such as yellow or green drainage.

- □ Avoid activities that increase IOP.
  - ▸ Bending over at the waist
  - ▸ Sneezing
  - ▸ Coughing
  - ▸ Straining
  - ▸ Head hyperflexion
  - ▸ Restrictive clothing, such as tight shirt collars
  - ▸ Sexual intercourse
- □ Limit activities.
  - ▸ Avoid tilting the head back to wash hair.
  - ▸ Limit cooking and housekeeping.
  - ▸ Avoid rapid, jerky movements, such as vacuuming.
  - ▸ Avoid driving and operating machinery.
  - ▸ Avoid sports.
- □ Report pain with nausea/vomiting – indications of increased IOP or hemorrhage.
- □ Best vision is not expected until 4 to 6 weeks following the surgery.
- □ The client should report if any changes occur, such as lid swelling, decreased vision, bleeding or discharge, a sharp, sudden pain in the eye, and/or flashes of light or floating shapes.

- • Client Outcomes
  - ○ The client will remain free from injury.
  - ○ The client will be free from infection.
  - ○ The client will be pain free.
  - ○ The client will have improved vision as result of cataract surgery.

Complications

- • Infection
  - ○ Infection can occur after surgery.
  - ○ Client Education
    - ■ Signs of infection that the client should report include yellow or green drainage, increased redness or pain, reduction in visual acuity, increased tear production, and/or photophobia.
- • Bleeding
  - ○ Bleeding is a potential risk several days following surgery.

○ Client Education

■ Clients should immediately report any sudden change in visual acuity or an increase in pain.

GLAUCOMA

 Overview

- Glaucoma is a disturbance of the functional or structural integrity of the optic nerve. Decreased fluid drainage or increased fluid secretion increases intraocular pressure (IOP) and can cause atrophic changes of the optic nerve and visual defects. An expected reference range for IOP is between 10 and 21 mm/Hg.

- There are two primary types of glaucoma:

  ○ Open-angle glaucoma – most common form of glaucoma. Open-angle refers to the angle between the iris and sclera. The aqueous humor outflow is decreased due to blockages in the eye's drainage system (Canal of Schlemm and trabecular meshwork) causing a rise in IOP.

  ○ Angle-closure glaucoma – less common form of glaucoma. IOP rises suddenly. With angle-closure glaucoma, the angle between the iris and the sclera suddenly closes causing a corresponding increase in IOP.

- Glaucoma is a leading cause of blindness. Early diagnosis and treatment is essential in preventing vision loss from glaucoma.

Health Promotion and Disease Prevention

- Encourage annual eye examinations and good eye health, especially adults over the age of 40.

- Educate the client about the disease and importance of adhering to a medication schedule to treat IOP.

Assessment

- Risk Factors

  ○ Age

  ○ Infection

  ○ Tumors

  ○ Diabetes mellitus

  ○ Genetic predisposition

- Subjective and Objective Data

  o Open-angle glaucoma

    - Loss of peripheral vision

    - Decreased accommodation

    - Elevated IOP (> 21 mm Hg)

  o Angle-closure glaucoma

    - Rapid onset of elevated IOP

    - Decreased or blurred vision

    - Seeing halos around lights

    - Pupils are nonreactive to light

    - Severe pain and nausea

    - Photophobia

  o Diagnostic Procedures

    - Visual assessments

      □ Decrease in visual acuity and peripheral vision

    - Tonometry

      □ Tonometry is used to measure IOP. IOP (expected reference range is 10 to 21 mm Hg) is elevated with glaucoma, especially angle-closure.

    - Gonioscopy

      □ Gonioscopy is used to determine the drainage angle of the anterior chamber of the eyes.

Collaborative Care

- Nursing Care

  o Monitor the client for increased IOP (> 21 mm Hg).

  o Monitor the client for decreased vision and light sensitivity.

  o Assess the client for aching or discomfort around the eye.

  o Explain the disease process to the client and allow him to express his feelings.

  o Treat severe pain and nausea that accompanies angle-closure glaucoma with analgesics and antiemetics.

- Medications

  o Pilocarpine (Isopto Carpine – ophthalmic solution)

    - Pilocarpine is a miotic, which constricts the pupil and allows for better circulation of the aqueous humor. Miotics can cause blurred vision.

- ○ Timolol (Timoptic – ophthalmic solution) and acetazolamide (Diamox – oral medication)
  - Beta-blockers (timolol) and carbonic anhydrase inhibitors (acetazolamide) decrease IOP by reducing aqueous humor production.
- ○ IV mannitol (Osmitrol)
  - IV mannitol is an osmotic diuretic used in the emergency treatment for angle-closure glaucoma to quickly decrease IOP.
- ○ Prednisolone acetate (Ocu-Pred – ophthalmic solution)
  - Prednisolone acetate is an ocular steroid used to decrease inflammation.

- Interdisciplinary Care

  - ○ Referral to an ophthalmologist may be indicated if surgery is necessary.

- Surgical Interventions

  - ○ Glaucoma surgery
    - Laser trabeculectomy, iridotomy, or the placement of a shunt are procedures used to improve the flow of the aqueous humor by opening a channel out of the anterior chamber of the eye.
    - Nursing Actions
      - □ IOP is checked 1 to 2 hr postoperatively by the surgeon.
      - □ Educate the client about the disease and importance of adhering to the medication schedule to treat IOP.
    - Client Education
      - □ Wear sunglasses while outside or in brightly lit areas.
      - □ Report signs of infection, such as yellow or green drainage.
      - □ Avoid activities that increase IOP.
        - ‣ Bending over at the waist
        - ‣ Sneezing
        - ‣ Coughing
        - ‣ Straining
        - ‣ Head hyperflexion
        - ‣ Restrictive clothing, such as tight shirt collars
        - ‣ Sexual intercourse
      - □ The client should not lie on the operative side and should report severe pain or nausea (possible hemorrhage).
      - □ The client should report if any changes occur, such as lid swelling, decreased vision, bleeding or discharge, a sharp, sudden pain in the eye and/or flashes of light or floating shapes.

- ☐ Limit activities.

  ▸ Avoid tilting head back to wash hair.

  ▸ Limit cooking and housekeeping.

  ▸ Avoid rapid, jerky movements, such as vacuuming.

  ▸ Avoid driving and operating machinery.

  ▸ Avoid sports.

- ☐ Report pain with nausea/vomiting – indications of increased IOP or hemorrhage.

- ☐ Final best vision is not expected until 4 to 6 weeks postoperative.

- ● Care after Discharge

  - ○ Set-up services such as community outreach programs, meals on wheels, and services for the blind.

- ● Client Outcomes

  - ○ The client will be free from injury.

  - ○ The client will be free from infection.

  - ○ The client will be pain free.

  - ○ The client will have decreased IOP due to the eye surgery.

Complications

- ● Blindness

  - ○ Blindness is a potential consequence of undiagnosed and untreated glaucoma.

  - ○ Client Education

    - ■ Encourage adults 40 or older to have an annual examination, including a measurement of IOP.

CHAPTER 13: DISORDERS OF THE EYE

(A) Application Exercises

Scenario: A nurse is caring for an older adult client who has diabetes mellitus. The client reports reduced vision.

1. What are some possible causes of the client's reduced vision?

2. If the client is also presbyopic, what visual deficit would the client report?

3. Which of the following client findings indicates an acute bleed has occurred as a result of a retinal detachment?

    A. Severe left eye pain

    B. Left palpebral edema

    C. Bilateral loss of vision

    D. Reporting a burst of black spots

4. What immediate action should be taken for a client with evidence of a retinal detachment?

Scenario: A nurse is caring for a client who has just been diagnosed with bilateral cataracts.

5. Which of the following client findings should the nurse anticipate? (Select all that apply.)

    _____   Eye pain

    _____   Floating spots

    _____   Blurred vision

    _____   White pupils

    _____   Bilateral red reflexes

    _____   Reduced visual acuity

6. The client is scheduled for surgical removal of the lens. Identify the purpose of the following preoperative medications:

MEDICATION	PURPOSE
Atropine (Isopto Atropine)	
Tobramycin with dexamethasone (TobraDex)	
Acetazolamide (Diamox)	

7. A client who is postoperative following cataract surgery reports nausea and severe eye pain. Which of the following actions should be taken?

   A. Notify the surgeon.

   B. Administer an analgesic.

   C. Administer an antiemetic.

   D. Turn the client onto the operative side.

CHAPTER 13: DISORDERS OF THE EYE

 Application Exercises Answer Key

Scenario: A nurse is caring for an older adult client who has diabetes mellitus. The client reports reduced vision.

1. What are some possible causes of the client's reduced vision?

   Presbyopia, cataracts, glaucoma, or retinal detachment

   Some possible causes of the client's reduced vision include presbyopia, cataracts, glaucoma, or a retinal detachment.

 NCLEX® Connection: Physiological Adaptation: Pathophysiology

2. If the client is also presbyopic, what visual deficit would the client report?

   The client will have an inability to focus on objects up close. Often, the client will report a headache and eye fatigue while focusing on objects up close to him. Instruct the client to hold reading materials at an arm's length.

 NCLEX® Connection: Physiological Adaptation: Pathophysiology

3. Which of the following client findings indicates an acute bleed has occurred as a result of a retinal detachment?

   A. Severe left eye pain

   B. Left palpebral edema

   C. Bilateral loss of vision

   D. Reporting a burst of black spots

   A sudden onset of flashes of bright light or dark floating spots (floaters) in the affected eye is a classic sign of detachment. The client will not experience left palpebral edema or bilateral loss of vision. Pain is generally not experienced since there are no pain fibers within the retina.

 NCLEX® Connection: Physiological Adaptation: Medical Emergencies

4. What immediate action should be taken for a client with evidence of a retinal detachment?

   Retinal detachment is a medical emergency and a provider should be sought immediately. Restrict activities (reading, writing) to prevent additional detachment. Cover the affected eye with an eye patch.

 NCLEX® Connection: Physiological Adaptation: Medical Emergencies

Scenario: A nurse is caring for a client who has just been diagnosed with bilateral cataracts.

5. Which of the following client findings should the nurse anticipate? (Select all that apply.)

_____ Eye pain

_____ Floating spots

__X__ **Blurred vision**

__X__ **White pupils**

_____ Bilateral red reflexes

__X__ **Reduced visual acuity**

A client who has bilateral cataracts will most likely have blurred vision, white pupils, and reduced visual acuity. Cataracts are generally not painful. Floating spots are characteristic of a retinal detachment. Red reflexes are generally absent.

 NCLEX® Connection: Reduction of Risk Potential: System Specific Assessment

6. The client is scheduled for surgical removal of the lens. Identify the purpose of the following preoperative medications:

MEDICATION	PURPOSE
Atropine (Isopto Atropine)	Cycloplegia (paralysis of ciliary muscle)
Tobramycin with dexamethasone (TobraDex)	Decrease infection and inflammation
Acetazolamide (Diamox)	Decrease IOP

 NCLEX® Connection: Pharmacological and Parenteral Therapies: Expected Actions/ Outcomes

7. Postoperative cataract surgery, the client reports nausea and severe eye pain. Which of the following actions should be taken?

A. Notify the surgeon.

B. Administer an analgesic.

C. Administer an antiemetic.

D. Turn the client onto the operative side.

Following cataract surgery, the surgeon should be notified if the client is experiencing nausea and severe pain. Turning the client on his operative side could cause more pain to the eye and worsen the nausea. Administering pain or an antiemetic medication should not be administered until the client is seen by the surgeon.

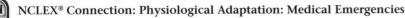 **NCLEX® Connection: Physiological Adaptation: Medical Emergencies**

UNIT 2	NURSING CARE OF CLIENTS WITH NEUROSENSORY DISORDERS
Section	Sensory Disorders
Chapter 14	Hearing Loss and Middle and Inner Ear Disorders

Overview

- Disorders related to hearing and balance can be caused by injury, disease, and/or the aging process.

- Auditory problems that nurses should be knowledgeable about include:

  ○ Hearing loss

  ○ Middle and inner ear disorders

HEARING LOSS

Overview

- Hearing loss is difficulty in hearing or accurately interpreting sounds due to a problem in either the middle or inner ear.

- There are two types of hearing loss:

  ○ Conductive hearing loss occurs when there is an alteration in the middle ear and sound waves are blocked before reaching the inner ear.

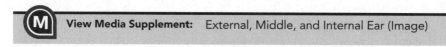

View Media Supplement: External, Middle, and Internal Ear (Image)

  ○ Sensorineural hearing loss occurs when there is an alteration in the inner ear that involves cranial nerve VIII and/or cochlear damage.

Health Promotion and Disease Prevention

- No objects should be placed in the ear, including cotton-tipped swabs.

- If a foreign object is present in the ear, have it removed by an otologist. If impacted cerumen is present, a commercial ceruminolytic (ear drops that soften cerumen) can be instilled. Irrigation with warm water may need to be done to complete removal.

- Ear protection should be worn for exposure to high-intensity noise and/or risk for ear trauma.

- The nose should be blown gently and with both nostrils unobstructed.

- When wearing headphones, volume should be kept as low as possible.

Assessment

- Risk Factors

  (G)

  - Risk for and degree of hearing loss progressively advances with aging.

  - Use of ototoxic medications (aminoglycosides, monobactams).

  - Conductive hearing loss

    - History of middle ear infections

    - Older age (otosclerosis)

  - Sensorineural hearing loss

    - Prolonged exposure to loud noises

    - Ototoxic medications

    - Infectious processes

    - Age-related (presbycusis – decreased ability to hear high-pitched sounds)

- Subjective and Objective Data

  - Conductive hearing loss

    - Subjective

      □ Reports hearing better in a noisy environment

    - Objective

      □ Client speaks softly

      □ Obstruction in external canal visualized (packed cerumen is very common)

      □ Abnormal tympanic membrane findings (holes, scarring)

      □ Rinne test that demonstrates that air conduction of sound is less than or equal to bone conduction (AC < or = to BC)

      □ Weber test that lateralizes to the affected ear

  - Sensorineural hearing loss

    - Subjective

      □ Tinnitus (ringing, roaring, or humming in ears)

      □ Dizziness

      □ Hears poorly in a noisy environment

    - Objective

      □ Client speaks loudly

      □ Otoscopic exam is normal

      □ Rinne test demonstrates normal response of air conduction is greater than bone conduction (AC > BC) but length of time is decreased for both.

☐ Weber test lateralizes to the unaffected ear.

☐ Diagnosis of acoustic neuroma (benign tumor cranial nerve VIII)

 View Media Supplement: Rinne and Weber Tests (Video)

○ Diagnostic Procedures

■ Audiometry

☐ An audiogram identifies if hearing loss is sensorineural and/or conductive.

☐ Nursing Actions

▸ Nurses may be required to use audiometry when screening for hearing loss in a school or older adult setting. The results will be more accurate in a room devoid of environmental sounds.

▸ Protocol should be followed to assess a client's ability to hear various frequencies (high versus low pitch) at various decibels (soft versus loud tones).

▸ The test should be done with the client wearing audiometer headphones and facing away from person performing test.

▸ The client should be instructed to indicate when a tone is heard and in which ear by raising the hand on the corresponding side. Responses are plotted on a graph for each ear and compared to expected findings based on age.

☐ Client Education

▸ Instruct client on how to respond when a tone is heard.

■ Tympanogram

☐ A tympanogram measures the mobility of the tympanic membrane and middle ear structures relative to sound.

☐ This test is effective in diagnosing disease of the middle ear.

■ Otoscopy

☐ An otoscope is used to examine the external auditory canal, the tympanic membrane (TM), and malleus bone visible through the TM.

 View Media Supplement: Otoscopic Examination (Video)

☐ Nursing Actions

▸ Otoscopic examination is done if audiometry results indicate a possible impairment or if a client is reporting ear pain.

▸ After selection of a properly sized speculum, an otoscope is introduced into the external ear.

- ▸ If the ear canal curves, pull up and back on the auricle of adults and down and back on the auricle of children to straighten out the canal and enhance visualization.

- ▸ The tympanic membrane should be a waxy gray color and intact. It should provide complete structural separation of the outer and middle ear structures.

- ▸ The light reflex should be visible from the center of the TM anteriorly (5 o'clock right ear; 7 o'clock left ear).

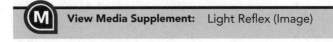

View Media Supplement: Light Reflex (Image)

- ▸ In the presence of fluid or infection in the middle ear, the tympanic membrane will become inflamed and may bulge from the pressure of the exudate. This will also displace the light reflex, a significant diagnostic finding.

- ▸ Avoid touching the lining of the ear canal, which causes pain due to sensitivity.

- □ Client Education

- ▸ Warn the client that to see the TM clearly, the auricle may need to be firmly pulled.

Collaborative Care

- • Nursing Care

  - ○ Monitor the client's functional ability.

  - ○ Communication

    - ■ Get the client's attention before speaking.

    - ■ Stand/sit facing the client in a well-lit, quiet room without distractions.

    - ■ Speak clearly and slowly to the client without shouting and without hands or other objects covering the mouth.

    - ■ Arrange for communication assistance (sign language interpreter, closed-captions, phone amplifiers, teletypewriter [TTY] capabilities) as needed.

  - ○ Check the hearing of clients receiving ototoxic medications for more than 5 days. Reduced renal function that occurs with aging increases the risk for ototoxicity. Ototoxic medications include:

    - ■ Multiple antibiotics – gentamicin (Garamycin), amikacin (Amikin), or metronidazole (Flagyl)

    - ■ Diuretics – furosemide (Lasix)

    - ■ NSAIDs – aspirin or ibuprofen (Advil)

    - ■ Chemotherapeutic agents – cisplatin (Abiplatin)

- Interdisciplinary Care

  o If abnormality is identified during audiometry, the client should be referred to audiologist for more sensitive testing.

- Therapeutic Procedures

  o Hearing aid – conductive hearing loss

    ▪ Hearing aids are effective in treating conductive hearing loss.

    ▪ Hearing aids amplify sounds, but do not help the client interpret what they are hearing.

    ▪ Amplification of sound in a loud environment can be distracting and disturbing.

  o Nursing Actions

    ▪ Clients should have hearing aids prescribed specifically for them.

    ▪ Hearing aids require special care.

    ▪ Use the lowest setting that allows hearing without feedback noise.

    ▪ To clean the ear mold, use mild soap and water while keeping hearing aid dry.

    ▪ When the hearing aid is not in use, make sure to turn it off to conserve the life of the batteries. Replacement batteries should always be kept on hand.

- Surgical Interventions

  o Tympanoplasty/myringoplasty – conductive hearing loss

    ▪ Tympanoplasty is a surgical reconstruction of the middle ear structures and myringoplasty is an eardrum repair.

    ▪ Nursing Actions

      ▫ Place sterile ear packing postoperatively.

      ▫ Position the client flat with the operative ear facing up for 12 hr.

    ▪ Client Education

      ▫ Avoid forceful straining, coughing, sneezing with the mouth closed, and air travel.

      ▫ Hair can be washed if the ear is covered with a dressing. No water should enter the ear.

      ▫ Remind the client that hearing will be impaired until packing is removed from the ear.

- Client Outcomes

  o The client will be able to accurately interpret speech and environmental sounds.

  o The client will demonstrate proper care of the ears and adaptive devices.

MIDDLE AND INNER EAR DISORDERS

Overview

- The middle ear consists of the tympanic membrane (eardrum), three bones (malleus, incus, and stapes), and connects to the oropharynx via the Eustachian tube.

- Middle ear infections are called otitis media.

- The inner ear consists of the oval window, cochlea (hearing organ) and the vestibular system – (organ responsible for balance, which includes the semicircular canals).

- Middle and inner ear disorders cause many of the same symptoms due to their close proximity and adjoining structures.

- Inner ear problems are characterized by tinnitus (continuous ringing in ear), vertigo (whirling sensation), and dizziness.

- Labyrinthitis and Ménière's disease are inner ear problems.

  - Labyrinthitis is an infection of the labyrinth, usually secondary to otitis media.

  - Ménière's disease is a vestibular disease characterized by a triad of symptoms: tinnitus, unilateral sensorineural hearing loss, and vertigo.

    - Benign paroxysmal vertigo (BPV) is a disorder that occurs in response to a change in position. It is thought to be due to a disturbance of crystals in the semicircular canals initiating vertigo that lasts from days to months.

- Visual, vestibular, and proprioceptive systems provide the brain with input regarding balance. Problems within any of these systems pose a risk for loss of balance.

Assessment

- Risk Factors

  - Middle ear disorders

    - Recurrent colds and otitis media

    - Enlarged adenoids

    - Trauma

    - Changes in air pressure (scuba diving, flying)

  - Inner ear disorders

    - Viral or bacterial infection

    - Ototoxic medications

- Subjective Data

  - Middle ear disorders

    - Hearing loss

    - Feeling of fullness and/or pain in the ear

- o   Inner ear disorders
    - ▪   Hearing loss
    - ▪   Tinnitus
    - ▪   Dizziness or vertigo
- •   Objective Data
    - o   Middle ear disorders
        - ▪   Red, inflamed ear canal and TM
        - ▪   Bulging TM
        - ▪   Fluid and/or bubbles behind TM
    - o   Inner ear disorders
        - ▪   Vomiting
        - ▪   Nystagmus
        - ▪   Poor balance
    - o   Diagnostic Procedures
        - ▪   Hearing acuity tests (Refer to tests performed for middle ear disorders.)
        - ▪   Electronystagmography (ENG)
            - □   ENG is done to determine the type of nystagmus elicited by the stimulation of the acoustic nerve.
            - □   Electrodes are placed around the eyes and movements of the eyes are recorded when the ear canal is stimulated with cold water instillation or injection of air. Recording of eye movements can be interpreted by a specialist as either normal or abnormal.
            - □   Nursing Actions
                - ‣   The client should be maintained on bed rest and NPO postprocedure until vertigo subsides.
            - □   Client Education
                - ‣   The client's preparation includes fasting immediately before the procedure and restricting caffeine, alcohol, sedatives, and antihistamines 24 hr prior to the test.
        - ▪   Caloric testing
            - □   Water (warmer or cooler than body temperature) is instilled in the ear in an effort to induce nystagmus.
            - □   The eyes' response to the instillation of cold and warm water is diagnostic of vestibular disorders.
            - □   This can be done concurrently with ENG.

- □ Nursing Actions
  - ▸ The client should follow the same restrictions as those for an ENG.
- □ Client Education
  - ▸ Inform the client of the above restrictions.

Collaborative Care

- Nursing Care
  - ○ Monitor the client's functional ability and balance. Take fall risk precautions as necessary.
  - ○ Check the hearing of clients receiving ototoxic medications for more than 5 days. Reduced renal function that occurs with aging increases the risk for ototoxicity. Ototoxic medications include:
    - Multiple antibiotics – gentamicin (Garamycin), amikacin (Amikin), or metronidazole (Flagyl)
    - Diuretics – furosemide (Lasix)
    - NSAIDs – aspirin or ibuprofen (Advil)
    - Chemotherapeutic agents – cisplatin (Abiplatin)
  - ○ Assist with ENG and/or caloric testing as needed.
  - ○ Administer antivertigo and antiemetic medications as needed.
- Medications
  - ○ Meclizine (Antivert)
    - Meclizine has antihistamine and anticholinergic effects and is used to treat the vertigo that accompanies inner ear problems.
    - Nursing Considerations
      - □ Restrict use in clients who have closed-angle glaucoma.
      - □ Observe the client for sedation and take appropriate precautions to ensure safe ambulation.
    - Client Education
      - □ Warn the client about the sedative effects of meclizine (avoid driving, operating heavy machinery).
  - ○ Antiemetics
    - Droperidol (Inapsine) is one of several antiemetics used to treat nausea and vomiting associated with vertigo.
    - Nursing Considerations
      - □ Observe the client for postural hypotension and tachycardia.
      - □ Tell the client to avoid abrupt changes in position.

- Client Education
  - □ Warn the client about the hypotensive effects of droperidol.
- o Diphenhydramine (Benadryl) and dimenhydrinate (Dramamine)
  - Antihistamines are effective in the treatment of vertigo and nausea that accompany inner ear problems.
  - Nursing Considerations
    - □ Observe the client for urinary retention.
    - □ Observe the client for sedation and take appropriate precautions to ensure safe ambulation.
  - Client Education
    - □ Warn the client about the sedative effects (avoid driving, operating heavy machinery).
    - □ Inform the client that dry mouth is to be expected.
- o Scopolamine (Transderm Scop)
  - Anticholinergics, such as scopolamine, are effective in the treatment of nausea that accompanies inner ear problems.
  - Nursing Considerations
    - □ Observe the client for urinary retention.
    - □ Observe the client for sedation and take appropriate precautions to ensure safe ambulation.
  - Client Education
    - □ Warn the client about the sedative effects antihistamines (avoid driving, heavy machinery).
    - □ Inform client that dry mouth is to be expected.
- o Diazepam (Valium)
  - Diazepam is a benzodiazepine that has antivertigo effects.
  - Nursing Considerations
    - □ Observe for sedation and take appropriate precautions to ensure safe ambulation.
    - □ Restrict use in clients who have closed-angle glaucoma.
  - Client Education
    - □ Warn the client about the sedative effects of diazepam (avoid driving, operating heavy machinery).
    - □ Inform the client of diazepam's addictive properties and appropriate use of the medication.

- Interdisciplinary Care

  o Vestibular rehabilitation is an option for clients who experience frequent episodes of vertigo and/or are incapacitated due to the vertigo. A team of health care providers is used to treat the cause and teach the client exercises that can help him adapt to and minimize the effects of vertigo. A combination of biofeedback, physical therapy, and stress management may be used. Postural education can teach the client positions to avoid as well as positional exercises that can terminate an attack of vertigo.

- Therapeutic Procedures

  o Vertigo reducing activities

    ▪ Client Education

        □ The client should be taught how to prevent stimulation/exacerbation of vertigo.

        □ Tell the client to space intake of fluids evenly throughout the day.

        □ Teach the client to decrease intake of salt and sodium-containing foods (processed meats, MSG).

        □ Have the client avoid caffeine and alcohol.

        □ Instruct the client to take a diuretic, if prescribed, to decrease the amount of fluid in semicircular canals.

        □ Tell the client to take these precautions when vertigo is present.

        □ Encourage the client to rest in a quiet, darkened environment when the symptoms are severe.

        □ Have the client use assistive devices as needed (cane, walker) for safe ambulation to assist with balance.

        □ Encourage the client to maintain a safe environment that is free of clutter.

- Surgical Interventions

  o Stapedectomy – conductive hearing loss

    ▪ A stapedectomy is a surgical procedure of the middle ear in which the stapes is removed and replaced with a prothesis.

    ▪ The procedure is done when otosclerosis has developed and the bones of the middle ear fuse together.

    ▪ Otosclerosis is one of the causes of conductive hearing loss in older adults.

    ▪ Nursing Actions

        □ The procedure is done through the external ear canal and TM.

        □ The stapes is completely or partially removed and replaced with a prosthesis.

        □ The TM is repaired and sterile ear packing is placed postoperatively.

        □ Assess the client for facial nerve damage.

        □ Intervene for vertigo, nausea, and vomiting (common findings following the procedure).

- Client Education

  □ Hearing is initially worse, but will improve as healing occurs.

  □ Avoid straining, coughing, sneezing with mouth closed, air travel, and rapid head movements.

  □ Hair can be washed if the ear is covered with a dressing. No water should enter the ear.

  ○ Cochlear implant – sensorineural hearing loss

  - Cochlear implants consist of a microphone that picks up sound, a speech processor, a transmitter and receiver that converts sounds into electric impulses, and electrodes that are attached to the auditory nerve.

  - The implant's transmitter is located outside the head behind the ear and connects via a magnet to the receiver located immediately below it, under the skin.

  - Young children and adults who lost their hearing after speech development adapt to cochlear implants more quickly than those who were totally deaf at birth. Intensive and prolonged language training is necessary for individuals who did not develop speech.

  - Nursing Actions

    □ Placement of an implant can be done on an outpatient basis.

  - Client Education

    □ Inform the client that immediately after surgery the unit is not turned on.

    □ Two to six weeks after surgery, the external unit is applied and the speech processor is programmed.

    □ Instruct the client on precautions to prevent infection.

    □ Instruct the client that MRIs must be avoided.

  ○ Labyrinthectomy

  - A labyrinthectomy is a surgical treatment for vertigo that involves removal of the labyrinthine portion of the inner ear.

  - Nursing Actions

    □ Client will have severe nausea and vertigo postoperatively. Take appropriate safety precautions and give antiemetics as needed.

  - Client Education

    □ Inform the client that hearing loss is to be expected in the affected ear.

- Client Outcomes

  ○ The client will have decreased episodes of vertigo.

  ○ The client will be free from injury.

CHAPTER 14: HEARING LOSS AND MIDDLE AND INNER EAR DISORDERS

(A) Application Exercises

Scenario: A nurse is caring for a client who has possible hearing loss.

1. Which of the following findings supports the diagnosis of sensorineural hearing loss in the left ear?

   A. Report of a humming sound in the left ear

   B. Weber test lateralizes to the right ear

   C. Rinne test that demonstrates air conduction less than bone conduction in the left ear

   D. Light reflex at 10 o'clock in the left ear

2. When performing the otoscopic examination, which of the following indicates an unexpected finding?

   A. Waxy, gray TM

   B. Malleus visible behind the TM

   C. Flaky skin in the external canal near the TM

   D. Black cerumen partially occluding the TM

3. Which of the following client findings are possible causative factors for the client's sensorineural hearing loss? (Select all that apply.)

   _____ Daily use of warfarin (Coumadin)

   _____ Age 85

   _____ Antibiotic therapy with reduced renal function

   _____ Employed as a ground crew member at a large airport

   _____ Presbyopia

   _____ Presbycusis

   _____ High doses of IV furosemide (Lasix) for heart failure exacerbation

   _____ Chronic use of NSAIDs for rheumatoid arthritis management

4. A client is newly fitted with a hearing aid. Which of the following client statements indicates a need for intervention by the nurse?

   A. "I have difficulty hearing in a loud environment."

   B. "I wash the earpiece of my hearing aid with alcohol."

   C. "I keep my hearing aid volume turned down low."

   D. "I turn my hearing aid off at night."

5. A client has been experiencing mild to moderate vertigo due to BPV for several weeks. Which of the following actions should the nurse recommend to help control the vertigo? (Select all that apply.)

_____ Request a prescription for meclizine (Antivert).

_____ Move head slowly when changing positions.

_____ Discontinue use of diuretics.

_____ Avoid fruits high in potassium.

_____ Use stress management techniques.

_____ Avoid smoking.

CHAPTER 14: HEARING LOSS AND MIDDLE AND INNER EAR DISORDERS

Ⓐ Application Exercises Answer Key

Scenario: A nurse is caring for a client who has possible hearing loss.

1. Which of the following findings supports the diagnosis of sensorineural hearing loss in the left ear?

   A. Report of a humming sound in the left ear

   B. Weber test lateralizes to the right ear

   C. Rinne test that demonstrates air conduction less than bone conduction in the left ear

   D. Light reflex at 10 o'clock in the left ear

   The Weber test is used to support the diagnosis of sensorineural hearing loss. Humming or tinnitus does not indicate hearing loss. The results of the Rinne test indicate possible conductive hearing loss of the left ear. Finally, the abnormal light reflex indicates that the tympanic membrane is displaced from air or fluid but does not indicate hearing loss.

   Ⓝ NCLEX® Connection: Reduction of Risk Potential: System Specific Assessment

2. When performing the otoscopic examination, which of the following indicates an unexpected finding?

   A. Waxy, gray TM

   B. Malleus visible behind the TM

   C. Flaky skin in the external canal near the TM

   D. Black cerumen partially occluding the TM

   Black cerumen that is packed and partially occluding the TM is an unexpected finding and indicates that the cerumen has been in the ear a long time. Its location and color may indicate that the client uses cotton-tipped swabs and is pushing the cerumen back into the ear against the TM. The other options are expected findings.

   Ⓝ NCLEX® Connection: Reduction of Risk Potential: System Specific Assessment

3. Which of the following client findings are possible causative factors for the client's sensorineural hearing loss? (Select all that apply.)

_____	Daily use of warfarin (Coumadin)
X	**Age 85**
X	**Antibiotic therapy with reduced renal function**
X	**Employed as a ground crew member at a large airport**
_____	Presbyopia
X	**Presbycusis**
X	**High doses of IV furosemide (Lasix) for heart failure exacerbation**
X	**Chronic use of NSAIDs for rheumatoid arthritis management**

   All of the above factors can contribute to sensorineural hearing loss except for the use of warfarin and presbyopia.

   Ⓝ NCLEX® Connection: Physiological Adaptation: Alterations in Body Systems

4. A client is newly fitted with a hearing aid. Which of the following client statements indicates a need for intervention by the nurse?

    A. "I have difficulty hearing in a loud environment."
    B. "I wash the earpiece of my hearing aid with alcohol."
    C. "I keep my hearing aid volume turned down low."
    D. "I turn my hearing aid off at night."

The earpiece of a hearing aid should be cleaned with mild soap and water, not alcohol. Clients who use hearing aids have difficulty hearing in loud environments because all sounds are amplified. Keeping the hearing aid's volume turned down low will prevent feedback and turning it off at night will enhance battery life.

NCLEX® Connection: Basic Care and Comfort: Assistive Devices

5. A client has been experiencing mild to moderate vertigo due to BPV for several weeks. Which of the following actions should the nurse recommend to help control the vertigo? (Select all that apply.)

    __X__   **Request a prescription for meclizine (Antivert).**
    __X__   **Move head slowly when changing positions.**
    _____   Discontinue use of diuretics.
    _____   Avoid fruits high in potassium.
    __X__   **Use stress management techniques.**
    _____   Avoid smoking.

Use of meclizine, an effective pharmacologic treatment for vertigo, moving the head slowly when changing positions, and stress management techniques can all lessen the incidence of vertigo. Diuretics are used in the treatment of vertigo and should be continued. Foods high in potassium and smoking have no effect on vertigo.

NCLEX® Connection: Physiological Adaptation: Illness Management

UNIT 2	NURSING CARE OF CLIENTS WITH NEUROSENSORY DISORDERS
Section	Neurologic Emergencies
Chapter 15	Head Injury

Overview

- Head injuries can be classified as open (skull integrity is compromised – penetrating trauma) or closed (skull integrity is maintained – blunt trauma). Head injuries are also classified as mild, moderate, or severe, depending upon Glasgow Coma Scale (GCS) ratings and the length of time the client was unconscious.

- Open-head injuries pose a high risk for infection.

- Skull fractures are often accompanied by brain injury. Damage to the brain tissue may be the result of decreased oxygen supply, or the direct impact from the skull fracture, which caused the trauma. The glucose levels in the brain are negatively affected, resulting in an alteration in neurological synaptic ability.

- Head injuries may or may not be associated with hemorrhage (epidural, subdural, and intracerebral). Cerebrospinal fluid leakage is also possible. Any collection of fluid, or foreign objects, that occupies the space within the skull consequently poses a risk for cerebral edema, cerebral hypoxia, and brain herniation.

- A cervical spine injury should always be suspected when a head injury occurs. A cervical spine injury must be ruled out prior to removing any devices used to stabilize the cervical spine.

Health Promotion and Disease Prevention

- Wear helmets when skateboarding, riding a bike or motorcycle, skiing, playing football and any other sport that could cause a head injury. Depending on the activity or sport, instruct the client to wear a helmet.

- Wear seat belts when driving or riding in a car.

- Avoid dangerous activities (speeding, driving under the influence of alcohol or drugs).

Assessment

- Risk Factors

  - Males under 25 years of age

  - Motor vehicle or motorcycle crashes

- ○ Drug and alcohol use
- ○ Sports injuries
- ○ Assault
- ○ Gunshot wounds
- ○ Falls
- • Subjective and Objective Data
  - ○ Presence of alcohol or illicit drugs at time of injury
  - ○ Amnesia (loss of memory) before or after the injury
  - ○ Loss of consciousness – Length of time the client is unconscious is significant
  - ○ Signs of increased intracranial pressure include:
    - ▪ Severe headache.
    - ▪ Deteriorating level of consciousness, restlessness, irritability.
    - ▪ Dilated or pinpoint pupils, slow to react or nonreactive.
    - ▪ Alteration in breathing pattern (Cheyne-Stokes respirations, central neurogenic hyperventilation, apnea).
    - ▪ Deterioration in motor function, abnormal posturing (decerebrate, decorticate, or flaccidity).
    - ▪ Cushing reflex is a late sign characterized by severe hypertension with a widening pulse pressure (systolic – diastolic) and bradycardia.
    - ▪ Cerebrospinal fluid leakage from the nose and ears ("halo" sign – yellow stain surrounded by blood on a paper towel; fluid tests positive for glucose).
    - ▪ Seizures.
  - ○ Laboratory Tests
    - ▪ ABGs
    - ▪ Alcohol level and drug screen
    - ▪ CBC with differential and BUN
      - □ BUN is used to determine the client's renal status. This information is needed prior to administration of radiology contrast media.
  - ○ Diagnostic Procedures
    - ▪ Cervical spine films are used to diagnose a cervical spine injury.
    - ▪ Computerized tomography (CT) and/or a magnetic resonance imaging (MRI) of the head and/or neck (with and without contrast if indicated).

Collaborative Care

- Nursing Care

  o There is a 1 hr "golden window" for treatment of head injuries. Emergency treatment provided during this time frame, especially for epidural hematomas, decreases the morbidity and mortality rates associated with these conditions.

  o Educate the client's family on effective ways to communicate with the client (touch, talk, and assist with care as appropriate).

  o Assess/monitor the client at regularly scheduled intervals:

    ▪ Respiratory status – the PRIORITY assessment

      □ The brain is dependent upon oxygen to maintain function and has little reserve available if oxygen is deprived. Brain function begins to diminish after 3 min of oxygen deprivation.

    ▪ Cranial nerve function (eye blink response, gag reflex, tongue and shoulder movement)

    ▪ Pupillary changes (PERRLA, pinpoint, fixed/nonresponsive, dilated)

    ▪ Signs of infection (nuchal rigidity occurs with meningitis)

    ▪ Sensory and/or motor responses if spinal injury is present

    ▪ Changes in level of consciousness, using the GCS, which provides the EARLIEST indication of neurological deterioration.

    ▪ Intracranial pressure (ICP)

      □ There are three ways to monitor ICP:

        ▸ Use a thin tube inserted into the lateral ventricle (intraventricular).

        ▸ Use a bolt or screw placed in the subarachnoid area (subarachnoid).

        ▸ Place a sensor in the epidural space (epidural).

      □ Expected reference range for ICP level is 10 to 15 mm Hg.

      □ ICP may be increased by:

        ▸ Hypercarbia which leads to cerebral vasodilation.

        ▸ Endotracheal or oral tracheal suctioning.

        ▸ Coughing.

        ▸ Blowing the nose forcefully.

        ▸ Extreme neck or hip flexion/extension.

        ▸ Maintaining the head of the bed at an angle less than 30°.

        ▸ Increasing intra abdominal pressure (restrictive clothing, Valsalva maneuver).

- □ Implement actions that will decrease ICP:
  - ▸ Elevate head to reduce ICP and to promote venous drainage.
  - ▸ Avoid extreme flexion, extension or rotation of the head, and maintain the body in a midline neutral position, with the head of the bed elevated 30°.
  - ▸ Maintain a patent airway. Provide mechanical ventilation as indicated.
  - ▸ Administer oxygen as indicated to maintain an oxygen saturation level of > 92.
  - ▸ Hyperventilate client to keep the $PaCO_2$ between 30 to 35 mm Hg (this reduces cerebral blood flow).
  - ▸ Maintain cervical spine stability until cleared by an x-ray.
  - ▸ Report presence of cerebrospinal fluid (CSF) from nose or ears to the provider.
  - ▸ Provide a calm, restful environment (limit visitors, minimize noise).
  - ▸ Implement measures to prevent complications of immobility (turn the client every 2 hr, footboard, and splints). Specialty beds can be used.
  - ▸ Monitor fluid and electrolyte values and osmolarity to detect changes in sodium regulation, the onset of diabetes insipidus, or severe hypovolemia.
  - ▸ Provide adequate fluids to maintain cerebral perfusion. When a large amount of IV fluids are prescribed, monitor the client carefully for excess fluid volume which could increase ICP.
  - ▸ Maintain client safety and seizure precautions (side rails up, padded side rails, call light within the client's reach).
  - ▸ Even if the level of consciousness is decreased, explain to the client the actions being taken and why.
    - ▹ Hearing is the last sense affected by a head injury

- Medications
  - ○ Corticosteroids – Dexamethasone (Decadron) and methylprednisolone (Solu-Medrol)
    - ■ Used to reduce cerebral edema
    - ■ Nursing Considerations
      - □ Use with caution in the presence of diabetes mellitus, hypertension, glaucoma, or renal impairment. If these conditions exist, additional monitoring is required as corticosteroids disrupt the stability of those conditions and can require alterations in care.

- ○ Mannitol (Osmitrol)
  - ■ Osmotic diuretic used to treat cerebral edema
  - ■ Nursing Considerations
    - □ Administer IV to treat acute cerebral edema.
    - □ Insert indwelling urinary catheter to monitor fluid and renal status.
- ○ Pentobarbital (Nembutal)
  - ■ Pentobarbital is used to induce a barbiturate coma to decrease cerebral metabolic demands.
  - ■ This treatment is performed when the ICP is refractory to treatment, has exceeded 25 mm Hg for 30 min, 30 mm Hg for 15 min, or 40 mm Hg for 1 min.
  - ■ A barbiturate coma is a treatment of last resort and aims to decrease elevated ICP by inducing vasoconstriction and decreasing cerebral metabolic demands.
  - ■ Nursing Considerations
    - □ Medication is administered in bursts to decrease cerebral activity. Dosages are controversial outside of the manufacturer's guidelines.
    - □ Protocols vary, but can begin with 10 mg/kg over 30 min, then 5 mg/kg every hour for 3 doses, with a maintenance dose of 1 mg/kg per hour.
    - □ Treatment continues until the ICP remains below 20 mm Hg for 48 hr.
    - □ Medication is then slowly withdrawn.
    - □ Nursing care during this treatment requires full physiological support for the client's body functions.
    - □ If treatment is not successful, a re-evaluation is completed if the client expressed a desire to donate his organs.
- ○ Phenytoin (Dilantin)
  - ■ Used prophylactically to prevent or treat seizures that can occur
    - □ Nursing Considerations
      - ▸ Dosing for this medication is client-specific and based on therapeutic blood levels.
      - ▸ Check for medication interactions.
- ○ Morphine sulfate or fentanyl (Sublimaze)
  - ■ Analgesics used to control pain and restlessness
  - ■ Nursing Considerations
    - □ Use opioids if client is receiving ventilation.
    - □ Avoid the use of opioids due to the CNS depressant effect that will make a neurological assessment difficult.

- Interdisciplinary Care

  o Care for a client with a head injury should include professionals from other disciplines as indicated. This may include a physical, occupational, recreational and/or speech therapist due to neurological deficits that may occur secondary to the area of the brain damaged.

  o Social services should be contacted to provide links to social service agencies and schools.

  o Rehabilitation facilities are frequently used to compress the time required to recover from a head injury and support re-emergence into society.

- Surgical Interventions

  o Craniotomy

    ▪ A craniotomy is the removal of nonviable brain tissue that allows for expansion and/or removal of epidural or subdural hematomas. It involves drilling a burr hole or creating a bone flap to permit access to the affected area. Treatment of intracranial hemorrhages require surgical evacuation.

    ▪ This is a life-saving procedure, and is associated with many potential complications, such as:

      □ Severe neurological impairment, infection, persistent seizures, neurological deficiencies, and/or death.

    ▪ Nursing Actions

      □ Postoperative treatment will depend upon the neurological status of the client after surgery.

      □ Initially, care will surround the prevention of complications, maximizing cerebral function and supporting other physiological systems.

- Client Outcomes

  o ICP will remain within the recommended reference range.

  o The client will be able to perform ADLs independently or with assistive devices.

  o The client will be able to ambulate independently or with assistive devices.

Complications

- Brain herniation

  o A brain herniation is the downward shift of brain tissue due to cerebral edema.

  o The brain consists of brain matter, cerebrospinal fluid, and intravascular blood.

  o The Monro-Kellie doctrine states that any alteration in the volume of one of these results in a compromise in the other components.

  o When trauma creates a shift in these components, and the other components are unable to accommodate, the brain shifts from the cranial vault, or herniates.

View Media Supplement: Brain Herniation (Image)

- ○ This can result in brain tissue moving downward, through the foramen magnum.

- ○ Clinical signs include fixed dilated pupils, deteriorating level of consciousness, Cheyne-Stokes respirations, hemodynamic instability, and abnormal posturing.

- ○ Recovery after this occurrence is rare, urgent medical mannitol (Osmitrol) and/or surgical (debulking) treatment is indicated.

- ○ With treatment, severe neurological impairment usually persists.

- ○ Nursing Actions

  - ▪ This situation should be prevented before treatment is needed.

  - ▪ Close monitoring of the client's vital signs and neurological status will allow early reporting of changes in the GCS score, an increase in the blood pressure, and an alteration in respiratory pattern and effort.

- ○ Client Education

  - ▪ Family members should be frequently updated on the health status of the client member.

  - ▪ The decision to surgically treat brain herniation is made in the presence of a critical situation.

  - ▪ Frequent updates and repeating medical information is often necessary to assure comprehension among family members.

  - ▪ Social service workers and/or pastoral personnel can be helpful to support the family, while reinforcing the medical situation.

CHAPTER 15: HEAD INJURY

 Application Exercises

1. A nurse is caring for a client who was recently admitted to the emergency department following a head-on motor vehicle crash. The client is unresponsive, has spontaneous respirations of 22/min, and a laceration on his forehead that is bleeding. Which of the following is the priority nursing action at this time?

    A. Keep neck stabilized.

    B. Insert NG tube.

    C. Monitor pulse and blood pressure frequently.

    D. Establish IV access and start fluid replacement.

2. An adolescent who has a gunshot wound to the head is being admitted to the critical care unit from the emergency department. Which of the following assessment findings are indicative of increased ICP? (Select all that apply.)

    _____ Headache

    _____ Dilated pupils

    _____ Tachycardia

    _____ Decorticate posturing

    _____ Hypotension

3. A nurse is caring for a client who has just been admitted from surgery for the evacuation of a subdural hematoma. Which of the following is the priority assessment?

    A. Glasgow Coma Scale

    B. Cranial nerve function

    C. Oxygen saturation level

    D. Pupillary response

4. A client who has a closed-head injury has had ICP readings that ranged between 16 to 22 mm Hg for the past 2 days. Which of the following actions should the nurse take to decrease the potential for raising the client's ICP? (Select all that apply.)

    _____ Suction endotracheal tube using a closed system.

    _____ Hyperventilate the client.

    _____ Elevate the client's head using two pillows.

    _____ Administer a stool softener.

    _____ Keep the client well hydrated.

5. A client who has increased ICP has been prescribed mannitol (Osmitrol) IV. For which of the following side effects should the nurse monitor?

    A. Hyperglycemia

    B. Hyponatremia

    C. Hypervolemia

    D. Oliguria

6. A client who has an open-head injury has been prescribed phenytoin (Dilantin) to reduce the risk of seizures. Concurrent use with which of the following medications should be reported to the provider due to the possibility of a medication interaction?

    A. Celecoxib (Celebrex)

    B. Ciprofloxacin (Cipro)

    C. Atorvastatin (Lipitor)

    D. Warfarin (Coumadin)

CHAPTER 15: HEAD INJURY

 Application Exercises Answer Key

1. A nurse is caring for a client who was recently admitted to the emergency department following a head-on motor vehicle crash. The client is unresponsive, has spontaneous respirations of 22/min, and a laceration on his forehead that is bleeding. Which of the following is the priority nursing action at this time?

   A. Keep neck stabilized.

   B. Insert NG tube.

   C. Monitor pulse and blood pressure frequently.

   D. Establish IV access and start fluid replacement.

   The greatest risk to the client is permanent damage to the spinal cord if a cervical injury does exist. The priority nursing intervention is to keep the neck immobile until damage to the cervical spine can be ruled out. Inserting an NG tube, monitoring pulse and blood pressure, and establishing IV access for fluid replacement are all important, but not the priority at this time.

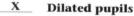 NCLEX® Connection: Physiological Adaptation, Medical Emergencies

2. An adolescent who has a gunshot wound to the head is being admitted to the critical care unit from the emergency department. Which of the following assessment findings are indicative of increased ICP? (Select all that apply.)

__X__	**Headache**
__X__	**Dilated pupils**
_____	Tachycardia
__X__	**Decorticate posturing**
_____	Hypotension

   Headache, dilated (or pinpoint) pupils, and decorticate (or decerebrate) posturing are signs of increased ICP. Bradycardia and hypertension with a widening pulse pressure are signs of increased ICP as opposed to tachycardia and hypotension.

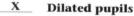 NCLEX® Connection: Reduction of Risk Potential, System Specific Assessment

3. A nurse is caring for a client who has just been admitted from surgery for the evacuation of a subdural hematoma. Which of the following is the priority assessment?

A. Glasgow Coma Scale

B. Cranial nerve function

C. Oxygen saturation level

D. Pupillary response

While all of the assessments are important in the care of this client, assessment of the client's oxygen saturation level is the highest priority. Brain tissue can only survive for 3 min without oxygen before permanent damage occurs.

 NCLEX® Connection: Physiological Adaptation, Unexpected Response to Therapies

4. A client who has a closed-head injury has had ICP readings that ranged between 16 to 22 mm Hg for the past 2 days. Which of the following actions should the nurse take to decrease the potential for raising the client's ICP? (Select all that apply.)

_____ Suction endotracheal tube using a closed system.

__X__ **Hyperventilate the client.**

_____ Elevate the client's head using two pillows.

__X__ **Administer a stool softener.**

_____ Keep the client well hydrated.

Hyperventilation of the client will prevent hypercarbia which can cause vasodilation with a secondary increase in ICP. Administration of a stool softener will also decrease the need to bear down (Valsalva maneuver) during bowel movements, which can increase ICP. Hyperflexion of the client's neck with pillows and overhydration all carry the risk of increasing ICP and should be avoided. Suctioning also increases ICP and should be done only when indicated.

 NCLEX® Connection: Physiological Adaptation, Unexpected Response to Therapies

5. A client who has increased ICP has been prescribed mannitol (Osmitrol) IV. For which of the following side effects should the nurse monitor?

A. Hyperglycemia

B. Hyponatremia

C. Hypervolemia

D. Oliguria

Mannitol is a powerful osmotic diuretic that carries the risk of fluid and electrolyte imbalances such as hyponatremia. Hyperglycemia is not a side effect of mannitol. Hypovolemia and polyuria are side effects as opposed to hypervolemia and oliguria.

 NCLEX® Connection: Physiological Adaptation, Unexpected Response to Therapies

6. A client who has an open-head injury has been prescribed phenytoin (Dilantin) to reduce the risk of seizures. Concurrent use with which of the following medications should be reported to the provider due to the possibility of a medication interaction?

    A. Celecoxib (Celebrex)

    B. Ciprofloxacin (Cipro)

    C. Atorvastatin (Lipitor)

    D. Warfarin (Coumadin)

Concurrent use of phenytoin and warfarin can lessen the effectiveness of warfarin. There are no interactions between phenytoin and celecoxib, ciprofloxacin, and atorvastatin.

NCLEX® Connection: Pharmacological and Parenteral Therapies, Adverse Effects/ Contraindications/Side Effects/Interactions

UNIT 2	NURSING CARE OF CLIENTS WITH NEUROSENSORY DISORDERS
Section	Neurologic Emergencies

Chapter 16   Cerebrovascular Accident

 Overview

- Cerebrovascular accidents (CVAs) or strokes involve a disruption in the cerebral blood flow secondary to ischemia, hemorrhage, or embolism.

- There are three causes of CVAs:

    o Hemorrhagic – These occur secondary to a ruptured artery or aneurysm. The prognosis for a client who has experienced a hemorrhagic CVA is poor due to the amount of ischemia and increased ICP caused by the expanding collection of blood. A CVA, if caught early and evacuation of the clot can be done with cessation of the active bleed, the prognosis of a hemorrhagic CVA improves significantly.

    o Thrombotic – These occur secondary to the development of a blood clot on an atherosclerotic plaque in a cerebral artery that gradually shuts off the artery and causes ischemia distal to the occlusion. Symptoms of a thrombotic CVA evolve over a period of several hours to days.

    o Embolic – These occur secondary to an embolus traveling from another part of the body to a cerebral artery. Blood to the brain distal to the occlusion is immediately shut off causing neurologic deficits or a loss of consciousness to instantly occur. An embolic CVA is very sensitive because many can be reversed if antiembolic medications such as alteplase (Activase, tPA) are administered within 4 to 6 hr of the initial symptoms.

> **View Media Supplement:**
> - Hemorrhagic Stroke (Image)
> - Thrombotic Stroke (Image)
> - Embolic Stroke (Image)

Health Promotion

- Health Promotion and Disease Prevention

    o Hypertension, diabetes mellitus, smoking, and other related disorders can increase a client's risk for a CVA.

    o Early treatment of hypertension, maintenance of blood glucose within expected range, and refraining from smoking will decrease these risk factors.

    o Maintaining a healthy weight and getting regular exercise can also decrease the risk of a CVA.

Assessment

- Risk Factors

  o Cerebral aneurysm

  o Arteriovenous malformation (AV)

  o Diabetes mellitus

  o Obesity

  o Hypertension

  o Atherosclerosis

  o Hyperlipidemia

  o Hypercoagulability

  o Atrial fibrillation

  o Use of oral contraceptives

  o Smoking

  o Cocaine use

- Subjective Data

  o Some clients report transient symptoms such as dizziness, slurred speech, and a weak extremity.

  o These symptoms may indicate a transient ischemic attack (TIA), which can be a warning of an impending CVA.

  o Antithrombotic medication and/or surgical removal of atherosclerotic plaques in the carotid artery can prevent the subsequent occurrence of a CVA.

- Objective Data

  o Physical Assessment Findings

    ▪ Symptoms will vary based on the area of the brain that is deprived of oxygenated blood.

      □ The left cerebral hemisphere is responsible for language, mathematic skills, and analytic thinking.

      □ Symptoms consistent with a left-hemispheric CVA include:

        ▸ Expressive and receptive aphasia (inability to speak and understand language respectively)

        ▸ Agnosia (unable to recognize familiar objects)

        ▸ Alexia (reading difficulty)

        ▸ Agraphia (writing difficulty)

        ▸ Right extremity hemiplegia (paralysis) or hemiparesis (weakness)

- ▸ Slow, cautious behavior

- ▸ Depression, anger, and quick to become frustrated

- ▸ Visual changes, such as hemianopsia (loss of visual field in one or both eyes)

 View Media Supplement: Hemianopsia (Image)

- □ The right cerebral hemisphere is responsible for visual and spatial awareness and proprioception.

  - ▸ Altered perception of deficits (overestimation of abilities)

  - ▸ One-sided neglect syndrome (ignore left side of the body – Cannot see, feel, or move affected side, so client unaware of its existence). Can occur with left-hemispheric CVAs, but is more common with right-hemispheric CVAs.

  - ▸ Loss of depth perception

  - ▸ Poor impulse control and judgment

  - ▸ Left hemiplegia or hemiparesis

  - ▸ Visual changes, such as hemianopsia

- ○ Diagnostic Procedures

  - ■ A magnetic resonance imaging (MRI), computed tomography (CT) imaging, and/or a computed axial tomography (CAT) scan may be used to identify edema, ischemia, and necrosis.

  - ■ A magnetic resonance angiography (MRA) or a cerebral angiography are used to identify the presence of a cerebral hemorrhage, abnormal vessel structures (AV malformation, aneurysms), vessel ruptures, and regional perfusion of blood flow in the carotid arteries and brain.

  - ■ A lumbar puncture is used to assess for the presence of blood in the cerebrospinal fluid (CSF). A positive finding is consistent with a cerebral hemorrhage or ruptured aneurysm.

  - ■ The Glasgow Coma Scale score is used when the client has a decreased level of consciousness or orientation. The risk for increased ICP exists related to the swelling of the brain that can occur secondary to ischemic insult.

Collaborative Care

- ● Nursing Care

  - ○ Monitor for changes in the client's level of consciousness (increased ICP sign).

  - ○ Elevate the client's head of the bed approximately 30° to reduce ICP and to promote venous drainage. Avoid extreme flexion or extension of the neck, and maintain the client's head in the midline neutral position.

  - ○ Institute seizure precautions.

- ○ Assist with the client's communication skills if his speech is impaired.

  - Assess the ability to understand speech by asking the client to follow simple commands.

  - Observe for consistently affirmative answers when the client actually does not comprehend what is being said.

  - Assess accuracy of yes/no responses in relation to closed-ended questions.

  - Supply the client with a picture board of commonly requested items/needs.

- ○ Assist with safe feeding.

  - Assess swallowing and gag reflexes before feeding. Speech therapy may be requested to do this during a swallowing study that can involve swallowing a barium substrate and radiography of the peristaltic activity of the esophagus.

  - If a swallowing deficit is identified, the client's liquids may need to be thickened with a commercial thickener to avoid aspiration.

  - Have the client eat in an upright position and swallow with the head and neck flexed slightly forward.

  - Place food in the back of the mouth on the unaffected side.

  - Have suction on standby.

  - Maintain a distraction-free environment during meals.

- ○ Maintain skin integrity.

  - Reposition the client frequently and use padding.

  - Monitor bony prominences, paying particular attention to the affected extremities.

  - If the client has one-sided neglect, teach him to protect and care for the affected extremity to avoid injuring it in the wheel of the wheelchair or hitting/smashing it against a doorway.

- ○ Encourage passive range of motion every 2 hr to the affected extremities and active range of motion every 2 hr to the unaffected extremities. Teach the client how to use the unaffected side to exercise the affected side of the body.

- ○ Elevate the affected extremities to promote venous return and reduce swelling. An elastic glove can be placed on the affected hand if swelling is severe. Teach the client to massage the affected hand by stroking it in a distal to proximal manner, encouraging fluid in the hand to move back into the wrist and arm.

- ○ Maintain a safe environment to reduce the risk of falls. Assistive devices should be used during transfers, such as transfer belts and sliding boards. Sit-to-stand lifts can also facilitate transfers and reduce strain on the care provider's body.

- ○ If the client has homonomous hemianopsia (loss of the same visual field in both eyes), instruct him to use a scanning technique (turning head from the direction of the unaffected side to the affected side) when eating and ambulating.

- o   To prevent deep vein thrombosis (DVT) from developing, provide preventive measures such as sequential compression stockings, frequent position changes, and mobilization.

- o   Provide assistance with ADLs as needed. Instruct the client to dress the affected side first and sit in a supportive chair that aids in balance. Have occupational therapy assess the client for adaptive aids, such as a plate guard, utensils with built-up handles, a reaching tool to pick things up, and shirts and shoes that have hook and loop fasteners/tape instead of buttons and ties.

- o   Prevent complications of immobility. While clients who have experienced CVAs are ambulated as soon as possible to prevent complications, during periods of inactivity, preventive measures related to complications of immobility should be implemented.

- o   Clients who have experienced CVAs have decreased endurance and impaired balance due to paralysis on one side of the body. Frequent rest periods from sitting in the wheelchair should be provided by returning the client to bed after therapies and meals. When sitting the client up in bed or in the wheelchair, leaning to the affected side typically occurs and should be countered with some manner of support.

- o   Shoulder subluxation can occur if the affected arm is not supported. The weight of the arm is such that it can actually cause a painful dislocation of the shoulder from its socket. Supporting the arm while in bed, the wheelchair, or during ambulation should be accomplished with an arm sling or strategically placed pillows.

- o   Support the client during periods of emotional lability and depression.

- Medications

  - o   Anticoagulants (aspirin, heparin sodium, enoxaparin [Lovenox], warfarin [Coumadin])

    - ▪   These medications are usually given to clients who have experienced an embolic CVA to prevent development of additional emboli.

  - o   Antiplatelets (ticlopidine [Ticlid], clopidogrel [Plavix])

    - ▪   These medications are usually given for clients who have experienced a thrombotic CVA to prevent extension of the CVA.

  - o   Thrombolytic medications alteplase (Activase, tPA)

    - ▪   Can be given within 3 hr of onset of symptoms to dissolve embolism.

  - o   Antiepileptic medications (phenytoin [Dilantin], gabapentin [Neurontin])

    - ▪   These medications are not commonly given following a CVA unless the client develops seizures.

    - ▪   Gabapentin can be given for paresthetic pain in an affected extremity.

- Interdisciplinary Care

  ○ Speech and language therapists can be consulted for language therapy and swallowing exercises.

  ○ Physical therapy can be consulted for assistance with re-establishment of ambulation with or without assistive devices (single or quad cane, walker) or wheelchair support. Wheelchair adaptations, such as an extended brake handle on the client's affected side of the wheelchair, may be necessary. Safety features, such as placing the brakes on when preparing to transfer and the use of a cushion on the seat, may also be integrated by physical therapy into the client's plan of care.

  ○ Occupational therapy can be consulted for assistance with re-establishment of partial or full function of the affected hand and arm. If function does not return to the extremity, measures, such as massage and elastic gloves will be prescribed by occupational therapy to prevent swelling of the extremity.

  ○ Social services can be consulted to make arrangements for rehabilitation services and temporary placement on a skilled rehabilitation unit or extended-care facility during provision of these services. Prior to discharge, the social worker may make a home visit with selected therapists and nurses to evaluate the need for environmental alterations in the home and adaptive equipment needed for ADLs.

- Therapeutic Procedures

  ○ Systemic or catheter-directed thrombolytic therapy restores cerebral blood flow. It must be administered within 3 hr of the onset of symptoms. It is contraindicated for treatment of a hemorrhagic CVA and for clients with an increased risk of bleeding due to anticoagulant therapy or other bleeding anomaly. Possibility of a hemorrhagic CVA is ruled out with an MRI prior to the initiation of thrombolytic therapy

- Surgical Interventions

  ○ Carotid endarterectomy is performed to open the artery by removing atherosclerotic plaque. This procedure is performed when the carotid artery is blocked or when the client is experiencing TIAs.

- Client Outcomes

  ○ The client's transient neurological deficits will cease and he will not experience a CVA.

  ○ The client will use adaptive devices to compensate for neurological deficits.

Complications

- Dysphagia and aspiration

  ○ Dysphagia can result from neurological involvement of the cranial nerves that innervate the face, tongue, soft palate, and throat. As a result, the client's risk of aspiration is great.

  ○ Not all client's who have experienced a CVA have dysphagia, but all should be evaluated prior to re-establishing oral nutrition and hydration.

- ○ Nursing Actions
  - Assess the client's gag reflex.
  - If the gag reflex is present, give the client a small sip of water to determine if choking occurs.
  - If the client exhibits some difficulty managing food or fluids, a swallowing evaluation should be done by a speech therapist.
  - Begin the client with a prescribed diet and observe closely for choking. Have the suction equipment available. Initial feedings should be done by an RN, so appropriate interventions can be taken if choking occurs.
  - Thicker liquids are usually tolerated better than thin liquids; therefore, thickener may need to be added to oral fluids. Use the appropriate amount of thickener to obtain the prescribed consistency.
- ○ Client Education
  - Teach the client's family how to thicken liquids to the proper consistency.

  - Instruct the client to flex his head forward when swallowing to decrease the risk of choking.

- Unilateral neglect
  - ○ Unilateral neglect is the loss of awareness of the side affected by the CVA. The client cannot see, feel, or move the affected side of his body; therefore, he forgets that it exists.

  - ○ This lack of awareness poses a great risk for injury to the neglected extremities and creates a self-care deficit.
  - ○ Nursing Actions
    - Observe the client's affected extremities for injury (bruises and abrasions of the affected hand and arm, hyperflexion of the foot from it falling off of the wheelchair during transport).
    - Apply an arm sling if the client is unable to remember to care for the affected extremity.
    - Ensure the foot rest is on the wheelchair and an ankle brace is on the affected foot.
  - ○ Client Education
    - Instruct the client to dress the affected side first.
    - Teach the client how to care for the affected side.
    - Use the unaffected hand to pull the affected extremity to midline and out of danger from the wheel of the wheelchair or from hitting or smashing it against a doorway.
    - Teach the client to scan the affected side.

CHAPTER 16: CEREBROVASCULAR ACCIDENT

(A) Application Exercises

Scenario: An older adult female client is brought to the emergency department after she fell from her chair during breakfast. The client has a Glasgow Coma Scale score of 5 and her blood pressure is 150/96 mm Hg, respirations are 16/min, pulse is 56/min, and a temperature of 38.3° C (101° F). Her admitting medical diagnosis is a suspected CVA. A CT scan is scheduled for the client.

1. Based on the CT results, the client is diagnosed with a right-hemispheric CVA of embolic origin. Which of the following neurological deficits should the nurse expect to find? (Select all that apply.)

    _____ Aphasia (receptive or expressive)

    _____ Right hemiplegia or hemiparesis

    _____ Lack of awareness of deficits

    _____ Impulse control difficulty

    _____ Slow, cautious behavior

    _____ Left hemiplegia or hemiparesis

2. The client is diagnosed with left homonymous hemianopsia. Which of the following actions is appropriate for the nurse to include in the client's plan of care?

    A. Teach the client to scan to the right to see objects on the right side of her body.

    B. Place the client's bedside table on the right side of the bed.

    C. Orient the client to the food on her plate using the clock method.

    D. Place the client's wheelchair on her left side.

3. When the client resumes dietary intake, which of the following actions should the nurse take? (Select all that apply.)

    _____ Have the suction equipment available for use.

    _____ Thicken liquids using a commercial thickener.

    _____ Place food on the client's unaffected side of her mouth.

    _____ Assign an assistive personnel to slowly feed the client.

    _____ Teach the client to swallow with her neck flexed.

    _____ Discontinue feeding the client if choking occurs.

4. A nurse has been assigned a client who is diagnosed with global aphasia (both receptive and expressive). Which of the following interventions are appropriate to include in the client's plan of care? (Select all that apply.)

_____ Speak to the client at a slower rate.

_____ Look directly at the client when speaking.

_____ Allow plenty of time for the client to answer.

_____ Complete sentences that the client cannot finish.

_____ Give instructions one step at a time.

_____ Speak louder if the client does not understand.

CHAPTER 16: CEREBROVASCULAR ACCIDENT

Ⓐ Application Exercises Answer Key

Scenario: An older adult female client is brought to the emergency department after she fell from her chair during breakfast. The client has a Glasgow Coma Scale score of 5 and her blood pressure is 150/96 mm Hg, respirations are 16/min, pulse is 56/min, and a temperature of 38.3° C (101° F). Her admitting medical diagnosis is a suspected CVA. A CT scan is scheduled for the client.

1. Based on the CT results, the client is diagnosed with a right-hemispheric CVA of embolic origin. Which of the following neurological deficits should the nurse expect to find? (Select all that apply.)

_____	Aphasia (receptive or expressive)
_____	Right hemiplegia or hemiparesis
X	**Lack of awareness of deficits**
X	**Impulse control difficulty**
_____	Slow, cautious behavior
X	**Left hemiplegia or hemiparesis**

A client who has experienced a right-hemispheric CVA will experience left-sided hemiplegia or hemiparesis along with impulsive behavior and a lack of awareness of deficits. This client poses a safety problem as she may impulsively respond to the urge to use the restroom or get a drink of water from across the room without assistance and fall. This is because she does not recognize her neurological deficits. Aphasia, right hemiplegia or hemiparesis and slow, cautious behavior is seen in clients who have had a left-hemispheric CVA.

Ⓝ NCLEX® Connection: Physiological Adaptation, Pathophysiology

2. The client is diagnosed with left homonymous hemianopsia. Which of the following actions is appropriate for the nurse to include in the client's plan of care?

A. Teach the client to scan to the right to see objects on the right side of her body.

B. Place the client's bedside table on the right side of the bed.

C. Orient the client to the food on her plate using the clock method.

D. Place the client's wheelchair on her left side.

A client who has left homonymous hemianopsia has lost the left visual field of both eyes. She is unable to visualize anything to the left of midline of her body. Placing the client's bedside table on the right side of her bed will allow her to easily visualize items on the table. Scanning to the right will decrease the client's field of vision, the clock method of food placement will be ineffective since only half of the plate can be seen, and the wheelchair should be placed on the right or unaffected side of the client.

Ⓝ NCLEX® Connection: Physiological Adaptation, Illness Management

3. When the client resumes dietary intake, which of the following actions should the nurse take? (Select all that apply.)

__X__	**Have the suction equipment available for use.**
__X__	**Thicken liquids using a commercial thickener.**
__X__	**Place food on the client's unaffected side of her mouth.**
_____	Assign an assistive personnel to slowly feed the client.
_____	Teach the client to swallow with her neck flexed.
__X__	**Discontinue feeding the client if choking occurs.**

The nurse caring for this client should have suction equipment available in case the client begins to choke. The client should be given thickened liquids, which are easier to swallow. Placing food on the unaffected side of the client's mouth will allow her to have better control of the food and again, reduce the risk of aspiration. Due to the risk of aspiration, an assistive personnel should not be assigned to the client because the client's swallowing ability needs to be assessed and suctioning may be needed if choking occurs. The client should also be taught to flex her neck, tucking the chin down and under, to close the epiglottis during swallowing. If choking during feedings occurs, the client should be made NPO and the provider should be notified.

NCLEX® Connection: Physiological Adaptation, Illness Management

4. A nurse has been assigned a client who is diagnosed with global aphasia (both receptive and expressive). Which of the following interventions are appropriate to include in the client's plan of care? (Select all that apply.)

__X__	**Speak to the client at a slower rate.**
__X__	**Look directly at the client when speaking.**
__X__	**Allow plenty of time for the client to answer.**
_____	Complete sentences that the client cannot finish.
__X__	**Give instructions one step at a time.**
_____	Speak louder if the client does not understand.

Clients who have global aphasia will have difficulty with both speaking and understanding speech. Strategies that can enhance understanding are speaking at a slower rate, looking at the client when speaking, giving instructions one step at a time, and allowing the client time to answer questions without trying to answer for him. Speaking louder to a client with receptive aphasia who does not have a hearing deficit will not enhance his understanding.

NCLEX® Connection: NCLEX Connection, Physiological Adaptation, Illness Management

UNIT 2	NURSING CARE OF CLIENTS WITH NEUROSENSORY DISORDERS
Section	Neurologic Emergencies
Chapter 17	Spinal Cord Injury

 Overview

- Spinal cord injuries (SCIs) involve the loss of motor function, sensory function, reflexes, and control of elimination. Injuries in the cervical region result in quadriplegia – Paralysis/paresis of all 4 extremities and trunk. Injuries below T1 result in paraplegia – Paralysis/paresis of the lower extremities. Truncal instability also results if the lesion is in the upper thoracic region.

- The level of cord involved dictates the consequences of spinal cord injury. For example, an injury at C4 or above poses a great risk for impaired spontaneous ventilation because of the involvement of the phrenic nerve.

(M) View Media Supplement: Spinal Cord and Cauda Equina (Image)

- Not all fractures of the vertebrae cause SCIs. Direct injury to the spinal cord secondary to the trauma or bone fragments in the spinal canal must occur for the spinal cord itself to become damaged.

- SCIs range from contusions or incomplete lesions of the spinal cord to complete lesions caused by a lesion that extends across the entire diameter of the cord, or an actual transection of the spinal cord. Complete lesions result in the loss of all voluntary movement and sensation below the level of the injury. Incomplete lesions result in varying losses of voluntary movement and sensation below the level of the injury.

Health Promotion and Disease Prevention

- Most SCIs are caused by trauma, such as motor vehicle crashes, diving accidents, and gunshot wounds.

- Hyperflexion injuries are caused by acceleration injuries that cause sharp, forward flexion of the spine (head-on collision, fall, or diving). Hyperextension injuries are caused by a backward snap of the spine (rear-end collision or a downward fall onto the chin).

Assessment

- Risk Factors

  o Males age 16 to 30

- o   High-risk activities (extreme sports or high-speed driving)
- o   Active in impact sports (football or diving)
- o   Acts of violence (gunshot and knife wounds)
- o   Alcohol and/or drug abuse
- o   Disease (metastatic cancer or arthritis of the spine)

- o   Falls, especially in older adults
- Subjective Data
  - o   Report of lack of sensation of dermatomes below the level of the lesion
  - o   Report of neck or back pain
- Objective Data
  - o   Physical Assessment Findings
    - ■   Inability to feel light touch when touched by a cotton ball, inability to discriminate between sharp and dull when touched with a safety pin or other sharp objects, and an inability to discriminate between hot and cold when touched with containers of hot and cold water.
    - ■   Absent deep tendon reflexes
    - ■   Flaccidity of muscles
    - ■   Hypotension that is more severe when the client is in sitting in an upright position
    - ■   Shallow respirations
    - ■   Dependent edema
    - ■   Spinal shock, which accompanies spinal trauma, causes a total loss of all reflexive and autonomic function below the level of the injury for a period of several days to weeks.
    - ■   Loss of temperature regulation: – Hyperthermia or hypothermia
  - o   Laboratory Tests
    - ■   Urinalysis, hemoglobin, ABGs
      - □   Used to monitor for undiagnosed internal bleeding (the client may not feel pain from internal injuries) and impaired respiratory exchange (due to phrenic nerve involvement and/or inability to voluntarily increase depth and rate of respirations).
  - o   Diagnostic Procedures
    - ■   X-rays, magnetic resonance imaging (MRI), and computed tomography (CT) imaging/computed axial tomography (CAT) scan can be used to assess the extent of the damage and the location of blood and bone fragments.

Collaborative Care

- Nursing Care
  - Respiratory status
    - Monitoring the client's respiratory status is the first priority. Involuntary respirations can be affected due to a lesion at or above the phrenic nerve or swelling from a lesion immediately below C4. Lesions in the cervical or upper thoracic area will also impair voluntary movement of muscles used in respiration (increase in depth or rate).
    - Provide the client with oxygen and suction as needed.
    - Assist with intubation and mechanical ventilation if necessary.
    - Assist the client to cough by applying abdominal thrusts when the attempting to cough.
  - Tissue perfusion – Spinal shock occurs after a SCI and can cause total loss of voluntary and autonomic function for several days to weeks. Hypotension, dependent edema, and loss of temperature regulation are common symptoms.
    - When in an upright position, clients who are in spinal shock will experience postural hypotension. Transferring the client to a wheelchair should occur in stages.
    - Raise the client's head of the bed and be ready to lower the angle if the client reports dizziness.
    - Transfer the client into a reclining wheelchair with the back of the wheelchair reclined.
    - Be ready to lock and lean the wheelchair back onto the knee to a fully reclined position if the client reports dizziness after the transfer. Do not attempt to return the client to the bed.
    - Monitor the client for signs of thrombophlebitis (swelling of extremity, absent/decreased pulses, and areas of warmth and/or tenderness). The client may be on anticoagulants to prevent development of lower extremity thrombi.
  - Intake and output – The client may be NPO for several days. Regulation of fluid balance and nutritional support is necessary. Maintain an adequate fluid intake for the client – fluid will aid in preventing urinary calculi, bladder infections, and maintain soft stools.
  - Neurological status – After determining the baseline, monitor for an increasing loss of neurological function.
  - Muscle strength and tone – After determining the baseline, monitor for an increasing loss of muscle strength in the affected extremities.
    - Clients who have upper motor neuron injuries (above L1 and L2) will convert to a spastic muscle tone after spinal shock.
    - Paraplegics who have lower motor neuron injuries (below L1 and L2) will convert to a flaccid type of paralysis.

- Since most lower motor neuron lesions involve the cauda equina, the motor and sensory deficits can be patchy with some areas of innervation and others without.

- Encourage active range-of-motion (ROM) exercises when possible and assist with passive ROM if the client lacks all motor function.

o Mobility – Clients who have complete injuries will not regain mobility. Clients who have incomplete injuries can regain some function that will allow mobility with various types of braces. However, functional mobility can still be best attained through the use of a wheelchair.

o Sensation – Varying degrees of loss of sensation will be experienced depending on whether the lesion is complete or incomplete. Care must be taken to prevent skin breakdown both in the bed and wheelchair. Various types of foam and air mattresses are available for beds and wheelchairs.

o Bowel and bladder function

- Spastic neurogenic bladder – Clients who have upper motor neuron injuries will develop a spastic bladder after the spinal shock resolves. Bladder management options for male clients include condom catheters and stimulation of the micturition reflex by tugging on the pubic hair. Female clients will need to use an indwelling urinary catheter due to the unpredictably of the release of urine.

- Flaccid neurogenic bladder – Clients who have lower motor neuron injuries will develop a flaccid bladder. Bladder management options for males and females include intermittent catheterization and Credé's method (downward pressure placed on the bladder to manually express the urine).

- Neurogenic bowel functioning does not differ a lot between upper and lower motor neuron injuries. Daily use of stool softeners or bulk forming laxatives is recommended to keep the stool soft. A bowel movement can be stimulated daily or every other day by administration of a bisacodyl (Dulcolax) suppository or digital stimulation (stimulation of the rectal sphincter with a gloved and lubricated finger).

- Development of a schedule as part of bladder and bowel training is critical for the establishment of a routine.

o Gastrointestinal function – An ileus can develop immediately after injury. Monitor for bowel sounds.

o Skin Integrity – Changing the client's position every 2 hr is critical (every 1 hr when in a wheelchair). Clients who have a SCI can neither move nor feel pain from prolonged pressure. Pressure-relief devices in both the bed and the wheelchair must be consistently used.

o Sexual Function – Teach the client about alterations in sexual function and possible adaptive strategies. Quadriplegics and other clients who have upper motor neuron lesions are usually capable of reflexogenic erections (erections secondary to manual manipulation). Ejaculation coordinated with emission may or may not occur. Clients who have lower motor neuron injuries are less able to have reflexogenic erections, but clients who have incomplete injuries may be able to have a combination of reflexogenic and psychogenic erections (erections stimulated by sexual thoughts and images). Administer medications as prescribed.

- Medications
  - Glucocorticoids
    - Adrenocortical steroids such as dexamethasone (Decadron) aid in decreasing swelling of the spinal cord, which can increase pressure on the spinal cord, and subsequently, areas of ischemia.
  - Vasopressors
    - Norepinephrine and dopamine are given to treat postural hypotension, particularly during spinal shock.
  - Plasma expanders
    - Dextran, a volume expander, is used to treat hypotension secondary to spinal shock.
    - Nursing Considerations
      - Observe the client for symptoms of fluid overload.
  - Muscle relaxants
    - Baclofen (Lioresal) and dantrolene sodium (Dantrium) – Given to clients who have severe muscle spasticity. Spasticity can be so severe that clients develop pressure ulcers, which can make sitting in a wheelchair very difficult.
  - Cholinergics
    - Bethanechol (Urecholine) – Decreases spasticity of the bladder, allowing for easier bladder training and fewer accidents.
    - Nursing Considerations
      - Observe the client for urinary retention. Measure residual periodically.
  - Analgesics
    - Opioids, non-opioids, and NSAIDs are given for pain. Clients may or may not be able to feel pain from spinal cord injury. Clients who do have muscle spasticity may report feeling discomfort from the muscle spasms.
  - Anticoagulants
    - Heparin or low-molecular-weight heparins used for deep vein thrombosis prophylaxis
    - Nursing Considerations
      - Monitor INR, PT, and aPTT for therapeutic levels of anticoagulation.
      - Observe for signs of gastrointestinal bleeding or bleeding secondary to unrecognized injury.
  - Stool softeners and bulk-forming laxatives
    - Docusate sodium (Colace) or polycarbophil (Fibercon) to prevent constipation and keep the stool soft.

- o Vasodilators

  - ■ Hydralazine (Apresoline) and nitroglycerin (Nitrostat) – Used PRN to treat episodes of hypertension during automatic dysreflexia.

- Interdisciplinary Care

  - o The client will need intensive occupational and physical therapy to learn how to perform ADLs, re-establish mobility using either a manual or electric wheelchair or braces and crutches. The client will also be fitted for splints to prevent contractures and/or provide wrist support for eating and manipulating joy stick on electric wheelchair.

  - o Social services will need to determine the client's financial resources, home care needs, and adaptations needed in the home prior to discharge.

  - o Referral of the client to an SCI support group can aid in emotionally adapting to changes in body image and role.

- Therapeutic Procedures

  - o Application of immobilization devices and traction

    - ■ Clients who have cervical fractures may be placed in a halo fixation device or cervical tongs. The purpose is to provide traction and/or immobilize the spinal column.

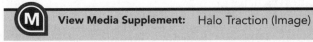

View Media Supplement: Halo Traction (Image)

    - ■ Nursing Actions

      - □ Maintain body alignment and ensure cervical tong weights hang freely.

      - □ Monitor skin integrity by providing pin care and assessing the skin under the halo fixation vest as appropriate.

    - ■ Client Education

      - □ If the client goes home with a halo fixation device on, provide instruction on pin and vest care.

      - □ Teach the client signs of infection and skin breakdown.

- Surgical Interventions

  - o Spinal Surgery

    - ■ Spinal fusion is commonly done when a spinal fracture creates an area of instability of the spine.

    - ■ Spinal fusions done in the cervical area are usually done using an anterior approach through the front of the neck.

    - ■ Spinal fusions done in the thoracic or lumbar areas are done using a posterior approach and can be combined with a decompressive laminectomy.

- A decompressive laminectomy is done by removing a section of lamina, accessing the spinal canal, and removing bone fragments, foreign bodies, or hematomas that may be placing pressure on the spinal cord.

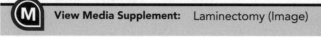

View Media Supplement: Laminectomy (Image)

- Donor bone is often obtained from the iliac crest and used to fuse together the vertebra that are unstable.

- Application of paravertebral rods can be used to mechanically immobilize several vertebral levels.

- Nursing Actions

  □ In clients who have undergone an anterior cervical fusion, monitor for possible airway compromise from swelling or hemorrhage. Observe for deviation of the trachea.

- Client Education

  □ Inform the client that an area of decreased range-of-motion will always exist in the area of fusion or paravertebral rods.

  □ Rods are usually not removed unless they cause pain. Removal can be done after the spine has restabilized.

- Care after Discharge

  ○ Clients who have experienced a SCI with subsequent loss of function will need varying levels of support upon discharge.

  ○ Clients who have quadriplegia will require a lengthy and extensive rehabilitative experience, which can occur on an outpatient or in-home basis.

  ○ Family members will need to be instructed on all aspects of the client's personal needs.

  ○ Referrals will need to be made, with the assistance of social services, for a home health nurse, home health aide, and in-home physical and occupational therapists.

  ○ Many adaptations may also need to be made to the home to make it wheelchair accessible.

  ○ While clients who have paraplegia will require less intensive therapy, all of the referrals and accommodations necessary for clients with quadriplegia will also be needed for clients with paraplegia.

  ○ Client Education

    - The client and family members will need to be taught all aspects of the client's care (ADLs, transfers, and medication regimen).

- Client Outcomes

  - The client will integrate physiological changes in his body into a new, positive body image.

  - The client will be free of urinary complications.

  - The client will develop a regular routine for bowel movements.

  - The client will not experience autonomic dysreflexia.

Complications

- Orthostatic hypotension

  - Occurs when the client changes position due to the interruption in functioning of the automatic nervous system and pooling of blood in lower extremities when the client is in an upright position.

  - Nursing Actions

    - Change the client positioning slowly and place the client in a wheelchair that reclines.

    - Use thigh-high elastic hose or elastic wraps to increase venous return. Elastic wraps may need to extend all the way up the client's legs and include the client's abdomen.

- Neurogenic shock

  - Neurogenic shock is a common response of the spinal cord following an injury.

  - Symptoms of bradycardia, hypotension, flaccid paralysis, loss of reflex activity below level of injury, and paralytic ileus accompany spinal shock due to the loss of autonomic function.

  - Nursing Actions

    - Monitor vital signs for hypotension and bradycardia.

    - Treat symptoms with appropriate medications (vasopressors or atropine).

- Autonomic dysreflexia

  - Occurs secondary to the stimulation of the sympathetic nervous system and inadequate compensatory response by the parasympathetic nervous system. Clients who have lesions below T6 do not experience dysreflexia because the parasympathetic nervous system is able to neutralize the sympathetic response.

  - Sympathetic stimulation is usually caused by a triggering stimulus in the lower part of the body (refer to list under Nursing Actions).

  - Stimulation of the sympathetic nervous system causes extreme hypertension, sudden severe headache, pallor below the level of the spinal cord's lesion dermatome, blurred vision, diaphoresis, restlessness, nausea, and piloerection (goose bumps).

- ○ Stimulation of the parasympathetic nervous system causes bradycardia, flushing above the corresponding dermatome to the spinal cord lesion (flushed face and neck), and nasal stuffiness.
- ○ Nursing Actions
  - ▪ Determine and treat the cause.
    - ☐ Sit the client up (to decrease blood pressure secondary to postural hypotension).
    - ☐ Notify the provider.
    - ☐ Determine the cause.
      - ‣ Distended bladder is the most common cause (kinked or blocked urinary catheter, urinary retention, or urinary calculi)
      - ‣ Fecal impaction
      - ‣ Cold stress or drafts on lower part of the body
      - ‣ Tight clothing
      - ‣ Undiagnosed injury or illness (kidney infection or stone, lower extremity fracture)
    - ☐ Treat the cause.
      - ‣ Relieve the kink in the catheter or irrigate to remove blockage.
      - ‣ Catheterize the client (use anesthetic ointment on the tip of the catheter).
      - ‣ Remove the impaction (use anesthetic ointment prior to removal).
      - ‣ Adjust the room temperature and block drafts.
      - ‣ Remove tight clothing.
      - ‣ Assess for injury, such as lower extremity fracture or kidney/bladder infection.
  - ▪ Monitor vital signs for severe hypertension and bradycardia.
  - ▪ Administer antihypertensives (nitrates or hydralazine).
- ○ Client Education
  - ▪ Provide client education regarding potential causes of dysreflexia.
  - ▪ Instruct the client to space out fluid intake and increase frequency of intermittent catheterizations if fluid intake is temporarily increased.
  - ▪ Provide a list of possible actions to pursue if an episode of dysreflexia does occur.

CHAPTER 17: SPINAL CORD INJURY

(A) Application Exercises

Scenario: A nurse is caring for a college student who experienced a T12 fracture while playing football resulting paraplegia. The client has no muscle control of his lower limbs, bowel, bladder, or genital area. The client is 1 week postoperative following spinal stabilization surgery.

1. During the acute phase following the SCI prevention of which of the following should be the nurse's highest priority when planning care for the client?

   A. Further damage to the spinal cord

   B. Contractures of the hands and extremities

   C. Skin breakdown of areas that lack sensation

   D. Postural hypotension when placing the client in a wheelchair

2. The client received a high dose of methylprednisolone (Solu-Medrol) when he was initially admitted to the neurosurgery unit. What effect does this type of medication have and what risks does it pose for the client?

3. A nurse is caring for a client who reports a severe headache and is sweating profusely. Upon taking the client's vital signs, the nurse finds that the client's blood pressure is 220/110 mm Hg, with a heart rate of 54/min. Which of the following actions the nurse should take first?

   A. Call the provider.

   B. Sit the client upright in bed.

   C. Check the client's catheter for blockage.

   D. Administer an antihypertensive.

4. Which of the following should be the nurse's primary concern when caring for a client who had a recent C4 injury?

   A. Spinal shock

   B. Paralytic ileus

   C. Stress ulcer

   D. Respiratory compromise

5. A nurse is caring for client who experienced a cervical spine injury 24 hr ago. Which of the following types of medications prescribed for the client by the provider should the nurse question?

   A. Glucocorticoids

   B. Plasma expanders

   C. H2 antagonists

   D. Muscle relaxants

6. A nurse is caring for a client who had a cervical spine injury 3 months ago. Which of the following types of bladder management methods is appropriate for this client?

    A. Condom catheter

    B. Intermittent catheterization

    C. Credé's method

    D. Indwelling urinary catheter

CHAPTER 17: SPINAL CORD INJURY

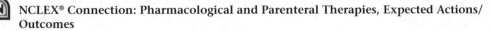 Application Exercises Answer Key

Scenario: A nurse is caring for a college student who experienced a T12 fracture while playing football resulting paraplegia. The client has no muscle control of his lower limbs, bowel, bladder, or genital area. The client is 1 week postoperative following spinal stabilization surgery.

1. During the acute phase following SCI prevention of which of the following should be the nurse's highest priority when planning care for the client?

   A. Further damage to the spinal cord

   B. Contractures of the hands and extremities

   C. Skin breakdown of areas that lack sensation

   D. Postural hypotension when placing the client in a wheelchair

   The greatest risk to the client during the acute phase of a SCI is further damage to the spinal cord. Therefore, when planning care the priority should be the prevention of further damage to the spinal cord. This should be done through the use of corticosteroids, minimal movement of the client until spinal stabilization is accomplished through either traction or surgery, and adequate oxygenation of the client to decrease ischemia of the spinal cord. Preventing contractures, skin breakdown, and postural hypotension are important, but they are not the highest priority.

   NCLEX® Connection: Physiological Adaptation, Medical Emergencies

2. The client received a high dose of methylprednisolone (Solu-Medrol) when he was initially admitted to the neurosurgery unit. What effect does this type of medication have and what risks does it pose for the client?

   Steroids reduce inflammation by suppressing the inflammatory process and subsequent swelling of the injured spinal cord. Steroids can pose a risk by increasing the client's susceptibility to infections, such as pulmonary, urinary tract, and wound.

   NCLEX® Connection: Pharmacological and Parenteral Therapies, Expected Actions/ Outcomes

3. A nurse is caring for a client who reports a severe headache and is sweating profusely. Upon taking the client's vital signs, the nurse finds that the client's blood pressure is 220/110 mm Hg, with a heart rate of 54/min. Which of the following actions the nurse should take first?

> A. Call the provider.
>
> **B. Sit the client upright in bed.**
>
> C. Check the client's catheter for blockage.
>
> D. Administer an antihypertensive.

> **The greatest risk to the client is experiencing a stroke secondary to blood pressure. The first thing the nurse should do is elevate the head of the bed until the client is in an upright position. This will naturally lower the blood pressure secondary to postural hypotension. The provider should then be notified and the cause of the episode determined. If the cause cannot be determined and resolved, an antihypertensive may need to be administered.**

 NCLEX® Connection: Physiological Adaptation, Medical Emergencies

4. Which of the following should be the nurse's primary concern when caring for a client who had a recent C4 injury?

> A. Spinal shock
>
> B. Paralytic ileus
>
> C. Stress ulcer
>
> **D. Respiratory compromise**

> **Using the airway, breathing, and circulation (ABC) priority setting framework, the greatest risk to the client with an SCI at the level of C4 is respiratory compromise secondary to involvement of the phrenic nerve. Maintenance of an airway and provision of ventilatory support, as needed, is the priority intervention. Spinal shock, paralytic ileus, and stress ulcers are also of concern, but are not the highest priority.**

 NCLEX® Connection: Physiological Adaptation, Medical Emergencies

5. A nurse is caring for client who experienced a cervical spine injury 24 hr ago. Which of the following types of medications prescribed for the client by the provider should the nurse question?

> A. Glucocorticoids
>
> B. Plasma expanders
>
> C. H2 antagonists
>
> **D. Muscle relaxants**

> **The client will still be in spinal shock 24 hr following the injury. The client will not experience muscle spasms until after the spinal shock has resolved, making muscle relaxants unnecessary at this time. The other medications are appropriate to provide at this time.**

 NCLEX® Connection: Pharmacological and Parenteral Therapies, Adverse Effects/ Contraindications/Side Effects/Interactions

6. A nurse is caring for a client who had a cervical spine injury 3 months ago. Which of the following types of bladder management methods is appropriate for this client?

   A. Condom catheter

   B. Intermittent catheterization

   C. Credé's method

   D. Indwelling urinary catheter

   A client who has a cervical spinal injury will also have an upper motor neuron injury, which will manifest itself by creating a spastic bladder. Since the bladder will empty on its own, a condom catheter is an appropriate method. It is noninvasive as opposed to an indwelling urinary catheter. The other two methods are appropriate for clients who have flaccid bladders.

   Ⓝ **NCLEX® Connection: Basic Care and Comfort, Elimination**

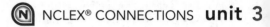

UNIT 3: NURSING CARE OF CLIENTS WITH RESPIRATORY DISORDERS

- Diagnostic and Therapeutic Procedures
- Respiratory System Disorders
- Respiratory Emergencies

NCLEX® CONNECTIONS

When reviewing the chapters in this unit, keep in mind the relevant sections of the NCLEX® outline, in particular:

CLIENT NEEDS: PHARMACOLOGICAL AND PARENTERAL THERAPIES	CLIENT NEEDS: REDUCTION OF RISK POTENTIAL	CLIENT NEEDS: PHYSIOLOGICAL ADAPTATION
Relevant topics/tasks include:	Relevant topics/tasks include:	Relevant topics/tasks include:

CLIENT NEEDS: PHARMACOLOGICAL AND PARENTERAL THERAPIES

Relevant topics/tasks include:
- Adverse Effects/Contraindications/Side Effects/Interactions
  - Manage the client experiencing side effects and adverse reactions of medication.
- Expected Actions/Outcomes
  - Evaluate the client's use of medications over time.
- Medication Administration
  - Educate the client on medication self-administration procedures.

CLIENT NEEDS: REDUCTION OF RISK POTENTIAL

Relevant topics/tasks include:
- Laboratory Values
  - Identify laboratory values for ABGs, BUN, cholesterol, glucose, hematocrit, hemoglobin, glycosylated hemoglobin, platelets, potassium, sodium, WBC, creatinine, PT, PTT and APTT, INR.
- Potential for Complications of Diagnostic Tests/Treatments/Procedures
  - Maintain tube patency.
- Therapeutic Procedures
  - Educate the client about home management of care (tracheostomy and ostomy).

CLIENT NEEDS: PHYSIOLOGICAL ADAPTATION

Relevant topics/tasks include:
- Alterations in Body Systems
  - Monitor and care for clients on a ventilator.
- Pathophysiology
  - Understand general principles of pathophysiology.
- Medical Emergencies
  - Apply knowledge of nursing procedures and psychomotor skills when caring for a client experiencing a medical emergency.

UNIT 3	NURSING CARE OF CLIENTS WITH RESPIRATORY DISORDERS
Section	Diagnostic and Therapeutic Procedures
Chapter 18	Respiratory Diagnostic Procedures

Overview

- Respiratory diagnostic procedures are used to evaluate a client's respiratory status by checking indicators such as the oxygenation of the blood, lung functioning, and the integrity of the airway.

- Respiratory diagnostic procedures that nurses should be knowledgeable about include:

  o Pulse oximetry

  o ABGs

  o Bronchoscopy

  o Thoracentesis

Pulse Oximetry

- Pulse oximetry is a noninvasive measurement of the oxygen saturation of the blood, but it is not a replacement for ABG measurement.

  o A pulse oximeter is a battery- or electric-operated device with a sensor probe that is attached securely onto the client's fingertip, toe, bridge of nose, earlobe, or forehead with a clip or band.

  o Pulse oximetry measures arterial oxygen saturation (SaO_2) via a wave of infrared light that measures light absorption by oxygenated and deoxygenated Hgb in arterial blood. SaO_2 and SpO_2 are used interchangeably.

- Indications

  o Pulse oximetry is indicated for conditions or situations in which a client's respiratory status should be monitored, such as during a continuous opioid epidural infusion.

  o Client Presentation

    ▪ The following signs and symptoms indicate oxygen saturation should be monitored in a client

      □ Increased work of breathing

      □ Wheezing

      □ Coughing

      □ Cyanosis

- Interpretation of Findings

  - The expected reference range for SaO_2 is 95% to 100%. Acceptable levels may range from 91% to 100%. Some illness states may even allow for an SaO_2 of 85% to 89%.

  - Values may be slightly lower in the older adult client and those with dark skin.

  - Additional reasons for low readings include hypothermia, poor peripheral blood flow, too much light (sun or infrared lamps), low Hgb levels, client movement, edema, and nail polish.

  - An SaO_2 below 91% requires interventions to help the client regain acceptable SaO_2 levels. An SaO_2 below 86% is an emergency. An SaO_2 below 80% is life-threatening. The lower the SaO_2 level, the less accurate the value.

  - Values obtained by pulse oximetry are unreliable in cardiac arrest, shock, and other states of low perfusion.

- Preprocedure

  - Nursing Actions

    - Perform hand hygiene and provide privacy.

    - Find an appropriate probe site. It must be dry and have adequate circulation.

    - Be sure the client is in a comfortable position, supporting the arm if a finger is used as a probe site.

- Intraprocedure

  - Nursing Actions

    - Apply the sensor probe to the site.

    - Press the power switch on the oximeter.

    - Note the pulse reading and compare it with the client's radial pulse. Any discrepancy warrants further assessment.

    - Allow time for the readout to stabilize, then record this value as the oxygen saturation.

    - Remove the probe, turn off the oximeter, and store it appropriately.

    - If continuous monitoring is required, make sure the alarms are set for a low and a high limit, they are functioning, and that the sound is audible.

- Postprocedure

  - Nursing Actions

    - Document the findings and report abnormal findings to the primary care provider.

    - If a client's SaO_2 is less than 90% (indicating hypoxemia):

      □ Confirm that the sensor probe is properly placed.

   ☐ Confirm that the oxygen delivery system is functioning and that the client is receiving prescribed oxygen levels.

   ☐ Place the client in a semi-Fowler's or Fowler's position to maximize ventilation.

   ☐ Encourage the client to deep breathe.

   ☐ Report significant findings to the primary care provider.

   ☐ Remain with the client and provide emotional support to decrease anxiety.

ABGs

- An ABG sample reports the status of oxygenation and acid-base balance of the blood.

  ○ An ABG measures:

  - pH – the amount of free hydrogen ions in the arterial blood (H^+).

  - PaO_2 – the partial pressure of oxygen.

  - $PaCO_2$ – the partial pressure of carbon dioxide.

  - HCO_3^- – the concentration of bicarbonate in arterial blood.

  - SaO_2 – percentage of oxygen bound to Hgb as compared to the total amount that can be possibly carried.

  ○ ABGs can be obtained by an arterial puncture or through an arterial line.

- Indications

  ○ Potential Diagnoses

  - Blood pH levels may be affected by any number of disease processes (respiratory, endocrine, or neurologic).

  - These assessments are helpful in monitoring the effectiveness of various treatments (such as acidosis interventions), in guiding oxygen therapy, and in evaluating client responses to weaning from mechanical ventilation.

- Interpretation of Findings

ABG MEASURE	NORMAL RANGE
pH	7.35 to 7.45
PaO_2	80 to 100 mm Hg
$PaCO_2$	35 to 45 mm Hg
HCO_3^-	22 to 26 mEq/L
SaO_2	95 to 100%

  ○ Blood pH levels below 7.35 reflect acidosis, while levels above 7.45 reflect alkalosis.

- Arterial Puncture

  ○ Preprocedure

    ■ Nursing Actions

      □ Obtain a heparinized syringe for the sample collection.

      □ Perform an Allen's test prior to arterial puncture to verify patent radial and ulnar circulation. The nurse should compress the ulnar and radial arteries simultaneously while instructing the client to form a fist. Then, have the client relax his hand while releasing pressure on the radial artery. His hand should turn pink quickly, indicating patency of the radial artery. Repeat this process for the ulnar artery.

      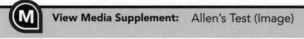
      View Media Supplement: Allen's Test (Image)

    ■ Client Education

      □ Explain and reinforce the procedure with the client. Clients often experience pain with repeated ABG level checks, but are often unaware of the purpose of the puncture.

  ○ Intraprocedure

    ■ Nursing Actions

      □ Perform an arterial puncture using surgical aseptic technique and collect a specimen into a heparinized syringe.

      □ Place the collected and capped specimen into a basin of ice and water to preserve pH levels and oxygen pressure. The specimen should be transported to the laboratory immediately.

      □ Accessing the radial artery for sampling may be more difficult with older adult clients because of impaired peripheral vasculature.

  ○ Postprocedure

    ■ Nursing Actions

      □ Immediately after an arterial puncture, hold direct pressure over the site for at least 5 min. Pressure must be maintained for at least 20 min if the client is receiving anticoagulant therapy. Ensure that bleeding has stopped prior to removing direct pressure.

      □ Monitor the ABG sampling site for bleeding, loss of pulse, swelling, and changes in temperature and color.

      □ Document all interventions and client response.

- □ Report results to the provider as soon as they are available.

- □ Administer oxygen as prescribed. Change ventilator settings as ordered or notify a respiratory therapist.

  - ■ Note: Arterial puncture is frequently done by a respiratory therapist in hospital settings.

- Arterial Line

  - ○ Preprocedure

    - ■ Nursing Actions

      - □ Verify that the arterial line may be used for specimen collection.

      - □ Obtain a heparinized syringe for the sample collection and a standard syringe for waste.

    - ■ Client Education

      - □ Explain and reinforce the procedure with the client.

  - ○ Intraprocedure

    - ■ Nursing Actions

      - □ Follow specific facility protocols for collection procedures.

      - □ Collect waste and specimen. Place both on ice for transport to the laboratory immediately.

      - □ Flush the arterial line with the preconnected flushing system.

  - ○ Postprocedure

    - ■ Nursing Actions

      - □ Assess the arterial waveform upon completion.

      - □ Document all interventions and the client's response.

      - □ Report results to the provider as soon as they are available.

      - □ Administer oxygen to the client as prescribed. Change the ventilator settings as ordered, or notify a respiratory therapist.

- Complications

  - ○ Hematoma, arterial occlusion

    - ■ A hematoma occurs when blood accumulates under the skin at the IV site.

    - ■ Nursing Actions

      - □ Observe the client for changes in temperature, swelling, color, loss of pulse, or pain.

      - □ Notify the primary care provider immediately if symptoms persist.

      - □ Apply pressure to the hematoma site.

- ○ Air embolism
  - ■ Air enters the arterial system during catheter insertion.
  - ■ Nursing Actions
    - ☐ Monitor the client for a sudden onset of shortness of breath, decreases in SaO_2 levels, chest pain, anxiety, and air hunger.
    - ☐ Notify the primary care provider immediately if symptoms occur, administer oxygen therapy, and obtain ABGs. Continue to assess the client's respiratory status for any deterioration.

Bronchoscopy

- Bronchoscopy permits visualization of the larynx, trachea, and bronchi through either a flexible fiberoptic bronchoscope or a rigid bronchoscope.
  - ○ Bronchoscopy can be performed as an outpatient procedure, in a surgical suite under general anesthesia, or at the bedside under local anesthesia and moderate sedation.
  - ○ Bronchoscopy can also be performed on clients who are receiving mechanical ventilation by inserting the scope through the client's endotracheal tube.
- Indications
  - ○ Potential Diagnoses
    - ■ Visualization of abnormalities such as tumors, inflammation, and strictures
    - ■ Biopsy of suspicious tissue (lung cancer)
      - ☐ Clients undergoing a bronchoscopy with biopsy have additional risks for bleeding and/or perforation.
    - ■ Aspiration of deep sputum or lung abscesses for culture and sensitivity and/or cytology (pneumonia)
  - ○ Note: Bronchoscopy is also performed for therapeutic reasons, such as removal of foreign bodies and secretions from the tracheobronchial tree, treating postoperative atelectasis, and to destroy and excise lesions.
- Preprocedure
  - ○ Nursing Actions
    - ■ Assess the client for allergies to anesthetic agents or routine use of anticoagulants.
    - ■ Ensure that a consent form is signed by the client prior to the procedure.
    - ■ Remove the client's dentures, if applicable, prior to the procedure.
    - ■ Maintain the client on NPO status prior to the procedure as ordered, usually 8 to 12 hr, to reduce the risk of aspiration when the cough reflex is blocked by anesthesia.
    - ■ Administer preprocedure medications as prescribed, such as viscous lidocaine or local anesthetic throat sprays.

- Intraprocedure
  - ○ Nursing Actions
    - ■ Position the client in a sitting position.
    - ■ Administer medications as prescribed, such as sedatives, antianxiety agents, and/or atropine to reduce oral secretions.
    - ■ Assist in the collecting and labeling of specimens. Ensure prompt delivery to the laboratory.
    - ■ Monitor the client's vital signs, respiratory pattern, and oxygenation status throughout the procedure.
    - ■ Sedation given to older adult clients with respiratory insufficiency may precipitate respiratory arrest.
- Postprocedure
  - ○ Nursing Actions
    - ■ Continuously monitor the client's respirations, blood pressure, pulse oximetry, heart rate, and level of consciousness during the recovery period.
      - □ Assess the client's level of consciousness while recognizing that older adult clients may develop confusion or lethargy due to the effects of medications given during the bronchoscopy.
    - ■ Assess the client's level of consciousness, presence of gag reflex, and ability to swallow prior to resuming oral intake (usually takes about 2 hr).
      - □ Allow adequate time for the cough and gag reflex to return prior to resuming oral intake. The cough reflex may be slower to return in older adult clients receiving local anesthesia due to impaired laryngeal reflex.
      - □ Once the cough reflex returns, the nurse may offer ice chips to the client and eventually fluids.
    - ■ Monitor the client for development of significant fever (mild fever for less than 24 hr is not uncommon), productive cough, significant hemoptysis indicative of hemorrhage (a small amount of blood-tinged sputum is expected), hypoxemia.
    - ■ Be prepared to intervene for unexpected responses and/or aspiration, laryngospasm.
    - ■ Provide oral hygiene to the client.
    - ■ Evaluate and document the client's response to the procedure (stable vital signs, return of gag reflex).
    - ■ For older adult clients, encourage coughing and deep breathing every 2 hr. There is an increased risk of respiratory infection and pneumonia in older adult clients due to decreased cough effectiveness and decreased secretion clearance. Respiratory infections may be more severe and last longer in older adult clients.
    - ■ The client is not discharged from the recovery room until adequate cough reflex and respiratory effort are present.

- ○ Client Education
  - Instruct clients that gargling with salt water or use of throat lozenges may provide comfort for soreness of the throat.
- Complications
  - ○ Laryngospasm
    - Laryngospasm is uncontrolled muscle contractions of the laryngeal cords (vocal cords) that impede the client's ability to inhale.
    - Nursing Actions
      - □ Continuously monitor the client for signs of respiratory distress.
      - □ Maintain a patent airway by repositioning the client or inserting an oral or nasopharyngeal airway as appropriate.
      - □ Administer oxygen therapy to the client as prescribed. Humidification can decrease the likelihood of laryngeal edema.
  - ○ Aspiration
    - Aspiration can occur if the client chokes on oral secretions.
    - Nursing Actions
      - □ Prevent aspiration in the client by withholding oral fluids or food until the gag reflex returns (usually 2 hr).
      - □ Perform suctioning as needed.

Thoracentesis

- Thoracentesis is the surgical perforation of the chest wall and pleural space with a large-bore needle. It is performed to obtain specimens for diagnostic evaluation, instill medication into the pleural space, and remove fluid (effusion) or air from the pleural space for therapeutic relief of pleural pressure.
  - ○ Thoracentesis is performed under local anesthesia by a primary care provider at the client's bedside, in a procedure room, or in a provider's office.
  - ○ Use of an ultrasound for guidance decreases the risk of complications.
- Indications
  - ○ Potential Diagnoses
    - Transudates (heart failure, cirrhosis, nephritic syndrome)
    - Exudates (inflammatory, infectious, neoplastic conditions)
    - Empyema
    - Pneumonia
    - Blunt, crushing or penetrating chest injuries/trauma or invasive thoracic procedures, such as lung and/or cardiac surgery

- o Client Presentation

  - ■ Large amounts of fluid in the pleural space compress lung tissue and can cause pain, shortness of breath, cough, and other symptoms of pleural pressure.

  - ■ Assessment of the effusion area may reveal decreased breath sounds, dull percussion sounds, and decreased chest wall expansion. Pain may occur due to inflammatory process.

- Interpretation of Findings

  - o Aspirated fluid is analyzed for general appearance, cell counts, protein and glucose content, the presence of enzymes such as lactate dehydrogenase (LDH) and amylase, abnormal cells, and culture.

- Preprocedure

  - o Percussion, auscultation, radiography, or sonography is used to locate the effusion and needle insertion site.

  - o Changes in fat deposition in many older adult clients may make it difficult for the provider to identify the landmarks for insertion of the thoracentesis needle.

  - o Nursing Actions

    - ■ Ensure that the client has signed the informed consent form.

    - ■ Gather all needed supplies.

    - ■ Obtain preprocedure x-ray as prescribed to locate pleural effusion and to determine needle insertion site.

    - ■ Position the client sitting upright with his arms and shoulders raised and supported on pillows and/or on an overbed table and with his feet and legs well-supported.

  - o Client Education

    - ■ Instruct the client to remain absolutely still (risk of accidental needle damage) during the procedure and to not to cough or talk unless instructed by the primary care provider.

- Intraprocedure

  - o Nursing Actions

    - ■ Assist the primary care provider with the procedure (strict surgical aseptic technique).

    - ■ Prepare the client for a feeling of pressure with needle insertion and fluid removal.

    - ■ Monitor the client's vital signs, skin color, and oxygen saturation throughout the procedure.

    - ■ Measure and record the amount of fluid removed from the client's chest.

    - ■ Label specimens at the bedside and promptly send them to the laboratory.

- o Note: The amount of fluid removed is limited to 1 L at a time to prevent cardiovascular collapse.

- Postprocedure
  - o Nursing Actions
    - Apply a dressing over the puncture site and position the client on the unaffected side for 1 hr.
    - Monitor the client's vital signs and respiratory status (respiratory rate and rhythm, breath sounds, oxygenation status) hourly for the first several hours after the thoracentesis.
    - Encourage the client to deep breathe to assist with lung expansion.
    - The client can usually resume normal activity after 1 hr if no signs of complications are present.
    - Obtain a postprocedure chest x-ray (check resolution of effusions, rule out pneumothorax).

- Complications
  - o Pneumothorax
    - Pneumothorax is a collapsed lung. It can occur due to injury to the lung during the procedure.
    - Nursing Actions
      - □ Monitor the client for signs and symptoms of pneumothorax, such as diminished breath sounds.
      - □ Monitor postprocedure chest x-ray results.
  - o Bleeding
    - Bleeding can occur if the client is moved during the procedure or is at an increased risk for bleeding.
    - Nursing Actions
      - □ Monitor the client for coughing and/or hemoptysis.
      - □ Monitor the client's vital signs and laboratory results for evidence of bleeding (hypotension, reduced Hgb level).
  - o Infection
    - Infection can occur due to the introduction of bacteria with the needle puncture.
    - Nursing Actions
      - □ Insure that sterile technique is maintained.
      - □ Monitor the client's temperature following the procedure.

CHAPTER 18: RESPIRATORY DIAGNOSTIC PROCEDURES

 Application Exercises

1. A nurse performs an ABG sampling at 0930 on a client who has a heparin drip infusing. At which of the following times will it be appropriate for the nurse to discontinue holding pressure on the puncture site?

    A. 0935

    B. 0940

    C. 0945

    D. 0950

2. Place the following steps for obtaining a client's ABGs in the correct order.

    _____ Immediately after an arterial puncture, hold direct pressure over the site for at least 5 min. Pressure must be maintained for at least 20 min if the client is receiving anti-coagulant therapy. Ensure that the bleeding has stopped prior to removing direct pressure.

    _____ Document all interventions and the client's response.

    _____ Explain and reinforce the procedure with the client.

    _____ Place the collected and capped specimen into a basin of ice and water to preserve pH levels and oxygen pressure. Ensure immediate transport to the laboratory.

    _____ Perform an Allen's test prior to arterial puncture to verify patent radial and ulnar circulation.

    _____ Perform an arterial puncture using a surgical aseptic technique, and collect a specimen into a heparinized syringe.

    _____ Obtain a heparinized syringe for the sample collection.

    _____ Report results to the primary care provider as soon as they are available.

    _____ Monitor the ABG sampling site for bleeding, loss of pulse, swelling, and changes in temperature and color.

3. Which of the following can cause a low pulse oximetry reading? (Select all that apply.)

    _____ Nail polish

    _____ Inadequate peripheral circulation

    _____ Hyperthermia

    _____ Increased Hgb level

    _____ Edema

4. A nurse is caring for a client following a bronchoscopy. Which of the following client findings should the nurse report to the primary care provider?

    A. Blood-tinged sputum

    B. Dry, nonproductive cough

    C. Sore throat

    D. Bronchospasms

5. A nurse is caring for a client who is scheduled for a thoracentesis at the bedside. Which of the following items should the nurse ensure is in client's room? (Select all that apply.)

    _____ Oxygen equipment

    _____ Incentive spirometer

    _____ Pulse oximeter

    _____ Thoracentesis tray

    _____ Suture removal kit

6. Which of the following are causes for concern following a thoracentesis? (Select all that apply.)

    _____ Dyspnea

    _____ Localized bloody drainage contained on the dressing

    _____ Fever

    _____ Hypotension

    _____ SaO_2 of 95%

    _____ Soreness around puncture site

CHAPTER 18: RESPIRATORY DIAGNOSTIC PROCEDURES

 Application Exercises Answer Key

1. A nurse performs an ABG sampling at 0930 on a client who has a heparin drip infusing. At which of the following times will it be appropriate for the nurse to discontinue holding pressure on the puncture site?

    A. 0935

    B. 0940

    C. 0945

    D. 0950

Immediately after arterial puncture, hold direct pressure over the site for at least 5 min. The pressure must be maintained for at least 20 min if the client is receiving anticoagulant therapy. Ensure that bleeding has stopped prior to removing direct pressure.

 NCLEX® Connection: Reduction of Risk Potential, Diagnostic Tests

2. Place the following steps for obtaining a client's ABGs in the correct order.

    __6__   Immediately after an arterial puncture, hold direct pressure over the site for at least 5 min. Pressure must be maintained for at least 20 min if the client is receiving anti-coagulant therapy. Ensure that the bleeding has stopped prior to removing direct pressure.

    __9__   Document all interventions and the client's response.

    __2__   Explain and reinforce the procedure with the client.

    __5__   Place the collected and capped specimen into a basin of ice and water to preserve pH levels and oxygen pressure. Ensure immediate transport to the laboratory.

    __3__   Perform an Allen's test prior to arterial puncture to verify patent radial and ulnar circulation.

    __4__   Perform an arterial puncture using a surgical aseptic technique, and collect a specimen into a heparinized syringe.

    __1__   Obtain a heparinized syringe for the sample collection.

    __8__   Report results to the primary care provider as soon as they are available.

    __7__   Monitor the ABG sampling site for bleeding, loss of pulse, swelling, and changes in temperature and color.

The following order are the steps in obtaining an ABG reading.

 NCLEX® Connection: Reduction of Risk Potential, Diagnostic Tests

3. Which of the following can cause a low pulse oximetry reading? (Select all that apply.)

   X   **Nail polish**

   X   **Inadequate peripheral circulation**

   _____   Hyperthermia

   _____   Increased Hgb level

   X   **Edema**

Nail polish, inadequate peripheral circulation, and edema can all generate a low reading. Hypothermia, rather than hyperthermia, and a decreased Hgb level rather, than an increased Hgb level, can result in a low reading.

 NCLEX® Connection: Reduction of Risk Potential, Diagnostic Tests

4. A nurse is caring for a client following a bronchoscopy. Which of the following client findings should the nurse report to the primary care provider?

   A. Blood-tinged sputum

   B. Dry, nonproductive cough

   C. Sore throat

   D. Bronchospasms

Bronchospasms may indicate difficulty maintaining a patent airway. This should be reported to the primary care provider immediately. Blood-tinged sputum, a dry, productive cough, and a sore throat are expected findings.

 NCLEX® Connection: Reduction of Risk Potential, Diagnostic Tests

5. A nurse is caring for a client who is scheduled for a thoracentesis at the bedside. Which of the following items should the nurse ensure is in client's room? (Select all that apply.)

   X   **Oxygen equipment**

   _____   Incentive spirometer

   X   **Pulse oximeter**

   X   **Thoracentesis tray**

   _____   Suture removal kit

Equipment to supply oxygen, a pulse oximeter, and a thoracentesis tray are all necessary for a thoracentesis. An incentive spirometer and suture removal kit are not indicated for this type of procedure.

 NCLEX® Connection: Reduction of Risk Potential, Therapeutic Procedures

6. Which of the following are causes for concern following a thoracentesis? (Select all that apply.)

 X **Dyspnea**

 _____ Localized bloody drainage contained on the dressing

 X **Fever**

 X **Hypotension**

 _____ SaO_2 of 95%

 _____ Soreness around puncture site

Dyspnea can indicate pneumothorax or reaccumulation of fluid. Fever can indicate infection. Hypotension can indicate intrathoracic bleeding. Localized bloody drainage contained on a dressing, and soreness around puncture site, are expected findings. An SaO_2 of 95% indicates good oxygenation.

Ⓝ **NCLEX® Connection: Reduction of Risk Potential, Potential for Complications of Diagnostic Tests/Treatments/Procedures**

UNIT 3   NURSING CARE OF CLIENTS WITH RESPIRATORY DISORDERS

Section   Diagnostic and Therapeutic Procedures

Chapter 19   Chest Tube Insertion and Monitoring

 Overview

- Chest tubes are inserted into the pleural space to drain fluid, blood, or air; reestablish a negative pressure; facilitate lung expansion; and restore normal intrapleural pressure.

- Chest tubes can be inserted in the emergency department, at the client's bedside, or in the operating room through a thoracotomy incision.

- Chest tubes are removed when the lungs have reexpanded and/or there is no more fluid drainage.

Chest Tube Systems

- Types of chest drainage systems:

  ○ Single chamber systems have a water seal and a drainage collection in the same chamber.

  ○ Two chamber systems have a water seal and a drainage collection in separate chambers, which allows for the collection of larger amounts of drainage.

  ○ Three chamber systems have a water seal, a drainage collection, and suction control in separate chambers.

  ○ Disposable chest tube drainage systems are now commonly used.

(M) View Media Supplement: Chest Tube Drainage System (Image)

- Water seals are created by adding sterile fluid to a chamber up to the 2 cm line. The water seal allows air to exit from the pleural space on exhalation and stops air from entering with inhalation.

  ○ To maintain the water seal, the chamber must be kept upright and below the chest tube insertion site at all times. The nurse should routinely monitor the water level due to the possibility of evaporation. The nurse should add fluid as needed to maintain the 2 cm water seal level.

- The height of the water in the suction control chamber determines the amount of suction transmitted to the pleural space. A suction pressure of –20 cm H_2O is common. The application of suction results in continuous bubbling in the suction chamber. The nurse should monitor the fluid level and add fluid as needed to maintain the prescribed level of suctioning.

- Tidaling (movement of the water level with respiration) is expected in the water seal chamber. With spontaneous respirations, the water level will rise with inspiration (increase in negative pressure in lung) and will fall with expiration. With positive-pressure mechanical ventilation, the water level will rise with expiration and fall with inspiration.

- Cessation of tidaling in the water seal chamber signals lung reexpansion or an obstruction within the system.

Chest Tube Insertion

- Indications
  - Diagnoses
    - Pneumothorax (collapsed lung)
    - Hemothorax (blood in lung)
    - Postoperative chest drainage (thoracotomy or open-heart surgery)
    - Pleural effusion (fluid in lung)
    - Lung abscess (necrotic lung tissue)
  - Client Presentation
    - Dyspnea
    - Distended neck veins
    - Poor circulation
    - Cough
- Client Outcomes
  - The client will maintain adequate gas exchange.
    - Poor oxygenation can quickly lead to serious consequences in older adult clients because many have decreased pulmonary reserves.
  - The client will be free from pain.
  - The client will remain free from infection.
- Preprocedure
  - Nursing Actions
    - Verify that the consent form is signed.
    - Reinforce client teaching. Breathing will improve when the chest tube is in place.

- ■ Assess for allergies to local anesthetics.

- ■ Assist the client into the desired position (supine or semi-Fowler's).

- ■ Prepare the chest drainage system prior to the insertion per the facilities protocol (fill the water seal chamber).

- ■ Administer pain and sedation medications as prescribed.

- ■ Prep the insertion site with povidone-iodine. Drape the insertion site.

- Intraprocedure

  - ○ Nursing Actions

    - ■ Assist the provider with insertion of the chest tube, application of a dressing to the insertion site, and set-up of the drainage system.

      - □ The chest tube tip is positioned up toward the shoulder (pneumothorax) or down toward the posterior (hemothorax or pleural effusion).

      - □ The chest tube is then sutured to the chest wall and an airtight dressing is placed over the puncture wound.

      - □ The chest tube is then attached to drainage tubing that leads to a collection device.

      - □ Place the chest tube drainage system below the client's chest level with the tubing coiled on the bed. Ensure that the tubing from the bed to the drainage system is straight to promote drainage via gravity.

    - ■ The nurse should continually monitor the client's vital signs and response to the procedure.

 View Media Supplement: Chest Tube (Image)

- Postprocedure

  - ○ Nursing Actions

    - ■ Assess the client's vital signs, breath sounds, SaO_2, color, and respiratory effort as indicated by the status of the client and at least every 4 hr.

    - ■ Encourage coughing and deep breathing every 2 hr.

    - ■ Keep the drainage system below the client's chest level, including during ambulation.

    - ■ Monitor the chest tube's placement and function.

      - □ Check the water seal level every 2 hr and add water as needed. The water level should fluctuate with respiratory effort.

      - □ Document the amount and color of drainage hourly for the first 24 hr and then at least every 8 hr. Mark the date, hour, and drainage level on the container at the end of each shift. Report excessive drainage (greater than 70 mL/hr) or drainage that is cloudy or red to the provider. Drainage will often increase with position changes or coughing.

□ Monitor the fluid in the suction control chamber and maintain the fluid level prescribed by the provider.

□ Check for expected findings of tidaling in the water seal chamber and continuous bubbling only in the suction chamber.

- Routinely monitor tubing for kinks, occlusions, or loose connections.

- Monitor the chest tube insertion site for redness, pain, infection, and crepitus (air leakage in subcutaneous tissue).

- Position the client in the semi-Fowler's to high-Fowler's position to promote optimal lung expansion and drainage of the fluid from the lungs.

- Administer pain medications as prescribed.

- Obtain a chest x-ray to verify the chest tube's placement.

- Keep two enclosed hemostats, a bottle of sterile water, and an occlusive dressing located at the bedside at all times.

- Due to the risk of causing a tension pneumothorax, chest tubes are only clamped when ordered by the provider in specific circumstances, such as an air leak, during drainage system change, accidental disconnection of tubing, or damage to the collection device.

- Do not strip or milk tubing routinely; only perform this action when prescribed by the provider. Stripping creates a high negative pressure and can damage the client's lung tissue.

- Complications

  ○ Air leaks

    - Air leaks can result if a connection is not taped securely.

    - Nursing Actions

      □ Monitor the water seal chamber for continuous bubbling (air leak finding). If observed, locate the source of the air leak and intervene accordingly (tighten the connection, replace drainage system).

        ▸ Check all of the connections.

        ▸ Cross clamp close to client's chest. If bubbling stops, the leak is at the insertion site or within the thorax. If bubbling doesn't stop, methodically move clamps down the drainage tubing toward the collection device, moving one clamp at a time. When the bubbling stops, the leak is within the section of tubing or at that connection distal to the clamp.

- ○ Accidental disconnection, system breakage, or removal
  - ■ These complications can occur at any time.
  - ■ Nursing Actions
    - □ If the tubing separates, the client is instructed to exhale as much as possible and to cough to remove air from the pleural space. The nurse should cleanse the tips and reconnect the tubing.
    - □ If the chest tube drainage system breaks, the nurse should immerse the end of the tube in sterile water to restore the water seal.
    - □ If a chest tube is accidentally removed, an occlusive dressing taped on only three sides should be immediately placed over the insertion site. This allows air to escape and reduces the risk for development of a tension pneumothorax.
- ○ Tension pneumothorax
  - ■ Sucking chest wounds, prolonged clamping of the tubing, kinks in the tubing, or obstruction may cause a tension pneumothorax.

Chest Tube Removal

- Provide pain medication 30 min before removing chest tubes.

- Assist the provider with sutures and chest tube removal.

- Instruct the client to take a deep breath, exhale, and bear down (Valsalva maneuver) or to take a deep breath and hold it (increases intrathoracic pressure and reduces risk of air emboli) during chest tube removal.

- Apply airtight sterile petroleum jelly gauze dressing. Secure in place with a heavy weight stretch tape.

- Obtain chest x-rays as prescribed. This is performed to verify continued resolution of the pneumothorax, hemothorax, or pleural effusion.

- Monitor the client for excessive wound drainage, signs of infection, or recurrent pneumothorax.

CHAPTER 19: CHEST TUBE INSERTION AND MONITORING

(A) Application Exercises

Scenario: A nurse is preparing to receive a client who has had a chest tube placed.

1. Which of the following items should the nurse have placed in the client's room? (Select all that apply.)

    _____ Oxygen

    _____ Sterile water

    _____ Enclosed hemostat clamps

    _____ Indwelling urinary catheter

    _____ Occlusive dressing

    _____ Suction source

    _____ Bladder scan machine

2. While assessing the client, the nurse notices that the client's chest tube has become dislodged. Which of the following actions should the nurse take first?

    A. Place the tubing into sterile water to restore the water seal.

    B. Apply sterile gauze to the site.

    C. Tape or clamp all connections.

    D. Assess the client's respiratory status.

3. A nurse is assessing the functioning of a client's chest drainage system. Which of the following are expected client findings? (Select all that apply.)

    _____ Continuous bubbling in the water seal chamber

    _____ Gentle constant bubbling in the suction control chamber

    _____ Rise and fall in the level of water in the water seal chamber with inspiration and expiration

    _____ Exposed sutures without dressing

    _____ Drainage system is upright at chest level

4. A nurse is assisting a provider with the removal of a chest tube. Which of the following should the nurse instruct the client to do?

    A. Lie on his left side during removal.

    B. Hold his breath.

    C. Inhale deeply during removal.

    D. Perform the Valsalva maneuver during removal.

CHAPTER 19: CHEST TUBE INSERTION AND MONITORING

 Application Exercises Answer Key

Scenario: A nurse is preparing to receive a client who has had a chest tube placed.

1. Which of the following items should the nurse have placed in the client's room? (Select all that apply.)

X	**Oxygen**
X	**Sterile water**
X	**Enclosed hemostat clamps**
	Indwelling urinary catheter
X	**Occlusive dressing**
X	**Suction source**
	Bladder scan machine

Oxygen, sterile water, hemostat clamps, an occlusive dressing, and a suction source are all indicated for this client. If the tubing becomes disconnected, the end connected to the client can be placed in sterile water to restore the water seal. The hemostat clamps should be used to check for air leaks. An indwelling urinary catheter and a bladder scan machine are not indicated for a client who has a chest tube.

 NCLEX® Connection: Reduction of Risk Potential, Potential for Complications of Diagnostic Tests/Treatments/Procedures

2. While assessing the client, the nurse notices that the client's chest tube has become dislodged. Which of the following actions should the nurse take first?

A. Place the tubing into sterile water to restore the water seal.

B. Apply sterile gauze to the site.

C. Tape or clamp all connections.

D. Assess the client's respiratory status.

Using the airway, breathing, and circulation (ABC) priority setting framework, the application of sterile gauze to the site should be the first action for the nurse to take. Placing the tubing into sterile water to restore the water seal is part of this process, but not the priority. Taping or clamping all connections is part of this process, but not the priority. Assessing the client's respiratory status is part of this process, but not the priority.

 NCLEX® Connection: Reduction of Risk Potential, Potential for Complications of Diagnostic Tests/Treatments/Procedures

3. A nurse is assessing the functioning of a client's chest drainage system. Which of the following are expected client findings? (Select all that apply.)

_____ Continuous bubbling in the water seal chamber

__X__ **Gentle constant bubbling in the suction control chamber**

__X__ **Rise and fall in the level of water in the water seal chamber with inspiration and expiration**

_____ Exposed sutures without dressing

_____ Drainage system is upright at chest level

Continuous bubbling in the water seal chamber indicates an air leak. The nurse should cover the insertion site with an airtight dressing. A dressing should be in place around the chest tube. The drainage system should be maintained upright and below the client's chest level. A rise and fall in the level of water in the water seal chamber indicates a good connection between the chest wall and the chamber. It also indicates that the system is working well. Gentle bubbling is an expected finding because air in the chest is being removed.

NCLEX® Connection: Reduction of Risk Potential, Therapeutic Procedures

4. A nurse is assisting a provider with the removal of a chest tube. Which of the following should the nurse instruct the client to do?

A. Lie on his left side during removal.

B. Hold his breath.

C. Inhale deeply during removal.

D. Perform the Valsalva maneuver during removal.

The client should be instructed to take a deep breath, exhale, and bear down (Valsalva maneuver) or to take a deep breath and hold it during tube removal. An airtight dressing is applied following removal. Placing the client on his left side during chest tube removal is not indicated.

NCLEX® Connection: Reduction of Risk Potential, Therapeutic Procedures

UNIT 3	NURSING CARE OF CLIENTS WITH RESPIRATORY DISORDERS
Section	Diagnostic and Therapeutic Procedures
Chapter 20	Airway Management

Overview

- Maintenance of a patent airway is critical when providing care to a client, and suctioning and tracheostomy care are procedures that nurses must be knowledgeable about to ensure a patent airway.

- Whenever possible, the client should be encouraged to cough. Coughing is more effective than artificial suctioning at moving secretions into the upper trachea or laryngopharynx.

- Airway suctioning involves the use of a suction machine and catheter to remove secretions from the airway.

- A tracheotomy is a sterile surgical incision into the trachea for the purpose of establishing an airway. A tracheostomy is the stoma/opening that results from a tracheotomy and the insertion and maintenance of a cannula.

Suctioning

- Suctioning can be accomplished orally, nasally, or endotracheally.

- Indications

  - Diagnoses

    - Hypoxemia

  - Client Presentation

    - Early signs of hypoxemia (restlessness, tachypnea, tachycardia), decreased SaO_2 levels, adventitious breath sounds, visualization of secretions, cyanosis, and absence of spontaneous cough.

- Client Outcomes

  - The client will maintain a patent airway.

  - The client will maintain an SaO_2 between 95% and 100%.

- Measures for all types of suctioning

  o Preprocedure

    ■ Nursing Actions

      □ Perform hand hygiene, provide privacy, and explain the procedure to the client.

      □ Don the required personal protective equipment.

      □ Assist the client to Fowler's or high-Fowler's position for suctioning if possible.

      □ Encourage the client to breathe deeply and cough in an attempt to clear the secretions without artificial suctioning.

      □ Obtain baseline breath sounds and vital signs, including SaO_2 by pulse oximeter. SaO_2 may be monitored continually during the procedure.

    ■ Client Education

      □ Explain the procedure to the clients, whether he is conscious or not.

  o Intraprocedure

    ■ Nursing Actions

      □ Use surgical aseptic technique when opening suction catheter kits.

      □ Use medical aseptic technique to suction the mouth (oropharyngeal)

      □ Use surgical aseptic technique for all other types of suctioning.

      □ Open the sterile suction package.

      □ Place a sterile drape or towel on the client's chest.

      □ Set up the container, touching only the outside.

      □ Pour approximately 100 mL of sterile water or 0.9% sodium chloride (NaCl) into the container.

      □ Don sterile gloves.

        ▸ The clean/nondominant hand should hold the connecting tube; this glove protects the nurse.

        ▸ The sterile/dominant hand should hold the sterile catheter; this glove protects the client.

      □ Connect the suction catheter to the wall unit's tubing.

      □ Set suction pressure to no more than 120 mm Hg.

      □ Test the suction setup by aspirating sterile water/0.9% NaCl solution from the cup. If the unit is operating properly, continue with the procedure.

      □ Limit each suction attempt to no longer than 10 to 15 seconds to avoid hypoxemia and the vagal response. Limit suctioning to two to three attempts.

- ☐ Once suctioning is complete, clear the suction tubing by aspirating sterile water 0.9% NaCl solution.

- ☐ Document pre and postassessment data (vital signs, SpO_2; breath sound, how the client tolerated the procedure; the color, consistency, and amount of secretions).

- Oropharyngeal suctioning

  - Preprocedure

    - Nursing Actions

      - ☐ Obtain baseline breath sounds and vital signs, including SaO_2 by pulse oximeter.

      - ☐ Use a Yankauer or tonsil-tipped rigid suction catheter for oropharyngeal suctioning.

  - Intraprocedure

    - Nursing Actions

      - ☐ Insert the catheter into the client's mouth.

      - ☐ Apply suction and move the catheter around the mouth, gumline, and pharynx.

      - ☐ Clear the catheter and tubing.

      - ☐ Repeat as needed.

      - ☐ Monitor the client's SaO_2 level.

  - Postprocedure

    - Nursing Actions

      - ☐ Replace the oxygen mask if applicable.

      - ☐ Store the catheter in a clean, dry place for reuse.

      - ☐ Allow the client to perform suctioning if possible.

      - ☐ Document the client's response.

- Nasopharyngeal and nasotracheal suctioning

  - Preprocedure

    - Nursing Actions

      - ☐ Perform suctioning with a flexible catheter.

      - ☐ Catheter size is based upon the diameter of the client's nostrils and the thickness of the secretions.

      - ☐ Hyperoxygenate the client during equipment preparation with 100% FiO_2.

□ Lubricate the distal 6 to 8 cm (2 to 3 in) of the suction catheter with a water-soluble lubricant.

□ Remove the oxygen delivery device with the nondominant hand if applicable.

○ Intraprocedure

■ Nursing Actions

□ Insert the catheter into the naris during inhalation.

□ Do not apply suction while inserting the catheter.

□ Follow the natural course of the nare and slightly slant the catheter downward as it is advanced.

□ Advance the catheter the approximate distance from the nose tip to the base of the earlobe.

□ Apply suction intermittently by covering and releasing the suction port with the thumb for 10 to 15 seconds.

□ Apply suction only while withdrawing the catheter and rotating it with the thumb and forefinger.

□ Clear the catheter and tubing.

□ Allow the client time for recovery (20 to 30 seconds) between sessions. Hyperoxygenate the client before each suctioning pass.

□ Repeat as necessary.

○ Postprocedure

■ Nursing Actions

□ Document the client's response.

□ Do not reuse the suction catheter.

• Endotracheal Suctioning (ETS)

○ Preprocedure

■ Nursing Actions

□ Perform ETS through a tracheostomy or endotracheal tube.

□ Ask for assistance if necessary.

□ Obtain a suction catheter with an outer diameter of no more than 1 cm (0.5 in) of the internal diameter of the endotracheal tube.

□ Hyperoxygenate the client using a bag-valve mask (BVM) or specialized ventilator function with an FiO_2 of 100%.

- ○ Intraprocedure
  - ■ Nursing Actions
    - □ Remove the BVM or ventilator from the tracheostomy or endotracheal tube and insert the catheter into the lumen of the airway. Advance the catheter until resistance is met. The catheter should reach the level of the carina (location of bifurcation into the main stem bronchi).
    - □ Pull the catheter back 1 cm (0.5 in) prior to applying suction to prevent mucosal damage.
    - □ Apply suction intermittently by covering and releasing the suction port with the thumb for 10 to 15 seconds.
    - □ Apply suction only while withdrawing the catheter and rotating it with the thumb and forefinger.
    - □ Reattach the BVM or ventilator and supply the client with 100% inspired oxygen.
    - □ Clear the catheter and tubing.
    - □ Allow time for client recovery between sessions.
    - □ Repeat as necessary.
- ○ Postprocedure
  - ■ Nursing Actions
    - □ Document the client's response.
- • Complications
  - ○ Hypoxemia
    - ■ A decrease in SaO_2 or cyanosis may occur during suctioning, indicating worsening hypoxemia.
    - ■ Nursing Actions
      - □ To reduce the risk of hypoxemia:
        - ▸ Limit each suction attempt to no longer than 10 to 15 seconds.
        - ▸ Limit suctioning to two to three attempts.
        - ▸ Allow the client time for recovery 20 to 30 seconds between sessions.
        - ▸ Hyperoxygenate the client before each suctioning pass.
        - ▸ Decrease suctioning times for older adult clients.
      - □ If the client shows signs or symptoms of hypoxemia, stop the procedure.
  - ○ Anxiety
    - ■ Clients undergoing suctioning may become anxious during the procedure.

■ Nursing Actions

    □ Explain the procedure to all clients prior to suctioning.

    □ Provide reassurance before, during, and after the procedure.

    □ Maintain a calm manner.

Artificial Airways and Tracheostomy Care

- A tracheotomy is a sterile surgical incision into the trachea through the skin and muscles made for the purpose of establishing an airway.

- A tracheotomy may be performed as an emergency procedure or as a scheduled surgical procedure; it may be temporary or permanent.

- Artificial airways can be placed in the mouth (orotracheal tube), the nose (nasotracheal tube), or through a tracheostomy.

- A tracheostomy is the stoma/opening that results from a tracheotomy to provide and secure a patent airway.

  ○ Tracheostomy tubes vary in composition (plastic or metal), number of parts, size (long versus short), and shape (50 to 90° angles).

  ○ There is no standard tracheostomy sizing system; however, the diameter of the tracheostomy tube must be smaller than the trachea.

  ○ The outside cannula has a flange or neck plate that sits against the skin of the neck and has holes on each side for attaching ties around the client's neck to stabilize the tracheostomy tube.

- Advantages of a tracheostomy for long-term therapy

  ○ Less risk of long-term damage to the airway

  ○ Increased client comfort because no tube is present in the mouth

  ○ Decreased incidence of pressure ulcers in the oral cavity and upper airway

  ○ Ability for the client to eat because the tube enters lower in the airway

  ○ Ability for the client to talk

- Air flow in and out of a tracheostomy without air leakage (a cuffed tracheostomy tube) bypasses the vocal cords resulting in an inability to produce sound or speech.

- Uncuffed tubes and fenestrated tubes that are in place or capped allow the client to speak. Clients with a cuffed tube, who can be off mechanical ventilation and breathe around the tube, can use a special valve to allow for speech. The cuff is deflated and the valve occludes the opening.

- Swallowing is possible with a tracheostomy tube in place; however, laryngeal elevation is affected and it is important to assess the client's risk for aspiration prior to intake.

TYPES OF TRACHEOSTOMY TUBES		
TUBE	CHARACTERISTICS	NURSING CONSIDERATIONS
Single lumen (cannula)	• Has a long, single-cannula tube • Is used for clients who have long or thick necks	• Do not use with clients who have excessive secretions.

Double lumen (cannula)	• Has three major parts:
	  ○ An outer cannula that fits into the stoma and keeps the airway open
	  ○ An inner cannula that fits snugly into the outer cannula and locks into place
	  ○ An obturator
	    ■ A thin, solid tool placed inside the tracheostomy and used as a guide for inserting the outer cannula
	    ■ Should be removed immediately after outer cannula insertion
		• This tube allows for the inner cannula to be removed, cleaned, and reused or discarded and replaced with a disposable inner cannula.
		• It is useful for clients who have excessive secretions.
		• Monitor the client for accidental decannulation and the need for reinsertion.

Cuffed tube	• Has a balloon that is inflated around the outside of the distal segment of the tube to protect the lower airway by producing a seal between the upper and lower airway	• This tube permits mechanical ventilation. • Cuffs do not hold the tube in place. • Assess cuff pressures to prevent tracheal tissue necrosis. • The client will be unable to speak.
Cuffless tube	• Has no balloon and is used for clients with long-term airway-management needs	• The client must be at low risk for aspiration. • Cuffless tubes are not used for clients receiving mechanical ventilation. • This device allows the client to speak.
Fenestrated tube with cuff	• Has one large or multiple openings (fenestrations) in the posterior wall of the outer cannula with a balloon around the outside of the distal segment of the tube • Has an inner cannula that is not fenestrated	• This device allows for mechanical ventilation when the inner cannula is in place. • Removing the inner cannula allows the fenestrations to permit air to flow through the openings. • This device allows the client to speak.

TYPES OF TRACHEOSTOMY TUBES		
TUBE	**CHARACTERISTICS**	**NURSING CONSIDERATIONS**
Fenestrated tube without cuff	• Has one larger or multiple openings (fenestrations) in the posterior wall of the outer cannula with no balloon • Has an inner cannula	• The holes in the tube help wean the client from the tracheostomy. • Remove the inner cannula to allow the fenestrations to permit air to flow through the openings. • This device allows the client to speak.

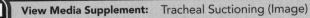

View Media Supplement: Tracheal Suctioning (Image)

- Indications

  - Diagnoses

    - Indications for insertion of a tracheostomy

      - Upper airway obstruction.

      - Edema (anaphylaxis, burns, trauma, head/neck surgery)

      - Copious secretions

      - The need for long-term mechanical ventilation

      - The need for reconstruction after laryngeal trauma or laryngeal cancer surgery

      - Obstructive sleep apnea refractory to conventional therapy

  - Client Presentation

    - Inability to oxygenate through the nasopharynx due to obstruction evidenced by dyspnea, poor SaO_2 and poor arterial blood gas (ABG) values

    - Inability to wean from mechanical ventilation within 2 weeks

    - Sleep apnea not improved by noninvasive mechanical ventilation (CPAP).

- Client Outcomes

  - The client will maintain a patent airway.

  - The client will maintain an SaO_2 between 95% and 100%.

- Nursing Actions

  - Preparation of the Client

    - Explain the procedure.

    - Place the client in semi-Fowler's or Fowler's position.

- Keep the following at the client's bedside: two extra tracheostomy tubes (one that is the client's size and one that is a size smaller, in case of accidental decannulation), the obturator for the existing tube, an oxygen source, suction catheters and a suction source, and a manual resuscitation bag.

- Provide the client with methods to communicate with staff (paper and pen, dry-erase board).

- Provide the client with an emergency call system, as well as a call light.

○ Ongoing Care

  - Assess/Monitor

    □ Oxygenation and ventilation (respiratory rate, effort, SaO_2) and vital signs hourly

    □ Thickness, quantity, odor, and color of mucous secretions

    □ Stoma and skin surrounding the stoma for signs of inflammation or infection (redness, swelling, drainage)

  - Provide adequate humidification and hydration to thin secretions and decrease risk of mucus plugging.

  - Do not suction routinely, because this may cause mucosal damage, bleeding, and bronchospasm.

  - Assess/monitor the need for suctioning. Suction on a PRN basis when assessment findings indicate it is needed (audible/noisy secretions, crackles, restlessness, tachypnea, tachycardia, mucus in the airway).

  - Maintain surgical aseptic technique when suctioning to prevent infection.

  - Provide emotional support to the client and family.

  - Give frequent oral care, usually every 2 hr.

  - For cuffed tubes, keep the pressure below 20 mm Hg to reduce the risk of tracheal necrosis due to prolonged compression of tracheal capillaries.

  - Provide tracheostomy care every 8 hr.

    □ Suction the tracheostomy tube if necessary, using sterile suctioning supplies.

    □ Remove old dressings and excess secretions.

    □ Apply the oxygen source loosely if the client desaturates during the procedure.

    □ Use cotton-tipped applicators and gauze pads to clean exposed outer cannula surfaces. Begin with half-strength (mixed with sterile 0.9% NaCl) or full-strength hydrogen peroxide followed by 0.9% NaCl. Clean in a circular motion from the stoma site outward.

    □ Use surgical aseptic technique to remove and clean the inner cannula (use half-strength or full-strength hydrogen peroxide solution to clean the cannula and sterile 0.9% NaCl to rinse it). Replace the inner cannula if it is disposable.

- □ Clean the stoma site and then the tracheostomy plate with half-strength or full-strength hydrogen peroxide solution followed by 0.9% NaCl saline.

- □ Place a split 4 in by 4 in dressing around the tracheostomy.

- □ Change tracheostomy ties if they are soiled. Secure new ties in place before removing soiled ones to prevent accidental decannulation.

- □ If a knot is needed, tie a square knot that is visible on the side of the neck. Check that one or two fingers fit between the tie tape and the neck.

- □ Document the type and amount of secretions, the general condition of the stoma and surrounding skin, the client's response to the procedure, and any teaching or learning that occurred.

- ■ Change nondisposable tracheostomy tubes every 6 to 8 weeks or per protocol.

- ■ Reposition the client every 2 hr to prevent atelectasis and pneumonia.

- ■ Minimize dust in the client's room; do not shake bedding.

- ■ If the client is permitted to eat, position the client in an upright position and tip the client's chin to her chest to enable swallowing. Assess for aspiration.

- ■ Administer prescribed medications.

  - □ Anti inflammatories to reduce edema

  - □ Antibiotics as indicated for prophylaxis or infection treatment

  - □ Aerosolized bronchodilators to relieve bronchospasm

  - □ Mucus liquefying agents

- ■ Considerations for older adult clients

  - □ There is an increased risk of respiratory infection and pneumonia in older adult clients due to the decrease in cough effectiveness and secretion clearance. Respiratory infections may be more severe and last longer.

  - □ Older adult clients may be at risk for dehydration (due to limited mobility, decrease in appetite, medications), contributing to thick, dried secretions that can occlude the airways.

  - □ Maintaining good hydration in older adult clients, as well as providing humidification (as ordered), is important to reduce the viscosity of secretions.

- ○ Client Education

  - ■ Provide discharge teaching.

    - □ Tracheostomy care

    - □ Signs and symptoms that the client should immediately report to the health care provider (signs of infection, copious secretions)

    - □ Ways to achieve good nutrition

  - ■ Consider referral of the client to a home health care agency and community support groups.

- Complications
  - o Accidental decannulation
    - Accidental decannulation in the first 72 hr after surgery is an emergency because the tracheostomy tract has not matured and replacement may be difficult.
    - Nursing Actions
      - □ Keep the tracheostomy obturator and a spare tracheostomy tube at the bedside.
      - □ Call for assistance.
      - □ If accidental decannulation occurs after the first 72 hr immediately hyperextend the neck and with the obturator inserted into the tracheostomy tube, quickly and gently replace the tube and remove the obturator.
  - o Damage to the trachea
    - Tracheal wall necrosis is tissue damage that results when the pressure of the inflated cuff impairs blood flow to the tracheal wall.
    - Tracheal stenosis is the narrowing of the tracheal lumen due to scar formation, resulting from irritation of the tracheal mucosa from the tracheal tube cuff.
    - Nursing Actions
      - □ Keep the cuff pressure between 14 and 20 mm Hg.
      - □ Check the cuff pressure at least once every 8 hr.
      - □ Keep the tube in the midline position and prevent pulling or traction on the tracheostomy tube.

CHAPTER 20: AIRWAY MANAGEMENT

(A) Application Exercises

1. Which of the following are indications that a nurse should suction a client? (Select all that apply.)

_____ Spontaneous cough

_____ Cyanosis

_____ SaO$_2$ greater than 95%

_____ Tachypnea

_____ Visualization of secretions

2. A nurse is caring for a client who has secretions in the airway. Which of the following is the most effective method for clearing the secretions?

A. Endotracheal suction

B. Oropharyngeal suction

C. Deep breathing and coughing

D. Nasopharyngeal suction

3. A nurse should measure a clients airway depth for nasopharyngeal and nasotracheal suctioning is by

A. determining the distance from the nares to the sternum.

B. determining the distance from the corner of the mouth to the earlobe.

C. determining the distance from the tip of the nose to the earlobe.

D. inserting the catheter until resistance is met.

4. A nurse is caring for a client who is being admitted following a tracheotomy. What equipment should a nurse make sure is in the room?

5. Write a brief nursing note documenting tracheostomy care.

6. A nurse is caring for a client following a tracheotomy 2 days ago. The nurse enters the room and notices that the tracheostomy tube is no longer in place. Describe the actions the nurse should take.

7. A nurse is caring for a client who has a tracheotomy. Which of the following interventions should the nurse include? (Select all that apply.)

_____ Use medical aseptic technique when performing tracheostomy care.

_____ Change tracheostomy ties each time tracheostomy care is given.

_____ Provide the client with materials for nonverbal communication.

_____ Keep pressure greater than 30 mm Hg.

_____ Clean the stoma site with half-strength hydrogen peroxide followed by 0.9% NaCl.

Scenario: A nurse is caring for a 36-year-old male client diagnosed with pneumonia and currently receiving mechanical ventilation. Initial assessment reveals crackles bilaterally and an SaO_2 of 92%. The client is coughing vigorously.

8. The nurse prepares to perform endotracheal suctioning. Which of the following are appropriate guidelines? (Select all that apply.)

_____ Set wall suction at 150 mm Hg to ensure adequate suction.

_____ Apply intermittent suction while inserting and withdrawing the catheter.

_____ Provide hyperoxygenation to the client with 100% FiO_2 before suctioning.

_____ Clear the catheter and tubing and save for later use.

_____ Maintain surgical aseptic technique.

9. What client findings indicate improved oxygenation as a result of suctioning?

CHAPTER 20: AIRWAY MANAGEMENT

 Application Exercises Answer Key

1. Which of the following are indications that a nurse should suction a client? (Select all that apply.)

_____	Spontaneous cough
__X__	**Cyanosis**
_____	SaO$_2$ greater than 95%
__X__	**Tachypnea**
__X__	**Visualization of secretions**

Cyanosis, tachypnea, and visualization of secretions are signs of respiratory distress and are indications of the need to suction the client. A spontaneous cough indicates that the client has the ability to clear secretions. An SaO$_2$ greater than 95% indicates adequate oxygenation.

 NCLEX® Connection: Physiological Adaptation, Alterations in Body Systems

2. A nurse is caring for a client who has secretions in the air way. Which of the following is the most effective method for clearing the secretions?

A. Endotracheal suction

B. Oropharyngeal suction

C. Deep breathing and coughing

D. Nasopharyngeal suction

Whenever possible, the client should be encouraged to cough. Coughing is more effective than artificial suctioning at moving secretions into the upper trachea or laryngopharynx. Also having the client deep breathe and cough is not invasive. Endotracheal, oropharyngeal, and nasopharyngeal suctioning require the use of invasive actions. The least invasive priority setting framework indicates that the lease invasive action takes priority.

 NCLEX® Connection: Physiological Adaptation, Alterations in Body Systems

3. A nurse should measure a clients airway depth for nasopharyngeal and nasotracheal suctioning by

A. determining the distance from the nares to the sternum.

B. determining the distance from the corner of the mouth to the earlobe.

C. determining the distance from the tip of the nose to the earlobe.

D. inserting the catheter until resistance is met.

By measuring the distance from the tip of the client's nose to the earlobe, the nurse can estimate how deeply the catheter should be inserted. The distance from the nares to the sternum or the distance from the corner of the mouth to the earlobe will not provide an accurate estimate. Inserting the catheter until resistance is met may damage the mucosa.

 NCLEX® Connection: Physiological Adaptation, Alterations in Body Systems

4. A nurse is caring for a client who is being admitted following a tracheotomy. What equipment should a nurse make sure is in the room?

Humidified oxygen, pulse oximeter, suction equipment and catheters, spare tracheostomy tube, extra tracheostomy ties, normal saline, split 4 x 4 dressings

 NCLEX® Connection: Reduction of Risk Potential, Potential for Complications of Diagnostic Tests/Treatments/Procedures

5. Write a brief nursing note documenting tracheostomy care.

The note should include date, time, care performed, description of secretions, and the appearance of the stoma.

Example:

Date & time: Tracheostomy care performed; Client has productive cough of thick, light-yellow secretions; Scant, thin, white secretions from stoma; Site cleansed with half-strength hydrogen peroxide and normal 0.9% NaCl; Sterile dressing applied; Tracheostomy ties changed; Stoma healing well without redness or edema.

 NCLEX® Connection: Reduction of Risk Potential, Therapeutic Procedures

6. A nurse is caring for a client following a tracheotomy 2 days ago. The nurse enters the room and notices that the tracheostomy tube is no longer in place. Describe the actions the nurse should take.

This is a medical emergency. The nurse should:

Call for assistance.

Assess respiratory rate and effort, SaO₂, and color/cyanosis.

Obtain an obturator and a spare tracheostomy tube from the head of the bed and reinsert, if possible.

If unable to insert a tracheostomy tube, administer oxygen through the stoma. If unable to administer oxygen through the stoma, occlude the stoma and use a mask or bag-valve-mask to administer through the nose and mouth.

 NCLEX® Connection: Physiological Adaptation, Medical Emergencies

7. A nurse is caring for a client who has a tracheotomy. Which of the following interventions should the nurse include? (Select all that apply.)

    _____ Use medical aseptic technique when performing tracheostomy care.

    _____ Change tracheostomy ties each time tracheostomy care is given.

    __X__ **Provide the client with materials for nonverbal communication.**

    _____ Keep pressure greater than 30 mm Hg.

    __X__ **Clean the stoma site with half-strength hydrogen peroxide followed by 0.9% sodium chloride (NaCl).**

Use surgical aseptic technique performing tracheostomy care. Suction pressures should be less than 20 mm Hg. Ties only need to be changed only when soiled. Half-strength hydrogen peroxide and 0.9% NaCl help to lift exudate from the stoma site.

 NCLEX® Connection: Reduction of Risk Potential, Therapeutic Procedures

---

Scenario: A nurse is caring for a 36-year-old male client diagnosed with pneumonia and currently receiving mechanical ventilation. Initial assessment reveals crackles bilaterally and an SaO_2 of 92%. The client is coughing vigorously.

---

8. The nurse prepares to perform endotracheal suctioning. Which of the following are appropriate guidelines? (Select all that apply.)

    _____ Set wall suction at 150 mm Hg to ensure adequate suction.

    _____ Apply intermittent suction while inserting and withdrawing the catheter.

    __X__ **Provide hyperoxygenation to the client with 100% FiO_2 before suctioning.**

    _____ Clear the catheter and tubing and save for later use.

    __X__ **Maintain surgical aseptic technique.**

Providing hyperoxygenation prior to suctioning the client minimizes the risk of hypoxia. Endotracheal suctioning requires surgical aseptic technique to prevent contamination of the respiratory tract. Suction pressure should be at 80 mm Hg. Intermittent suction is applied only when the catheter is withdrawn. A sterile catheter is required for each suctioning attempt.

 NCLEX® Connection: Physiological Adaptation, Alterations in Body Systems

9. What client findings indicate improved oxygenation as a result of suctioning?

SaO_2 > 95%

Decrease or absence of crackles

Cessation of coughing

Decrease in client anxiety

NCLEX® Connection: Reduction of Risk Potential, Potential for Alterations in Body Systems

UNIT 3	NURSING CARE OF CLIENTS WITH RESPIRATORY DISORDERS
Section	Diagnostic and Therapeutic Procedures
Chapter 21	Oxygen Therapy and Mechanical Ventilation

Overview

- Oxygen is a tasteless and colorless gas that accounts for 21% of atmospheric air.

- Oxygen is used to maintain adequate cellular oxygenation. It is used in the treatment of many acute and chronic respiratory problems.

- Oxygen is administered in an attempt to maintain an SaO_2 of at least 95% to 100% by using the lowest amount of oxygen without putting the client at risk for complications.

- Clients who cannot spontaneously breathe on their own require mechanical ventilation.

Oxygen Delivery Devices

- Supplemental oxygen can be delivered by a variety of methods based on the client's particular circumstances. The percentage of oxygen delivered to the client is expressed as the fraction of inspired oxygen (FiO_2).

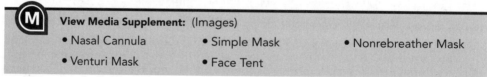

M **View Media Supplement:** (Images)
- Nasal Cannula
- Simple Mask
- Nonrebreather Mask
- Venturi Mask
- Face Tent

- Low-flow oxygen delivery systems deliver varying amounts of oxygen based on the method and the client's breathing pattern.

  ○ Nasal cannula – A length of tubing with two small prongs for insertion into the nares

    ▪ FiO_2 – 24% to 44% at flow rates of 1 to 6 L/min

    ▪ Advantages

      □ It is safe, easy to apply, comfortable, and well tolerated.

      □ The client is able to eat, talk, and ambulate.

    ▪ Disadvantages

      □ The FiO_2 varies with the flow rate and the client's rate and depth of breathing.

      □ Extended use can lead to skin breakdown and dry the mucous membranes.

      □ The tubing is easily dislodged.

- Nursing Interventions
  - Assess the patency of the nares.
  - Ensure that the prongs fit in the nares properly.
  - Use water-soluble gel to prevent dry nares.
  - Provide humidification for flow rates of 4 L/min and above.
- Simple face mask (covers the client's nose and mouth)
  - FiO_2 – 40% to 60% at flow rates of 1 to 6 L/min (the minimum flow rate is 5 L/min to ensure flushing of CO_2 from the mask).
  - Advantages
    - A face mask is easy to apply and may be more comfortable than a nasal cannula.
  - Disadvantages
    - Flow rates of 5 L/min or lower can result in rebreathing of CO_2.
    - This device is poorly tolerated by clients who have anxiety or claustrophobia.
    - Eating, drinking, and talking are impaired.
    - Use caution with clients who have a high risk of aspiration or airway obstruction.
  - Nursing Interventions
    - Assess proper fit to ensure a secure seal over the nose and mouth.
    - Ensure that the client wears a nasal cannula during meals.
- Partial rebreather mask (covers the client's nose and mouth)
  - FiO_2 – 60% to 75% at flow rates of 6 to 11 L/min
  - Advantages
    - The mask has a reservoir bag attached with no valve, which allows the client to rebreathe up to $1/3$ of exhaled air together with room air.
  - Disadvantages
    - Complete deflation of the reservoir bag during inspiration causes CO_2 buildup.
    - The FiO_2 varies with the client's breathing pattern.
    - This device is poorly tolerated by clients who have anxiety or claustrophobia.
    - Eating, drinking, and talking are impaired.
    - Use with caution for clients who have a high risk of aspiration or airway obstruction.

- ■ Nursing Interventions
  - □ Keep the reservoir bag from deflating by adjusting the oxygen flow rate to keep it inflated.
  - □ Use with caution for clients at high risk of aspiration or airway obstruction.
  - □ The FiO_2 varies with the client's breathing pattern.
  - □ Assess proper fit to ensure a secure seal over the nose and mouth.
  - □ Ensure that the client uses a nasal cannula during meals.
- ○ Nonrebreather mask (covers the client's nose and mouth)
  - ■ FIO_2 – 80% to 95% at flow rates of 10 to 15 L/min to keep the reservoir bag $^2/_3$ full during inspiration and expiration
  - ■ Advantages
    - □ Delivers the highest O_2 concentration possible (except for intubation).
    - □ A one-way valve situated between the mask and reservoir allows the client to inhale maximum O_2 from the reservoir bag. The two exhalation ports have flaps covering them that prevent room air from entering the mask.
  - ■ Disadvantages
    - □ The valve and flap on the mask must be intact and functional during each breath.
    - □ Poorly tolerated by clients who have anxiety or claustrophobia.
    - □ Eating, drinking, and talking are impaired.
  - ■ Nursing Interventions
    - □ Perform an hourly assessment of the valve and flap.
    - □ Assess proper fit to ensure a secure seal over the nose and mouth.
    - □ Use with caution for clients who have a high risk of aspiration or airway obstruction.
    - □ Ensure that the client uses a nasal cannula during meals.
- • High-flow oxygen delivery systems deliver precise amounts of oxygen when properly fitted.
  - ○ Venturi mask (covers the client's nose and mouth)
    - ■ FIO_2 – 24% to 55% at flow rates of 2 to 10 L/min via different sized adaptors
    - ■ Advantages
      - □ Delivers the most precise oxygen concentration.
      - □ Humidification is not required.
      - □ Best suited for clients who have chronic lung disease.
    - ■ Disadvantages
      - □ The use of a Venturi mask is expensive.

- ■ Nursing Interventions
    - □ Assess frequently to ensure an accurate flow rate.
    - □ Make sure the tubing is free of kinks.
- ○ Aerosol mask, face tent (fits loosely around the face and neck), and tracheostomy collar (a small mask that covers a surgically created opening in the trachea)
    - ■ FiO_2 – 24% to 100% at flow rates of at least 10 L/min (they provide high humidification with oxygen delivery)
    - ■ Advantages
        - □ Good for clients who do not tolerate masks well.
        - □ Useful for clients who have facial trauma, burns, and/or thick secretions.
    - ■ Disadvantages
        - □ High humidification requires frequent monitoring.
    - ■ Nursing Interventions
        - □ Empty condensation from the tubing often.
        - □ Ensure that there is adequate water in the humidification canister.
        - □ Ensure that the aerosol mist leaves from the vents during inspiration and expiration.
        - □ Make sure the tubing does not pull on the tracheostomy.
- ○ T-piece
    - ■ FiO_2 – 24% to 100% at flow rates of at least 10 L/min
    - ■ Advantages
        - □ This device can be used for clients who have tracheostomies, laryngectomies, or endotracheal tubes (ET).
    - ■ Disadvantages
        - □ High humidification requires frequent monitoring.
    - ■ Nursing Interventions
        - □ Ensure that the exhalation port is open and uncovered.
        - □ Make sure that the T-piece does not pull on the tracheostomy or ET tube.
        - □ Ensure that the mist is evident during inspiration and expiration.

Oxygen Therapy

- ● Indications
    - ○ Diagnoses
        - ■ Hypoxemia and hypoxia

☐ Hypoxemia is an inadequate level of oxygen in the blood. Hypovolemia, hypoventilation, and interruption of arterial flow can lead to hypoxemia.

○ Client Presentation

EARLY FINDINGS	LATE FINDINGS
Tachypnea	Confusion and stupor
Tachycardia	Cyanotic skin and mucous membranes
Restlessness	Bradypnea
Pale skin and mucous membranes	Bradycardia
Elevated blood pressure	Hypotension
Symptoms of respiratory distress (use of accessory muscles, nasal flaring, tracheal tugging, and adventitious lung sounds)	Cardiac dysrhythmias

- Client Outcomes

    ○ The client maintains an oxygen saturation of 95% to 100%.

    ○ The client maintains a patent airway.

- Nursing Actions

    ○ Preparation of the Client

        ▪ Explain all procedures to the client.

        ▪ Place the client in semi-Fowler's or Fowler's position to facilitate breathing and promote chest expansion.

        ▪ Ensure that all equipment is working properly.

    ○ Ongoing Care

        ▪ Provide oxygen therapy at the lowest flow that will correct hypoxemia.

        ▪ Assess/monitor respiratory rate, rhythm and effort, and lung sounds to determine the client's need for supplemental oxygen.

            ☐ Signs and symptoms of hypoxemia are shortness of breath, anxiety, tachypnea, tachycardia, restlessness, pallor, or cyanosis of the skin and/or mucous membranes, adventitious breath sounds, and confusion.

            ☐ Signs and symptoms of hypercarbia (elevated levels of CO_2) are restlessness, hypertension, and headache.

        ▪ Assess/monitor oxygenation status with pulse oximetry and ABGs.

        ▪ Apply the oxygen delivery device prescribed. Assess the fit of the mask to ensure a secure seal over the client's nose and mouth.

        ▪ Promote good oral hygiene and provide as needed.

        ▪ Promote turning, coughing, deep breathing, use of incentive spirometer, and suctioning.

- Promote rest and decrease environmental stimuli.

- Provide emotional support for clients who appear anxious.

- Assess nutritional status; provide supplements as prescribed.

- Assess/monitor the client's skin integrity; provide moisture and pressure-relief devices as indicated.

- Assess/monitor and document the client's response to oxygen therapy.

- Titrate oxygen to maintain prescribed oxygen saturation.

- Discontinue supplemental oxygen gradually.

○ Interventions

- Monitor for signs and symptoms of respiratory depression such as decreased respiratory rate and decreased level of consciousness; notify the provider if these findings are present.

- For respiratory distress:

  □ Position the client for maximum ventilation (Fowler's or semi-Fowler's position).

  □ Complete a focused respiratory assessment.

  □ Promote deep breathing and use supplemental oxygen as prescribed.

  □ Stay with the client and provide emotional support to decrease anxiety.

  □ Promote airway clearance by encouraging coughing and oral/oropharyngeal suctioning if necessary.

- Complications

  ○ Oxygen toxicity

    - Oxygen toxicity can result from high concentrations of oxygen (typically above 50%), long durations of oxygen therapy (typically more than 24 to 48 hr), and the client's degree of lung disease.

    - Signs and symptoms include a nonproductive cough, substernal pain, nasal stuffiness, nausea, vomiting, fatigue, headache, sore throat, and hypoventilation.

    - Nursing Actions

      □ Use the lowest level of oxygen necessary to maintain an adequate SaO_2.

      □ Monitor the ABGs and notify the provider if SaO_2 levels are outside of the expected reference range.

      □ Use an oxygen mask with continuous positive airway pressure (CPAP), bilevel positive airway pressure (BiPAP), or positive end expiratory pressure (PEEP) as prescribed while the client is on a mechanical ventilator to help decrease the amount of needed oxygen.

○ Oxygen-induced hypoventilation

■ Oxygen-induced hypoventilation can develop in clients who have COPD and chronic hypoxemia and hypercarbia. Clients who have COPD rely on low levels of arterial oxygen as their primary drive for breathing. Providing supplemental oxygen at high levels can decrease or eliminate their respiratory drive.

■ Nursing Actions

□ Monitor the client's respiratory rate and pattern, level of consciousness, and SaO_2.

□ Provide oxygen therapy at the lowest flow that corrects hypoxemia.

□ If the client tolerates it, use a Venturi mask to deliver precise oxygen levels.

□ Notify the provider of impending respiratory depression, such as a decreased respiratory rate and a decreased level of consciousness.

○ Combustion

■ Oxygen is combustible.

■ Nursing Actions

□ Post "No Smoking" or "Oxygen in Use" signs to alert others of a fire hazard.

□ Know where the closest fire extinguisher is located.

□ Educate the client and others about the fire hazard of smoking during oxygen use.

□ Have the client wear a cotton gown, because synthetic or wool fabrics can generate static electricity.

□ Ensure that all electric devices (razors, hearing aids, radios) are working well.

□ Ensure electric machinery (monitors, suction machines) are well-grounded.

□ Do not use volatile, flammable materials (alcohol or acetone) near clients who are receiving oxygen.

Mechanical Ventilation

- Mechanical ventilation provides breathing support until lung function is restored, delivering warm (body temperature 37° C [98.6° F]), 100% humidified oxygen at FiO_2 levels between 21% to 100%.

View Media Supplement: Mechanical Ventilation (Video)

○ Positive-pressure ventilators deliver air to the lungs under pressure throughout inspiration and/or expiration to keep the alveoli open during inspiration and to prevent alveolar collapse during expiration. The benefits include:

■ Forced/enhanced lung expansion

■ Improved gas exchange (oxygenation)

■ Decreased work of breathing

    ○   Mechanical ventilation can be delivered via:

- An endotracheal tube
- A tracheostomy tube
- A nasal or face mask (non-invasive modes such as CPAP, BiPAP)

    ○   Mechanical ventilators can be cycled based on pressure, volume, time, and/or flow.

| COMMON MODES OF VENTILATION ||
VENTILATION MODE	DESCRIPTION
Assist-control (AC)	Preset ventilator rate and tidal volume. The client can initiate breaths; however, the ventilator takes over and delivers a preset tidal volume. Hyperventilation can result in respiratory alkalosis. The client may require sedation to decrease respiratory rate.
Synchronized intermittent mandatory ventilation (SIMV)	Preset ventilator rate and tidal volume. For client-initiated breaths, tidal volume depends on the client's effort. Ventilator-initiated breaths are synchronized to reduce competition between the ventilator and the client. SIMV is used as a regular mode of ventilation and as a weaning mode (rate decreased to allow more spontaneous ventilation). It can increase the work of breathing and respiratory muscle fatigue.
Pressure support ventilation (PSV)	Preset pressure delivered during spontaneous inspiration to reduce work of breathing. The client controls rate and tidal volume. Often used as a weaning mode. PSV decreases the work of breathing and promotes respiratory muscle conditioning. No ventilator breaths are delivered. PSV does not guarantee minimal minute ventilation. It is often combined with other modes of ventilation (SIMV, AC).
Positive end expiratory pressure (PEEP)	Positive pressure applied at the end of expiration to increase functional residual capacity and improve oxygenation by opening collapsed alveoli. PEEP must be used in conjunction with AC or SIMV; it cannot be used alone. PEEP decreases cardiac output and can cause volutrauma (trauma to lung tissue caused by tidal volumes that are too high) and increased intracranial pressure (ICP).
Volume assured pressure support ventilation (VAPSV)	Similar to PSV with a minimal set tidal volume for each breath. VAPSV optimizes inspiratory flow, reduces the work of breathing, decreases volutrauma, and ensures minimal minute ventilation. VAPSV is used with clients who have severe respiratory disease or those who are having difficulty weaning.
Independent lung ventilation (ILV)	Double lumen endotracheal tube allows each lung to be ventilated separately. ILV is used in clients who have unilateral lung disease. It requires two ventilators, sedation, and/or neuromuscular blocking agents.

COMMON MODES OF VENTILATION	
VENTILATION MODE	**DESCRIPTION**
High-frequency ventilation	Delivers a small amount of gas at very rapid rates (60 to 3,000 cycles/min). High-frequency ventilation is used frequently in children. The client must be sedated and/or receiving neuromuscular blocking agents. Breath sounds are difficult to assess.
Inverse ratio ventilation (IRV)	Lengthens inspiratory phase of respiration to maximize oxygenation. IRV is used for hypoxemia refractory to PEEP. It is uncomfortable for clients and requires sedation and/or neuromuscular blocking agents. There is a high risk of volutrauma and decreased cardiac output due to air trapping.
Continuous positive airway pressure (CPAP)	Positive pressure supplied during spontaneous breaths. No ventilator breaths are delivered unless they are in conjunction with SIMV. Risks include volutrauma, decreased cardiac output, and increased ICP. CPAP can be invasive or noninvasive. It is often used for obstructive sleep apnea.
Bilevel positive airway pressure (BiPAP)	Positive pressure delivered during spontaneous breaths. Different pressures are delivered for inspiration and expiration. No spontaneous breaths are delivered. BiPAP is a noninvasive mode.

- Indications
  - Diagnoses
    - Hypoxemia, hypoventilation with respiratory acidosis
      - Airway trauma
      - Exacerbation of COPD
      - Acute pulmonary edema due to myocardial infarction or heart failure
      - Asthma attack
      - Head injuries, cerebrovascular accident, or coma
      - Neurological disorders (multiple sclerosis, myasthenia gravis, Guillain-Barré)
      - Obstructive sleep apnea
    - Respiratory support following surgery (decrease workload)
    - Respiratory support while under general anesthesia or heavy sedation
- Client Outcomes
  - The client will maintain an oxygen saturation of 95% to 100%.
  - The client will maintain a patent airway.
- Nursing Actions
  - Preparation of the Client
    - Explain the procedure to the client.

- Establish a method for communication, such as asking yes/no questions, providing writing materials, using a dry erase board and/or a picture communication board, or lip reading.

○ Ongoing Care

- Maintain a patent airway.
  □ Assess the position and placement of tube.
  □ Document the tube placement in centimeters at the client's teeth or lips.
  □ Use two staff members for repositioning and resecuring the tube.
  □ Apply protective barriers (soft wrist restraints) according to hospital protocol to prevent self-extubation.
  □ Use caution when moving the client.
  □ Suction oral and tracheal secretions to maintain tube patency.
  □ Support ventilator tubing to prevent mucosal erosion and displacement.

- Assess respiratory status every 1 to 2 hr: breath sounds, respiratory effort, and spontaneous breaths.

- Monitor and document ventilator settings hourly.
  □ Rate, FiO_2, and tidal volume
  □ Mode of ventilation
  □ Use of adjuncts (PEEP, CPAP)
  □ Plateau or peak inspiratory pressure (PIP)
  □ Alarm settings

- Monitor the ventilator alarms, which signal if the client is not receiving the correct ventilation.
  □ Never turn off the ventilator alarms.
  □ There are three types of ventilator alarms: volume, pressure, and apnea alarms.
    ▸ Volume (low pressure) alarms indicate a low exhaled volume due to a disconnection, cuff leak, and/or tube displacement.
    ▸ Pressure (high pressure) alarms indicate excess secretions, client biting the tubing, kinks in the tubing, client coughing, pulmonary edema, bronchospasm, and/or pneumothorax.
    ▸ Apnea alarms indicate that the ventilator does not detect spontaneous respiration in a preset time period.

- Maintain adequate (but not excessive) volume in the cuff of the endotracheal tube.
  □ Assess the cuff pressure at least every 8 hr. Maintain the cuff pressure below 20 mm Hg to reduce the risk of tracheal necrosis.

- ☐ Assess for an air leak around the cuff (client speaking, air hissing, or decreasing SaO_2). Inadequate cuff pressure can result in inadequate oxygenation and/or accidental extubation.

- ■ Administer medications as prescribed.

  - ☐ Analgesics – morphine and fentanyl (Sublimaze)

  - ☐ Sedatives – propofol (Diprivan), diazepam (Valium), lorazepam (Ativan), midazolam (Versed), and haloperidol (Haldol)

    - ‣ Clients receiving mechanical ventilation may require sedation or paralytic agents to prevent competition between extrinsic and intrinsic breathing and the resulting effects of hyperventilation.

  - ☐ Neuromuscular blocking agents – pancuronium bromide (Pavulon), atracurium (Tracrium), and vecuronium (Norcuron)

  - ☐ Ulcer-preventing agents – famotidine (Pepcid) or lansoprazole (Prevacid)

  - ☐ Antibiotics for established infections

- ■ Reposition the oral endotracheal tube every 24 hr or according to protocol. Assess for skin breakdown.

  - ☐ Older adult clients have fragile skin and are more prone to skin and mucous membrane breakdown. Older adult clients have decreased oral secretions. They require frequent, gentle skin and oral care.

- ■ Provide adequate nutrition.

  - ☐ Assess gastrointestinal functioning every 8 hr.

  - ☐ Monitor bowel habits.

  - ☐ Administer enteral or parenteral feedings as prescribed.

- ■ Continually monitor the client during the weaning process and watch for signs of weaning intolerance.

  - ☐ Respiratory rate greater than 30/min or less than 8/min

  - ☐ Blood pressure or heart rate changes more than 20% of baseline

  - ☐ SaO_2 less than 90%

  - ☐ Dysrhythmias, elevated ST segment

  - ☐ Significant decrease in tidal volume

  - ☐ Labored respirations, increased use of accessory muscles, and diaphoresis

  - ☐ Restlessness, anxiety, and decreased level of consciousness

- ■ Suction the oropharynx and trachea prior to extubation.

- ■ Following extubation, monitor the client for signs of respiratory distress or airway obstruction, such as ineffective cough, dyspnea, and stridor.

- ■ Suction the tracheal tube to clear secretions, as needed. Reposition the client to promote mobility of secretions.

- Older adult clients have decreased respiratory muscle strength and chest wall compliance, which makes them more susceptible to aspiration, atelectasis, and pulmonary infections. The older adult client will require more frequent position changes to promote mobility of secretions.

- Complications

  - Fluid retention

    - Fluid retention in clients who are receiving mechanical ventilation is due to decreased cardiac output, activation of renin-angiotensin-aldosterone system, and/or ventilator humidification.

    - Nursing Actions

      □ Monitor the client's intake and output and weight.

  - Oxygen toxicity

    - Oxygen toxicity can result from high concentrations of oxygen (typically above 50%), long durations of oxygen therapy (typically more than 24 to 48 hr), and/or the client's degree of lung disease.

    - Nursing Actions

      □ Monitor for signs (fatigue, restlessness, severe dyspnea, tachycardia, tachypnea, crackles, and cyanosis).

  - Hemodynamic compromise

    - Mechanical ventilation has a risk of increased thoracic pressure (positive pressure), which can result in decreased venous return.

    - Nursing Actions

      □ Monitor for tachycardia, hypotension, urine output less than or equal to 30 mL/hr, cool, clammy extremities, decreased peripheral pulses, and a decreased level of consciousness.

  - Aspiration

    - Keep the head of the bed elevated 30° at all times to decrease the risk of aspiration.

    - Nursing Actions

      □ Check residuals every 4 hr if the client is receiving enteral feedings to decrease the risk of aspiration.

  - Gastrointestinal ulceration (stress ulcer)

    - Gastric ulcers can be evident in clients receiving mechanical ventilation.

    - Nursing Actions

      □ Monitor gastrointestinal drainage and stools for occult bleeding.

      □ Administer ulcer prevention medications (sucralfate and histamine$_2$ blockers) as prescribed.

CHAPTER 21: OXYGEN THERAPY AND MECHANICAL VENTILATION

Ⓐ Application Exercises

1. Match each of the following oxygen delivery devices with the appropriate description.

_____ Nasal cannula

_____ Simple face mask

_____ Nonrebreather mask

_____ Venturi mask

_____ Face tent

A. Delivers an FiO_2 of 24% to 55% at flow rates of 2 to 10 L/min via different sized adaptors

B. Delivers an FiO_2 of 24% to 100% at flow rates of at least 10 L/min and provides high humidification of oxygen

C. Delivers an FiO_2 of 24% to 44% at a flow rate of 1 to 6 L/min via tubing with two small prongs for insertion into the nares

D. Delivers an FiO_2 of 40% to 60% at flow rates of 5 to 8 L/min for short-term oxygen therapy

E. Delivers an FiO_2 of 80% to 95% at flow rates of 10 to 15 L/min to keep the reservoir bag $^2/_3$ full during inspiration and expiration

2. Differentiate between early (E) and late (L) signs of hypoxemia.

_____ Confusion and stupor

_____ Pale skin and mucous membranes

_____ Bradycardia

_____ Hypotension

_____ Elevated blood pressure

_____ Restlessness

_____ Cyanotic skin and mucous membranes

3. A nurse is caring for a client who has dyspnea. In which of the following positions should the nurse place the client?

A. Supine

B. Dorsal recumbent

C. Fowler's

D. Lateral

4. Which of the following oxygen delivery devices is used when a precise amount of oxygen must be delivered?

A. Nonrebreather mask

B. Venturi mask

C. Nasal cannula

D. Simple face mask

5. Which of the following modes of ventilation can increase conditioning of the respiratory muscles? (Select all that apply.)

_____ Assist-control

_____ Synchronized intermittent mandatory ventilation

_____ Continuous positive airway pressure

_____ Pressure support ventilation

_____ Independent lung ventilation

6. A nurse is training a newly licensed nurse who is caring for a client who is receiving mechanical ventilation. The ventilator has been placed on pressure support ventilation (PSV) mode. The newly licensed nurse demonstrates an understanding of PSV by stating that, "Pressure support maintains the amount of pressure

A. in the lungs to open alveoli and prevent atelectasis."

B. on spontaneous ventilation to decrease the work of breathing."

C. on spontaneous ventilation to increase the work of breathing."

D. on continuous ventilation to decrease the work of breathing."

7. A nurse is orientating a newly licensed nurse on how to complete a routine assessment for a client who is receiving mechanical ventilation. Which of the following should be included in the newly licensed nurse's assessment of the client?

A. Assess blood pressure every 6 to 8 hr.

B. Assess blood pressure every 2 to 4 hr.

C. Assess breath sounds every 6 to 8 hr.

D. Assess breath sounds every 2 to 4 hr.

CHAPTER 21: OXYGEN THERAPY AND MECHANICAL VENTILATION

(A) Application Exercises Answer Key

1. Match each of the following oxygen delivery devices with the appropriate description.

__C__	Nasal cannula	A. Delivers an FiO$_2$ of 24% to 55% at flow rates of 2 to 10 L/min via different sized adaptors
__D__	Simple face mask	B. Delivers an FiO$_2$ of 24% to 100% at flow rates of at least 10 L/min and provides high humidification of oxygen
__E__	Nonrebreather mask	C. Delivers an FiO$_2$ of 24% to 44% at a flow rate of 1 to 6 L/min via tubing with two small prongs for insertion into the nares
__A__	Venturi mask	D. Delivers an FiO$_2$ of 40% to 60% at flow rates of 5 to 8 L/min for short-term oxygen therapy
__B__	Face tent	E. Delivers an FiO$_2$ of 80% to 95% at flow rates of 10 to 15 L/min to keep the reservoir bag $^2/_3$ full during inspiration and expiration

(N) **NCLEX® Connection: Reduction of Risk Potential, Therapeutic Procedures**

2. Differentiate between early (E) and late (L) signs of hypoxemia.

__L__	Confusion and stupor
__E__	Pale skin and mucous membranes
__L__	Bradycardia
__L__	Hypotension
__E__	Elevated blood pressure
__E__	Restlessness
__L__	Cyanotic skin and mucous membranes

Signs of early hypoxemia include: pale skin and mucous membranes, elevated blood pressure, and restlessness. Signs of later hypoxemia include: confusion and stupor, bradycardia, hypotension, restlessness, and cyanotic skin and mucous membranes.

(N) **NCLEX® Connection: Physiological Adaptation, Pathophysiology**

3. A nurse is caring for a client who has dyspnea. In which of the following positions should the nurse place the client?

    A. Supine

    B. Dorsal recumbent

    C. Fowler's

    D. Lateral

Fowler's position facilitates maximal lung expansion and thus optimizes breathing. Supine, dorsal recumbent, and lateral positions would suppress optimal breathing.

 NCLEX® Connection: Reduction of Risk Potential, Potential for Complications of Diagnostic Tests/Treatments/Procedures

4. Which of the following oxygen delivery devices is used when a precise amount of oxygen must be delivered?

    A. Nonrebreather mask

    B. Venturi mask

    C. Nasal cannula

    D. Simple face mask

A Venturi mask incorporates an adaptor that allows a precise amount of oxygen to be delivered. The other oxygen delivery systems deliver an approximated amount of oxygen.

 NCLEX® Connection: Reduction of Risk Potential, Therapeutic Procedures

5. Which of the following modes of ventilation can increase conditioning of the respiratory muscles? (Select all that apply.)

    _____   Assist-control

    __X__   **Synchronized intermittent mandatory ventilation**

    __X__   **Continuous positive airway pressure**

    __X__   **Pressure support ventilation**

    _____   Independent lung ventilation

Synchronized intermittent mandatory ventilation, continuous positive airway pressure, and pressure support ventilation all require the client to generate the force to take spontaneous breaths. Assist-control mode takes over the work of breathing. Independent lung ventilation mode is used for unilateral lung disease to ventilate the lung individually.

 NCLEX® Connection: Reduction of Risk Potential, Therapeutic Procedures

6. A nurse is training a newly licensed nurse who is caring for a client who is receiving mechanical ventilation. The ventilator has been placed on pressure support ventilation (PSV) mode. The newly licensed nurse demonstrates an understanding of PSV by stating that, "Pressure support maintains the amount of pressure

    A. in the lungs to open alveoli and prevent atelectasis."

    B. on spontaneous ventilation to decrease the work of breathing."

    C. on spontaneous ventilation to increase the work of breathing."

    D. on continuous ventilation to decrease the work of breathing."

Pressure support ventilation provides pressure on spontaneous ventilation to decrease the work of breathing. The other options are incorrect.

 NCLEX® Connection: Reduction of Risk Potential, Therapeutic Procedures

7. A nurse is orientating a newly licensed nurse on how to complete a routine assessment for a client who is receiving mechanical ventilation. Which of the following should be included in the newly licensed nurse's assessment of the client?

    A. Assess blood pressure every 6 to 8 hr.

    B. Assess blood pressure every 2 to 4 hr.

    C. Assess breath sounds every 6 to 8 hr.

    D. Assess breath sounds every 2 to 4 hr.

Breath sounds should be monitored every 2 to 4 hr, and blood pressure should be monitored hourly for a client who is receiving mechanical ventilation.

NCLEX® Connection: Reduction of Risk Potential, System Specific Assessment

UNIT 3	NURSING CARE OF CLIENTS WITH RESPIRATORY DISORDERS
Section	Respiratory System Disorders
Chapter 22	Asthma

Overview

- Asthma is a chronic inflammatory disorder of the airways that results in intermittent and reversible airflow obstruction of the bronchioles.

    o The obstruction occurs either by inflammation or airway hyperresponsiveness.

    o Asthma can occur at any age.

    o The cause of asthma is unknown.

- Manifestations of asthma

    o Mucosal edema

    o Bronchoconstriction

    o Excessive mucus production

    M   View Media Supplement: Normal and Asthmatic Lung Changes (Image)

- Asthma diagnoses are based on symptoms and classified into one of the following four categories.

    o Mild intermittent – Symptoms occur less than twice a week.

    o Mild persistent – Symptoms arise more than twice a week but not daily.

    o Moderate persistent – Daily symptoms occur in conjunction with exacerbations twice a week.

    o Severe persistent – Symptoms occur continually, along with frequent exacerbations that limit the client's physical activity and quality of life.

Health Promotion and Disease Prevention

- If the client smokes, promote smoking cessation.

- Advise the client to use protective equipment (mask) and ensure proper ventilation while working in environments that contain carcinogens or particles in the air.

- Encourage influenza and pneumonia vaccinations for all clients who have asthma and especially for the older adult.

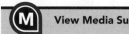

- Instruct the client how to recognize and avoid triggering agents, such as:

  o Environmental factors, such as changes in temperature (especially warm to cold) and humidity

  o Air pollutants

  o Strong odors (perfume)

  o Seasonal allergens (grass, tree, and weed pollens) and perennial allergens (mold, feathers, dust, roaches, animal dander, foods treated with sulfites)

  o Stress and emotional distress

  o Medications (aspirin, NSAIDS, beta-blockers, cholinergics)

  o Enzymes, including those in laundry detergents

  o Chemicals (household cleaners)

  o Sinusitis with postnasal drip

  o Viral respiratory tract infection

- Instruct the client how to properly self-administer medications (nebulizers and inhalers).

> **(M)** **View Media Supplement:** Asthmatic Breathing – Metered-Dose Inhaler (Video)

- Educate the client regarding infection prevention techniques.

- Encourage regular exercise as part of asthma therapy.

  o Promotes ventilation and perfusion.

  o Maintains cardiac health.

  o Enhances skeletal muscle strength.

  o Clients may require pre-medication.

Assessment

- Risk Factors

  o Older adult clients have decreased pulmonary reserves due to physiologic lung changes that occur with the aging process.

    ■ Older adult clients are more susceptible to infections.

    ■ The sensitivity of beta-adrenergic receptors decreases with age. As the beta receptors age and lose sensitivity, they are less able to respond to agonists, which can result in bronchospasms.

    ■ Clients who have mild to moderate asthma can experience few or no symptoms between asthma attacks. During attacks, monitor for signs and symptoms.

- Subjective Data

  ○ Dyspnea

  ○ Chest tightness

  ○ Anxiety and/or stress

- Objective Data

  ○ Physical Assessment Findings

    ▪ Coughing

    ▪ Wheezing

    ▪ Mucus production

    ▪ Use of accessory muscles

    ▪ Poor oxygen saturation (low SaO_2)

    ▪ Barrel chest or increased chest diameter

  ○ Obtain the client's history regarding current and previous asthma exacerbations.

    ▪ Onset and duration

    ▪ Precipitating factors (stress, exercise, exposure to irritant)

    ▪ Changes in medication regimen

    ▪ Medications that relieve symptoms

    ▪ Other medications taken

    ▪ Self-care methods used to relieve symptoms

 View Media Supplement: Metered-Dose Inhaler (Animation)

  ○ Laboratory Tests

    ▪ ABGs

      □ Hypoxemia (decreased PaO_2 < 80 mm Hg)

      □ Hypocarbia (decreased $PaCO_2$ < 35 mm Hg – early in attack)

      □ Hypercarbia (increased $PaCO_2$ > 45 mm Hg – later in attack)

    ▪ Sputum cultures

      □ Bacteria can indicate infection.

    o   Diagnostic Procedures

- Pulmonary function tests (PFTs) are the most accurate tests for diagnosing asthma and its severity.

  □ Forced vital capacity (FVC) is the volume of air exhaled from full inhalation to full exhalation.

  □ Forced expiratory volume in the first second (FEV1) is the volume of air blown out as hard and fast as possible during the first second of the most forceful exhalation after the greatest full inhalation.

  □ Peak expiratory rate flow (PERF) is the fastest airflow rate reached during exhalation.

  □ A decrease in FEV1 or PERF by 15% to 20% below the expected value is common in clients who have asthma. An increase in these values by 12% following the administration of bronchodilators is diagnostic for asthma.

- A chest x-ray is used to diagnose changes in the client's chest structure over time.

Collaborative Care

- Nursing Care

  o Position the client to maximize ventilation (high-Fowler's = 90°).

  o Administer oxygen therapy as prescribed.

  o Monitor cardiac rate and rhythm for changes during an acute attack (can be irregular, tachycardic, or with PVCs).

  o Initiate and maintain IV access.

  o Maintain a calm and reassuring demeanor.

  o Provide rest periods for older adult clients who have dyspnea. Design room and walkways with opportunities for rest. Incorporate rest into ADLs.

  o Encourage prompt medical attention for infections and appropriate vaccinations.

  o Administer medications as prescribed.

- Medications

  o Bronchodilators (inhalers)

  - Short-acting beta$_2$ agonists, such as albuterol (Proventil, Ventolin), provide rapid relief of acute symptoms and prevent exercise-induced asthma.

  - Anticholinergic medications, such as ipratropium (Atrovent), block the parasympathetic nervous system. This allows for the sympathetic nervous system effects of increased bronchodilation and decreased pulmonary secretions.

  - Methylxanthines, such as theophylline (Theo-Dur), require close monitoring of serum medication levels due to a narrow therapeutic range.

- **Nursing Considerations**
  - Theophylline – Monitor the client's serum levels for toxicity. Side effects will include tachycardia, nausea, and diarrhea.
  - Albuterol – Watch the client for tremors and tachycardia.
  - Ipratropium – Observe the client for dry mouth.
- **Client Education**
  - Ipratropium – Advise the client to suck on hard candies to help relieve dry mouth.

- Anti-inflammatory agents
  - These are used to decrease airway inflammation, and they include:
    - Corticosteroids, such as fluticasone (Flovent) and prednisone (Deltasone)
    - Leukotriene antagonists, such as montelukast (Singulair), mast cell stabilizers, such as cromolyn sodium (Intal), and monoclonal antibodies, such as omalizumab (Xolair)
  - Nursing Considerations
    - Watch the client for decreased immunity function.
    - Monitor for hyperglycemia.
    - Advise the client to report black, tarry stools.
    - Observe the client for fluid retention and weight gain. This can be common.
    - Monitor the client's throat and mouth for aphthous lesions (cold sores).
  - Client Education
    - Encourage the client to drink plenty of fluids to promote hydration.
    - Encourage the client to take prednisone with food.

- Combination agents (bronchodilator and anti-inflammatory)
  - Ipratropium and albuterol (Combivent)
  - Fluticasone and salmeterol (Advair)
  - If prescribed separately for inhalation administration at the same time, administer the bronchodilator first in order to increase the absorption of the anti-inflammatory agent.

- Interdisciplinary Care
  - Respiratory services should be consulted for inhalers and breathing treatments for airway management.
  - Nutritional services can be contacted for weight loss or gain related to medications or diagnosis.
  - Rehabilitation care can be consulted if the client has prolonged weakness and needs assistance with increasing level of activity.

- Client Outcomes

  o The client will maintain adequate gas exchange.

  o The client will prevent acute attacks.

  o The client will have relief of symptoms.

  o The client will adhere to the medication regimen.

Complications

- Respiratory failure

  o Persistent hypoxemia related to asthma can lead to respiratory failure.

  o Nursing Actions

    ▪ Monitor oxygenation levels and acid-base balance.

    ▪ Prepare for intubation and mechanical ventilation as indicated.

- Status asthmaticus

  o This is a life-threatening episode of airway obstruction that is often unresponsive to common treatment. It involves extreme wheezing, labored breathing, use of accessory muscles, distended neck veins, and creates a risk for cardiac and/or respiratory arrest.

  o Nursing Actions

    ▪ Prepare for emergency intubation.

    ▪ As prescribed, administer oxygen, bronchodilators, epinephrine, and initiate systemic steroid therapy.

CHAPTER 22: ASTHMA

 Application Exercises

Scenario: A nurse is caring for a client who presented to the emergency department with an admitting diagnosis of an acute asthma attack.

1. Which of the following parameters indicate deterioration in the client's respiratory status? (Select all that apply.)

_____ SaO_2 95%

_____ Wheezing

_____ Retraction of sternal muscles

_____ Warm and pink extremities and mucous membranes

_____ Premature ventricular complexes (PVCs)

_____ Respiratory rate of 34/min

_____ Anxiety

2. Two hours after arriving on the medical-surgical unit, the client develops dyspnea. SaO_2 is 91%, and the client is exhibiting audible wheezing and use of accessory muscles. Which of the following medications should the nurse expect to administer?

    A. Antibiotic

    B. Beta-blocker

    C. Antiviral

    D. Beta$_2$ agonist

3. A nurse is completing discharge teaching with a client who has a new prescription for prednisone (Deltasone) for asthma. Which of the following client statements indicates a need for further teaching?

    A. "I will drink plenty of fluids while taking this medication."

    B. "I will tell the doctor if I have black, tarry stools."

    C. "I will take my medication on an empty stomach."

    D. "I will monitor my mouth for cold sores."

CHAPTER 22: ASTHMA

 Application Exercises Answer Key

Scenario: A nurse is caring for a client who presented to the emergency department with an admitting diagnosis of an acute asthma attack.

1. Which of the following parameters indicate deterioration in the client's respiratory status? (Select all that apply.)

_____	SaO$_2$ 95%
X	**Wheezing**
X	**Retraction of sternal muscles**
_____	Warm and pink extremities and mucous membranes
X	**Premature ventricular complexes (PVCs)**
X	**Respiratory rate of 34/min**
X	**Anxiety**

Wheezing, retraction of sternal muscles, PVCs, a respiratory rate of 34/min, and anxiety are all related to a declining respiratory status. Warm and pink extremities and mucous membranes along with an SaO$_2$ of 95% are expected findings within the respiratory system and exhibit no signs of distress.

 NCLEX® Connection: Reductions of Risk Potential, System Specific Assessment

2. Two hours after arriving on the medical-surgical unit, the client develops dyspnea. SaO$_2$ is 91%, and the client is exhibiting audible wheezing and use of accessory muscles. Which of the following medications should the nurse expect to administer?

   A. Antibiotic

   B. Beta-blocker

   C. Antiviral

   D. Beta$_2$ agonist

   The nurse should expect to administer a beta$_2$ agonist. Beta$_2$ agonists are used for relief of acute symptoms. Neither an antibiotic, an antiviral, nor a beta blocker are indicated for this condition.

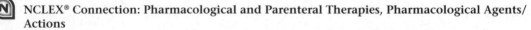 **NCLEX® Connection: Pharmacological and Parenteral Therapies, Pharmacological Agents/ Actions**

3. A nurse is completing discharge teaching with a client who has a new prescription for prednisone (Deltasone) for asthma. Which of the following client statements indicates a need for further teaching?

    A. "I will drink plenty of fluids while taking this medication."

    B. "I will tell the doctor if I have black, tarry stools."

    C. "I will take my medication on an empty stomach."

    D. "I will monitor my mouth for cold sores"

The third statement, "I will take my medication on an empty stomach," indicates a need for further teaching. Prednisone can cause an upset stomach, so it should be taken with food. The other options are all correct statements regarding this medication.

Ⓝ NCLEX® Connection: Physiological Adaptation, Illness Management

UNIT 3	NURSING CARE OF CLIENTS WITH RESPIRATORY DISORDERS
Section	Respiratory System Disorders
Chapter 23	Chronic Obstructive Pulmonary Disease

Ⓞ Overview

- Chronic obstructive pulmonary disease (COPD) encompasses two diseases: emphysema and chronic bronchitis. Most clients who have emphysema also have chronic bronchitis. COPD is irreversible.

- Emphysema is characterized by the loss of lung elasticity and hyperinflation of lung tissue. Emphysema causes destruction of the alveoli, leading to a decreased surface area for gas exchange, carbon dioxide retention, and respiratory acidosis.

- Chronic bronchitis is an inflammation of the bronchi and bronchioles due to chronic exposure to irritants.

Ⓖ
- COPD typically affects middle age to older adults.

Health Promotion and Disease Prevention

- Promote smoking cessation.

- Use protective equipment, such as a mask, and ensure proper ventilation while working in environments that contain carcinogens or particles in the air.

Ⓖ
- Influenza and pneumonia vaccinations are important for all clients who have COPD, but especially for the older adult client.

- Older adult clients have a decreased pulmonary reserve due to normal lung changes.

Assessment

- Risk Factors

  ○ Advanced age

  ○ Cigarette smoking is the primary risk factor for the development of COPD.

  ○ Alpha1-antitrypsin (AAT) deficiency

  ○ Exposure to air pollution

- Subjective Data

  ○ Chronic dyspnea

- Objective Data

  - Physical Assessment Findings

    - Dyspnea upon exertion

    - Productive cough that is most severe upon rising in the morning

    - Respiratory acidosis and compensatory metabolic alkalosis

    - Crackles and wheezes

    - Rapid and shallow respirations

    - Use of accessory muscles

    - Barrel chest or increased chest diameter (with emphysema)

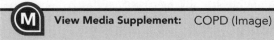

View Media Supplement: COPD (Image)

    - Hyperresonance on percussion due to "trapped air" (with emphysema)

    - Irregular breathing pattern

    - Thin extremities and enlarged neck muscles

    - Dependent edema secondary to right-sided heart failure

    - Clubbing of fingers and toes

    - Pallor and cyanosis of nail beds and mucous membranes (late stages of the disease)

    - Decreased oxygen saturation levels (expected reference range is 95% to 100%)

    - In clients who have dark-colored skin or in older adults, oxygen saturation levels can be slightly lower.

  - Laboratory Tests

    - An increased hematocrit level is due to low oxygenation levels.

    - Use sputum cultures and WBC counts to diagnose acute respiratory infections.

  - Diagnostic Procedures

    - Pulmonary function tests

      - These tests are used for diagnosis, as well as determining the effectiveness of therapy.

      - Comparisons of forced expiratory volume (FEV) to forced vital capacity (FVC) are used to classify COPD as mild to very severe.

      - As COPD advances, the FEV to FVC ratio decreases. The expected reference range is 100%. For mild COPD, the FEV/FVC ratio is decreased to < 70%. As the disease progresses to moderate and severe, the ratio decreases to < 50%.

- Chest x-ray

  □ Reveals hyperinflation of alveoli and flattened diaphragm in the late stages of emphysema.

  □ It is often not useful for the diagnosis of early or moderate disease.

 View Media Supplement: X-ray of Lungs with Emphysema (Image)

- Arterial blood gases (ABGs)

  □ Hypoxemia (decreased PaO_2 < 80 mm Hg)

  □ Hypercarbia (increased $PaCO_2$ > 45 mm Hg)

  □ Respiratory acidosis, metabolic alkalosis compensation

- Pulse oximetry

  □ Clients who have COPD usually have oxygen levels less than the expected reference range of 95% to 100%

- AAT (alpha₁ antitrypsin) levels used to assess for AAT deficiency

  □ A deficiency in a special enzyme produced by the liver that helps regulate other enzymes (that help breakdown pollutants) from attacking lung tissue.

Collaborative Care

- Nursing Care

  ○ Position the client to maximize ventilation (high-Fowler's is 90°).

  ○ Encourage effective coughing, or suction to remove secretions.

  ○ Encourage deep breathing and use of an incentive spirometer.

  ○ Administer breathing treatments and medications as prescribed.

  ○ Administer oxygen as prescribed.

  ○ Monitor for skin breakdown around the nose and mouth from the oxygen device.

  ○ Promote adequate nutrition.

    - Increased work of breathing increases caloric demands.

    - Proper nutrition aids in the prevention of infection.

    - Encourage fluids to promote adequate hydration.

    - Dyspnea decreases energy available for eating, so soft, high-calorie foods should be encouraged.

  ○ Monitor current weight and note any changes.

- o Instruct the client to practice breathing techniques to control dyspneic episodes.
  - For diaphragmatic, or abdominal, breathing, instruct the client to:
    - □ Take breaths deep from the diaphragm.
    - □ Lie on back with knees bent.
    - □ Rest hand over abdomen to create resistance.
    - □ If the client's hand rises and lowers upon inhalation and exhalation, the breathing is being performed correctly.
  - For pursed lip breathing, instruct the client to:
    - □ Form the mouth as if preparing to whistle.
    - □ Take a breath in through the nose and out through the lips/mouth.
    - □ Do not puff the cheeks.
    - □ Take breaths deep and slow.
- o Incentive spirometry
  - This is used to monitor optimal lung expansion.
  - Nursing Actions
    - □ Show the client how to use the incentive spirometry machine.
  - Client Education
    - □ Instruct the client to keep a tight mouth seal around mouthpiece and to inhale and hold breath for 3 to 5 seconds. As the client inhales, the needle of the spirometry machine will rise. This promotes lung expansion.
- o Clients who have COPD may need 2 to 4 L/min of oxygen via nasal cannula or up to 40% via Venturi mask.
  - Clients who have chronically increased $PaCO_2$ levels usually require 1 to 2 L/min of oxygen via nasal cannula.
  - It is important to recognize that low arterial levels of oxygen serve as the primary drive for breathing.
- o Determine the client's physical limitations and structure activity to include periods of rest.
- o Provide rest periods for older adult clients who have dyspnea. Design the room and walkways with opportunities for relaxation.
- o Provide support to the client and family.
  - Talk about disease and lifestyle changes, including homecare services such as portable oxygen.
- o Encourage verbalization of feelings.
- o Increase fluid intake.
  - Encourage the client to drink 2 to 3 L/day to liquify mucus.

- Medications
  - Bronchodilators (inhalers)
    - Short-acting beta$_2$ agonists, such as albuterol (Proventil, Ventolin) provide rapid relief.
    - Cholinergic antagonists (anticholinergic medications), such as ipratropium (Atrovent), block the parasympathetic nervous system. This allows for the sympathetic nervous system effects of increased bronchodilation and decreased pulmonary secretions.
    - Methylxanthines, such as theophylline (Theo-Dur), relax smooth muscles of the bronchi. These medications require close monitoring of serum medication levels due to narrow therapeutic ranges.
    - Nursing Considerations
      - Monitor the client's serum levels for toxicity when taking theophylline. Side effects will include tachycardia, nausea, and diarrhea.
      - Watch the client for tremors and tachycardia when taking albuterol.
      - Observe the client for dry mouth when taking ipratropium.
    - Client Education
      - Encourage the client to suck on hard candies to help moisten dry mouth while taking ipratropium.
  - Anti-inflammatory agents
    - These medications decrease airway inflammation.
    - If corticosteroids, such as fluticasone (Flovent) and prednisone (Deltasone), are given systemically, monitor for serious side effects (immunosuppression, fluid retention, hyperglycemia, hypokalemia, poor wound healing).
    - Leukotriene antagonists, such as montelukast (Singulair); mast cell stabilizers, such as cromolyn sodium (Intal); and monoclonal antibodies, such as omalizumab (Xolair), can be used.
    - Nursing Considerations
      - Watch the client for a decrease in immunity function.
      - Monitor the client for hyperglycemia.
      - Advise the client to report black, tarry stools.
      - Observe the client for fluid retention and weight gain. This is common.
      - Check the client's throat and mouth for aphthous lesions (cold sores).
    - Client Education
      - Encourage the client to drink plenty of fluids to promote hydration.
      - Encourage the client to take glucocorticoids (Prednisone) with food.

- Interdisciplinary Care

  o Respiratory services should be consulted for inhalers, breathing treatments, and suctioning for airway management.

  o Nutritional services should be contacted for weight loss or gain related to medications or diagnosis.

  o Rehabilitative care can be consulted if the client has prolonged weakness and needs assistance with increasing level of activity.

- Therapeutic Procedures

  o Chest physiotherapy uses percussion and vibration to mobilize secretions.

  o Raising the foot of the bed slightly higher than the head can facilitate optimal drainage and removal of secretions by gravity.

- Care after Discharge

  Ⓖ

  o COPD is debilitating for older adult clients. Referrals to assistance programs, such as food delivery services, can be indicated.

  o Set-up referral services, including homecare services such as portable oxygen.

  o Client Education

    ▪ Encourage the client to eat high-calorie foods to promote energy.

    ▪ Encourage rest periods as needed.

    ▪ Promote hand hygiene to prevent infection.

    ▪ Reinforce the importance of taking medications (inhalers, oral medications) as prescribed.

    ▪ Promote smoking cessation if the client is a smoker.

    ▪ Encourage immunizations, such as influenza and pneumonia, to decrease the risk of infection.

    ▪ Clients should use oxygen as prescribed. Inform other caregivers not to smoke around the oxygen due to flammability.

    ▪ Provide support to the client and family.

- Client Outcomes

  o The client will maintain adequate gas exchange.

  o The client will be able to keep a patent airway.

  o The client will remain free from infection.

  o The client will be able to maintain 10% of ideal body weight.

Complications

- Respiratory infection

  - Respiratory infections result from increased mucus production and poor oxygenation levels.

  - Nursing Actions

    - Administer oxygen therapy.

    - Monitor oxygenation levels.

    - Administer antibiotics and other medications as prescribed.

- Right-sided heart failure (cor pulmonale)

  - Air trapping, airway collapse, and stiff alveoli lead to increased pulmonary pressures.

  - Blood flow through the lung tissue is difficult. This increased workload leads to enlargement and thickening of the right atrium and ventricle.

  - Manifestations include:

    - Low oxygenation levels

    - Cyanotic lips

    - Enlarged and tender liver

    - Distended neck veins

    - Dependent edema

  - Nursing Actions

    - Monitor respiratory status and administer oxygen therapy.

    - Monitor heart rate and rhythm.

    - Administer medications as prescribed.

    - Administer IV fluids and diuretics to maintain fluid balance.

CHAPTER 23: CHRONIC OBSTRUCTIVE PULMONARY DISEASE

 Application Exercises

1. Match the interventions listed below with the appropriate COPD management techniques in the table.

AIRWAY MANAGEMENT	COUGH ENHANCEMENT	OXYGEN THERAPY	ENERGY MANAGEMENT

   A. Encourage the client to take deep breaths.

   B. Monitor the position of the oxygen delivery device.

   C. Promote bedrest.

   D. Position the client to maximize ventilation potential.

   E. Assist with incentive spirometry.

   F. Determine the client's physical limitations.

   G. Instruct the client to breathe deeply, hold breath for 3 to 5 seconds, and then cough two to three times.

2. A middle-aged client presents to the emergency department with symptoms of dyspnea, chronic cough, and sputum production. The client is newly diagnosed with emphysema. She currently smokes one pack of cigarettes a day and has been smoking since she was 19. When the nurse talks about smoking cessation programs, the client doesn't believe quitting will help because the damage is already done. How should the nurse respond to the client?

3. When discharging a client home who is on oxygen, which of the following is most important for the nurse to teach?

   A. Smoking cessation

   B. Equipment maintenance

   C. Incorporating rest into ADLs

   D. Anger management

4. A nurse is caring for a client who has COPD. Upon discharge, the client is concerned that he will never be able to leave his house now that he has been placed on continuous oxygen. Which of the following statements should the nurse make?

    A. "There are portable oxygen delivery systems that you can take with you."

    B. "When you go out, you can remove the oxygen and then reapply it when you get home."

    C. "You probably will not be able to go out as much as you used to."

    D. "Home health services will come to you so you will not need to get out."

CHAPTER 23: CHRONIC OBSTRUCTIVE PULMONARY DISEASE

(A) Application Exercises Answer Key

1. Match the interventions listed below with the appropriate COPD management techniques in the table.

AIRWAY MANAGEMENT	COUGH ENHANCEMENT	OXYGEN THERAPY	ENERGY MANAGEMENT
D. Position the client to maximize ventilation potential. E. Assist with incentive spirometry.	A. Encourage the client to take deep breaths. G. Instruct the client to breathe deeply, hold breath for 3 to 5 seconds, and then cough two to three times.	B. Monitor the position of the oxygen delivery device.	C. Promote bedrest. F. Determine the client's physical limitations.

      A. Encourage the client to take deep breaths.

      B. Monitor the position of the oxygen delivery device.

      C. Promote bedrest.

      D. Position the client to maximize ventilation potential.

      E. Assist with incentive spirometry.

      F. Determine the client's physical limitations.

      G. Instruct the client to breathe deeply, hold breath for 3 to 5 seconds, and then cough two to three times.

(N) **NCLEX® Connection: Physiological Adaptation, Illness Management**

2. A middle-aged client presents to the emergency department with symptoms of dyspnea, chronic cough, and sputum production. The client is newly diagnosed with emphysema. She currently smokes one pack of cigarettes a day and has been smoking since she was 19. When the nurse talks about smoking cessation programs, the client doesn't believe quitting will help because the damage is already done. How should the nurse respond to the client?

      The nurse should inform the client that smoking cessation at any point will improve her prognosis.

 NCLEX® Connection: Physical Adaptation, Pathophysiology

3. When discharging a client home who is on oxygen, which of the following is most important for the nurse to teach?

    A. Smoking cessation

    B. Equipment maintenance

    C. Incorporating rest into ADLs

    D. Anger management

    Using the safety/risk reduction priority setting framework, keeping the client free from injury and harm is the first priority. Oxygen enhances combustion; therefore, all flames, including lit cigarettes and candles, should be kept away from the oxygen flow. Equipment maintenance, incorporating rest into ADLs, and anger management are all part of this process but are not the priority at this time.

 NCLEX® Connection: Physiological Adaptation, Illness Management

4. A nurse is caring for a client who has COPD. Upon discharge, the client is concerned that he will never be able to leave his house now that he has been placed on continuous oxygen. Which of the following statements should the nurse make?

    A. "There are portable oxygen delivery systems that you can take with you."

    B. "When you go out, you can remove the oxygen and then reapply it when you get home."

    C. "You probably will not be able to go out as much as you used to."

    D. "Home health services will come to you so you will not need to get out."

    The client should be informed that there are portable oxygen systems that he can use to leave the house. This should allay his anxiety. The other responses are not therapeutic.

 NCLEX® Connection: Physiological Adaptation, Alterations in Body Systems

UNIT 3	NURSING CARE OF CLIENTS WITH RESPIRATORY DISORDERS
Section	Respiratory System Disorders
Chapter 24	Pneumonia

Overview

- Pneumonia is an inflammatory process in the lungs that produces excess fluid. Pneumonia is triggered by infectious organisms or by the aspiration of an irritant, such as fluid or a foreign object.

- The inflammatory process in the lung parenchyma results in edema and exudate that fills the alveoli.

- Pneumonia can be a primary disease or a complication of another disease or condition. It affects people of all ages, but the young, older adult clients, and clients who are immunocompromised are more susceptible. Immobility can be a contributing factor in the development of pneumonia.

- There are two types of pneumonia. Community acquired pneumonia (CAP) is the most common type and often occurs as a complication of influenza. Hospital acquired pneumonia (HAP), also known as nosocomial pneumonia, has a higher mortality rate and is more likely to be resistant to antibiotics. It usually takes 24 to 48 hr from the time the client is exposed to acquire HAP.

- Older adult clients are more susceptible to infections and have decreased pulmonary reserves due to normal lung changes, including decreased lung elasticity and thickening alveoli.

Health Promotion and Disease Prevention

- Encourage older adult clients, especially those who have chronic illnesses, to receive immunizations for influenza and pneumonia.

- Promote smoking cessation.

- Perform frequent hand hygiene to prevent the spread of infection.

Assessment

- Risk Factors
    - Advanced age
    - Recent exposure to viral or influenza infections
    - Tobacco use

- ○ Substance abuse (alcohol, cocaine)

- ○ Chronic lung disease (asthma, emphysema)

- ○ Conditions that increase the risk of aspiration (dysphagia)

- ○ Mechanical ventilation (ventilator acquired pneumonia)

- ○ Impaired ability to mobilize secretions (decreased level of consciousness, immobility, recent abdominal or thoracic surgery)

- ○ Immunocompromised status

- ○ Older adult clients have a weak cough reflex and decreased muscle strength. Therefore, they have trouble expectorating, which can lead to difficulty in breathing and make specimen retrieval more difficult.

- ○ Inactivity and immobility

- **Subjective Data**

  - ○ Anxiety

  - ○ Fatigue

  - ○ Weakness

  - ○ Chest discomfort

  - ○ Confusion from hypoxia is the most common manifestation of pneumonia in older adult clients.

- **Objective Data**

  - ○ Physical Assessment Findings

    - ▪ Fever

    - ▪ Chills

    - ▪ Flushed face

    - ▪ Diaphoretic

    - ▪ Shortness of breath or difficulty breathing

    - ▪ Tachypnea

    - ▪ Pleuritic chest pain (sharp)

    - ▪ Sputum production (yellow-tinged)

    - ▪ Crackles and wheezes

    - ▪ Coughing

    - ▪ Dull chest percussion over areas of consolidation

    - ▪ Decreased oxygen saturation levels (expected reference range is 95% to 100%)

    - ▪ Fever, cough, and yellow-tinged sputum are often absent in clients who have pneumonia.

- o Laboratory Tests
  - CBC
    - □ Elevated WBC count (may not be present in older adult clients)
  - Sputum culture and sensitivity
    - □ Obtain specimen before starting antibiotic therapy.
    - □ Obtain specimen by suctioning if the client is unable to cough.
    - □ The responsible organism is only identified about 50% of the time.
    - □ Older adult clients have a weak cough reflex and decreased muscle strength. Therefore, older adult clients have trouble expectorating, which can lead to difficulty in breathing and make specimen retrieval more difficult.
  - ABGs
    - □ Hypoxemia (decreased $PaO_2 < 80$ mm Hg)
- o Diagnostic Procedures
  - Chest x-ray
    - □ A chest x-ray will show consolidation (solidification, density) of lung tissue.
    - □ A chest x-ray is an important diagnostic tool because the early signs and symptoms of pneumonia are often vague in older adult clients.

  View Media Supplement: Pneumonia (Image)

  - Pulse Oximetry
    - □ Clients who have pneumonia usually have oximetry levels less than the expected reference range of 95% to 100%.

Collaborative Care

- Nursing Care
  - o Position the client to maximize ventilation (high-Fowler's = 90%).
  - o Encourage coughing or suction to remove secretions.
  - o Administer breathing treatments and medications as prescribed.
  - o Administer oxygen therapy as prescribed.
  - o Monitor for skin breakdown around the nose and mouth from the oxygen device.
  - o Encourage deep breathing with an incentive spirometer to prevent alveolar collapse.
  - o Determine the client's physical limitations and structure activity to include periods of rest.
  - o Promote adequate nutrition.

- ○ An increased work of breathing increases caloric demands.

- ○ Proper nutrition aids in the prevention of secondary respiratory infections.

- ○ Encourage fluid intake of 2 to 3 L/day to promote hydration and thinning of secretions, unless contraindicated due to another condition.

Ⓖ
- ○ Provide rest periods for older adult clients who have dyspnea.

- ○ Reassure the client who is experiencing respiratory distress.

- Medications

  - ○ Antibiotics

    - Antibiotics are given to destroy infectious pathogens, and commonly used antibiotics include penicillins and cephalosporins.

    - Antibiotics are often initially given via IV and then switched to an oral form as the client's condition improves.

    - It is important to obtain any culture specimens prior to giving the first dose of an antibiotic. Once the specimen has been obtained, the antibiotics can be given while waiting for the results of the ordered culture.

    - Nursing Considerations

      - □ Observe clients taking cephalosporins for frequent stools.

      - □ Monitor clients kidney function, especially older adults who are taking penicillins and cephalosporins.

    - Client Education

      - □ Encourage clients to take penicillins and cephalosporins with food. Some penicillins should be taken 1 hr before meals or 2 hr after.

  - ○ Bronchodilators

    - Bronchodilators are given to reduce bronchospasms and reduce irritation.

      - □ Short-acting beta$_2$ agonists, such as albuterol, provide rapid relief.

      - □ Cholinergic antagonists (anticholinergic medications), such as ipratropium (Atrovent), block the parasympathetic nervous system, allowing for increased bronchodilation and decreased pulmonary secretions.

      - □ Methylxanthines, such as theophylline (Theo-Dur), require close monitoring of serum medication levels due to the narrow therapeutic range.

    - Nursing Considerations

      - □ Monitor serum medication levels for toxicity for clients taking theophylline. Side effects will include tachycardia, nausea, and diarrhea.

      - □ Watch for tremors and tachycardia for clients taking albuterol.

      - □ Observe for dry mouth for clients taking ipratropium.

- Client Education
  - Encourage clients to suck on hard candies to help moisten dry mouth while taking ipratropium.
- Anti-inflammatories
  - Anti-inflammatories decrease airway inflammation.
  - Glucocorticosteroids, such as fluticasone (Flovent) and prednisone (Deltasone), can be prescribed to help with inflammation. Monitor for immunosuppression, fluid retention, hyperglycemia, hypokalemia, and poor wound healing.
  - Nursing Considerations
    - Monitor the client for decreased immunity function.
    - Monitor the client for hyperglycemia.
    - Advise the client to report black, tarry stools.
    - Observe the client for fluid retention and weight gain. This can be common.
    - Monitor the client's throat and mouth for aphthous lesions (cold sores).
  - Client Education
    - Encourage the client to drink plenty of fluids to promote hydration.
    - Encourage the client to take glucocorticosteroids with food.

- Interdisciplinary Care
  - Respiratory services should be consulted for inhalers, breathing treatments, and suctioning for airway management.
  - Nutritional services can be contacted for weight loss or gain of the client related to medications or diagnosis.
  - Rehabilitation care can be consulted if the client has prolonged weakness and needs assistance with increasing level of activity.

- Care after Discharge
  - Client Education
    - Educate the client on the importance of continuing medications for treatment of pneumonia.
    - Encourage rest periods as needed.
    - Encourage the client to maintain hand hygiene to prevent infection.
    - Encourage the client to avoid crowded areas to reduce the risk of infection.
    - Remind the client that treatment and recovery from pneumonia can take time.
    - Encourage immunizations for influenza and pneumonia.
    - Promote smoking cessation if the client is a smoker.

- o Client Outcomes
  - The client is able to maintain adequate gas exchange.
  - The client is able to keep a patent airway.
  - The client remains free from infection.

Complications

- Atelectasis
  - o Airway inflammation and edema lead to alveolar collapse and increase the risk of hypoxemia.
  - o The client might report shortness of breath and exhibit signs of hypoxemia.
  - o The client might have diminished or absent breath sounds over the affected area.
  - o A chest x-ray will show an area of density.
- Bacteremia (sepsis)
  - o This can occur if pathogens enter the bloodstream from the infection in the lungs.

CHAPTER 24: PNEUMONIA

 Application Exercises

1. Which of the following clients have an increased risk for developing pneumonia? (Select all that apply.)

_____ Client who has dysphagia

_____ Client who has AIDS

_____ Client who was vaccinated for pneumococcus and influenza 6 months ago

_____ Client who is postoperative and has received local anesthesia

_____ Client who has a closed head injury and is receiving ventilation

_____ Client who has myasthenia gravis

Scenario: A nurse is caring for a 76-year-old female client brought in to an outpatient clinic by her husband. The husband states that his wife woke up this morning and did not recognize him or know where she was. The client reports chills and chest pain that worsens with inspiration.

---

2. Which of the following is the highest priority nursing task?

A. Obtain baseline vital signs and oxygen saturation.

B. Obtain a sputum culture.

C. Obtain a complete history from the client.

D. Provide a pneumococcal vaccination.

3. Further assessment yields the following vital signs: temperature 37.3° C (99.1° F), respiratory rate 30/min, blood pressure 130/76 mm Hg, pulse 110/min, and SaO_2 91% on room air. Using a scale of 1 to 4 with 1 being the highest priority, prioritize the following nursing interventions.

_____ Administer antibiotics as prescribed.

_____ Administer oxygen therapy.

_____ Perform a sputum culture.

_____ Administer an antipyretic medication to promote client comfort.

---

4. A nurse is caring for a client who has pneumonia and has a prescription for prednisone (Deltasone). The nurse should monitor the client for which of the following? (Select all that apply.)

_____ Fluid retention

_____ Tremors

_____ Hyperglycemia

_____ Fever

_____ Black, tarry stools

CHAPTER 24: PNEUMONIA

 Application Exercises Answer Key

1. Which of the following clients have an increased risk for developing pneumonia? (Select all that apply.)

__X__	**Client who has dysphagia**
__X__	**Client who has AIDS**
_____	Client who was vaccinated for pneumococcus and influenza 6 months ago
_____	Client who is postoperative and has received local anesthesia
__X__	**Client who has a closed head injury and is receiving ventilation**
__X__	**Client who has myasthenia gravis**

A client who has difficulty swallowing has an increased risk of aspiration, which increases the risk of pneumonia. A client who has AIDS is immunocompromised, which increases the risk of opportunistic infections, such as pneumonia. Mechanical ventilation is invasive and increases the risk of respiratory infections. A client who has myasthenia gravis has generalized weakness and will have difficulty clearing secretions from the airway, which increases the risk of infection. A client who has recently been vaccinated in the past few months is least likely to acquire pneumonia. A client who is postoperative should not be immunosuppressed, since he has just received surgery.

Ⓝ NCLEX® Connection: Physiological Adaptation, Alterations in Body Systems

---

Scenario: A nurse is caring for a 76-year-old female client brought in to an outpatient clinic by her husband. The husband states that his wife woke up this morning and did not recognize him or know where she was. The client reports chills and chest pain that worsens with inspiration.

---

2. Which of the following is the highest priority nursing task?

A. Obtain baseline vital signs and oxygen saturation.

B. Obtain a sputum culture.

C. Obtain a complete history from the client.

D. Provide a pneumococcal vaccination.

Assessment is the first step of the nursing process and is an essential first step in planning client care. It is important in prioritizing care to meet the client's physiologic needs first, which is the respiratory system in this case.

Ⓝ NCLEX® Connection: Reduction of Risk Potential, System Specific Assessment

3. Further assessment yields the following vital signs: temperature 37.3° C (99.1° F), respiratory rate 30/min, blood pressure 130/76 mm Hg, pulse 110/min, and SaO$_2$ 91% on room air. Using a scale of 1 to 4 with 1 being the highest priority, prioritize the following nursing interventions.

    __3__   Administer antibiotics as prescribed.

    __1__   Administer oxygen therapy.

    __2__   Perform a sputum culture.

    __4__   Administer an antipyretic medication to promote client comfort.

The client's respiratory and heart rates are elevated, and her oxygen saturation level is 91% on room air. These signs indicate that her oxygenation needs are not being met. Therefore, according to the ABC priority framework, providing oxygen is the highest priority. After starting the oxygen, it is important to obtain the sputum specimen before starting the antibiotics and administering an antipyretic.

Ⓝ **NCLEX® Connection: Physiological Adaptation, Illness Management**

4. A nurse is caring for a client who has pneumonia and has a prescription for prednisone (Deltasone). The nurse should monitor the client for which of the following? (Select all that apply.)

    __X__   **Fluid retention**

    _____   Tremors

    __X__   **Hyperglycemia**

    __X__   **Fever**

    __X__   **Black, tarry stools**

Fluid retention and hyperglycemia are adverse effects of prednisone. The immunosuppressive action of prednisone places the client at risk for infection which can be signaled by the presence of fever. Prednisone can cause a peptic ulcer which may cause tarry stools. Tremors are a side effect of albuterol and theophylline (Theo-Dur), but not prednisone.

Ⓝ **NCLEX® Connection: Pharmacological and Parenteral Therapies, Adverse Effects/Contraindications/Side Effects/Interactions**

UNIT 3	NURSING CARE OF CLIENTS WITH RESPIRATORY DISORDERS
Section	Respiratory System Disorders

Chapter 25   Tuberculosis

Overview

- Tuberculosis (TB) is an infectious disease caused by *Mycobacterium tuberculosis*.

- TB is transmitted through aerosolization (airborne route).

- Once inside the lung, the body encases the TB bacillus with collagen and other cells. This may appear as a Ghon tubercle on a chest x-ray.

- Only a small percentage of people infected with TB actually develop an active form of the infection. The TB bacillus may lie dormant for many years before producing the disease.

- TB primarily affects the lungs but can spread to any organ in the blood.

- The risk of transmission decreases after 2 to 3 weeks of antibiotic therapy.

- An intradermal TB test is a common screening tool to assess for TB infection. A client's TB test will be positive within 2 to 10 weeks of exposure to the infection.

- Early detection and treatment are vital. TB has a slow onset, and the client may not be aware until the symptoms and disease are advanced. TB diagnosis should be considered for any client with a persistent cough, weight loss, anorexia, hemoptysis, dyspnea, fever, night sweats, or chills.

- Increasing the percentage of clients who complete treatment for TB should be a goal.

- Individuals who have been exposed to TB but have not developed the disease may have latent TB. This means that the mycobacterium tuberculosis in the body, but the body has been able to fight off the infection. If not treated, it can lie dormant for several years and then become active as the individual becomes older or immunocompromised.

Health Promotion and Disease Prevention

- Clients who live in high risk areas for tuberculosis should be screened on a yearly basis.

- Family members of clients diagnosed with tuberculosis should be screened.

Assessment

- Risk Factors

  o Frequent and close contact with an untreated individual

- ○ Lower socioeconomic status and homelessness

- ○ Immunocompromised status (HIV, chemotherapy)

- ○ Poorly ventilated, crowded environments (prisons, long-term care facilities)

- ○ Advanced age

- ○ Recent travel outside of the United States to areas where TB is endemic

- ○ Substance abuse

- ○ Health care occupation that involves performance of high-risk activities (respiratory treatments, suctioning, coughing procedures)

- Subjective Data

  - ○ Persistent cough

  - ○ Purulent sputum, possibly blood-streaked

  - ○ Fatigue and lethargy

  - ○ Weight loss and anorexia

  - ○ Night sweats and low-grade fever in the afternoon

- Objective Data

  - ○ Physical Assessment Findings

    - ■ Older adult clients often present with atypical symptoms of the disease (altered mentation or unusual behavior, fever, anorexia, weight loss).

  - ○ Laboratory Tests

    - ■ QuantiFERON-TB Gold

      - □ Blood test that detects release of interferon-gamma (IFN-g) in fresh heparinized whole blood from sensitized people

      - □ Diagnostic for infection, whether it is active or latent

  - ○ Diagnostic Procedures

    - ■ Mantoux test (should be read in 48 to 72 hr)

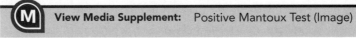

View Media Supplement: Positive Mantoux Test (Image)

      - □ An intradermal injection of an extract of the tubercle bacillus is made.

      - □ An induration (palpable, raised, hardened area) of 10 mm or greater in diameter indicates a positive skin test.

      - □ An induration of 5 mm is considered a positive test for immunocompromised clients.

        □ A positive Mantoux test indicates that the client has developed an immune response to TB. It does not confirm that active disease is present. Clients who have been treated for TB may retain a positive reaction.

        □ Individuals who have latent TB may have a positive Mantoux test and may receive treatment to prevent development of an active form of the disease.

        □ Clients who have received a Bacillus Calmette-Guerin (BCG) vaccine within the past 10 years may have a false-positive Mantoux test. These clients will need a chest x-ray to evaluate the presence of active TB infection.

        □ Clients who are HIV positive should be tested for TB.

        □ Client Education

            ▸ Reinforce to the client the importance of returning for a reading of the injection site by a health care personnel within 48 to 72 hr.

- A chest x-ray may be ordered to detect active lesions in the lungs.

- Acid-fast bacilli smear and culture

        □ A positive acid-fast test suggests an active infection.

        □ The diagnosis is confirmed by a positive culture for *Mycobacterium tuberculosis*.

        □ Nursing Actions

            ▸ Three early morning sputum samples are obtained.

            ▸ Wear personal protective equipment when obtaining specimens.

            ▸ Samples should also be obtained in a negative airflow room.

Collaborative Care

- Nursing Care

    ○ Administer heated and humidified oxygen therapy as prescribed.

    ○ Prevent infection transmission.

        ■ Wear an N95 or HEPA respirator when caring for clients who are hospitalized with TB.

        ■ Place the client in a negative airflow room and implement airborne precautions.

        ■ Use barrier protection when the risk of hand or clothing contamination exists.

        ■ Have the client wear a mask if transportation to another department is necessary. The client should be transported using the shortest and least busy route.

        ■ Teach the client to cough and expectorate sputum into tissues that are disposed of by the client into provided sacks.

    ○ Administer medications as prescribed.

    ○ Promote adequate nutrition.

        ■ Encourage fluid intake and a well-balanced diet for adequate caloric intake.

- Encourage foods that are rich in protein, iron, and vitamin C.
  - Provide emotional support.
- Medications
  - Due to the resistance that is developing against the anti-tuberculin medications, combination therapy of up to four medications at a time is presently recommended.
  - Since these medications must be taken for 6 to 12 months, medication noncompliance is a major contributing factor in the development of resistant strains of TB.
  - The current four-medication regimen includes isoniazid (Nydrazid), rifampin (Rifadin), pyrazinamide, and ethambutol hydrochloride (Myambutol).
  - Isoniazid
    - Isoniazid, commonly referred to as INH, is bactericidal and inhibits growth of mycobacteria by preventing synthesis of mycolic acid in the cell wall.
    - Nursing Considerations
      - This medication should be taken on an empty stomach.
      - Monitor for hepatotoxicity and neurotoxicity, such as tingling of the hands and feet.
      - Vitamin B_6 (pyridoxine) is used to prevent neurotoxicity from isoniazid
    - Client Education
      - Advise the client not to drink alcohol while taking isoniazid, because it may increase the risk for hepatotoxicity.
  - Rifampin
    - Rifampin, commonly referred to as RIF, is a bacteriostatic and bactericidal antibiotic that inhibits DNA-dependent RNA polymerase activity in susceptible cells.
    - Nursing Considerations
      - Observe for hepatotoxicity.
    - Client Education
      - Inform the client that urine and other secretions will be orange.
      - Advise the client to report yellowing of the skin, pain or swelling of joints, loss of appetite, or malaise immediately.
      - Inform the client this medication may interfere with the efficacy of oral contraceptives.
  - Pyrazinamide
    - Pyrazinamide, commonly referred to as PZA, is a bacteriostatic and bactericidal, and its exact mechanism of action is unknown.
    - Nursing Considerations
      - Observe for hepatotoxicity.

- Client Education
    - Instruct the client to drink a glass of water with each dose and increase fluids during the day.
    - Advise the client to report yellowing of the skin, pain or swelling of joints, loss of appetite, or malaise immediately.
    - Advise the client to avoid using alcohol while taking pyrazinamide.
  - Ethambutol
    - Ethambutol, commonly referred to as EMB, is a bacteriostatic and works by suppressing RNA synthesis, subsequently inhibiting protein synthesis.
    - Nursing Considerations
        - Obtain baseline visual acuity tests.
        - Determine color discrimination ability.
        - This medication should not be given to children under 13 years of age.
    - Client Education
        - Instruct the client to report changes in vision immediately.
  - Streptomycin sulfate (Streptomycin)
    - Streptomycin sulfate is an aminoglycoside antibiotic. It potentiates the efficacy of macrophages during phagocytosis.
    - Nursing Considerations
        - Due to its high level of toxicity, this medication should only be used in clients who have multi-drug resistance TB (MDR-TB).
        - It can cause ototoxicity, so monitor hearing function and tolerance often.
        - Report significant changes in urine output and renal function studies.
    - Client Education
        - Advise the client to drink at least 2 to 3 L of fluid daily.
        - Advise the client to notify the provider if hearing declines.
- Interdisciplinary Care
  - Contact social services if the client will need assistance in obtaining prescribed medications.
  - Refer the client to a community clinic as necessary for follow-up appointments to monitor medication regimen and status of disease.

o   Client Education

- Provide the client and family education because TB is often treated in the home setting.

  □   Exposed family members should be tested for TB.

  □   Educate the client and family to continue medication therapy for its full duration of 6 to 12 months. Emphasize that failure to take the medications may lead to a resistant strain of TB.

  □   Instruct the client to continue with follow-up care for 1 full year.

  □   Inform the client that sputum samples are needed every 2 to 4 weeks to monitor therapy effectiveness. Clients are no longer considered infectious after three negative sputum cultures.

  □   Encourage proper hand hygiene.

  □   Instruct the client to cover her mouth and nose when coughing or sneezing.

  □   Inform the client that contaminated tissues should be disposed of in plastic bags.

  □   Advise clients with active TB to wear masks when in public places.

o   Client Outcomes

- The client will adhere with the medication regimen.

- The client's sputum will test negative for TB.

Complications

- Military TB

  o   The organism invades the blood stream and can spread to multiple body organs with complications including:

  - Headaches, neck stiffness, and drowsiness (can be life-threatening)

  - Pericarditis

    □   Dyspnea, swollen neck veins, pleuritic pain, and hypotension due to an accumulation of fluid in pericardial sac that inhibits the heart's ability to pump effectively

  o   Nursing Actions

  - Treatment is the same as for pulmonary TB.

CHAPTER 25: TUBERCULOSIS

 Application Exercises

Scenario: A home health nurse is caring for an older adult client who has active tuberculosis. The client lives at home with her husband. She is prescribed the following medication regimen: Isoniazid (Nydrazid) 250 mg PO daily, Rifampin (Rifadin) 500 mg PO daily, Pyrazinamide 750 mg PO daily, and Ethambutol (Myambutol) 1 g PO daily.

1. Which of the following statements indicate that the client understands appropriate care measures? (Select all that apply.)

   _____ "It is okay to substitute one medication for another when I run out because they all fight the infection."

   _____ "I will wash my hands each time I cough or sneeze."

   _____ "I will increase my intake of citrus fruits, red meats, and whole grains."

   _____ "I am glad that I don't have to collect any more sputum specimens."

   _____ "I will make sure that I wear a mask when I am in a public place."

   _____ "I do not need to worry about where I go once I start taking my medications."

2. Should the client's husband be tested for TB?

3. A client recently diagnosed with tuberculosis is placed on a multi-medication regimen. Which of the following instructions should the nurse give the client in regard to ethambutol (Myambutol)?

   A. "Your urine may turn a dark orange."

   B. "Watch for a change in the color of your sclera."

   C. "Watch for any changes in vision."

   D. "Take vitamin B$_6$ daily."

CHAPTER 25: TUBERCULOSIS

 Application Exercises Answer Key

Scenario: A home health nurse is caring for an older adult client who has active tuberculosis. The client lives at home with her husband. She is prescribed the following medication regimen: Isoniazid (Nydrazid) 250 mg PO daily, Rifampin (Rifadin) 500 mg PO daily, Pyrazinamide 750 mg PO daily, and Ethambutol (Myambutol) 1 g PO daily.

1. Which of the following statements indicate that the client understands appropriate care measures? (Select all that apply.)

   _____ "It is okay to substitute one medication for another when I run out because they all fight the infection."

   __X__ **"I will wash my hands each time I cough or sneeze."**

   __X__ **"I will increase my intake of citrus fruits, red meats, and whole grains."**

   _____ "I am glad that I don't have to collect any more sputum specimens."

   __X__ **"I will make sure that I wear a mask when I am in a public place."**

   _____ "I do not need to worry about where I go once I start taking my medications."

   The correct statements demonstrate understanding by the client on how to prevent infection and promote nutrition. The remaining statements are direct contradictions for appropriate care practices, such as adhering to the medication regimen and continuing sputum collection to monitor disease progression.

   Ⓝ NCLEX® Connection: Physiological Adaptation, Alterations in Body Systems

2. Should the client's husband be tested for TB?

   Yes, any exposed family members should be tested for TB.

   Ⓝ NCLEX® Connection: Physiological Adaptation, Alterations in Body Systems

3. A client recently diagnosed with tuberculosis is placed on a multi-medication regimen. Which of the following instructions should the nurse give the client in regard to ethambutol (Myambutol)?

   A. "Your urine may turn a dark orange."

   B. "Watch for a change in the color of your sclera."

   C. "Watch for any changes in vision."

   D. "Take vitamin B_6 daily."

   Clients taking ethambutol will need to watch for changes in vision due to optic neuritis. Clients receiving isoniazid should take vitamin B_6 daily and observe for signs of hepatotoxicity. Clients receiving rifampin should expect their urine to turn a dark orange to brown.

   Ⓝ NCLEX® Connection: Pharmacological and parenteral Therapies, Adverse Effects/ Contraindications/Side Effects/Interactions

UNIT 3	NURSING CARE OF CLIENTS WITH RESPIRATORY DISORDERS
Section	Respiratory System Disorders
Chapter 26	Laryngeal Cancer

Overview

- Laryngeal cancer can be devastating because of its impact on a client's ability to breath, eat, and speak, as well as the impact on the client's appearance.

- Men are three times more likely to be affected than women, and most cancers occur after 60 years of age.

- Most laryngeal cancers are slow-growing squamous cell carcinomas.

- Treatment includes laryngectomy, radiation, and/or chemotherapy.

Health Promotion/Disease Prevention

- Advise the client to refrain from smoking and excessive alcohol intake.

Assessment

- Risk Factors

  o Tobacco and alcohol use are the primary risk factors. Their effects are synergistic when used in combination.

  o Chronic exposure to harmful chemicals, (asbestos, metals, wood, paint fumes, tar products also increases risk.)

- Subjective Data

  - Persistent or recurrent hoarseness or sore throat

  - Lump in throat, mouth, or neck

  - Dysphagia

  - Persistent, unilateral ear pain

  - Weight loss and anorexia

  - Foul breath

- Objective Data
  - Physical Assessment Findings
    - Hard, immobile lymph nodes in the neck (if metastasis has occurred)
    - Hoarse, raspy voice
    - Dyspnea (if tumor is in an advanced stage)
  - Laboratory Tests
  - Tumor mapping may be done by taking multiple biopsy samples.
  - Mapping verifies where the tumor is located, its margins, and type.
  - Staging is done using this information.
  - Diagnostic Procedures
    - X-rays of skull, sinuses, neck, and chest; CT scan and magnetic resonance imaging (MRI) scan
      - These help to determine the extent and exact location of the tumor and level of soft tissue invasion
    - Indirect and direct laryngoscopy
      - An indirect laryngoscopy is initially done to see if the tumor can be visualized. The client is awake and a topical anesthetic is applied to the tongue and throat. Visualization is done using a laryngeal mirror or fiberoptic laryngoscope.
      - Direct laryngoscopy is used to visualize the tumor more closely and to obtain biopsy, which will definitively determine cell type and staging.
      - Nursing Actions
        - Prepare the client for the procedure as appropriate (informed consent, NPO).
        - Monitor the client and maintain the client safety following the procedure (vital signs, return of gag reflex). A small amount of bloody sputum is normal.
      - Client Education
        - Inform clients that after the topical anesthetic is applied, they may feel like they cannot swallow. Encourage clients to relax and spit out secretions if they cannot be swallowed.
    - Bone scan and positron emission tomography (PET) scan
      - Determines presence of metastasis

Collaborative Care

- Nursing Care

  - Maintain a patent airway.

    - Suction the client's mouth, throat, and airway as needed. Use aseptic technique when suctioning the airway.

    - Position the client upright to facilitate ventilation.

  - Administer medications as prescribed.

    - Crush pills to aid in swallowing.

    - Obtain elixirs when possible.

  - Provide pain relief.

    - Administer analgesics as prescribed.

    - Consider alternative/adjunctive pain relief methods, such as a humidifier, cough and throat lozenges, and salt water or antiseptic/anesthetic gargles or throat sprays.

  - Provide oral care.

  - Provide emotional support.

    - Encourage verbalization of feelings regarding the prognosis and changes in self-image.

    - Provide information regarding support groups.

- Interdisciplinary Care

  - If surgical removal of the larynx it done, initiate a speech therapy consult to discuss communication options.

  - Refer the client and family to support groups.

  - Initiate a social work consult for the client if outpatient radiation or chemotherapy is ordered.

- Surgical Interventions

  - Laryngectomy

    - May be a partial (removal of one or part of one larynx) or total laryngectomy (removal of both larynx)

      - If the cancer is advanced, all or part of the epiglottis may need to be removed.

    - Temporary tracheostomies may be established for clients who require only a partial laryngectomies. Permanent tracheal stomas are created for clients who have undergone total laryngectomies.

- A laryngectomy tube is inserted into the stoma immediately after the surgery. This prevents contractures from forming while the stoma is healing. Care is the same as caring for any other type of tracheostomy tube.

- Nursing Actions

  □ Provide preoperative teaching.

  □ Determine the preferred alternate form of communication (dry erase board, pen and paper, alphabet board, picture board). Determine the client's preference, and don't assume the client is literate or that handwriting and spelling is legible.

    ▸ Inform the client about care of the airway, including tracheostomy care and suctioning techniques.

    ▸ Discuss pain control methods that will be used postoperatively.

    ▸ Assess the client's anxiety level and provide psychological support.

  □ Postoperative care

    ▸ Elevate the head of the bed.

    ▸ Monitor airway patency and vital signs. Anticipate the need for frequent suctioning, but suction gently to prevent trauma to fragile tissue. Oral suctioning may need to be done and can be accomplished by giving the client a catheter or tonsil sucker attached to suction.

    ▸ Monitor hemodynamic status and observe the surgical site and mucus suctioned from the trachea for bleeding.

    ▸ Place the call light within easy reach of the client.

    ▸ Monitor the client's pain level and administer analgesics as prescribed.

    ▸ Cleanse and dress wounds as prescribed. If the client had radiation therapy prior to the surgery, wound breakdown is a potential postoperative complication. Notify the provider at the first sign of wound breakdown.

    ▸ Initiate nutritional intake as ordered. Nasogastric feedings are usually provided for the first few days until the surgical site has had a chance to heal. Interruption of the surgical site can cause a fistula to form that will be very hard to close.

    ▸ If a nodal neck dissection ("radical neck") is done, additional care must be rendered.

    ▸ The eleventh cranial nerve may be cut, resulting in shoulder drop following surgery.

    ▸ A skin flap may have been used to cover the defect, which will need to be monitored for adequate circulation.

- Client Education

  □ Clients undergoing total laryngectomies will lose their natural voice.

◻ Tracheoesophageal fistula, esophageal speech, and electrolarynx devices are methods of speech communication that may be explored and developed following a total laryngectomy. These will allow the client to speak, but the quality of the client's speech will always sound different.

View Media Supplement:

Electrolarynx and Tracheoesophageal Fistula (Video)

○ A cordectomy or hemilaryngectomy (excision of one vocal cord) may be performed.

▪ Nursing Actions

◻ The risk for aspiration is greater during eating and drinking.

◻ The client will need to be taught to tuck the chin under when swallowing.

◻ An epiglottidectomy (excision of epiglottis) involves the removal of the epiglottis, leaving the trachea open to swallowed fluids.

◻ If the client had all or part of the epiglottis removed, the client must learn how to swallow without aspirating. Instruct the client to tuck the chin under when swallowing. Arching the tongue in the back of the mouth when swallowing may also be effective.

▪ Care After Discharge

▪ Client Education

◻ Instruct the client about the importance of smoking cessation if applicable. Provide nicotine replacement as prescribed.

◻ Instruct the client about appropriate techniques for stoma care and suctioning.

◻ Instruct the client to:

▸ Use saline and cotton-tipped swabs to cleanse the stoma.

▸ Use a humidifier and/or saline atomizer to moisten the environment and stoma frequently during the day.

▸ Wear a buttoned cotton shirt or a stoma covering (crocheted bib, scarf or bandana) to keep dust and other particles out of the lungs.

▸ Wear a shower shield over the stoma when taking a shower.

▸ Report any signs of incisional or lung infection (fever, purulent drainage, redness, four odor, swelling).

▸ Consume a diet high in protein and calories.

▸ Avoid water sports. All other activities are allowed, but lifting may be more difficult because the client will be unable to perform the Valsalva maneuver with an open airway.

● Client Outcomes

○ The client will maintain a patent airway.

o   The client will be able to swallow food and fluids without choking.

o   The client will relearn how to speak using an alternate method of vocalization.

Complications

- Airway obstruction

  o   Following a laryngectomy, the client may have copious amounts of secretions. If secretions are not removed, mucous plugs may form and can occlude a client's airway.

  o   Nursing Actions

   ▪   Monitor respiratory status (SaO$_2$, breath sounds).

   ▪   Maintain humidity in the form of aerosolized oxygen or room air. Supplement with a saline atomizer as needed to keep secretions thin.

   ▪   Suction the client when needed and be sure to oxygenate prior to suctioning.

   ▪   Encourage deep breathing and coughing to aid in secretion removal.

- Aspiration

  o   Clients who have had one vocal cord or the epiglottis removed are at an increased risk for aspiration.

  o   Aspiration may lead to the development of pneumonia.

  o   Clients who have had total laryngectomies (removal of both vocal cords) will not be able to aspirate due to the surgical separation of the trachea from the esophagus.

  o   Nursing Actions

   ▪   Maintain clients in an upright position. Have clients tuck the chin down when swallowing.

   ▪   Use thickened liquids.

   ▪   Cut food into small pieces, and instruct the client to chew well before swallowing. Mechanical soft/pureed diets may be better tolerated than full liquid or soft diets.

   ▪   Provide foods that can be formed into a bolus before swallowing (meats, bread).

   ▪   Notify the health care provider if aspiration is suspected. Place the client on NPO status until swallowing ability can be determined.

  o   Client Education

   ▪   Have the client follow previously described methods of swallowing.

   ▪   Instruct the client to notify the health care provider if symptoms of aspiration or pneumonia develop (fever, shortness of breath, fatigue).

CHAPTER 26: LARYNGEAL CANCER

 Application Exercises

Scenario: A nurse is admitting a client whose main symptom is hoarseness that has persisted for more than 2 months. The client reports that he has had difficulty swallowing due to the feeling that he has a lump in his throat. A CT scan reveals a subglottic lesion with lymph node enlargement on the right side of the neck. A direct laryngoscopy reveals a lesion involving both vocal cords and biopsies confirm the presence of malignancy. The client is diagnosed with laryngeal cancer and is admitted for a total laryngectomy with a right radical neck dissection.

1. The client asks the nurse if he will be able to speak after the surgery. Which of the following is an appropriate response by the nurse?

    A. "There is a good chance that you will be able to speak in your natural voice."

    B. "You will have to use a written form of communication for the rest of your life."

    C. "You will not be able to speak again with your natural voice, but there are options for re-establishing speech."

    D. "The primary concern at this time is to remove the cancer, so you shouldn't worry about your voice at this time."

2. The client returns from surgery with a tracheostomy tube in his permanent stoma and a nasogastric tube. The client's spouse asks why the client has a nasogastric tube. She also asks if he will have difficulty eating in the future. How should the nurse respond to the spouse's inquiries?

3. The client reports that he is having difficulty raising his right arm above his head when dressing. Which of the following responses is appropriate?

    A. "I will call your provider and let her know that your right arm is weak."

    B. "This sometimes occurs as a complication after a radical neck dissection."

    C. "It is normal for you to be weak after this type of surgery."

    D. "You may need to wear your arm in a sling the rest of your life."

4. Which of the following are at an increased risk for the development of laryngeal cancer? (Select all that apply.)

    _____ A client who paints houses for a living

    _____ A client who uses chewing tobacco

    _____ A radiology technician who takes x-rays of clients daily

    _____ A client who smokes only cigars, not cigarettes

    _____ A client who lives with a spouse who smokes cigarettes

CHAPTER 26: LARYNGEAL CANCER

(A) Application Exercises Answer Key

Scenario: A nurse is admitting a client whose main symptom is hoarseness that has persisted for more than 2 months. The client reports that he has had difficulty swallowing due to the feeling that he has a lump in his throat. A CT scan reveals a subglottic lesion with lymph node enlargement on the right side of the neck. A direct laryngoscopy reveals a lesion involving both vocal cords and biopsies confirm the presence of malignancy. The client is diagnosed with laryngeal cancer and is admitted for a total laryngectomy with a right radical neck dissection.

---

1. The client asks the nurse if he will be able to speak after the surgery. Which of the following is an appropriate response by the nurse?

    A. "There is a good chance that you will be able to speak in your natural voice."

    B. "You will have to use a written form of communication for the rest of your life."

    C. "You will not be able to speak again with your natural voice, but there are options for re-establishing speech."

    D. "The primary concern at this time is to remove the cancer, so you shouldn't worry about your voice at this time."

    There are several methods and devices (electrolarynx devices, esophageal speech) that may be used to help the client re-establish communication. Because both vocal cords are being removed, the client will never be able to speak with his normal voice again. Initially, the client may need to use written communication or a communication board, but other options are available once healing has occurred. Telling the client not to worry about his voice at this time is not a therapeutic response.

(N) NCLEX® Connection: Physiological Adaptation, Alterations in Body Systems

2. The client returns from surgery with a tracheostomy tube in his permanent stoma and a nasogastric tube. The client's spouse asks why the client has a nasogastric tube. She also asks if he will have difficulty eating in the future. How should the nurse respond to the spouse's inquiries?

    The nurse should inform the spouse that the NG tube will be used for nutrition as the incision in the throat heals. It will be removed within 7 to 10 days, and oral nutrition will be re-established. Because the client had a total laryngectomy, the trachea has been brought through a permanent stoma in his neck, which no longer communicates with his esophagus. Subsequently, after the NG tube is removed, the client will no longer be at risk for aspiration and he will be able to re-establish normal eating habits.

(N) NCLEX® Connection: Reduction of Risk Potential, Therapeutic Procedures

3. The client reports that he is having difficulty raising his right arm above his head when dressing. Which of the following responses is an appropriate?

    A. "I will call your provider and let her know that your right arm is weak."

    B. "This sometimes occurs as a complication after a radical neck dissection."

    C. "It is normal for you to be weak after this type of surgery."

    D. "You may need to wear your arm in a sling the rest of your life."

During a radical neck dissection, the nerves and muscles in the neck may be damaged, resulting in numbness and decreased function of distal structures. Weakness of the arm on the surgical side of the body may result. Through the use of muscle strengthening exercises, the client will regain much of the strength in the affected arm.

Ⓝ NCLEX® Connection: Reduction of Risk Potential, Therapeutic Procedures

---

4. Which of the following clients are at an increased risk for the development of laryngeal cancer? (Select all that apply.)

    __X__   **A client who paints houses for a living**

    __X__   **A client who uses chewing tobacco**

    _____   A radiology technician who takes x-rays of clients daily

    __X__   **A client who smokes only cigars, not cigarettes**

    __X__   **A client who lives with a spouse who smokes cigarettes**

Clients who use tobacco of any kind, use alcohol, are exposed to second hand smoke, or are exposed to harmful chemicals (paint) are at risk for laryngeal cancer. A radiology technician is not at risk due to the use of lead aprons, gloves, and other shielding devices. Instruments that monitor exposure to radiation are also worn and records are kept on cumulative lifetime dosage

Ⓝ NCLEX® Connection: Reduction to Risk Potential, Potential for Complications

Overview

- Lung cancer is one of the leading causes of cancer-related deaths for both men and women. It most commonly occurs between the ages of 45 and 70.

- Prognosis of lung cancer is poor because it is often diagnosed in an advanced stage, when metastasis has occurred. Palliative care or treatment geared toward relieving symptoms is often the focus at the advanced stage.

- Bronchogenic carcinomas (arising from the bronchial epithelium) account for 90% of primary lung cancers.

- Histologic cell type determines lung cancer classification. Categories include:

  o Non-small cell lung cancer (NSCLC)

    ▪ Most lung cancers are from this category.

    ▪ They include squamous, adeno, and large cell carcinomas.

  o Small cell lung cancer (SCLC)

    ▪ Fast-growing

    ▪ Almost always associated with a history of cigarette smoking

- Staging of lung cancer is defined with the TMN system.

  o T = Tumor

  o N = Nodes

  o M = Metastasis

- Chemotherapy is the primary choice of treatment for lung cancers. It is often used in combination with radiation and/or surgery.

Health Promotion and Disease Prevention

- Promote smoking cessation.

- Use protective equipment (mask) and ensure proper ventilation while working in environments that can contain carcinogens or particles in the air.

Assessment

- Risk Factors

  - Cigarette smoking (both first and secondhand smoke)

  - Radiation exposure

  - Chronic exposure to inhaled environmental irritants (air pollution, asbestos, other talc dusts)

   Older adult clients have decreased pulmonary reserves due to normal lung changes, including decreased lung elasticity and thickening alveoli. This contributes to impaired gas exchange.

  - Structural changes in the skeletal system decrease diaphragmatic expansion thereby therefore restricting ventilation.

- Subjective Data

  - Chronic cough

  - Chronic dyspnea

- Objective Data

  - Clients who have lung cancer may experience few symptoms early in the disease. Monitor for signs and symptoms that often appear late in the disease.

    - Persistent cough, with or without hemoptysis (rust-colored or blood-tinged sputum)

    - Hoarseness

    - Dyspnea

    - Unilateral wheezing (if the airway is obstructed)

    - Chest wall pain

    - Chest wall masses

    - Muffled heart sounds

    - Fatigue, weight loss, or anorexia

    - Clubbing of fingers

  - Diagnostic Procedures

    - Chest x-ray and computed tomography (CT) scan

      - Provides initial identification of the tumor

        (M) View Media Supplement: Lung Cancer Chest X-ray (Image)

- Bronchoscopy
  - □ Can provide direct visibility of the tumor
  - □ Allows for specimen and biopsy collection
  - □ Nursing Actions
    - ▸ Prepare the client for the procedure as appropriate (informed consent, NPO), monitor the client, and maintain client safety following the procedure (vital signs, return of gag reflex, sedatives and supplemental oxygen as needed).
  - □ Client Education
    - ▸ Inform the client he can have nothing to eat or drink after the procedure until the gag reflex returns.
    - ▸ Inform the client that his throat may be sore after the procedure.

Collaborative Care

- Nursing Care
  - o Determine the client's history regarding use of tobacco products.
  - o Determine the pack-year history, which is the number of packs of cigarettes smoked per day times the number of years smoked.
  - o Evaluate the client's use of other tobacco products (cigars, pipes, and chewing tobacco).
  - o Ask about exposure to secondhand smoke.
  - o Monitor for a cough that changes in pattern.
  - o Monitor nutritional status, weight loss, and anorexia.
    - ▪ Promote adequate nutrition to provide needed calories for increased work of breathing and prevention of infection.
    - ▪ Encourage intake of soft, high-calorie foods.
    - ▪ Encourage fluids to promote adequate hydration.
  - o Maintain a patent airway and suction as needed.
  - o Position the client in Fowler's position to maximize ventilation.
  - o Determine the client's physical limitations and provide periods of rest.
  - o Provide emotional support to the client and family. Encourage verbalization of feelings about the disease.
  - o Discuss the topic of death and dying with the client (if cancer is terminal), and encourage the client to express feelings.
  - o A fever may be present along with one or two other symptoms.

- Medications
  - Chemotherapy agents
    - Chemotherapy is the treatment of choice for lung cancer. The purpose of these medications is to destroy cancer cells, as well as healthy cells, to prevent DNA formation. Platinum compounds such as cisplatin (Platinol AQ) are commonly used.
    - Nursing Considerations
      - Watch the client for a decrease in immunity function.
      - Observe the client for nausea and vomiting.
      - Monitor the client for fatigue.
      - Assess the client for shortness of breath.
      - Assess the client's throat and mouth for aphthous (cold sore) lesions.
    - Client Education
      - Encourage the client to inform the nurse if nausea and vomiting persists.
      - Encourage the client to use frequent oral hygiene and use a soft-bristled toothbrush. Advise the client to avoid alcohol-based mouthwashes.
      - Inform the client that hair loss (alopecia) occurs 7 to 10 days after treatment begins. Encourage the client to select a hairpiece before treatment starts.
  - Opioid agonists (Pain medication)
    - Morphine sulfate (MS Contin), oxycodone (OxyContin), and fentanyl (Duragesic) are opioid agents used to treat moderate to severe pain, caused by an illness. These medications act on the mu and kappa receptors that help to alleviate pain.
    - Activation of these receptors produces analgesia (pain relief), respiratory depression, euphoria, sedation, and decrease in gastrointestinal motility.
    - Use cautiously with clients who have asthma or emphysema due to the risk of respiratory depression.
    - Nursing Considerations
      - Assess the client's pain every 4 hr.
      - Remind clients receiving the fentanyl patch that the initial patch takes several hours to take effect. A short-acting pain medication will be administered for breakthrough pain.
      - Watch the client for signs of respiratory depression, especially in older adult clients. If respirations are 12/min or less, stop the medication and notify the health care provider immediately.
      - Monitor the client's vital signs closely for signs of hypotension and decreased respirations.

- □ Observe the client for nausea and vomiting.
- □ Assess the client's level of sedation (drowsiness, (level of consciousness).
- □ Encourage fluid intake and activity related to a decrease in gastric motility.
- □ Monitor intake and output and for signs of fluid retention. This is common in clients who have an enlarged prostate.
- Client Education
  - □ Encourage the client to suck on hard candies to help with dry mouth.
  - □ Encourage the client to drink plenty of fluids to help prevent constipation.
  - □ Advise the client to increase fiber intake to help with constipation.
  - □ Advise the client to notify the nurse if nausea and vomiting persists.
  - □ Advise the client to avoid driving while taking the medication
  - □ Teach the client to use a patient-controlled analgesia (PCA) pump if applicable. The client is the only person that is to push the medication administration button. Reassure the client that the safety lockout mechanism on the PCA prevents overdosing of medication.
  - □ Bronchodilators and corticosteroids can be given to help decrease inflammation and to dry secretions.
- Interdisciplinary Care
  - ○ Respiratory services should be consulted for inhalers, breathing treatments, and suctioning for airway management.
  - ○ Pain management services can be consulted if pain is persists and/or is uncontrolled.
  - ○ Radiology and oncology services may be contacted to treat the cancer.
  - ○ Nutritional services may be contacted for weight loss related to medications or diagnosis.
  - ○ Rehabilitation care may be consulted if the client has prolonged weakness and needs assistance with increasing the level of activity.
  - ○ Hospice care may be contacted if the client's cancer is terminal.
- Therapeutic Procedures
  - Palliative care
    - □ Includes medication, radiation, and laser therapy; thoracentesis; pain management; and hospice referral and care
- Surgical Interventions
  - ○ The goal of surgery is to remove all tumor cells, including involved lymph nodes.
    - Often involves removal of a lung (pneumonectomy), lobe (lobectomy), segment (segmentectomy), or peripheral lung tissue (wedge resection)

- o Nursing Actions
  - Receive consent from the client prior to the procedure.
  - Assess the client's pain and administer pain medication as prescribed.
  - Monitor vital signs, oxygenation (SaO_2, ABG values), and for signs of hemorrhage.
  - Manage the chest tube and drainage system.
  - Administer oxygen and manage the ventilator if appropriate.
- o Client Education
  - Teach the client about the surgical procedure and chest tube placement.
  - Relieve client anxiety and encourage verbalization of feelings.
- Care After Discharge
  - Set up referral services, including home health, hospice, or respiratory services such as portable oxygen.
  - Contact community outreach programs, such as food delivery services or cancer support groups.
- o Client Education
  - Encourage the client to take rest periods as needed.
  - Encourage the client to eat high-calorie foods to promote energy.
  - Encourage the client to perform hand hygiene to prevent infection.
  - Encourage the client to avoid crowded areas to reduce the risk of infection.
  - Promote smoking cessation if the client smokes.
  - Educate the client and family about the illness and encourage them to express their feelings.
  - Discuss the topic of death and dying (if the cancer is terminal) with the client, and encourage the client to express his feelings.
- Client Outcomes
  - o The client will be able to keep a patent airway.
  - o The client will remain free from pain.
  - o The client will remain free from infection.
  - o The client will be able to maintain within 10% of ideal body weight.

Complications

- Superior vena cava syndrome

    - Superior vena cava syndrome results from pressure placed on the vena cava by a tumor. It is a medical emergency.

    o Nursing Actions

        - Monitor for signs.

            □ Early signs include facial edema, edema in neck, nosebleeds, peripheral edema, and dyspnea.

            □ Late signs include mental status changes, cyanosis, hemorrhage, and hypotension.

        - Notify the health care provider immediately.

        - Radiation and stent placement provide temporary relief. Prepare the client for the procedure (informed consent, NPO if possible, client transport).

        - Monitor the client's status (vital signs, oxygenation) during and after the procedure.

- Metastasis

    - Metastasis to the bones can cause bone pain and increase the risk of pathologic fractures.

    - Metastasis to the central nervous system can lead to changes in mentation, lethargy, and bowel and bladder malfunction.

    o Nursing Actions

        - Encourage the client to ambulate carefully.

        - Reorient the client as needed.

CHAPTER 27: LUNG CANCER

 Application Exercises

Scenario: A nurse in an emergency department is caring for a client who reports dyspnea and rust-colored sputum that has persisted for nearly 3 weeks. Lung cancer is suspected, and diagnostic tests are ordered. A CT scan reveals the presence of a mass at the base of the bronchial tree. The client is expected to undergo a bronchoscopy.

1. The client asks, "What is a bronchoscopy?" An appropriate response by the nurse is, "A bronchoscopy is when

   A. a needle is inserted between two ribs and a piece of the tumor is aspirated."

   B. a set of x-rays are taken that provide a three-dimensional picture of your lungs."

   C. magnetic fields and radio waves are used to obtain sectional pictures of your lungs that outline the tumor."

   D. a flexible tube is inserted through your mouth and into your lungs to see the tumor and obtain a biopsy."

Scenario: A nurse in an emergency department is caring for a client who has advanced lung cancer. The client reports dyspnea on exertion and at rest, and her family states that she has become disoriented over the last 72 hr. A chest x-ray reveals a baseball-sized mediastinal tumor. Vital signs are as follows: heart rate 104, blood pressure 88/42 mm Hg, respiratory rate 38/min, and temperature 37.9° C (100.2° F). The client's SaO_2 is 89% on room air.

2. Which of the following do these findings indicate?

   A. Cardiac tamponade

   B. Sick sinus syndrome

   C. Superior vena cava syndrome

   D. Right heart block

3. Which of the following interventions should the nurse implement first?

   A. Notify the health care provider.

   B. Obtain a CT scan to determine the exact location of the tumor.

   C. Administer oxygen.

   D. Provide family support.

CHAPTER 27: LUNG CANCER

 Application Exercises Answer Key

Scenario: A nurse in an emergency department is caring for a client who reports dyspnea and rust-colored sputum that has persisted for nearly 3 weeks. Lung cancer is suspected, and diagnostic tests are ordered. A CT scan reveals the presence of a mass at the base of the bronchial tree. The client is expected to undergo a bronchoscopy.

1. The client asks, "What is a bronchoscopy?" An appropriate response by the nurse is, "A bronchoscopy is when

    A. a needle is inserted between two ribs and a piece of the tumor is aspirated."

    B. a set of x-rays are taken that provide a three-dimensional picture of your lungs."

    C. magnetic fields and radio waves are used to obtain sectional pictures of your lungs that outline the tumor."

    D. a flexible tube is inserted through your mouth and into your lungs to see the tumor and obtain a biopsy."

A bronchoscopy is a diagnostic test that is performed by inserting a flexible tube through the mouth and into the lungs to visualize and biopsy a tumor. Inserting a needle between two ribs and aspirating the tumor describes a needle biopsy, taking x-rays to provide a three dimensional picture describes a CAT scan, and using magnetic fields and radio waves to obtain sectional pictures describes an MRI.

 NCLEX® Connection: Reduction of Risk Potential, Diagnostic Tests

Scenario: A nurse in an emergency department is caring for a client who has advanced lung cancer. The client reports dyspnea on exertion and at rest, and her family states that she has become disoriented over the last 72 hr. A chest x-ray reveals a baseball-sized mediastinal tumor. Vital signs are as follows: heart rate 104, blood pressure 88/42 mm Hg, respiratory rate 38/min, and temperature 37.9° C (100.2° F). The client's SaO_2 is 89% on room air.

2. Which of the following do these findings indicate?

    A. Cardiac tamponade

    B. Sick sinus syndrome

    C. Superior vena cava syndrome

    D. Right heart block

These symptoms indicate that the client is experiencing superior vena cava syndrome, which is a medical emergency. Cardiac tamponade, sick sinus syndrome, and right heart block do not relate to the client findings.

 NCLEX® Connection: Physiological Adaptation, Medical Emergencies

3. Which of the following interventions should the nurse implement first?

    A. Notify the health care provider.

    B. Obtain a CT scan to determine the exact location of the tumor.

    C. Administer oxygen.

    D. Provide family support.

Notifying the provider, obtaining a CT scan, and providing family support are all actions the nurse should take, but administering oxygen is the most important intervention, according to the ABC priority setting framework.

Ⓝ **NCLEX® Connection: Physiological Adaptation, Medical Emergencies**

UNIT 3	NURSING CARE OF CLIENTS WITH RESPIRATORY DISORDERS
Section	Respiratory Emergencies
Chapter 28	Pulmonary Embolism

 Overview

- A pulmonary embolism (PE) occurs when a substance (solid, gaseous, or liquid) enters venous circulation and forms a blockage in the pulmonary vasculature.

- Emboli originating from deep vein thrombosis (DVT) are the most common cause. Tumors, bone marrow, amniotic fluid, and foreign matter can also become emboli.

(M) **View Media Supplement:** Pulmonary Embolism (Image)

- Increased hypoxia to pulmonary tissue and impaired blood flow can result from a large embolus. A PE is a medical emergency.

- Prevention, rapid recognition, and treatment of a PE are essential for a positive outcome.

Health Promotion and Disease Prevention

- Promote smoking cessation.

- Encourage maintenance of appropriate weight for height and body frame.

- Encourage a healthy diet and physical activity.

- Prevent deep vein thrombosis (DVT) by encouraging clients to do leg exercises, wear compression stockings, and avoid sitting for long periods of time.

Assessment

- Risk Factors

  o Long-term immobility

  o Oral contraceptive use and estrogen therapy

  o Pregnancy

  o Tobacco use

  o Hypercoagulability (elevated platelet count)

- o   Obesity

- o   Surgery (especially orthopedic surgery of the lower extremities or pelvis)

- o   Heart failure or chronic atrial fibrillation

- o   Autoimmune hemolytic anemia (sickle cell)

- o   Long bone fractures

- o   Advanced age

- o   Older adult clients have decreased pulmonary reserves due to normal lung changes, including decreased lung elasticity and thickening alveoli. Older adult clients can decompensate more quickly.

- o   Certain pathological conditions and procedures that predispose clients to DVT formation (peripheral vascular disease, hypertension, hip and knee orthoplasty) are more prevalent in older adults.

- o   Many older adult clients experience decreased physical activity levels, thus predisposing them to DVT formation and pulmonary emboli.

- • Subjective Data

  - o   Anxiety

  - o   Feelings of impending doom

  - o   Pressure in chest

  - o   Pain upon inspiration

  - o   Dyspnea and air hunger

- • Objective Data

  - o   Physical Assessment Findings

    - ▪ Pleurisy

    - ▪ Tachycardia

    - ▪ Hypotension

    - ▪ Tachypnea

    - ▪ Adventitious breath sounds (crackles) and cough

    - ▪ Heart murmur in S_3 and S_4

    - ▪ Diaphoresis

    - ▪ Decreased oxygen saturation levels (the expected reference range is 95% to 100%)–low SaO_2 Petechiae (red dots under the skin), cyanosis

    - ▪ Petechiae (red dots under the skin) and cyanosis

    - ▪ Pleural effusion (fluid in the lungs)

- o Laboratory Tests
  - ■ ABG analysis
    - □ PaCO$_2$ levels are low (the expected reference range is 35 to 45 mm Hg) due to initial hyperventilation (respiratory alkalosis).
    - □ As hypoxemia progresses, respiratory acidosis occurs.
  - ■ CBC analysis
    - □ D-dimer
      - ▸ Is elevated above expected reference range in response to clot formation and release of fibrin degradation products (the expected reference range is 0.43 to 2.33 mcg/mL).
- o Diagnostic Procedures
  - ■ Chest x-ray and computed tomography (CT) scan
    - □ These provide initial identification of a PE. A CT scan is most commonly used. A chest x-ray can show a large PE.
  - ■ Ventilation and perfusion scan (V/Q scan)
    - □ Images show the circulation of air and blood in the lungs and can detect a PE.
  - ■ Pulmonary Angiography
    - □ This is the most thorough test to detect a PE, but it is invasive and costly. A catheter is inserted into the vena cava to visually see a PE.
    - □ Pulmonary angiography is a higher risk procedure than a V/Q scan.
    - □ Nursing Actions
      - ▸ Verify that informed consent has been obtained.
      - ▸ Monitor the client's status (vital signs, SaO$_2$, anxiety, bleeding with angiography) during and after the procedure.

Collaborative Care

- • Nursing Care
  - o Administer oxygen therapy as prescribed to relieve hypoxemia and dyspnea.
    - ■ Position the client to maximize ventilation (high-Fowler's = 90%)
  - o Initiate and maintain IV access.
  - o Administer medications as prescribed.
  - o Provide emotional support and comfort to control client anxiety.
  - o Monitor changes in level of consciousness and mental status.

- Medications
  - Anticoagulants: Enoxaparin (Lovenox), heparin, and warfarin (Coumadin)
    - Anticoagulants are used to prevent clots from getting larger or other clots from forming.
    - Nursing Considerations
      - Assess for contraindications (active bleeding, peptic ulcer disease, history of stroke, recent trauma).
      - Monitor bleeding times – Prothrombin time (PT) and international normalized ratio (INR) for warfarin, partial thromboplastin time (a PTT) for heparin, and complete blood count (CBC)
      - Monitor for side effects of anticoagulants (e.g., thrombocytopenia, anemia, hemorrhage).
  - Thrombolytic therapy– Alteplase (Activase) and streptokinase (Streptase)
    - Used to dissolve blood clots and restore pulmonary blood flow
    - Similar side effects and contraindications as anticoagulants
    - Nursing Considerations
      - Assess for contraindications (known bleeding disorders, uncontrolled hypertension, active bleeding, peptic ulcer disease, history of stroke, recent trauma or surgery, pregnancy).
      - Monitor for evidence of bleeding, thrombocytopenia, and anemia.
      - Give streptokinase slowly to prevent hypotension.
- Interdisciplinary Care
  - Cardiology and pulmonary services should be consulted to manage a PE and treatment.
  - Respiratory services should be consulted for oxygen therapy, breathing treatments, and ABGs.
  - Radiology should be consulted for diagnostic studies to determine PE.
- Surgical Interventions
  - Embolectomy
    - Surgical removal of embolus
    - Nursing Actions
      - Prepare the client for the procedure (NPO status, informed consent).
      - Monitor postoperatively (vital signs, SaO_2, incision drainage, pain management).

- ○ Vena cava filter

  - □ Insertion of a filter in the vena cava to prevent further emboli from reaching the pulmonary vasculature

- ■ Nursing Actions

  - □ Prepare the client for the procedure (NPO status, informed consent).

  - □ Monitor postoperatively (vital signs, SaO_2, incision drainage, pain management).

- Care After Discharge

  - ■ If the client is homebound, set up home care services to perform weekly blood draws.

  - ■ Set up referral services to supply portable oxygen for clients who have severe dyspnea.

- ○ Client Education

  - ■ Provide education to the client for the treatment and prevention of a PE.

    - □ Promote smoking cessation if the client smokes.

    - □ Encourage the client to avoid long periods of immobility.

    - □ Encourage physical activity such as walking.

    - □ Encourage the client to wear compression stockings to promote circulation.

    - □ Encourage the client to avoid crossing his legs.

  - ■ Advise the client to monitor intake of foods high in vitamin K (green, leafy vegetables) if taking warfarin. Vitamin K can reduce the anticoagulant effects of warfarin.

  - ■ Advise the client to adhere to a schedule for monitoring PT and INR, follow instructions regarding medication dosage adjustments (for clients on warfarin), and adhere with the need for weekly blood draws.

  - ■ Remind the client of the increased risk for bruising and bleeding.

    - □ Instruct the client to avoid taking aspirin products, unless specified by health care provider.

    - □ Encourage the client to check his mouth and skin daily for bleeding and bruising.

    - □ Encourage the client to use electric shavers and soft-bristled toothbrushes.

    - □ Instruct the client to avoid blowing his nose hard, and if nose bleeds occur, gently apply pressure.

- Client Outcomes

  - ○ The client will adhere with anticoagulant therapy.

  - ○ The client will maintain adequate gas exchange.

  - ○ The client will be free from severe bleeding incidences.

- o The client will be pain free.

- o The client will maintain an appropriate weight for height and body frame.

Complications

- • Decreased cardiac output

  - o The amount of blood pumped by the heart is decreased.

  - o Nursing Actions

    - ▪ Monitor for hypotension, tachycardia, cyanosis, jugular venous distention, and syncope.

    - ▪ Assess for the presence of S_3 or S_4 heart sounds.

    - ▪ Initiate and maintain IV access.

    - ▪ Monitor urinary output (output should be 30 mL/hr or more).

    - ▪ Administer IV fluids (crystalloids) to replace vascular volume.

    - ▪ Continuously monitor the ECG.

    - ▪ Monitor pulmonary pressures. IV fluids can contribute to pulmonary hypertension for clients who have right-sided heart failure (cor pulmonale).

    - ▪ Administer inotropic agents (milrinone [Primacor], dobutamine [Dobutrex]), to increase myocardial contractility.

    - ▪ Vasodilators may be needed if pulmonary artery pressure is high enough that it interferes with cardiac contractility.

- • Hemorrhage

    - ▪ Receiving anticoagulant therapy increases the risk for bleeding.

  - o Nursing Actions

    - ▪ Assess for oozing, bleeding, or bruising from injection and surgical sites.

    - ▪ Monitor cardiovascular status (blood pressure, heart rate and rhythm).

    - ▪ Monitor CBC (hemoglobin, hematocrit, platelets) and bleeding times (PT, aPTT, INR).

    - ▪ Administer IV fluids and blood products as required.

    - ▪ Test stools, urine, and vomit for occult blood.

    - ▪ Monitor for internal bleeding (measure abdominal girth and abdominal or flank pain).

CHAPTER 28: PULMONARY EMBOLISM

Ⓐ Application Exercises

1. A nurse is caring for several clients. Which of the following clients are at risk for a pulmonary embolism? (Select all that apply.)

_____ A woman who is taking birth control pills

_____ A woman who is postmenopausal

_____ A client who has a fractured femur

_____ A client who smokes one pipe daily

_____ A client who is a marathon runner

_____ A client who has heart failure and chronic atrial fibrillation

2. A nurse is caring for a middle adult female client who is admitted to the coronary care unit with acute dyspnea and diaphoresis. The client states that she is anxious because she feels that she cannot get enough air. Vital signs are as follows: heart rate 117/min, respiratory rate 38/min, temperature 38.4° C (101.2° F), and blood pressure 100/54 mm Hg. Which of the following actions is the highest priority?

A. Obtain an ABG.

B. Initiate a heparin drip.

C. Administer oxygen therapy.

D. Obtain a spiral CT scan.

3. A nurse is caring for the client who has a new prescription for heparin therapy. Which of the following statements by a client should pose an immediate concern for the nurse?

A. "I am allergic to morphine."

B. "I take antacids several times a day."

C. "I had a blood clot in my leg several years ago."

D. "It hurts to take a deep breath."

4. Match each of the following interventions with its associated rationale.

_____ Administer crystalloids.   A. Improves cardiac contractility

_____ Administer dobutamine.   B. Restores intravascular volume

_____ Monitor platelet count.   C. Assesses for thrombocytopenia

5. A nurse is caring for a client who is to receive fibrinolytic thrombolytic therapy. Which of the following should the nurse recognize as a contraindication to the therapy?

A. Hip arthroplasty 2 weeks ago

B. Elevated sedimentation rate

C. Incident of exercise-induced asthma 1 week ago

D. Elevated platelet count

CHAPTER 28: PULMONARY EMBOLISM

(A) Application Exercises Answer Key

1. A nurse is caring for several clients. Which of the following clients are at risk for a pulmonary embolism? (Select all that apply.)

   __X__   **A woman who is taking birth control pills**

   _____   A woman who is postmenopausal

   __X__   **A client who has a fractured femur**

   __X__   **A client who smokes one pipe daily**

   _____   A client who is a marathon runner

   __X__   **A client who has heart failure and chronic atrial fibrillation**

Estrogen use and smoking can cause hypercoagulability, which increases the risk of a blood clot. A client with turbulent blood flow in the heart, such as with a dysrhythmia, is also at increased risk of a blood clot. A fractured bone, particularly in a long bone such as the femur, increases the risk of fat emboli. A client who is postmenopausal and a client who is a marathon runner are not at risk for developing a PE.

(N) **NCLEX® Connection: Reduction of Risk Potential, System Specific Assessment**

2. A nurse is caring for a middle adult female client who is admitted to the coronary care unit with acute dyspnea and diaphoresis. The client states that she is anxious because she feels that she cannot get enough air. Vital signs are as follows: heart rate 117/min, respiratory rate 38/min, temperature 38.4° C (101.2° F), and blood pressure 100/54 mm Hg. Which of the following actions is the highest priority?

A. Obtain an ABG.

B. Initiate a heparin drip.

C. Administer oxygen therapy.

D. Obtain a spiral CT scan.

Using the ABC priority setting framework, meeting the client's oxygenation needs is the highest priority. The nurse should administer oxygen as needed.

(N) **NCLEX® Connection: Physiological Adaptation, Illness Management**

3. A nurse is caring for a client who has a new prescription for heparin therapy. Which of the following statements by the client should pose an immediate concern for the nurse?

> A. "I am allergic to morphine."
> **B. "I take antacids several times a day."**
> C. "I had a blood clot in my leg several years ago."
> D. "It hurts to take a deep breath."

The greatest risk to this client is the possibility of bleeding from a peptic ulcer. Further assessment should be completed and the nurse should notify the health care provider of the findings.

 NCLEX® Connection: Pharmacological and Parenteral Therapies, Adverse Effects/Contraindications/Side Effects/Interactions

4. Match each of the following interventions with its associated rationale.

> **__B__** Administer crystalloids.   A. Improves cardiac contractility
> **__A__** Administer dobutamine.   B. Restores intravascular volume
> **__C__** Monitor platelet count.   C. Assesses for thrombocytopenia

Crystalloids will help restore fluid volume and prevent shock. Dobutamine can be used if cardiac output is low and IV therapy is not effective in preventing shock. A decreasing platelet count could be related to heparin-induced thrombocytopenia.

 NCLEX® Connection: Physiological Adaptation, Illness Management

5. A nurse is caring for a client who is to receive fibrinolytic thrombolytic therapy. Which of the following should the nurse recognize as a contraindication to the therapy?

> **A. Hip arthroplasty 2 weeks ago**
> B. Elevated sedimentation rate
> C. Incident of exercise-induced asthma 1 week ago
> D. Elevated platelet count

Clients who have undergone a major surgical procedure within the last 3 weeks should not receive thrombolytic therapy because of the risk of hemorrhage from the surgical site. An elevated sedimentation rate, an elevated platelet count, or an incident of exercise-induced asthma does not place the client at risk for hemorrhage.

NCLEX® Connection: Pharmacological and Parenteral Therapies, Adverse Effects/Contraindications/Side Effects/Interactions

UNIT 3	NURSING CARE OF CLIENTS WITH RESPIRATORY DISORDERS
Section	Respiratory Emergencies
Chapter 29	Pneumothorax and Hemothorax

Overview

- A pneumothorax is the presence of air or gas in the pleural space that causes lung collapse.

- A tension pneumothorax occurs when air enters the pleural space during inspiration through a one-way valve and is not able to exit upon expiration. The trapped air causes pressure on the heart and the lung. As a result, the increase in pressure compresses blood vessels and limits venous return, leading to a decrease in cardiac output. Death can be a result if not treated immediately.

    o   As a result of a tension pneumothorax, air and pressure continue to rise in the pleural cavity, which cause a mediastinal shift.

- A hemothorax is an accumulation of blood in the pleural space.

- A spontaneous pneumothorax can occur when there has been no trauma. A small bleb on the lung ruptures and air enters the pleural space.

Assessment

- Risk Factors

    o   Blunt chest trauma

    o   Penetrating chest wounds

    o   Closed/occluded chest tube

    o   Older adult clients have decreased pulmonary reserves due to normal lung changes, including decreased lung elasticity and thickening alveoli.

    o   Older adult clients are more susceptible to infections.

- Subjective Data

    o   Anxiety

    o   Pleuritic pain

- Objective Data
  - Physical Assessment Findings
    - Signs of respiratory distress (tachypnea, tachycardia, hypoxia, cyanosis, dyspnea, and use of accessory muscles)
    - Tracheal deviation to the unaffected side (tension pneumothorax)
    - Reduced or absent breath sounds on the affected side
    - Asymmetrical chest wall movement
    - Hyperresonance on percussion due to trapped air (pneumothorax)
    - Dull percussion (hemothorax)
    - Subcutaneous emphysema (air accumulating in subcutaneous tissue)
  - Laboratory Tests
    - ABGs
      - Hypoxemia (PaO_2 less than 80 mm Hg)
  - Diagnostic Procedures
    - Chest x-ray
      - Used to confirm pneumothorax or hemothorax

View Media Supplement:
- Pneumothorax (Image)
- Hemothorax (Image)

    - Thoracentesis may be used to confirm hemothorax.
      - Thoracentesis is the surgical perforation of the chest wall and pleural space with a large-bore needle.
      - Nursing Actions
        - Ensure that informed consent has been obtained.
        - Make sure the client understands the importance of remaining still during the procedure.
        - Assist with client positioning and specimen transport. Monitor the client's status (vital signs, SaO_2, injection site). Assist the client to at the edge of the bed and lean over a bedside table.
        - Inform the client he will feel discomfort when the local anesthetic solution is injected, and when the needle is inserted into the lung, some pressure may be felt, but no pain.

Collaborative Care

- Nursing Care

    o Administer oxygen therapy.

    o Document ventilator settings hourly if the client is receiving ventilation.

    o Check ABGs, SaO$_2$, CBC, and chest x-ray results.

    o Position the client to maximize ventilation (high-Fowler's = 90%).

    o Provide emotional support to the client and family.

    o Monitor chest tube drainage.

    o Administer medications as prescribed.

    o Encourage prompt medical attention when signs of infection occur.

- Medications

    o Benzodiazepines (sedatives)

        □ Lorazepam (Ativan) or midazolam (Versed) may be used to decrease the client's anxiety.

        ■ Nursing Considerations

            □ Monitor the client's vital signs (benzodiazepines may cause hypotension and respiratory distress).

            □ The medications have amnesiac effect.

            □ Watch for paradoxical effects (euphoria, rage)

        ■ Client Education

            □ Remind the client that medications will have amnesic effect and cause drowsiness.

    o Opioid agonists (pain medications)

        □ Morphine sulfate and fentanyl (Duragesic) are opioid agents used to treat moderate to severe pain. These medication acts on the mu and kappa receptors that help alleviate pain.

        □ Activation of these receptors produces analgesia (pain relief), respiratory depression, euphoria, sedation, and a decrease in gastrointestinal motility.

        ■ Nursing Considerations

            □ Use cautiously with clients who have asthma or emphysema, due to the risk of respiratory depression.

            □ Assess the client's pain every 4 hr.

            □ Remind clients who are receiving the fentanyl patch that the initial patch takes several hours to take effect. A short-acting pain medication will be administered for breakthrough pain.

- □ Watch clients, especially older adults for signs of respiratory depression. If respirations are 12/min or less, stop the medication and notify health care provider immediately.

- □ Monitor the client's vital signs closely for sign of hypotension and decreased respirations.

- □ Observe the client for nausea and vomiting.

- □ Assess the client's level of sedation (drowsiness, level of consciousness).

- □ Watch for signs of constipation.

- □ Encourage fluid intake and activity related to a decrease in gastric motility.

- □ Monitor intake and output and for signs of fluid retention (common in clients who have an enlarged prostate).

- ■ Client Education

  - □ Encourage clients who do not have fluid restrictions due to other conditions to drink plenty of fluids to help prevent constipation.

  - □ Teach the client how to use a patient controlled analgesia pump if applicable. The client is the only person who should push the medication administration button. Reassure the client that the safety lockout mechanism on the PCA prevents overdosing of medication.

  - □ If the client is receiving ventilation, the above nursing considerations and client education may vary.

- • Interdisciplinary Care

  - ○ Respiratory services should be consulted for ABGs, breathing treatments, and suctioning for airway management.

  - ○ Pulmonary services may be consulted for chest tube management and pulmonary care of the client.

  - ○ Pain management services may be consulted if pain persists and/or is uncontrolled.

  - ○ Rehabilitation care may be consulted if the client has prolonged weakness and needs assistance with an increasing level of activity.

- • Surgical Interventions

  - ○ Chest tube insertion

    - □ Chest tubes are inserted in the pleural space to drain fluid, blood, or air; re-establish a negative pressure; facilitate lung expansion; and restore normal intrapleural pressure.

- Nursing Actions
  - Obtain informed consent, gather supplies, monitor the client's status (vital signs, SaO$_2$, chest tube drainage), report abnormalities to the health care provider, and administer pain medications.
  - Continually monitor vital signs and the client's response to the procedure.
  - Monitor chest tube placement and function.

- Care After Discharge

  - Set up referral services (home health, respiratory services) to provide portable oxygen if needed.

  o Client Education

  - Encourage the client to take rest periods as needed.

  - Remind the client to use proper hand hygiene to prevent infection.

  - Encourage immunizations for influenza as well as pneumonia.

  - Remind the client that recovery from a pneumothorax/hemothorax may be lengthy.

  - Educate the client and family about the illness, and encourage them to express their feelings.

  - Encourage smoking cessation if the client currently smokes.

  - Stress the importance of follow-up care and instruct the client to report the following to the provider:
    - Upper respiratory infection
    - Fever
    - Cough
    - Difficulty breathing
    - Sharp chest pain

- Client Outcomes

  o The client will maintain a patent airway.

  o The client will maintain adequate gas exchange.

  o The client will remain free from pain.

  o The client will remain free from infection.

  o The client will remain free from anxiety.

  o The client will gradually increase exercise and activity to previous levels.

Complications

- Decreased cardiac output

    - The amount of blood pumped by the heart is decreased.
    - This is a result of intrathoracic pressures rising.
    - Hypotension develops.

  o Nursing Actions

    - Administer IV fluids and blood products as prescribed.
    - Monitor heart rate and rhythm.
    - Monitor intake and output (chest tube drainage).

- Respiratory failure

    - Inadequate gas exchange due to lung collapse

  o Nursing Actions

    - Prepare for mechanical ventilation.
    - Continue respiratory assessment.

CHAPTER 29: PNEUMOTHORAX AND HEMOTHORAX

(A) Application Exercises

Scenario: A nurse in an emergency department is caring for a young adult male client who was admitted with a gunshot wound. The client has a of blood pressure 108/55 mm Hg, a heart rate of 124/min, a respiratory rate of 36/min, a temperature of 38.6° C (101.4° F), and an SaO_2 of 95% on 15 L/min via a nonrebreather mask. The client reports dyspnea and pain.

1. The nurse reassesses the client 30 min later. Which of the following assessment findings should the nurse report to the health care provider? (Select all that apply.)

   _____ SaO_2 of 90%

   _____ Tracheal deviation

   _____ Headache

   _____ Blood pressure of 104/54 mm Hg

   _____ Heart rate of 154/min

   _____ Hemoptysis

   _____ Distended neck veins

   _____ Nausea

2. A chest x-ray is performed, and tracheal deviation is observed. The client's vital signs are now as follows: blood pressure 82/48 mm Hg, heart rate 158/min, respiratory rate 42/min, temperature 38.7° C (101.6° F), and SaO_2 87%. What do these vital signs indicate?

3. Prioritize the following provider orders from most important to least. Designate "1" as the most important intervention.

   _____ Document interventions.

   _____ Obtain a large-bore IV needle for decompression.

   _____ Administer lorazepam (Ativan).

   _____ Prepare for chest tube insertion.

4. A nurse is caring for a client who has a tension pneumothorax. The nurse knows that, as a result of the tension pneumothorax, air continues to accumulate and the intrapleural pressure rises, which

   A. causes small blebs to develop in the lung on the affected side.

   B. allows air to flow freely through the chest wall during inspiration and expiration.

   C. causes less air to enter on inspiration and exceed the barometric pressure.

   D. will cause the mediastinum to shift away from the affected side and decrease venous return.

CHAPTER 29: PNEUMOTHORAX AND HEMOTHORAX

Ⓐ Application Exercises Answer Key

Scenario: A nurse in an emergency department is caring for a young adult male client who was admitted with a gunshot wound. The client's has a blood pressure of 108/55 mm Hg, a heart rate of 124/min, a respiratory rate of 36/min, a temperature of 38.6° C (101.4° F), and an SaO_2 of 95% on 15 L/min via a nonrebreather mask. The client reports dyspnea and pain.

1. The nurse reassesses the client 30 min later. Which of the following assessment findings should the nurse report to the health care provider? (Select all that apply.)

__X__	**SaO_2 of 90%**
__X__	**Tracheal deviation**
_____	Headache
_____	Blood pressure of 104/54 mm Hg
__X__	**Heart rate of 154/min**
__X__	**Hemoptysis**
__X__	**Distended neck veins**
_____	Nausea

An SaO_2 of 90%, tracheal deviation, heart rate of 154/min, hemoptysis, and distended neck veins are all signs that indicate the client's condition is worsening and needs to be reported to the health care provider. Nausea and a blood pressure of 104/54 mm Hg are expected findings. The report of a headache does not have clinical significance in this situation.

 NCLEX® Connection: Physiological Adaptation, Medical Emergencies

2. A chest x-ray is performed, and tracheal deviation is observed. The client's vital signs are now as follows: blood pressure 82/48 mm Hg, heart rate 158/min, respiratory rate 42/min, temperature 38.7° C (101.6° F), and SaO_2 87%. What do these vital signs indicate?

The client is experiencing a tension pneumothorax. The tracheal deviation is a definitive sign of tension pneumothorax. The hypotension, tachycardia, tachypnea, and decreasing SaO_2 indicate that the client is progressing toward respiratory failure.

Ⓝ NCLEX® Connection: Physiological Adaptation, Medical Emergencies

3. Prioritize the following provider orders from most important to least. Designate "1" as the most important intervention.

   4   Document interventions.

   1   Obtain a large-bore IV needle for decompression.

   3   Administer lorazepam (Ativan).

   2   Prepare for chest tube insertion.

Establishing and maintaining the client's respiratory function are the highest priority. The health care provider should insert a large-bore needle into the second intercostal space. The nurse should obtain the supplies to do an immediate needle aspiration or decompression. After the provider completes the needle aspiration, she will insert a chest tube. The next action the nurse should take is to prepare for chest tube insertion. The client will likely be anxious, and a benzodiazepine medication may be prescribed. Finally, the nurse should document the interventions.

Ⓝ **NCLEX® Connection: Physiological Adaptation, Medical Emergencies**

4. A nurse is caring for a client who has a tension pneumothorax. The nurse knows that, as a result of the tension pneumothorax, air continues to accumulate and the intrapleural pressure rises, which

    A. causes small blebs to develop in the lung on the affected side.

    B. allows air to flow freely through the chest wall during inspiration and expiration.

    C. causes less air to enter on inspiration and exceed the barometric pressure.

    D. will cause the mediastinum to shift away from the affected side and decrease venous return.

A tension pneumothorax causes air to be trapped in the pleural space, which compresses the local blood vessels and ultimately decreases venous return. Small blebs cause a spontaneous pneumothorax. With an open pneumothorax, air flows through the chest wall during inspiration and expiration. With tension pneumothorax, air enters the pleural space with each inspiration; therefore less air entering on inspiration is incorrect.

Ⓝ **NCLEX® Connection: Physiological Adaptation, Pathophysiology**

UNIT 3	NURSING CARE OF CLIENTS WITH RESPIRATORY DISORDERS
Section	Respiratory Emergencies
Chapter 30	Respiratory Failure

Overview

- Acute respiratory failure (ARF)

    o ARF is caused by failure to adequately ventilate and/or oxygenate.

    o Ventilatory failure is due to a mechanical abnormality of the lungs or chest wall, impaired muscle function (the diaphragm), or a malfunction in the respiratory control center of the brain.

    o Oxygenation failure can result from a lack of perfusion to the pulmonary capillary bed (a pulmonary embolism) or a condition that alters the gas exchange medium (pulmonary edema, pneumonia).

    o Both inadequate ventilation and oxygenation can occur in individuals with diseased lungs (asthma, emphysema). Diseased lung tissue can cause oxygenation failure and increased work of breathing, eventually resulting in respiratory muscle fatigue and ventilatory failure.

    o Criteria for acute respiratory failure are based on ABG values.

    o ABGs that indicate ARF

        ▪ Room air, PaO_2 less than 60 mm Hg, and SaO_2 less than 90% or

        ▪ $PaCO_2$ greater than 50 mm Hg in conjunction with a pH less than 7.30

- Acute respiratory distress syndrome (ARDS)

    o ARDS is a state of acute respiratory failure with a mortality rate of 25% to 40%.

    o Indicators present with ARDS

        ▪ Dyspnea

        ▪ Bilateral noncardiogenic pulmonary edema

        ▪ Reduced lung compliance

        ▪ Diffuse patchy bilateral pulmonary infiltrates

        ▪ Severe hypoxemia despite administration of 100% oxygen

    o A systemic inflammatory response injures the alveolar-capillary membrane. It becomes permeable to large molecules, and the lung space is filled with fluid.

    o A reduction in surfactant weakens the alveoli, which causes collapse or filling of fluid, leading to worsening edema.

- Severe acute respiratory syndrome (SARS)

  ○ SARS is the result of a viral infection from a mutated strain of the coronaviruses, a group of viruses that also cause the common cold.

  ○ The virus invades the pulmonary tissue, which leads to an inflammatory response.

  ○ The virus is spread easily through airborne droplets from sneezing, coughing, or talking.

  ○ The virus does not spread to the bloodstream because it flourishes at temperatures slightly below normal core body temperature.

(G) - Older adult clients have decreased pulmonary reserves due to normal lung changes, including decreased lung elasticity and thickening alveoli. Older adult clients may decompensate more quickly.

Assessment

- Risk Factors

  ○ ARF

  ○ Ventilatory failure

    ▪ COPD

    ▪ Pulmonary embolism and pneumothorax

    ▪ ARDS

    ▪ Asthma

    ▪ Pulmonary edema

    ▪ Fibrosis of lung tissue

    ▪ Neuromuscular disorders, (multiple sclerosis, Guillain-Barré syndrome), spinal cord injuries, and cerebrovascular accident, that impair the client's rate and depth of respiration

    ▪ Elevated intracranial pressure (closed-head injuries, cerebral edema, hemorrhagic stroke)

  ○ Oxygenation failure

    ▪ Pneumonia

    ▪ Hypoventilation

    ▪ Hypovolemic shock

    ▪ Pulmonary edema

    ▪ Low hemoglobin

    ▪ Low concentrations of oxygen (carbon monoxide poisoning, high altitude, smoke inhalation)

- o ARDS
  - May result from localized lung damage or from the effects of other systemic problems
  - Aspiration
  - Pulmonary emboli (fat, amniotic fluid)
  - Pneumonia and other pulmonary infections
  - Sepsis
  - Near-drowning accident
  - Trauma
  - Damage to the central nervous system
  - Smoke or toxic gas inhalation
  - Drug ingestion/overdose (heroin, opioids, salicylates)
- o SARS
  - Exposure to an infected individual
  - Immunocompromised individuals (chemotherapy, AIDS)
- o Subjective Data
  - ARF, ARDS, and SARS
  - Shortness of breath
  - Dyspnea with or without exertion
  - Orthopnea (difficulty breathing lying flat)
- o Objective Data
  - Physical Assessment Findings
    - □ ARF, ARDS, and SARS
    - □ Rapid, shallow breathing
    - □ Cyanotic, mottled, dusky skin
    - □ Tachycardia
    - □ Hypotension
    - □ Substernal or suprasternal retractions
    - □ Decreased SaO_2 (less than 90%)
    - □ Adventitious breath sounds (wheezing, rales)
    - □ Cardiac arrhythmias
    - □ Confusion
    - □ Lethargy

- ○ Laboratory Tests
  - ■ ARF, ARDS, and SARS
  - ■ ABG sample
  - ■ Room air, PaO_2 less than 60 mm Hg, SaO_2 less than 90%
  - ■ $PaCO_2$ greater than 50 mm Hg and pH less than 7.30 (hypoxemia, hypercarbia)
  - ■ Sputum culture (used to rule out or diagnose an infection)
  - ■ CBC (elevated WBC count may indicate infection or inflammation)
- ○ Diagnostic Procedures
  - ■ Chest x-ray
    - □ Results may include:
      - ▸ Pulmonary edema (ARF, ARDS)
      - ▸ Cardiomegaly (ARF)
      - ▸ Diffuse infiltrates and white-out or ground-glass appearance (ARDS)
      - ▸ Infiltrates (SARS)
    - □ Nursing Actions
      - ▸ Assist with client positioning before and after the x-ray.
      - ▸ Interpret and communicate the results to the appropriate personnel in a timely manner.
  - ■ Electrocardiogram (ECG)
    - □ Used to rule out cardiac involvement
  - ■ Hemodynamic monitoring
    - □ A Swan-Ganz catheter is placed to measure pulmonary artery pressures and cardiac output. Pulmonary capillary wedge pressure with ARDS is usually low or within the expected reference range (4 to12 mm Hg). Continuous hemodynamic monitoring is important for fluid management.
    - □ Nursing Actions
      - ▸ Monitor the ECG during catheter insertion.
      - ▸ Have resuscitation medications and equipment ready.
      - ▸ Monitor hemodynamic waveforms and readings.
      - ▸ Confirm catheter placement using a chest x-ray.

Collaborative Care

- • Nursing Care
  - ○ Maintain a patent airway and monitor respiratory status every hour as needed.
  - ○ Suction the client as needed.

- o Assess and document sputum color, amount, and consistency.

- o Oxygenate before suctioning secretions to prevent further hypoxemia.

- o Mechanical ventilation is often required. Positive-end expiratory pressure (PEEP) is often used to prevent alveolar collapse during expiration. Follow facility protocol for monitoring and documenting ventilator settings.

- o Monitor for pneumothorax (a high PEEP may cause the lungs to collapse).

- o Obtain ABGs as prescribed and following each ventilator setting adjustment.

- o Maintain continuous ECG monitoring for changes that may indicate increased hypoxemia, especially when repositioning and applying suction.

- o Continually monitor vital signs, including SaO_2.

- o Position the client to facilitate ventilation and perfusion.

- o Prevent infection

  - Perform frequent hand hygiene.

  - Use appropriate suctioning technique.

  - Provide oral care every 2 hr and as needed.

  - Wear protective clothing (gown, gloves, mask) when appropriate.

- o Promote nutrition

  - Assess bowel sounds.

  - Monitor elimination patterns.

  - Obtain daily weights.

  - Record urine output.

  - Administer enteral and/or parenteral feedings as prescribed.

  - Prevent aspiration with enteral feedings (elevate the head of the bed 30 to 45°).

    - □ Confirm nasogastric (NG) tube placement prior to feeding.

- o Provide emotional support to the client and family.

  - Encourage verbalization of feelings.

  - Provide alternative communication means (dry erase board, pen and paper).

- Medications

PHARMACOLOGIC AGENTS	ACTIONS	NURSING CONSIDERATIONS
Benzodiazepines • Lorazepam (Ativan) • Midazolam (Versed)	• Reduces anxiety and resistance to ventilation and decreases oxygen consumption	• Monitor respirations on clients who are not ventilated. • Monitor blood pressure and SaO_2. • Use cautiously in conjunction with opioid narcotics.
General anesthesia • Propofol (Diprivan)	• Used to induce and maintain anesthesia • May be used to sedate clients who are to be placed on mechanical ventilation	• Contraindicated for clients with hyperlipidemia and egg allergies. • Administer only to clients that are intubated and ventilated. • Monitor ECG, blood pressure, and sedation levels. • IV rate must be slowed to assess the client's neurological status (follow institution protocol). • Monitor for hypotension. • Titrate to desired sedation.
Opioid analgesics • Morphine sulfate • Fentanyl citrate (Sublimaze)	• Provides pain management	• Monitor respirations on clients who are not ventilated. • Monitor blood pressure, heart rate, and SaO_2. • Monitor ABGs (hypercapnia can result from depressed respirations). • Use cautiously in conjunction with hypnotic sedatives. • Assess the client's pain level and response to medication. • Document the client's pain level. • Have naloxone hydrochloride (Narcan) and resuscitation equipment available for severe respiratory depression in clients who are not receiving ventilation.

PHARMACOLOGIC AGENTS	ACTIONS	NURSING CONSIDERATIONS
Neuromuscular blocking agents • Vecuronium (Norcuron)	• Facilitate ventilation and decreases oxygen consumption • Often used with painful ventilatory modes (inverse ratio ventilation and PEEP)	• Give only to clients that are intubated and ventilated. • Monitor ECG, blood pressure, and muscle strength. • Give pain medication and sedatives with neuromuscular blocking agents. • Neuromuscular blocking agents do not sedate or relieve pain (the client may be awake and frightened). • Have neostigmine methylsulfate (Prostigmin) and atropine sulfate (Atropair) available to reverse the effects of the neuromuscular blocking agent. • Have resuscitation equipment available. • Reassure the client that paralysis is medication induced. • Explain all procedures to the client.
Corticosteroids • Cortisone acetate (Cortistan) • Methylprednisolone sodium succinate (Solu-Medrol) • Dexamethasone sodium phosphate (Decadron)	• Reduces WBC migration, decreases inflammation, and help stabilize the alveolar-capillary membrane during ARDS	• Discontinue the medication gradually. • Administer with an anti-ulcer medication to prevent peptic ulcer formation. • Monitor weight and blood pressure. • Monitor glucose and electrolytes. • Advise the client to take oral doses with food and avoid stopping the medication suddenly.
Antibiotics sensitive to cultured organism(s) • Vancomycin (Vancocin)	• Treats identified organisms	• Culture sputum prior to administration of first dose. • Monitor for a hypersensitivity reaction. • Give IV doses slowly. • Monitor the IV site for infiltration. • Do not give with other medications. • Monitor coagulopathy and renal function. • Advise client to take oral doses with food and finish the prescribed dose.

- Interdisciplinary Care
  - Respiratory therapy
    - The respiratory therapist typically manages the ventilator, adjusts the settings, and provides chest physical therapy to improve ventilation and chest expansion.
    - The respiratory therapist may also suction the endotracheal tube and administer inhalation medications, such as bronchodilators.
  - Physical therapy
    - Indicated for extended ventilatory support and rehabilitation
  - Nutritional therapy
    - Enteral or parenteral feeding
    - Nutritional support following extubation
- Therapeutic Procedures
  - Intubation and mechanical ventilation
    - Artificial airway insertion with mechanical ventilation
    - Nursing Actions
      - Monitor ECG, SaO_2, breath sounds, and color.
      - Sedate as needed.
      - Provide reassurance to calm the client.
      - Have suction equipment, manual resuscitation bag, and face mask available at all times.
      - Suction secretions as needed.
      - Preintubation
        - Oxygenate with 100% oxygen.
        - Assist ventilation with manual resuscitation bag and face mask.
        - Have emergency resuscitation equipment readily available.
      - Postintubation
        - Assess bilateral breath sounds, symmetrical chest movement, and chest x-ray to confirm placement of the endotracheal tube.
        - Secure the endotracheal tube per institutional guidelines.
        - Assess the balloon cuff for air leaks periodically.
      - PEEP
        - Positive pressure is applied at the end of expiration to keep the alveoli expanded.
        - PEEP is added to the ventilator setting to increase oxygenation and improve lung expansion.

- Client Education
  - Explain all procedures to the client.
  - Reassure and calm the client.
  - Explain to the client and family that the client will be unable to speak while the endotracheal tube is in place.
- Kinetic therapy
  - A special kinetic bed that rotates laterally alters client positioning to reduce atelectasis and improve ventilation.
  - Nursing Actions
    - Begin slowly and gradually increase the degree of rotation as tolerated.
    - Monitor ECG, SaO_2, breath sounds, and blood pressure.
    - Stop rotation if the client becomes distressed.
    - Provide routine skin care to prevent breakdown.
    - Sedate as needed.
  - Client Education
    - Explain all procedures to the client.

- Client Outcomes
  - The client will be able to breathe independently with no respiratory assistance.
  - The client will be able to maintain an SaO_2 greater than 90% on room air.
  - The client will be free of infection.
  - The client will maintain optimal physical and mental functioning.

Complications

- Endotracheal tube
  - Trauma during intubation or long-term intubation
    - Can cause damage to trachea and vocal cords
    - Nursing Actions
      - Consider a tracheostomy for long-term ventilation.
  - Aspiration pneumonia
    - Nursing Actions
      - Check the cuff on the endotracheal tube for leaks.
      - Assess suction contents for gastric secretions.
      - Verify NG tube placement.

- o Infection
  - ▪ Nursing Actions
    - ☐ Prevent infection by using proper hand hygiene and suctioning technique.
    - ☐ Assess color, amount, and consistency of secretions.
  - ▪ Blocked endotracheal tube
    - ☐ The high-pressure alarm on the ventilator may indicate a blocked endotracheal tube.
  - ▪ Nursing Actions
    - ☐ Suction secretions to relieve a mucous plug or insert an oral airway to prevent biting on the tube.
  - ▪ Altered position of endotracheal tube
  - ▪ Nursing Actions
    - ☐ Check tube positioning every 1 to 2 hr.
    - ☐ Assess breath sounds, SaO_2, and chest movement.
    - ☐ Secure endotracheal tube per institution's guidelines to maintain tube placement.
- • Mechanical Ventilation
  - o Increased intrathoracic pressure
    - ▪ Positive pressure (PEEP) increases intrathoracic pressure, which can cause a decreased blood return to the heart, decreased cardiac output and/or hypotension.
    - ▪ Decreased cardiac output can activate the renin-angiotensin-aldosterone system, leading to fluid retention and/or decreased urine output.
    - ▪ Nursing Actions
      - ☐ Monitor input and output, weight, and hydration status.
    - ▪ Client Education
      - ☐ Advise the client to avoid using the Valsalva maneuver (straining with bowel movement), because it can further increase intrathoracic pressure.
  - o Barotrauma
    - ▪ Ventilation with positive pressure causes damage to the lungs (pneumothorax, subcutaneous emphysema).

- Nursing Actions
  - Monitor oxygenation status and chest x-ray.
  - Assess for subcutaneous emphysema (crackles and/or air movement felt under skin).
  - Document all ventilator changes made.
    - A high pressure ventilator alarm may indicate pneumothorax.
- Immobilization
  - Can result in muscle atrophy, pneumonia, and pressure sores
  - Nursing Actions
    - Reposition and suction every 2 hr.
    - Provide routine skin care.
    - Implement range-of-motion exercises to prevent muscle atrophy.

CHAPTER 30: RESPIRATORY FAILURE

(A) Application Exercises

Scenario: A nurse in an emergency department is caring for a 40-year-old male client who was admitted following a motor vehicle crash. Physical assessment reveals absent breath sounds in the left lower lobe. The client is dyspneic, has a blood pressure of 111/68 mm Hg, a heart rate of 124/min, a respiratory rate of 38/min, a temperature of 38.6° C (101.4° F), and an SaO_2 of 92% on room air.

1. Which of the following actions should the nurse take first?

   A. Obtain a chest x-ray.

   B. Prepare for chest tube insertion.

   C. Administer oxygen via a high-flow mask.

   D. Obtain IV access.

2. The client is now receiving 15 L/min of oxygen via a non rebreather mask. The client's ABG results are as follows: pH 7.25, PaO_2 55 mm Hg, $PaCO_2$ 58 mm Hg, and HCO_3^- 34 mEq/L. Interpret this ABG.

3. What medical intervention should the nurse anticipate next?

4. The client is started on mechanical ventilation. Explain why positive-end expiration pressure would be useful for this client.

5. This client is receiving vecuronium (Norcuron). Which of the following medications should the nurse anticipate administering? (Select all that apply.)

   _____ Fentanyl (Duragesic)

   _____ Furosemide (Lasix)

   _____ Midazolam (Versed)

   _____ Famotidine (Pepcid)

   _____ Dexamethasone (Decadron)

6. Which of the following clients are at risk for the development of acute respiratory failure (ARF) and/ or acute respiratory distress syndrome (ARDS)? (Select all that apply.)

   _____ A 14-year-old boy who received 2 min of CPR following a near-drowning incident

   _____ A client who is post coronary artery bypass graft with two chest tubes

   _____ A client with a hemoglobin level of 14.5 mg/dL

   _____ A client with an exacerbation of cystic fibrosis

   _____ A client with dysphagia

   _____ A client with a sinus infection

7. A nurse is caring for a client who has severe acute respiratory syndrome. Treatment for this client may include

_____ antibiotics.

_____ supplemental oxygen.

_____ antiviral medications.

_____ bronchodilators.

_____ intubation.

CHAPTER 30: RESPIRATORY FAILURE

 Application Exercises Answer Key

Scenario: A nurse in an emergency department is caring for a 40-year-old male client who was admitted following a motor vehicle crash. Physical assessment reveals absent breath sounds in the left lower lobe. The client is dyspneic has a blood pressure of 111/68 mm Hg, a heart rate 124/min, a respiratory rate of 38/min, a temperature of 38.6° C (101.4° F), and an SaO$_2$ of 92% on room air.

1. Which of the following actions should the nurse take first?

    A. Obtain a chest x-ray.

    B. Prepare for chest tube insertion.

    C. Administer oxygen via high-flow mask.

    D. Obtain IV access.

    According to the airway, breathing, and circulation (ABC) priority setting framework, administering oxygen via a high-flow mask is the first priority. Obtaining a chest x-ray, preparing for chest tube insertion, and obtaining IV access are also important actions, but none of them is the priority.

    Ⓝ **NCLEX® Connection: Physiological Adaptation, Medical Emergencies**

2. The client is now receiving 15 L/min of oxygen via a non rebreather mask. The client's ABG results are as follows: pH 7.25, PaO$_2$ 55 mm Hg, PaCO$_2$ 58 mm Hg, and HCO$_3^-$ 34 mEq/L. Interpret this ABG.

CLIENT ABGS	REFERENCE RANGE	INDICATION
pH 7.25	7.35 to 7.45	A low pH indicates acidosis.
PaCO$_2$ 58	35 to 45	A high PaCO$_2$ indicates respiratory (hypoventilation)
HCO$_3^-$ 34	22 to 26	A high HCO$_3^-$ indicates metabolic alkalosis or compensated respiratory acidosis (depending on the pH).

    This client is in a state of partially compensated respiratory acidosis.

    Ⓝ **NCLEX® Connection: Physiological Adaptation, Fluid and Electrolyte Imbalances**

3. What medical intervention should the nurse anticipate next?

    The nurse should prepare the client for endotracheal intubation and mechanical ventilation.

    Ⓝ **NCLEX® Connection: Physiological Adaptation, Fluid and Electrolyte Imbalances**

4. The client is started on mechanical ventilation. Explain why positive-end expiration pressure would be useful for this client.

> PEEP exerts pressure at the end of expiration to prevent alveolar collapse and improve gas exchange.

 NCLEX® Connection: Physiological Adaptation, Medical Emergencies

5. This client is receiving vecuronium (Norcuron). Which of the following medications should the nurse anticipate administering? (Select all that apply.)

__X__	**Fentanyl (Duragesic)**
_____	Furosemide (Lasix)
__X__	**Midazolam (Versed)**
_____	Famotidine (Pepcid)
_____	Dexamethasone (Decadron)

> Pain medication and sedation (fentanyl, midazolam) are often used when a client is on a ventilator along with a neuromuscular blocking agent, because a neuromuscular blocking agent does not block pain impulses. The client may be in pain and anxious but unable to communicate these feelings. Furosemide, famotidine, and dexamethasone are not medications used to help block pain or help sedate a client.

 NCLEX® Connection: Pharmacological and Parenteral Therapies, Pharmacological Pain Management

6. Which of the following clients are at risk for the development of acute respiratory failure (ARF) and/or acute respiratory distress syndrome (ARDS)? (Select all that apply.)

__X__	**A 14-year-old boy who received 2 min of CPR following a near-drowning incident**
__X__	**A client who post coronary artery bypass graft with two chest tubes**
_____	A client with a hemoglobin level of 14.5 mg/dL
__X__	**A client with an exacerbation of cystic fibrosis**
__X__	**A client with dysphagia**
_____	A client with a sinus infection

> Clients that are at risk for developing ARF and/or ARDS include anyone who has a lung injury or is at risk for developing a lung injury, such as from aspiration, near drowning, dysphagia, cystic fibrosis, or a coronary artery bypass graft.

 NCLEX® Connection: Reduction of Risk Potential, System Specific Assessment

7. A nurse is caring for a client who has severe acute respiratory syndrome. Treatment for this client may include

   _____   antibiotics.

   __X__   **supplemental oxygen.**

   _____   antiviral medications.

   __X__   **bronchodilators.**

   __X__   **intubation.**

SARS is caused by the coronavirus. Treatment involves supplemental oxygen, bronchodilators, and mechanical ventilation. Antibiotics may indicate for a secondary infection. There are no effective antiviral medications to treat the coronavirus at this time.

Ⓝ NCLEX® Connection: Physiological Adaptation, Medical Emergencies

UNIT 4: NURSING CARE OF CLIENTS WITH CARDIOVASCULAR DISORDERS

- Diagnostic and Therapeutic Procedures
- Cardiac Disorders
- Vascular Disorders

NCLEX® CONNECTIONS

When reviewing the chapters in this unit, keep in mind the relevant sections of the NCLEX® outline, in particular:

CLIENT NEEDS: PHARMACOLOGICAL AND PARENTERAL THERAPIES	CLIENT NEEDS: REDUCTION OF RISK POTENTIAL	CLIENT NEEDS: PHYSIOLOGICAL ADAPTATION
Relevant topics/tasks include:	Relevant topics/tasks include:	Relevant topics/tasks include:

CLIENT NEEDS: PHARMACOLOGICAL AND PARENTERAL THERAPIES

Relevant topics/tasks include:
- Adverse Effects/ Contraindications/Side Effects/Interactions
  - Identify a contraindication to the administration of a medication to the client.
- Central Venous Access Devices
  - Provide care for the client with a central venous access device.
- Parenteral/Intravenous Therapy
  - Apply knowledge and concepts of mathematics/nursing procedures/psychomotor skills when caring for a client receiving intravenous and parenteral therapy.

CLIENT NEEDS: REDUCTION OF RISK POTENTIAL

Relevant topics/tasks include:
- Diagnostic Tests
  - Apply knowledge of related nursing procedures and psychomotor skills when caring for clients undergoing diagnostic testing.
- Changes/Abnormalities in Vital Signs
  - Evaluate invasive monitoring data.
- System Specific Assessment
  - Assess the client for abnormal peripheral pulses after a procedure or treatment.

CLIENT NEEDS: PHYSIOLOGICAL ADAPTATION

Relevant topics/tasks include:
- Alterations in Body Systems
  - Assist with invasive procedures.
- Hemodynamics
  - Identify cardiac rhythm strip abnormalities.
- Unexpected Responses to Therapies
  - Assess the client for unexpected adverse responses to therapy.

UNIT 4	NURSING CARE OF CLIENTS WITH CARDIOVASCULAR DISORDERS
Section	Diagnostic and Therapeutic Procedures
Chapter 31	Cardiovascular Diagnostic and Therapeutic Procedures

Overview

- Cardiovascular diagnostic procedures evaluate the functioning of the heart by monitoring for enzymes in the blood; using ultrasound to visualize the heart; determining the heart's response to exercise; and using catheters to determine blood volume, perfusion, fluid status, how the heart is pumping, and degree of artery blockage.

- Cardiovascular diagnostic procedures that nurses should be familiar with include:

  o Cardiac enzymes and lipid profile

  o Echocardiogram

  o Stress testing

  o Hemodynamic monitoring

  o Angiography

  o Vascular Access

Cardiac Enzymes and Lipid Profile

- Cardiac enzymes are released into the bloodstream when the heart muscle suffers ischemia. A lipid profile provide information regarding cholesterol levels and is used for early detection of heart disease.

- Cardiac enzymes are a specific marker in diagnosing an MI.

- Indications

  o Angina

  o MI

  o Heart disease

  o Hyperlipidemia

- Interpretation of Findings

CARDIAC ENZYME	EXPECTED REFERENCE RANGE	ELEVATED LEVELS FIRST DETECTABLE FOLLOWING MYOCARDIAL INJURY	EXPECTED DURATION OF ELEVATED LEVELS
Creatine kinase MB isoenzyme (CK-MB) – more sensitive to myocardium	0% of total CK (30 to 170 units/L)	4 to 6 hr	3 days
Troponin T	< 0.2 ng/L	3 to 5 hr	14 to 21 days
Troponin I	< 0.03 ng/L	3 hr	7 to 10 days
Myoglobin	< 90 mcg/L	2 hr	24 hr

TEST	EXPECTED REFERENCE RANGE	PURPOSE
Cholesterol (total)	< 200 mg/dL	Screening test for heart disease
HDL	• Females – 35 to 80 mg/dL • Males – 35 to 65 mg/dL	"Good" cholesterol produced by the liver
LDL	< 130 mg/dL	"Bad" cholesterol can be up to 70% of total cholesterol
Triglycerides	< 150 mg/dL	Evaluating test for atherosclerosis

- Preprocedure

  - Nursing Actions

    - Explain the reason for the test to the client.

- Intraprocedure

  - A blood specimen is drawn from client via venipuncture.

- Postprocedure

  - Lab findings will be discussed with the client by the provider, and choice of treatment will be determined.

Echocardiogram

- An echocardiogram is an ultrasound of the heart. The test is used to diagnose valve disorders and cardiomyopathy.

- Indications

  - Cardiomyopathy

  - Heart failure

- ○ Angina

- ○ Myocardial infarction

- Preprocedure

  - ○ Nursing Actions

    - Explain the reason for the test to the client. The test is pain free and takes up to 1 hr.

- Intraprocedure

  - ○ Nursing Actions

    - Instruct the client to lie on left side and remain still.

- Postprocedure

  - ○ Nursing Actions

    - Inform the client that the results of the test and a plan for follow-up care will be provided by the provider. There is no specific postprocedure instructions that need to be followed.

Stress Testing

- The cardiac muscle is exercised by the client walking on a treadmill. This provides information regarding the workload of the heart. Once the client's heart rate reaches a certain rate, the test is discontinued.

  - ○ Clients sometimes become too tired and are unable to finish the test. The provider can reorder the test to be done as a pharmacological stress test.

- Indications

  - ○ Angina

  - ○ Heart Failure

  - ○ Myocardial Infarction

  - ○ Dysrhythmia

- Preprocedure

  - ○ Nursing Actions

    - Ensure that informed consent has been obtained.

    - Explain to the client that he will be walking on a treadmill, and comfortable shoes and clothing are recommended.

    - If the client is disabled or unable to be physically challenged, the provider can order the test be a pharmacological stress test, where a drug, such as adenosine (Adenocard), is given to stress the heart instead of walking on the treadmill.

    - The client is instructed to fast 2 to 4 hours before the procedure according to agency policy and to avoid tobacco, alcohol, and caffeine before the test.

- Intraprocedure
  - Nursing Actions
    - Remind the client that once the heart reaches a certain rate, the test will be discontinued.
- Postprocedure
  - Nursing Actions
    - The client is monitored by ECG and his blood pressure is checked frequently until he is stable.
    - The provider will discuss findings with client. There are no specific postprocedure considerations for this test.

Hemodynamic Monitoring

- Hemodynamic monitoring involves special indwelling catheters to provide information about blood volume and perfusion, fluid status, and how well the heart is pumping.

 View Media Supplement: Hemodynamic Monitoring (Image)

  - Hemodynamic status is assessed with several parameters.
    - Central venous pressure (CVP)
    - Pulmonary artery pressure (PAP)
    - Pulmonary artery wedge pressure (PAWP)
    - Cardiac output (CO)
    - Intra arterial pressure
  - Mixed venous oxygen saturation (SvO_2) indicates the balance between oxygen supply and demand. It is measured by a pulmonary artery catheter with fiberoptics.
  - A pressure-monitoring system comprised of a catheter with an infusion system, a transducer, and a monitor is used to display a client's hemodynamic information.
  - Components of Hemodynamic Monitoring Systems
    - Pressure transducer
    - Pressure tubing
    - Monitor
    - Pressure bag and flush device
  - Arterial Lines
    - Arterial lines are placed in the radial (most common), brachial, or femoral artery

- Arterial lines provide continuous information about changes in blood pressure and permit the withdrawal of samples of arterial blood. Intra-arterial pressures can differ from cuff pressures.

- The integrity of the arterial waveform should be assessed to verify the accuracy of blood pressure readings.

- Monitor circulation in the limb with the arterial line (capillary refill, temperature, color).

- Arterial lines are not to be used for intravenous fluid infusion.

  ○ Pulmonary Artery Catheters

- Pulmonary artery (PA) catheters have multiple ports and components that enable a variety of hemodynamic measurements, the collection of blood samples, and the infusion of intravenous fluids.

- The PA catheter is inserted into a large vein (internal jugular, femoral, subclavian, brachial) and threaded through the right atria and ventricle into a branch of the pulmonary artery.

- Pulmonary artery catheters have multiple lumens.

  □ Proximal lumen can be used to measure right atrial pressure (CVP), infuse intravenous fluids, and to obtain venous blood samples.

  □ Distal lumen can be used to measure pulmonary artery pressures (PA systolic, PA diastolic, mean pulmonary artery pressure, and pulmonary artery wedge pressure). This lumen is not to be used for intravenous fluid infusion.

  □ Balloon inflation port is intermittently used for PAWP measurements. When not in use, it should be left deflated and in the 'locked' position.

  □ Thermistor measures temperature differences between the right atrium and the pulmonary artery in order to determine cardiac output.

  □ Additional infusion ports may be indicated, depending on the brand.

- Indications

  ○ Serious or critical illness

  ○ Heart failure

  ○ Post coronary artery bypass graft (CABG) clients

  ○ ARDS

  ○ Acute renal failure

  ○ Burn victims

  ○ Trauma victims

- Interpretation of Findings

  o Normal Values of Hemodynamic Readings

Central Venous Pressure (CVP)	1-8 mm Hg
Pulmonary Artery Systolic (PAS)	15-26 mm Hg
Pulmonary Artery Diastolic (PAD)	5-15 mm Hg
Pulmonary Artery Wedge Pressure (PAWP)	4-12 mm Hg
Cardiac Output (CO)	4-6 L/min
Mixed Venous Oxygen Saturation (SvO$_2$)	60% to 80%

  o The intravascular volume in older adult clients is often reduced; therefore, the nurse should anticipate lower hemodynamic readings, particularly if dehydration is a complication.

- Preprocedure

  o Nursing Actions

    ■ Line Insertion

      □ Ensure the client's understanding of the procedure prior to obtaining consent.

      □ Assemble the pressure monitoring system. Purge all air from system.

      □ Maintain sterility of connections.

      □ Place the client in supine or Trendelenburg position.

      □ Administer sedation and pain medications as prescribed.

      □ Level transducer with phlebostatic axis (4th intercostal space, mid-axillary line).

      □ Zero system with atmospheric pressure.

      □ Hemodynamic pressure lines must be calibrated to read atmospheric pressure as zero, and the transducer should be positioned at the right atrium (phlebostatic axis).

      □ Obtain initial readings as prescribed. Compare arterial blood pressure to non-invasive cuff pressure (NIBP).

      □ Document the client's response.

- Intraprocedure

  - Monitor for symptoms of altered hemodynamics.

PRELOAD		AFTERLOAD	
Right heart – CVP Left heart – PAWP		Right heart – Pulmonary Vascular Resistance (PVR) Left heart – Systemic Vascular Resistance (SVR)	
Elevated	Decreased	Elevated	Decreased
• Crackles in lungs • Jugular vein distention • Hepatomegaly • Peripheral edema • Taut skin turgor	• Poor skin turgor • Dry mucous membranes	• Cool extremities • Weak peripheral pulses	• Warm extremities • Bounding peripheral pulses

- Postprocedure

  - Nursing Actions

    - Obtain chest x-ray following the procedure to confirm catheter placement.

    - Continually monitor respiratory and cardiac status (vital signs, heart rhythm, SaO_2).

      - Observe respiratory pattern and effort.

      - Compare NIBP to arterial blood pressure.

    - Maintain line placement and integrity.

      - Observe and document waveforms. Report changes in waveforms to the provider, as this can indicate catheter migration or displacement.

      - Document catheter placement each shift and as needed (after movement for transport).

      - Monitor and secure connections between pressure tubing, transducers, and catheter ports.

    - Obtain readings from hemodynamic catheter as prescribed.

      - Place the client in supine position prior to recording hemodynamic values. Head of bed can be elevated 15° to 30°.

      - Level the transducer at the phlebostatic axis before readings and with all position changes.

      - Zero system to atmospheric pressure.

      - Compare hemodynamic findings to physical assessment.

      - Monitor trends in values obtained over time.

- Complications
  - Infection/Sepsis
    - Infection at insertion site can occur if aseptic technique is not used carefully.
    - Nursing Actions
      - Change dressings per hospital protocol and as needed.
      - Use surgical aseptic technique with all dressing changes (mask, sterile gloves, maintain sterile field).
      - Monitor for evidence of infection (elevated WBC count or temperature).
      - Perform thorough handwashing.
      - Collect specimens (blood cultures, catheter tip cultures) and deliver to the laboratory.
      - Administer antibiotic therapy as prescribed.
      - Administer intravenous fluids for intravascular support.
      - Administer vasopressors (dopamine) for vasodilation secondary to sepsis.
  - Embolism
    - Plaque or a clot can become dislodged during the procedure.
    - Nursing Actions
      - Use heparinized solution for flushing system to prevent thromboembolism.
      - Avoid introduction of air into flushing system to prevent air embolism.
      - Recognize that there is a risk of pneumothorax with insertion of the line.
      - Recognize that there is a risk of dysrhythmias with insertion/movement of the line.

Angiography

- A coronary angiogram, also called a cardiac catheterization, is an invasive diagnostic procedure used to evaluate the presence and degree of coronary artery blockage.
  - Angiography can also be done on the lower extremities to determine blood flow and areas of blockage.
  - Angiography involves the insertion of a catheter into a femoral (sometimes a brachial) vessel and threading it into the right or left side of the heart. Coronary artery narrowings and/or occlusions are identified by the injection of contrast media under fluoroscopy.

 View Media Supplement: Cardiac Catheter (Image)

- Indications

- o Unstable angina and ECG changes (T wave inversion, ST segment elevation, depression)

- o Confirm and determine location and extent of heart disease.

- Preprocedure

  - o Nursing Actions

    - Ensure that the consent form is signed.

    - Maintain the client on NPO status for at least 8 hr (risk for aspiration when lying flat for the procedure).

    - Assess that the client and family understand the procedure.

    - Assess for iodine/shellfish allergy (contrast media).

    - Assess renal function prior to introduction of contrast dye.

    - Administer premedications as prescribed [methylprednisone (Solu-Medrol), diphenhydramine (Benadryl)].

  - o Client Education

    - Instruct the client that he can be awake and sedated during procedure. A local anesthetic should be used. A small incision is made, often in the groin to insert the catheter. The client can feel warmth and flushed when the dye is inserted. After the procedure, the client must keep the affected leg straight. Pressure (a sandbag) can be placed on the incision to prevent bleeding.

- Intraprocedure

  - o Nursing Actions

    - Administer sedatives and analgesia as prescribed.

    - Continually monitor vital signs and heart rhythm.

    - Be prepared to intervene for dysrhythmias.

    - Have resuscitation equipment and emergency medications readily available.

- Postprocedure

  - o Nursing Actions

    - Assess vital signs every 15 min x 4, every 30 min x 2, every hour x 4, and then every 4 hr (follow hospital protocol).

    - Assess the groin site at the same intervals for:

      - □ Bleeding and hematoma formation

      - □ Thrombosis; document pedal pulse, color, temperature

    - Maintain bedrest in supine position with extremity straight for prescribed time.

      - □ A vascular closure devise may be used to hasten hemostasis following catheter removal.

Ⓖ

- □ Older adult clients can have arthritis, which can make lying in bed for 4 to 6 hr after the procedure painful. The provider can be notified for prescribed medication.
- Conduct continuous cardiac monitoring for dysrhythmias (reperfusion following angioplasty can cause dysrhythmias).
- Administer antiplatelet or thrombolytic agents as prescribed to prevent clot formation and restenosis.
  - □ Aspirin
  - □ Clopidogrel (Plavix), ticlopidine (Ticlid)
  - □ Heparin
  - □ Low molecular weight heparin (Enoxaparin, Lovenox)
  - □ GP IIb/IIIa inhibitors, such as eptifibatide (Integrilin)
- Administer anxiolytics (Ativan) and analgesia (morphine) as needed.
- Monitor urine output and administer IV fluids for hydration.
  - □ Contrast media acts as an osmotic diuretic.
- Perform/assist with sheath removal from vessel.
  - □ Apply pressure to arterial/venous sites for the prescribed period of time (varies depending upon the method used for vessel closure).
  - □ Observe for vagal response (hypotension, bradycardia) from compression of nerves.
  - □ Apply pressure dressing.
  - ○ Client Education
    - Instruct the client to:
      - □ Avoid strenuous exercise for the prescribed period of time.
      - □ Immediately report bleeding from the insertion site, chest pain, shortness of breath, and changes in the color or temperature of the extremity.
      - □ Restrict lifting (< 10 lb) for the prescribed period of time.
    - Clients with stent placement will receive anticoagulation therapy for 6 to 8 weeks. Instruct the client to:
      - □ Take the medication at the same time each day.
      - □ Have regular laboratory tests to determine therapeutic levels.
      - □ Avoid activities that could cause bleeding (use soft toothbrush, wear shoes when out of bed).
    - Encourage the client to follow lifestyle guidelines (manage weight, consume a low-fat/low-sodium diet, get regular exercise, stop smoking, decrease alcohol intake).
  - • Complications

- o Cardiac Tamponade
  - Cardiac tamponade can result from fluid accumulation in the pericardial sac.
    - □ Signs include hypotension, jugular venous distention, muffled heart sounds, and paradoxical pulse (variance of 10 mm Hg or more in systolic blood pressure between expiration and inspiration).
    - □ Hemodynamic monitoring will reveal intracardiac and pulmonary artery pressures similar and elevated (plateau pressures).
  - Nursing Actions
    - □ Notify the provider immediately.
    - □ Administer IV fluids to combat hypotension as prescribed.
    - □ Obtain a chest x-ray or echocardiogram to confirm diagnosis.
    - □ Prepare the client for pericardiocentesis (informed consent, gather materials, administer medications as appropriate).
      - ▸ Monitor hemodynamic pressures as they normalize.
      - ▸ Monitor heart rhythm; changes indicate improper positioning of the needle.
      - ▸ Monitor for reoccurrence of signs after the procedure.
- o Hematoma Formation
  - Blood clots may form near the insertion site.
  - Nursing Actions
    - □ Assess the groin at prescribed intervals and as needed.
    - □ Hold pressure for uncontrolled oozing/bleeding.
    - □ Monitor peripheral circulation.
    - □ Notify the primary care provider.
- o Restenosis of Treated Vessel
  - Clot reformation in the coronary artery can occur immediately or several weeks after procedure.
  - Nursing Actions
    - □ Assess ECG patterns and for occurrence of chest pain.
    - □ Notify the provider immediately.
    - □ Prepare the client for return to the cardiac catheterization laboratory.
- o Retroperitoneal Bleeding
  - Bleeding into retroperitoneal space (abdominal cavity behind the peritoneum) can occur due to femoral artery puncture.
  - Nursing Actions
    - □ Assess for flank pain and hypotension.

□ Notify the provider immediately.

□ Administer IV fluids and blood products as prescribed.

Vascular Access

- The site and type of vascular access is determined by the characteristics of the prescribed therapy (medication type, pH and osmolality, length of time for therapy). The goal is to minimize the number of catheter insertions and the risk for adverse reactions.

  ○ Age-related loss of skin turgor and poor vein conditions pose challenges to vascular access. Using hand veins is not appropriate for older adult clients.

- Central Catheters

  ○ Central catheters are appropriate for any fluids due to rapid hemodilution in the superior vena cava (SVC).

  ○ They require x-ray verification of tip placement prior to use.

  ○ All central catheters must be inserted by a provider with the exception of PICC lines, which may be inserted by a specially trained nurse. Insertion occurs in the OR, the client's hospital room, or in an outpatient facility.

  ○ Tunneled and implanted catheters require surgical removal.

  ○ Central catheter types include nontunneled percutaneous central catheter (triple lumen), peripherally inserted central catheter (PICC), tunneled percutaneous central catheter (Hickman, Groshong), and implanted port.

    ■ Nontunneled percutaneous central catheter

      □ Description – 15 to 20 cm in length with 1 to 3 lumens

      □ Length of use – Up to 3 months

      □ Insertion location – Subclavian vein, jugular vein; tip in the distal third of the superior vena cava

      □ Indications – Administration of blood, long-term administration of chemotherapeutic agents, antibiotics, and total parenteral nutrition

    ■ Peripherally inserted central catheter

      □ Description – 40 to 65 cm with single or multiple lumens

      □ Length of use – Up to 12 months

      □ Insertion location – Basilic or cephalic vein at least one finger's breadth below or above the antecubital fossa; the catheter should be advanced until the tip is positioned in the lower one-third of the superior vena cava.

      □ Indications – Administration of blood, long-term administration of chemotherapeutic agents, antibiotics, and total parenteral nutrition

      □ Preprocedure

        ► PICCs may be inserted by specially trained nurses.

- ▸ Apply local anesthetic at insertion site and insert the catheter using surgical aseptic technique.
  - ☐ Postprocedure
    - ▸ Apply an initial dressing of gauze and replace with a transparent dressing within 24 hr.
    - ▸ An initial x-ray should be taken to ensure proper placement.
    - ▸ Care of a PICC line includes:
      - ▷ Assessing the site at least every 8 hr. Note redness, swelling, drainage, tenderness, and condition of the dressing.
      - ▷ Changing the tube and positive pressure cap per facility protocol (usually a minimum of every 3 days for the hospitalized client).
      - ▷ Using 10 mL or larger syringe to flush the line.
      - ▷ Cleaning the insertion port with alcohol for 3 seconds and allowing it to dry completely prior to accessing it.
      - ▷ Performing flush for intermittent medication administration per facility protocol, usually with 10 mL of 0.9 % sodium chloride before, between, and after medications.
      - ▷ Obtaining blood samples by withdrawing 10 mL of blood and discarding; taking a second syringe and withdrawing 10 mL of blood for sample; taking a third syringe and flushing with 10 mL of 0.9% sodium chloride (follow facility protocol for specific flushing guidelines).
      - ▷ Using transparent dressing. Follow facility protocol for dressing changes, usually every 7 days and when indicated (wet, loose, soiled).
      - ▷ Advising the client not to immerse his arm in water. To shower, covering dressing site to avoid water exposure.
      - ▷ Educating the client not to have blood pressure taken in arm with PICC line.
- ■ Tunneled percutaneous central catheter
  - ☐ Description – 48 to 104 cm (19 to 41 in) in length
  - ☐ For long-term use
  - ☐ Insertion location – A portion of the catheter lies in a subcutaneous tunnel separating the point where the catheter enters the vein from where it enters the skin with a cuff. Tissue granulates into the cuff to provide a mechanical barrier to organisms and an anchoring for the catheter.
  - ☐ Indications – Frequent and long-term need for vascular access

□ No dressing is needed since entrance into skin and vein are separate and tissue granulates into catheter cuff, providing a barrier. Groshong catheters have pressure-sensitive valves to prevent blood reflux and do not require a clamp.

■ Implanted port

□ Description – Port is comprised of a small reservoir covered by a thick septum.

□ Insertion location – Port is surgically implanted into chest wall pocket; the catheter is inserted into the subclavian vein with the tip in the superior vena cava.

□ Indications – Long-term (a year or more) need for vascular access; commonly used for chemotherapy

□ Preprocedure

▸ To access an implanted port:

▹ Apply local anesthetic to skin if indicated. Palpate skin to locate the port body septum to ensure proper insertion of the needle.

▹ Clean the skin with alcohol for at least 3 seconds and allow to dry prior to insertion of the needle.

▹ Access with a noncoring (Huber) needle.

□ Postprocedure

▸ Flush (with 10 mL 0.9% sodium chloride or per facility protocol) after every use and at least once per month.

● Complications

○ Phlebitis

■ Phlebitis can be chemical (osmolarity or pH is different, veins too small for substance), bacterial, or mechanical irritation (excess IV manipulation).

■ Nursing Actions

□ Monitor for signs and symptoms.

▸ Erythema at the site (usual initial sign)

▸ Pain or burning at the site and the length of the vein

▸ Discomfort when the skin over the tip is touched

▸ Warmth over the site

▸ Edema at the site

▸ Vein indurated (hard), red streak, and/or cordlike

▸ Slowing infusion rate

▸ Temperature elevation of 1° F or more

▸ Infection appearing 7-10 days after insertion

□ Take preventive measures.

▸ Observe the site every 2 hr for signs of infection or infiltration.

▸ Nontunneled catheters require an intact sterile dressing (tunneled catheters do not).

▸ Use the smallest gauge in the largest vein possible to minimize mechanical and chemical irritation to the vein wall.

▸ Clean the site with 2% chlorhexidine-based preparation, 70% alcohol, or tincture of iodine per protocol with friction. Let preparation air dry before insertion.

▸ Change IV sites every 3 days.

□ Provide treatment.

▸ Discontinue the IV.

▸ Apply warm compresses.

▸ Restart with new tubing/infusate.

○ Occlusion

■ Occlusion is a blockage in the access device that impedes flow.

■ Nursing Actions

□ Flush the line at least every 12 hr (3 mL for peripheral, 10 mL for central lines) to maintain patency.

▸ Studies show that 0.9% sodium chloride is as effective as heparinized flush solutions to maintain catheter patency. Follow facility policy.

□ Flush ports after every use and at least once a month while implanted.

□ Administer urokinase (Abbokinase) to lyse obstructions per protocol.

○ Catheter Thrombosis/Emboli

■ Blood can become coagulated and cause an occlusion.

■ Nursing Actions

□ Flush the line per facility protocol.

□ Do not force fluid if resistance is encountered (may dislodge thrombosis).

□ Use a large-barrel syringe (10 cc or bigger) to avoid excess pressure per square inch (PSI) that could cause catheter fracture/rupture.

○ Infiltration and Extravasation

■ Infiltration is fluid leaking into surrounding subcutaneous tissue, and extravasation is unintentional infiltration of a vesicant medication that causes tissue damage.

- Causes
  - □ Improper IV insertion
  - □ Improper vein selection (too small, too fragile, poor location)
  - □ Irritating infusates that weaken and rupture the vein wall
  - □ Overmanipulation of the IV catheter
  - □ Improper taping that allows IV catheter movement and vein compromise
  - □ Tape too tight, becoming a tourniquet
- Nursing Actions
  - □ Monitor for signs and symptoms.
    - ▸ Swelling around the site and proximal or distal to the IV
    - ▸ Edema "puffiness" in the dependent area underneath
    - ▸ Skin taut or rigid with blanching
    - ▸ Sensation of coolness
  - □ Check the client and the system.
    - ▸ Putting pressure on the vein just beyond the tip of the catheter should stop the IV flow. If flow is not affected, the fluid is probably going into the subcutaneous tissue.
    - ▸ The IV alarm may sound due to occlusion. (Do not rely on the pump alarm because pressure must be significant to activate.)
    - ▸ If there is "leaking" at the site after confirming tube connections, this indicates a problem.
    - ▸ Blood return is not considered a reliable indicator.
  - □ Take preventive measures.
    - ▸ Do not use arm with MLC or PICC for blood pressure or phlebotomy.
    - ▸ Do not use hand veins in older adult clients who have lost subcutaneous tissue.
    - ▸ Do not use hand veins for vesicant medication.
    - ▸ Use a hand board for sites affected by the motion of a joint.
  - □ Provide treatment.
    - ▸ Remove using direct pressure with gauze sponge until bleeding stops.
    - ▸ Apply cool, compresses.
    - ▸ Elevation is now considered optional.
    - ▸ Avoid starting a new IV site in the same extremity.

○ Air Embolism

- Vascular access can result in gas bubbles being introduced into the vascular system.

- Nursing Actions

  □ Leave central lines clamped when not in use.

  □ Have the client hold breath while the tubing is changed.

  □ If the client has sudden shortness of breath, place in Trendelenburg on left side, give oxygen, and notify the provider (to trap and aspirate air).

○ Mechanical Complications

- Mechanical complications include accidental dislodgement, mesh damage on port catheters, and catheter migration.

- Nursing Actions

  □ To prevent accidental dislodgement:

    ▸ Cover the extremity site with stretch netting.

    ▸ Wrap a washcloth folded in thirds around the arm before applying a needed restraint. This prevents the restraint from sliding and dislodging the catheter.

    ▸ Only tape the catheter hub to minimize manipulation.

    ▸ When removing the dressing, pull from distal to proximal.

    ▸ If the skin is oily, "defat" oils with alcohol and air-dry before antiseptic cleansing.

  □ Use only a noncoring (Huber) needle to avoid damaging the mesh on port catheters.

  □ Note the length to help detect catheter migration. Notify the provider of any changes in length.

CHAPTER 31: CARDIOVASCULAR DIAGNOSTIC AND THERAPEUTIC PROCEDURES

 Application Exercises

1. Place "P" for "preload" or "A" for "afterload" next to the following hemodynamic pressures.

_____ PAWP

_____ SVR

_____ PVR

_____ CVP

2. Which of the following actions are necessary to obtain an accurate hemodynamic reading? (Select all that apply.)

_____ Place the client in high-Fowler's position, with the head elevated no more than 30°.

_____ Level transducer to phlebostatic axis.

_____ Zero transducer to room air.

_____ Record readings.

_____ Compare readings to physical assessment.

3. Why is it imperative that a client lie still for 6 hr following an angiography?

A. Risk of increased blood pressure

B. Risk of infection

C. Anesthesia risks

D. Risk for bleeding

4. A nurse receives an order to administer 0.9% sodium chloride IV at 50 mL/hr. Which of the following lines can be used for administration? (Select all that apply.)

_____ Peripheral IV site

_____ Arterial line

_____ Proximal (CVP) lumen of PA catheter

_____ Distal lumen of PA catheter

5. A nurse has just obtained the following hemodynamic readings for a client:

PAS 34 mm Hg

PAD 21 mm Hg

PAWP 16 mm Hg

CVP 12 mm Hg

Which of the following conditions support these hemodynamic values? (Select all that apply.)

_____ Heart failure

_____ Cor pulmonale

_____ Hypovolemic shock

_____ Pulmonary hypertension

CHAPTER 31: CARDIOVASCULAR DIAGNOSTIC AND THERAPEUTIC PROCEDURES

 Application Exercises Answer Key

1. Place "P" for "preload" or "A" for "afterload" next to the following hemodynamic pressures.

    P   PAWP

    A   SVR

    A   PVR

    P   CVP

Hemodynamic pressures that would be preload are PAWP and CVP. Afterload would be SVR and PVR.

 NCLEX® Connection: Physiological Adaptation, Hemodynamics

2. Which of the following actions are necessary to obtain an accurate hemodynamic reading? (Select all that apply.)

        Place the client in high-Fowler's position, with the head elevated no more than 30°.

    X   **Level transducer to phlebostatic axis.**

    X   **Zero transducer to room air.**

    X   **Record readings.**

    X   **Compare readings to physical assessment.**

Level transducer to phlebostatic axis, zero transducer to room air, record readings, and compare readings to physical assessment would all needed to obtain accurate hemodynamic readings. Placing a client in high-Fowler's position with the head elevated no more than 30° is not appropriate for this scenario.

 NCLEX® Connection: Physiological Adaptation, Hemodynamics

3. Why is it imperative that a client lie still for 6 hr following an angiography?

    A. Risk of increased blood pressure

    B. Risk of infection

    C. Anesthesia risks

    D. Increased risk for bleeding

Following angiography, the client must lie still for 6 hr due to the increased risk for bleeding. A risk for increased blood pressure or infection or risks related to anesthesia are not necessarily related to the client lying still following angiography.

 NCLEX® Connection: Reduction of Risk Potential, Potential for Complications of Diagnostic Tests/Treatments/Procedures

4. A nurse receives an order to administer 0.9% sodium chloride IV at 50 mL/hr. Which of the following lines can be used for administration? (Select all that apply.)

__X__ **Peripheral IV site**

_____ Arterial line

__X__ **Proximal (CVP) lumen of PA catheter**

_____ Distal lumen of PA catheter

Arterial lines and the distal lumens of pulmonary artery catheters are used for hemodynamic measurements and the collection of blood samples. They are not to be used for intravenous fluid administration.

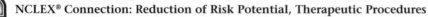 NCLEX® Connection: Reduction of Risk Potential, Therapeutic Procedures

5. A nurse has just obtained the following hemodynamic readings for a client:

PAS 34 mm Hg

PAD 21 mm Hg

PAWP 16 mm Hg

CVP 12 mm Hg

Which of the following conditions support these hemodynamic values? (Select all that apply.)

__X__ **Heart failure**

__X__ **Cor pulmonale**

_____ Hypovolemic shock

__X__ **Pulmonary hypertension**

These elevated hemodynamic measurements are consistent with left ventricular failure and pulmonary problems. Hypovolemic shock is characterized by low hemodynamic values.

 NCLEX® Connection: Physiological Adaptation, Hemodynamics

UNIT 4	NURSING CARE OF CLIENTS WITH CARDIOVASCULAR DISORDERS
Section	Diagnostic and Therapeutic Procedures

Chapter 32   Electrocardiography and Dysrhythmia Monitoring

 Overview

- Cardiac electrical activity can be monitored by using an ECG. The heart's electrical activity can be monitored by a standard 12-lead ECG (resting ECG), ambulatory ECG (Holter monitoring), continuous cardiac monitoring, or by telemetry.

> **(M)** **View Media Supplement:**   ECG Strip (Image)

- Cardiac dysrhythmias are heartbeat disturbances (beat formation, beat conduction, or myocardial response to beat).

- Nurses should be familiar with cardioversion and defibrillation procedures for treating dysrhythmias.

Electrocardiography

- Electrocardiography uses an electrocardiograph to record the electrical activity of the heart over time. The electrocardiograph is connected by wires (leads) to skin electrodes placed on the chest and limbs of a client.

  ○ Continuous cardiac monitoring requires the client to be in close proximity to the monitoring system.

  ○ Telemetry allows the client to ambulate while maintaining proximity to the monitoring system.

- Indications

> **(M)** **View Media Supplement:**   (Images)
> - Premature Atrial Contractions
> - Ventricular Tachycardia
> - Premature Ventricular Contractions
> - Atrial Fibrillation

  ○ Diagnoses

    ▪ Bradycardia

    ▪ Heart block

- Atrial fibrillation
- Supraventricular tachycardia
- Ventricular tachycardia
- Ventricular fibrillation
  - ○ Client presentation
    - Cardiovascular disease
    - MI
    - Hypoxia
    - Acid-base imbalances
    - Electrolyte disturbances
    - Chronic renal failure, liver, or lung disease
    - Pericarditis
    - Drug or alcohol abuse
    - Hypovolemia
    - Shock
- Preprocedure
  - ○ Nursing actions
    - Prepare the client for a 12-lead ECG by:
      - □ Positioning the client in a supine position with chest exposed.
      - □ Washing the client's skin to remove oils.
      - □ Attaching one electrode to each of the client's extremities by applying electrodes to flat surfaces above the wrists and ankles and the other six electrodes to the chest, avoiding chest hair. (Chest hair may need to be shaved on male clients).

 View Media Supplement: ECG Lead Placement (Image)

- Intraprocedure
  - ○ Nursing actions
    - Instruct the client to remain still and breathe normally while the 12-lead ECG is performed.
    - Monitor the client for signs and symptoms of dysrhythmia (chest pain, decreased level of consciousness, and shortness of breath) and hypoxia.

- Postprocedure

  - Nursing actions

    - Remove leads from client, print ECG report, and notify the primary care provider.

    - Apply a Holter monitor if the client is on a telemetry unit and/or needs continuous cardiac monitoring.

    - Continue to monitor the client for symptoms of dysrhythmia (chest pain, decreased level of consciousness, and shortness of breath) and hypoxia.

    - Dysrhythmia treatment is based on the client's symptoms and the cardiac rhythm, which can require cardioversion or defibrillation after an ECG has been completed and a diagnosis has been found.

Dysrhythmias

- Dysrhythmias are classified by the:

  - Site of origin – sinoatrial (SA) node, atria, atrioventricular (AV) node, or ventricle.

    - Electrophysiological study determines the area of the heart causing the dysrhythmia. Ablation of the area is possible.

  - Effect on the rate and rhythm of the heart – bradycardia, tachycardia, heart block, premature beat, flutter, fibrillation, or asystole.

- Dysrhythmias can be benign or life-threatening.

- The life-threatening effects of dysrhythmias are generally related to decreased cardiac output and ineffective tissue perfusion.

- Cardiac dysrhythmias are a primary cause of death in clients suffering acute MI and other sudden death disorders.

- Rapid recognition and treatment of serious dysrhythmias is essential to preserve life.

DYSRHYTHMIA	MEDICATION	ELECTRICAL MANAGEMENT
Bradycardia (any rhythm < 60/min) Treat if the client is symptomatic	Atropine and isoproterenol	Pacemaker
Atrial fibrillation, supraventricular tachycardia (SVT), or ventricular tachycardia with pulse	Amiodarone, adenosine, and verapamil	Synchronized cardioversion
Ventricular tachycardia without pulse or ventricular fibrillation	Amiodarone, lidocaine, and epinephrine	Defibrillation

- Dysrhythmias can present atypically in older adult clients.

- Risks for heart disease, hypertension, dysrhythmias, and atherosclerosis increase with age.

Cardioversion and Defibrillation

- Cardioversion is the delivery of a synchronized, direct countershock to the heart.

- Defibrillation is the delivery of an unsynchronized, direct countershock to the heart. Defibrillation stops all electrical activity of the heart, allowing the SA node to take over and re-establish a perfusing rhythm.

- Indications

  o Cardioversion – elective treatment of atrial dysrhythmias, supraventricular tachycardia, and ventricular tachycardia with a pulse. Cardioversion is the treatment of choice for clients who are symptomatic.

  o Defibrillation – ventricular fibrillation or pulseless ventricular tachycardia.

- Client Outcome

  o The client's heart will return to a normal rhythm.

- Preprocedure

  o Clients who have atrial fibrillation of unknown duration must receive adequate anticoagulation prior to cardioversion therapy to prevent dislodgement of thrombi into the bloodstream.

  o Nursing actions

    ▪ Prepare the client for cardioversion, if prescribed.

    ▪ Explain the procedure to the client and obtain consent.

    ▪ Administer oxygen.

    ▪ Document preprocedure rhythm.

    ▪ Have emergency equipment available.

- Intraprocedure

  o Nursing actions

    ▪ Administer sedation as prescribed.

    ▪ Administer a prescribed antidysrhythmic agent or other prescribed medications.

    ▪ Monitor the client in a lead that provides an upright QRS complex.

    ▪ All staff must stand clear of the client, equipment connected to the client, and the bed when a shock is delivered.

    ▪ Cardioversion requires activation of the synchronizer button in addition to charging the machine. This allows the shock to be in sync with the client's underlying rhythm. Failure to synchronize can lead to development of a lethal dysrhythmia, such as ventricular fibrillation.

    ▪ Perform CPR for cardiac asystole or other pulseless rhythms.

    ▪ Defibrillate the client immediately for ventricular fibrillation.

    ▪ Monitor the client for pulmonary or systemic emboli following cardioversion.

- Postprocedure
  - Nursing actions
    - After cardioversion or defibrillation, check the client's vital signs, assess airway patency, and obtain an ECG.
    - Provide the client/family with reassurance and emotional support.
    - Document
      - Postprocedure rhythm
      - Number of defibrillation or cardioversion attempts, energy settings, time, and response
      - The client's condition and state of consciousness following the procedure
      - Skin condition under the electrodes
  - Client education
    - Teach the client and family how to assess pulse.
    - Advise the client to report palpitations or irregularities.
- Complications
  - Embolism
    - Cardioversion can dislodge blood clots, potentially causing:
      - A pulmonary embolism (evidenced by dyspnea, chest pain, air hunger, and decreasing SaO_2)
      - A cerebrovascular accident (evidenced by decreased level of consciousness, slurred speech, and muscle weakness/paralysis).
      - An MI (evidenced by chest pain and ST segment depression or elevation).
    - Nursing actions
      - Provide therapeutic anticoagulation for clients who have dysrhythmias.
  - Decreased cardiac output and heart failure
    - Cardioversion may damage some heart tissue and impair heart function.
    - Nursing actions
      - Monitor the client for signs of decreased cardiac output (hypotension, syncope, and increased heart rate) and heart failure (dyspnea, productive cough, edema, and venous distention).
      - Provide medications to increase output (inotropic agents) and to decrease cardiac workload.

CHAPTER 32: ELECTROCARDIOGRAPHY AND DYSRHYTHMIA MONITORING

(A) Application Exercises

Scenario: A nurse is caring for a client who reports feeling lightheaded. Assessment of his vital signs reveals a heart rate at 144/min and irregular, blood pressure of 84/49 mm Hg, and an SaO_2 reading of 95%. An ECG reveals atrial fibrillation with a rapid ventricular response. Synchronized cardioversion is performed at 50 joules.

1. Which of the following observations should the nurse include in documentation? (Select all that apply.)

   _____ The client feels lightheaded

   _____ The client is short of breath.

   _____ The client's ECG reveals atrial fibrillation with a rapid ventricular response

   _____ The client's vital signs are within the expected reference range

   _____ The client is synchronized with cardioversion at 50 joules

   _____ The client's oxygen saturation is 95%

2. Two hours after the client's cardioversion he develops ventricular fibrillation. What is the expected treatment?

3. Which of the following clients are at risk for the development of dysrhythmias? (Select all that apply.)

   _____ Metabolic alkalosis

   _____ A client who has a serum potassium level of 4.3 mEq/L

   _____ A client who has an SaO_2 of 96%

   _____ A client who has COPD

   _____ A client who is 3 hr post MI

CHAPTER 32: ELECTROCARDIOGRAPHY AND DYSRHYTHMIA MONITORING

 Application Exercises Answer Key

Scenario: A nurse is caring for a client who reports feeling lightheaded. Assessment of his vital signs reveals a heart rate at 144/min and irregular, blood pressure of 84/49 mm Hg, and an SaO_2 reading of 95%. An ECG reveals atrial fibrillation with a rapid ventricular response. Synchronized cardioversion is performed at 50 joules.

1. Which of the following observations should the nurse include in documentation? (Check all that apply.)

__X__	**The client feels lightheaded**
_____	The client is short of breath.
__X__	**The client's ECG reveals atrial fibrillation with a rapid ventricular response**
_____	The client's vital signs are within the expected reference range
__X__	**The client is synchronized with cardioversion at 50 joules**
__X__	**The client's oxygen saturation is 95%**

The client who is feeling lightheaded, an ECG revealing atrial fibrillation with rapid ventricular response, a client who is synchronized with cardioversion at 50 joules, and a client who has an oxygen saturation of 95% would all be included in the nurse's documentation. A client who reports shortness of breath and vital signs that are within expected reference range are inaccurate findings and should not be documented by the nurse.

NCLEX® Connection: Reduction of Risk Potential, Therapeutic Procedures

2. Two hours after the client's cardioversion he develops ventricular fibrillation. What action should the nurse take first?

When a client has a lethal rhythm such as ventricular fibrillation, the first intervention should be defibrillation.

NCLEX® Connection: Physiological Adaptation, Hemodynamics

3. Which of the following clients are at risk for the development of dysrhythmias? (Select all that apply.)

   X   **Metabolic alkalosis**

   _____   A client who has a serum potassium level of 4.3 mEq/L

   _____   A client who has an SaO$_2$ of 96%

   X   **A client who has COPD**

   X   **A client who is 3 hr post MI**

These ABG results, COPD, and a recent MI are risk factors for developing a dysrhythmia. A potassium level of 4.3 mEq/L (expected reference range) and an oxygen saturation of 96% (expected reference range) do not increase the risk for developing dysrhythmias.

NCLEX® Connection: Physiological Adaptation, Hemodynamics

UNIT 4   NURSING CARE OF CLIENTS WITH CARDIOVASCULAR DISORDERS

Section   Diagnostic and Therapeutic Procedures

Chapter 33   Pacemakers

 Overview

- An artificial pacemaker is a battery-operated device that electrically stimulates the heart when the natural pacemaker of the heart fails to maintain an acceptable rhythm.

 View Media Supplement: Pacemaker (Image)

- Pacemakers may be temporary or permanent.

- Pacemakers are composed of two parts:

  o   The pulse generator houses the energy source (battery) and the control center.

  o   The electrodes are wires that attach to the myocardial muscle on one side and connect to the pulse generator on the other.

- Nurses should be familiar with the various types of pacemakers, how they function, and the care involved with their placement/insertion.

- Conduction of electrical impulses through the sinoatrial (SA) node may be slowed with aging, causing bradycardia and conduction defects.

Types of Pacemakers

- Temporary Pacemakers (the energy source is provided by an external battery pack)

  o   External (transcutaneous)

    ▪   Pacing energy is delivered transcutaneously through the thoracic musculature to the heart via two electrode patches placed on the skin.

    ▪   It requires large amounts of electricity, which can be painful for a client.

    ▪   It is only used in emergency resuscitation of a client who does not have pacing wires inserted.

- o Epicardial

    - Pacemaker leads are attached directly to the heart during open heart surgery. Wires run externally through the chest incision and may be attached to an external impulse generator if needed.

    - It is commonly used during and immediately following open heart surgery.

- o Endocardial (transvenous)

    - Pacing wires are threaded through a large central vein (subclavian, jugular, or femoral) and lodged into the wall of the right ventricle (ventricular pacing), right atrium (atrial pacing), or both chambers (dual chamber pacing).

- • Permanent Pacemakers (contain an internal pacing unit)

    - o Indicated for chronic or recurrent dysrhythmias due to sinus or atrioventricular (AV) node malfunction

    - o Can be programmed to pace the atria, ventricles, or both (AV sequential pacing)

    - o Pacemaker modes

        - Fixed rate (asynchronous) – fires at a constant rate without regard for the heart's electrical activity

        - Demand mode (synchronous) – detects the heart's electrical impulses and fires at a preset rate only if the heart's intrinsic rate is below a certain level

        - Antidysrhythmic function – can overpace a tachydysrhythmia or deliver an electrical shock

    - o Inter-Society Commission for Heart Disease (ICHD) codes are used to identify pacemaker function. The five-letter coding system is used in the following manner:

        - First letter – chamber paced

        - Second letter – chamber sensed

        - Third letter – mode of response (response to sensing determines the pacemaker's activity when intrinsic activity is sensed):

            - □ Inhibited – pacemaker activity is inhibited/does not fire.

            - □ Triggered – pacemaker activity is triggered/fires when intrinsic activity is sensed.

        - Fourth letter – programmable functions

        - Fifth letter – tachydysrhythmia functions

            - □ Often, the first three letters are used to describe the pacemaker function. For example, in a VVI mode, the ventricle is paced, sensed, and inhibited. If no QRS complex is sensed within the desired time interval, the pacemaker fires. The pacemaker is inhibited, or does not fire, if the intrinsic cardiac heart rate is above a set rate.

FIVE-LETTER SYSTEM TO IDENTIFY PACEMAKER FUNCTION				
CHAMBER PACED	CHAMBER SENSED	RESPONSE MODE	PROGRAMMABLE FUNCTIONS	TACHY-DYSRHYTHMIC FUNCTIONS
O – None	O – None	O – None	O – None	O – None
A – Atria	A – Atria	T – Triggered	P – Simple Programmable	P- Pacing (anti-tachydysrhythmia)
V – Ventricle	V – Ventricle	I – Inhibited	M – Multiple Programmable	S – Shock
D – Dual (AV)	D – Dual (AV)	D – Dual (AV)	C – Communicating	D – Dual (P + S)
			R – Rate Modulation	

Pacemaker Placement

- Indications

    o Diagnoses

        ▪ Symptomatic bradycardia

        ▪ Complete heart block

        ▪ Sick sinus syndrome

        ▪ Sinus arrest

        ▪ Asystole

        ▪ Atrial tachydysrhythmias

        ▪ Ventricular tachydysrhythmias

    o Client presentation

        ▪ Symptoms

            □ Dizziness

            □ Palpitations (racing heart)

            □ Chest pain or pressure

            □ Anxiousness

            □ Fatigue

            □ Nausea

            □ Breathing difficulties

        ▪ Signs

            □ Bradycardia

            □ Tachycardia

- □ Abnormal ECG

- □ Dyspnea, tachypnea

- □ Restlessness

- □ Distended jugular vein

- □ Vomiting

- □ Hypotension

- □ Diaphoresis

- □ Decreased cardiac output

- Client Outcomes

  - ○ The client will be able to tolerate activities of daily living free of cardiac symptoms.

  - ○ The client will use strategies to reduce stress and improve cardiac health.

  - ○ The client will recognize cardiac symptoms and seek medical attention immediately when needed.

- Preprocedure

  - ○ Nursing actions

    - ▪ Assess the client's knowledge of the procedure and need for pacemaker (if nonemergent situation).

    - ▪ Obtain written consent from the client.

    - ▪ Transcutaneous pacing

      - □ Cleanse the client's skin with soap and water. Do not shave, rub, or apply alcohol to the skin. Trim excess hair.

      - □ Apply the posterior electrode between the client's spine and the left scapula. Avoid placing it over bone, as bone is a poor conductor of electricity.

      - □ Place the anterior electrode over the heart, between the V_2 and V_5 positions. Shift female breast tissue to position the electrode under the breast.

  - ○ Client education

    - ▪ Teach the client about the type of pacemaker that is to be inserted and information about the procedure.

      - □ Temporary pacemaker

        - ▸ Explain that wires and a pacemaker box will be on the client's chest after the procedure.

        - ▸ Instruct the client not to touch the dials on the pacemaker box.

        - ▸ The wires and box will need to be kept dry. The client will not be able to shower.

- □ Permanent pacemaker
  - ▸ Explain that a small incision will be made using a local anesthetic and IV sedation.
  - ▸ The pacemaker may be reprogrammed externally after the procedure.

- Intraprocedure
  - ○ Nursing actions
    - Monitor the client's status (vital signs, SaO_2, and comfort).
    - Administer medications as prescribed (analgesia, anxiolytics, and anti-arrhythmics).
    - Set pacemaker settings as prescribed. Establish a threshold (lowest stimulation that achieves capture).

- Postprocedure
  - ○ Nursing actions
    - Document the time and date of insertion, model (permanent pacemaker), settings, rhythm strip, presence of adequate pulse and blood pressure, and client response.
    - Continually monitor heart rate and rhythm.
    - Obtain chest x-ray as prescribed to assess lead placement and for pneumothorax, hemothorax, or pleural effusion.
    - Provide analgesia as prescribed.
    - Minimize shoulder movement initially and provide a sling (if prescribed) to allow leads to anchor.
    - Maintain the client's safety.
      - □ Ensure that all electrical equipment has grounded connections.
      - □ Remove any electrical equipment that is damaged.
      - □ For a temporary pacemaker
        - ▸ Wear gloves when handling pacemaker leads.
        - ▸ Insulate pacemaker terminals and leads with nonconductive material when not in use (rubber gloves).
        - ▸ Keep spare generator, leads, and batteries at the client's bedside.
        - ▸ Secure the pacemaker battery pack. Take care when moving the client and ensure that there is enough wire slack.

□ For a permanent pacemaker

▸ Provide the client with a pacemaker identification card including the manufacturer's name, model number, mode of function, rate parameters, and expected battery life.

■ Assess the client for hiccups, which may indicate that the generator is pacing the diaphragm.

○ Client education

■ Temporary pacemakers are only used in a controlled facility-like environment with telemetry for continuous ECG monitoring. If needed, a permanent pacemaker is inserted before discharge to home.

■ Permanent pacemaker discharge teaching

□ Instruct the client to carry a pacemaker identification card at all times.

□ Teach the client that batteries last 10 years on average.

□ Tell the client to wear a sling when out of bed, if prescribed.

□ Teach the client not to raise the arm on the surgical side above the shoulder for 1 to 2 weeks.

□ Teach the client to take pulse daily at the same time.

□ Teach the client to set the rate of the pacemaker. Notify the provider if the heart rate is less than 5 beats below the pacer rate.

□ Report signs of dizziness, fainting, fatigue, weakness, chest pain, hiccupping, or palpitations.

□ For clients with pacer-defibrillators, inform the client and family that anyone touching the client when the device delivers a shock will feel a slight electrical impulse but that the impulse will not harm the person.

□ The client should follow activity restrictions as prescribed, including no contact sports or heavy lifting for 2 months.

□ The client should avoid direct blows or injury to the generator site.

□ The client can resume sexual activity as desired, avoiding positions that put stress on the incision site.

□ Household appliances should not affect pacemaker function unless held directly over pacer generator. This includes garage door openers, burglar alarms, microwave ovens, and antitheft devices.

□ Pacemakers will set off airport security detectors and officials should be notified. The airport security device should not affect pacemaker functioning.

□ Instruct the client to inform other providers and dentists about the pacemaker. Some tests, such as magnetic resonance imaging and therapeutic diathermy (heat therapy), may be contraindicated.

- Complications
  - Pacemaker insertion complications
    - Infection or hematoma
      - The insertion site can develop an infection or hematoma.
      - Nursing actions
        ‣ Assess the incision site for redness, pain, drainage, or swelling.
        ‣ Treat an infection with antibiotics as prescribed.
        ‣ Monitor coagulation and CBC.
    - Pneumothorax or hemothorax
      - Trauma during the procedure can cause a pneumothorax or hemothorax.
      - Nursing actions
        ‣ Monitor the client's breath sounds and chest movement.
        ‣ Monitor oxygen saturation.
        ‣ Obtain a chest x-ray after the procedure.
    - Arrhythmias
      - Irritation of a ventricle from a pacing electrode may cause ectopic beats, such as premature ventricular contractions.
      - Nursing actions
        ‣ Monitor ECG and blood pressure.
        ‣ Give antiarrhythmics as prescribed.
        ‣ Have emergency resuscitation equipment and medications readily available.
  - Pacemaker complications
    - Failure to capture
      - The pacemaker initiates a stimulus, but depolarization of the myocardium does not happen.
        ‣ An ECG shows pacing spikes without the expected P wave or QRS complex.
        ‣ Failure to capture causes include dislodgement of the electrode, MI ischemia or infarction, antidysrhythmic medications, electrolyte imbalances (hypokalemia, hyperkalemia), and too low of a voltage (mA).
        ‣ Treatment depends on the cause. A dislodged electrode may reattach by turning the client onto his left side. The primary care provider may need to increase the voltage delivered if the voltage is too low to capture.

- Failure to sense

  □ The pacemaker fails to sense the heart's intrinsic electrical activity, resulting in the delivery of an unnecessary stimulus.

  ▸ An ECG shows pacemaker spikes at intervals different from the programmed interval.

  ▸ Discharge of an impulse during the T wave can lead to life-threatening ventricular dysrhythmias.

  ▸ Treatment involves decreasing the amplitude at which the pacemaker recognizes intrinsic electrical activity (mV).

- Failure to pace (no output)

  □ Failure to pace may be caused by a broken lead wire.

  ▸ Treatment involves replacing the battery or lead.

- Oversensing

  □ The pacemaker is oversensitive and sensing excessive electrical activity.

  ▸ The primary care provider may need to increase the voltage delivered (mA) to reduce sensitivity.

- Stimulation of chest wall or diaphragm

  □ The pacemaker's electrical charge may stimulate the client's chest wall or diaphragm.

  ▸ Stimulation is indicated by muscle twitching or hiccups.

  ▸ It is often caused by lead wire perforation with high electrical current.

  ▸ Stimulation can lead to cardiac tamponade.

  □ Nursing actions

  ▸ Monitor the client for signs of cardiac tamponade such as dyspnea, chest pain, hypotension, and distended neck veins.

  □ Client education

  ▸ Instruct the client to notify the primary care provider with symptoms of chest muscle twitching or hiccups. The pacemaker wires may need to be repositioned.

- Microshock

  □ A small electrical current is sent through unattached external pacemaker wires and may cause cardiac arrhythmias or ventricular fibrillation. This may occur with pacemaker wires that are not attached to a pacemaker generator.

□ Nursing actions

▸ Cover wires with nonconductive insulation (rubber gloves) and nonconductive tape.

▸ Made sure all equipment is grounded with a three-pronged plug. Contact the engineering department for all ungrounded or unsafe electrical equipment (frayed wires).

▸ Wear rubber gloves when handling pacing wires. Static electricity may be transmitted to the pacing wires from hands, causing serious arrhythmias.

□ Client education

▸ Instruct the client not to touch the pacemaker wires. If wires are exposed, the client should alert a primary care provider to secure them.

▸ Tell the client not to plug in or unplug electrical items. Advise the client not to use an electric razor or blow dryer.

CHAPTER 33: PACEMAKERS

Ⓐ Application Exercises

Scenario: A nurse is caring for a client who has been admitted to the coronary care unit from the emergency department. The client's vital signs are: heart rate of 34/min, blood pressure of 83/48 mm Hg, respiratory rate of 30/min, and temperature of 38.6° C (101.4° F). The client is lethargic and unable to complete sentences. The heart rhythm strip indicates complete heart block.

1. List the safety measures to implement when a client has a temporary pacemaker in place.

2. Which of the following interventions should the nurse perform first?

    A. Obtain informed consent.

    B. Prepare the client for insertion of a permanent pacemaker.

    C. Attach transcutaneous pacing pads.

    D. Obtain a 12-lead ECG to confirm heart rhythm.

3. A temporary venous pacemaker is inserted until a permanent pacemaker can be inserted. It is set as a VVI pacemaker at a rate of 70/min. Which of the following signs and symptoms pose a concern for the nurse? (Select all that apply.)

    _____ Cool and clammy foot with capillary refill of 5 seconds

    _____ Observed pacing spike followed by a QRS complex

    _____ Twitching of intercostal muscle

    _____ Heart rate of 84/min

    _____ Blood pressure of 104/62 mm Hg

4. The client has now received a permanent pacemaker. Which of the following statements indicates a need for further teaching?

    A. "I will notify the airport screeners about my pacemaker."

    B. "I will call if I notice hiccups or muscle twitching."

    C. "I will have to disconnect my garage door opener."

    D. "I will take my pulse every morning when I awake."

CHAPTER 33: PACEMAKERS

(A) Application Exercises Answer Key

Scenario: A nurse is caring for a client who has been admitted to the coronary care unit from the emergency department. The client's vital signs are: heart rate of 34/min, blood pressure of 83/48 mm Hg, respiratory rate of 30/min, and temperature of 38.6° C (101.4° F). The client is lethargic and unable to complete sentences. The heart rhythm strip indicates complete heart block.

1. List the safety measures to implement when a client has a temporary pacemaker in place.

Wear rubber gloves when touching exposed wires.

Check that all electrical equipment has adequate grounding.

Limit motion of the extremity near the insertion site.

Secure the battery pack.

Make sure wires are loose enough to reposition the client.

Keep spare batteries at bedside.

(N) NCLEX® Connection: Reduction of Risk Potential, Therapeutic Procedures

2. Which of the following interventions should the nurse perform first?

    A. Obtain informed consent.

    B. Prepare the client for insertion of a permanent pacemaker.

    C. Attach transcutaneous pacing pads.

    D. Obtain 12-lead ECG to confirm heart rhythm.

This client is symptomatic, so transcutaneous pacing should be used to stabilize the client's heart rate, rhythm, and blood pressure. Note, the pacemaker may need to be turned on and the threshold established by the primary care provider, depending on the guidelines of the facility.

(N) NCLEX® Connection: Reduction of Risk Potential, Therapeutic Procedures

3. A temporary venous pacemaker is inserted until a permanent pacemaker can be inserted. It is set as a VVI pacemaker at a rate of 70/min. Which of the following signs and symptoms pose a concern for the nurse? (Select all that apply.)

   X   **Cool and clammy foot with capillary refill of 5 seconds**

_____ Observed pacing spike followed by a QRS complex

   X   **Twitching of intercostal muscle**

_____ Heart rate of 84 beats/min

_____ Blood pressure of 104/62 mm Hg

Pacing spike followed by a QRS complex, heart rate of 84/min, and blood pressure of 104/62 mm Hg are expected findings. A cool and clammy foot may be an indication of a hematoma secondary to insertion via the femoral vein. Twitching of intercostal muscle may be a sign of lead wire perforation and stimulation of the diaphragm.

 NCLEX® Connection: Reduction of Risk Potential, System Specific Assessment

4. The client has now received a permanent pacemaker. Which of the following statements indicates a need for further teaching?

A. "I will notify the airport screeners about my pacemaker."

B. "I will call if I notice hiccups or muscle twitching."

C. "I will have to disconnect my garage door opener."

D. "I will take my pulse every morning when I awake."

This indicates that the client does not understand that household appliances, such as microwaves and garage door openers, will not affect his pacemaker.

 NCLEX® Connection: Physiological Adaptation, Illness Management

UNIT 4	NURSING CARE OF CLIENTS WITH CARDIOVASCULAR DISORDERS
Section	Diagnostic and Therapeutic Procedures
Chapter 34	Invasive Cardiovascular Procedures

 Overview

- Cardiovascular procedures covered in this chapter are invasive methods used to improve blood flow for arteries and veins that have become occluded.

- Invasive cardiovascular procedures are indicated if symptoms persist after non-invasive interventions have been tried, such as diet, exercise and medications.

- Invasive cardiovascular procedures that nurses should be knowledgeable about include:

   o Angioplasty

   o Coronary artery bypass grafts

   o Peripheral bypass grafts

Angioplasty

- Percutaneous transluminal coronary angioplasty (PTCA) involves inflating a balloon to dilate the arterial lumen and the adhering plaque, thus widening the arterial lumen. A stent (mesh-wire device) is often placed to prevent restenosis of the artery.

> **(M) View Media Supplement:** Stent Placement (Animation)

- Indications

   o PTCA can be performed on an elective basis to treat coronary artery disease when there is greater than 50% occlusion of one to two coronary arteries. The area of occlusion is confined, not scattered, and easy to access (proximal).

   o PTCA may reduce ischemia during the occurrence of an acute MI, and it is most effective if it is done within 90 min of chest pain.

   o PTCA may be used as an alternative to coronary artery bypass graft.

   o PTCA with stent placement, to prevent artery reocclusion, may be used to dilate the left main coronary artery, which supplies blood flow to a large area of the heart.

- o Client Presentation
  - ▪ Subjective Data
    - □ Chest pain may occur with or without exertion. Pain may radiate to the jaw, left arm, through the back, or to the shoulder. Symptoms may increase in cold weather or with exercise. Other symptoms may include dyspnea, nausea, fatigue, and diaphoresis.
  - ▪ Objective Data
    - □ ECG changes may include ST elevation, depression, or nonspecific ST changes. Other signs may include, bradycardia, tachycardia, hypotension, elevated blood pressure, vomiting, and mental disorientation.
- • Client Outcomes
  - o The client will be able to perform activities of daily living free of pain or shortness of breath.
  - o The client will use strategies to reduce stress and modify lifestyle habits.
- • Preprocedure
  - o Nursing Actions
    - ▪ Ensure that the client signs the consent form.
    - ▪ Maintain the client on NPO status for at least 8 hr if possible (risk for aspiration when lying flat for the procedure).
    - ▪ Assess that the client and family understand the procedure.
    - ▪ Assess the client for an iodine/shellfish allergy (Use contrast dye instead of contrast media for consistency.).
    - ▪ Assess renal function prior to introduction of contrast dye.
    - ▪ Administer premedications as prescribed (antiplatelet medications).
  - o Client Education
    - ▪ Instruct the client that he may be awake and sedated for the procedure. A local anesthetic should be used. A small incision is made, often in the groin to insert the catheter. The client may feel warmth and flushed when the dye is inserted. After the procedure, the client will be asked to keep the affected leg straight. Pressure (a sandbag) may be placed on the incision to prevent bleeding.
- • Intraprocedure
  - o Nursing Actions
    - ▪ Administer sedatives, such as midazolam (Versed), and analgesia, such as fentanyl (Sublimaze) as prescribed.
    - ▪ Monitor the client for chest pain.
    - ▪ Continually monitor vital signs and heart rhythm.

- ⓢ
  - Have resuscitation equipment and emergency medications readily available.
  - Be prepared to intervene for dysrhythmias.
- Postprocedure
  - Nursing Actions
    - Assess the client's vital signs every 15 min x 4, every 30 min x 2, every hour x 4, and then every 4 hr (or per facility protocol).
    - Assess the groin site at the same intervals for:
      - □ Bleeding and hematoma formation.
      - □ Thrombosis – document pedal pulse, color, and temperature.
    - Maintain bed rest in a supine position with leg straight for a prescribed time.
      - □ Older adult clients may have arthritis, which can make lying in bed for 4 to 6 hr after the procedure painful.
    - Conduct continuous cardiac monitoring for dysrhythmias (reperfusion following angioplasty may cause dysrhythmias).
    - Administer antiplatelet or thrombolytic agents as prescribed to prevent clot formation and restenosis.
      - □ Aspirin
      - □ Clopidogrel (Plavix), tirofiban (Aggrastat)
      - □ Heparin
      - □ Low molecular weight heparin enoxaparin (Lovenox)
      - □ Glycoprotein (GP IIb/IIIa) inhibitors (antiplatelet), such as eptifibatide (Integrilin)
    - Administer anxiolytics and analgesia as needed.
    - Monitor urine output and administer IV fluids for hydration.
      - □ Contrast dye acts as an osmotic diuretic.
    - Assist with sheath removal from the insertion site (artery or vein).
      - □ The catheter sheath is a short hollow tube placed inside the artery or vein at the insertion site. It is used as a guide for the balloon catheter. After the angioplasty, the catheter sheath may be left in for access, so that the angioplasty may be repeated, if needed (for restenosis or perforation).
      - □ Apply pressure to arterial/venous sites for the prescribed period of time (varies depending upon the method used for vessel closure).
      - □ Observe for vagal response (hypotension, bradycardia) from compression of vagus nerve.
      - □ Apply a pressure dressing.

- ○ Client Education
  - ■ Instruct the client to:
    - □ Avoid strenuous exercise for the prescribed period of time.
    - □ Immediately report bleeding from the insertion site, chest pain, shortness of breath, and changes in the color or temperature of the extremity.
    - □ Restrict lifting (< 10 lb) for the prescribed period of time.
  - ■ Clients with stent placement will receive anticoagulation therapy for 6 to 8 weeks. Instruct the client to:
    - □ Take the medication at the same time each day.
    - □ Have regular laboratory tests to determine therapeutic levels.
    - □ Avoid activities that could cause bleeding (use a soft toothbrush, wear shoes when out of bed).
  - ■ Encourage the client to follow lifestyle guidelines (manage weight, consume a low-fat/low-cholesterol diet, exercise regularly, stop smoking, and decrease alcohol intake).
- • Complications
  - ○ Artery dissection
    - ■ Perforation of an artery by the catheter may cause cardiac tamponade or require emergency bypass surgery.
    - ■ Artery dissection findings include severe hypotension and tachycardia, and may require extended occlusion of perforation with a balloon catheter and reversal of anticoagulants.
  - ○ Cardiac tamponade
    - ■ Cardiac tamponade can result from fluid accumulation in the pericardial sac.
      - □ Signs include hypotension, jugular venous distention, muffled heart sounds, and paradoxical pulse (variance of 10 mm Hg or more in systolic blood pressure between expiration and inspiration).
      - □ Hemodynamic monitoring will reveal that intracardiac and pulmonary artery pressures are similar and elevated (plateau pressures) and that cardiac output is decreased.
    - ■ Nursing Actions
      - □ Notify the primary care provider immediately.
      - □ Administer IV fluids to manage hypotension as prescribed.
      - □ Obtain a chest x-ray or echocardiogram to confirm diagnosis.
      - □ Prepare the client for pericardiocentesis or return to surgical suite (informed consent, gather materials, administer medications as appropriate).
        - ‣ Monitor hemodynamic pressures and heart rhythm for reoccurrence of signs after the procedure.

- ○ Hematoma formation
  - ■ A blood clot may form near the insertion site.
  - ■ Nursing Actions
    - □ Monitor for sensation, color, and peripheral pulses in the extremity distal to the insertion site.
    - □ Assess the groin for signs of a hematoma at prescribed intervals and as needed.
    - □ Hold pressure for uncontrolled oozing/bleeding.
    - □ Notify the primary care provider.
- ○ Allergic reaction
  - ■ Some clients can have an allergic reaction to the contrast dye. Signs and symptoms may include chills, fever, rash, wheezing, tachycardia, and bradycardia.
  - ■ Nursing Actions
    - □ Monitor for an allergic reaction.
    - □ Have resuscitation equipment readily available.
    - □ Administer diphenhydramine or epinephrine if prescribed.
- ○ External bleeding
  - ■ Bleeding at the insertion site is a possible complication.
  - ■ Nursing Actions
    - □ Monitor the insertion site for bleeding or swelling.
    - □ Apply pressure to the site.
    - □ Keep the client's leg straight.
- ○ Embolism
  - ■ Plaque or a clot could become dislodged.
  - ■ Nursing Actions
    - □ Monitor the client for chest pain during and after the procedure.
    - □ Monitor the client's vital signs and SaO_2.
- ○ Retroperitoneal bleeding
  - ■ Bleeding into the retroperitoneal space (abdominal cavity behind the peritoneum) can occur due to femoral artery puncture.
  - ■ Nursing Actions
    - □ Assess for flank pain and hypotension.
    - □ Notify the primary care provider immediately.
    - □ Administer IV fluids and blood products as prescribed.

- Client Education

  □ Advise the client that pressure will be applied to the insertion site.

  □ Remind the client to keep his leg straight.

  □ Advise the client to report any chest pain, shortness of breath, or cardiac symptoms.

○ Restenosis of treated vessel

- Clot reformation in the coronary artery may occur immediately or several weeks after the procedure.

- Nursing Actions

  □ Assess ECG patterns and for the occurrence of chest pain.

  □ Notify the primary care provider immediately.

  □ Prepare the client for return to the cardiac catheterization laboratory.

- Client Education

  □ Advise the client to notify the primary care provider of cardiac symptoms and to take all medications as prescribed.

Coronary Artery Bypass Grafts

- Coronary artery bypass grafting (CABG) is an invasive surgical procedure that aims to restore vascularization of the myocardium.

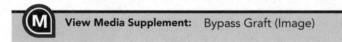

View Media Supplement: Bypass Graft (Image)

○ Performed to bypass an obstruction in one or more of the coronary arteries, CABG does not alter the atherosclerotic process but improves the quality of life for clients restricted by painful coronary artery disease.

○ The procedure is most effective when a client has sufficient ventricular function (ejection fraction greater than 40% to 50%).

○ Older adult clients are more likely to experience transient neurological changes, toxic effects from cardiac medications, and dysrhythmias.

- Indications

○ Diagnoses

- Over 50% blockage of the left main coronary artery with anginal episodes (blockage inaccessible to angioplasty and stenting)

- Significant two-vessel disease with unstable angina

- Triple-vessel disease with or without angina

- Persistent ischemia or likely MI following coronary angiography, percutaneous transluminal coronary angioplasty (PTCA), or stent placement

- Heart failure or cardiogenic shock with acute MI or ischemia (may not be reasonable for clients with poor ejection fractions)
- Coronary arteries that are unable to be accessed or treated by angioplasty and stent placement (narrow or calcified)
- Coronary artery disease nonresponsive to medical management
- Heart valve disease

○ Client Presentation

- Subjective Data
  □ Chest pain may occur with or without exertion. Pain may radiate to the jaw, left arm, through the back, or to the shoulder. Symptoms may increase in cold weather or with exercise. Other symptoms may include dyspnea, nausea, fatigue and diaphoresis.
- Objective Data
  □ ECG changes may include ST elevation, depression, or nonspecific ST changes. Other signs may include, bradycardia, tachycardia, hypotension, elevated blood pressure, vomiting, and mental disorientation.

- Client Outcomes
  ○ The client will be able to perform activities of daily living free of pain or shortness of breath.
  ○ The client will use strategies to reduce stress and modify lifestyle habits.

- Preprocedure
  ○ Nursing Actions
    - A CABG may be an elective procedure or done as an emergency. When planned, preparation begins before the client comes to the facility for the procedure.
    - Verify that the client has signed the informed consent form.
    - Confirm that recent chest x-ray, ECG, and blood work results are available if needed.
    - Administer preoperative medications as prescribed.
      □ Anxiolytics, such as lorazepam (Ativan) and diazepam (Valium)
      □ Prophylactic antibiotics
      □ Anticholinergics, such as scopolamine, to reduce secretions
    - Provide safe transport of the client to the operating suite. Monitor heart rate and rhythm, oxygenation, and other vital indicators.
  ○ Client Education
    - Provide instruction to the client and family about the procedure and the postsurgical environment.

□ Inform the client of the importance of coughing and deep breathing after the procedure to prevent complications.

□ Instruct the client to splint the incision when coughing and deep breathing. Allow the client to provide a return demonstration.

□ Instruct the client to report any pain to the nursing staff. The majority of pain stems from the harvest site for the vein.

□ Inform the client and family to expect the following postoperatively

▸ Endotracheal tube and mechanical ventilator for airway management for several hours following surgery

▸ Inability to talk while the endotracheal tube is in place

▸ Sternal incision and possible leg incision

▸ One to 2 chest tubes

▸ Indwelling urinary catheter

▸ Pacemaker wires

▸ Hemodynamic monitoring devices (pulmonary artery catheter, arterial line)

□ Instruct the client to alter or discontinue regular medications as prescribed by the primary care provider.

▸ Medications frequently discontinued for CABG

▹ Diuretics 2 to 3 days before surgery

▹ Aspirin and other anticoagulants 1 week before surgery

▸ Medications often continued for CABG

▹ Potassium supplements

▹ Scheduled antidysrhythmics, such as amiodarone (Cordarone)

▹ Scheduled antihypertensives, such as metoprolol (Lopressor), a beta-blocker, and diltiazem (Cardizem), a calcium-channel blocker

▹ Insulin (clients who have diabetes mellitus and are insulin-dependent usually receive half the regular insulin dose)

□ Assess the client and family anxiety levels surrounding the procedure.

▸ Encourage the client to verbalize his feelings.

● Intraprocedure

○ An extracardiac vein (saphenous vein), artery (usually the mammary artery), or synthetic graft is used to bypass an obstruction in one or more of the coronary arteries.

○ Most often, a median sternotomy incision is made to visualize the heart and the great vessels.

o   The client is placed on cardiopulmonary bypass, and the client's core temperature may be lowered to decrease the rate of metabolism and the demand for oxygen. A normal core temperature may be maintained during cardiopulmonary bypass to improve postoperative myocardial function and reduce postoperative complications.

o   A cardioplegic solution is used to stop the heart. This prevents myocardial ischemia and allows for a motionless operative field.

o   The artery or vein to be used is harvested. When a saphenous vein is used, it is reversed to prevent the valves from interfering with blood flow.

o   The harvested vessel is anastomosed from the aorta to the affected coronary artery distal to the occlusion.

o   Once the bypass is complete, the hypothermic client is rewarmed by the heat exchanges on the bypass machine. The grafts are monitored for patency and leakage as the client is weaned from the bypass machine and blood is redirected through the coronary vasculature.

o   Lastly, the pacemaker wires may be sutured into the myocardium and chest tubes are placed. The incision is closed with wire sutures, and the client is transported to the intensive care unit.

o   Nursing Actions

- Provide padding to bony prominences to provide comfort and prevent skin breakdown.

- Communicate surgical progress to family members, if appropriate.

- Assist in monitoring urine output and blood loss.

- Document appropriate surgical events.

- Assist in arranging intensive care unit placement and communicate client postoperative needs.

- Postprocedure

  o   Nursing Actions

  - Maintain a patent airway and adequate ventilation.

    □   Monitor respiratory rate and effort.

    □   Auscultate breath sounds. Report crackles.

    □   Monitor SaO_2.

    □   Document ventilator settings.

    □   Suction as needed.

    □   Assist with extubation.

  - Encourage the client to splint the incision while deep breathing and coughing.

  - Dangle and turn the client from side to side as tolerated within 2 hr following extubation. Assist the client to a chair within 24 hr. Ambulate the client 25 to 100 ft by the first postoperative day.

- Continually monitor the client's heart rate and rhythm. Treat dysrhythmias per protocol.

- Maintain an adequate circulating blood volume.

  ▫ Monitor blood pressure.

    ▸ Hypotension may result in graft collapse.

    ▸ Hypertension may result in bleeding from the grafts and sutures.

    ▸ Titrate IV drips (dopamine [Intropin], dobutamine [Dobutrex], milrinone [Primacor], sodium nitroprusside [Nipride]) (per protocol to control blood pressure and/or increase cardiac output).

  ▫ Monitor hemodynamic pressures, and monitor catheter placement. Observe waveforms and markings on the catheter.

  ▫ Monitor the client's level of consciousness. Assess neurological status every 30 to 60 min until the client awakens from anesthesia, then every 2 to 4 hr, or per facility policy.

  ▫ Notify the surgeon of significant changes in values.

- Monitor chest tube patency and drainage.

  ▫ Measure drainage at least once an hour.

  ▫ Volume exceeding 150 mL/hr could be a sign of possible hemorrhage and should be reported to the surgeon.

  ▫ Avoid dependent loops in tubing to facilitate drainage.

- Assess and control pain.

  ▫ Determine the source of the pain (angina, incisional pain).

    ▸ Anginal pain often radiates and is unaffected by breathing.

    ▸ Incisional pain is localized, sharp, aching, burning, and often worsens with deep breathing.

- Administer analgesia as prescribed (morphine, fentanyl).

  ▫ Pain will stimulate the sympathetic nervous system, resulting in increased heart rate and systemic vascular resistance.

  ▫ Provide frequent and adequate doses to control pain. Maintain around-the-clock administration.

- Monitor fluid and electrolyte status.

  ▫ Fluid administration is determined by blood pressure, pulmonary artery wedge pressure, right atrial pressure, cardiac output and index, systemic vascular resistance, blood loss, and urine output.

  ▫ Follow provider or unit-specific orders for fluid administration.

  ▫ Monitor the client for electrolyte imbalances, especially for hypokalemia and hyperkalemia.

- Prevent and monitor for infection.

- Practice proper hand hygiene.

- Use surgical aseptic technique during the procedures such as dressing changes and suctioning.

- Administer antibiotics.

- Monitor WBC counts, incisional redness and drainage, and fever.

- Monitor the client's temperature and provide warming measures if indicated.

- Client Education

  - Instruct the client to monitor and report signs of infection such as fever, incisional drainage, and redness.

  - Instruct the client to treat angina.

    - Maintain a fresh supply of sublingual nitroglycerin.

    - Store the nitroglycerin in a light-resistant container.

    - Discontinue activity and rest with the onset of pain. Follow directions for treating anginal pain.

  - Instruct the client to adhere to the pharmacological regimen.

  - Instruct clients who have diabetes mellitus to closely monitor blood glucose levels.

  - Encourage the client to consume a heart-healthy diet (low-fat, low-cholesterol, high-fiber, low-salt).

  - Encourage the client to quit smoking if applicable. Provide resources on smoking cessation.

  - Encourage physical activity. Consult the cardiac rehabilitation program or a physical therapist to devise a specific program.

  - Instruct the client to remain home during the first week after surgery and to resume normal activities slowly.

    - Week 2 – possible return to work part time, increase in social activities

    - Week 3 – lifting of up to 15 lb, avoidance of heavier lifting for 6 to 8 weeks

  - Clients can resume sexual activity based on the advice of the primary care provider.

    - Walking 1 block or climbing 2 flights of stairs symptom-free generally indicates that it is safe for the client to resume normal sexual activity.

  - Encourage the client to verbalize his feelings.

- Complications

  - Pulmonary complications

    - Atelectasis is a primary complication of a CABG. Other complications include pneumonia and pulmonary edema.

- Nursing Actions
    - While the client is intubated, suction every 1 to 2 hr and as needed.
    - Turn the client every 2 hr and advance him out of bed as soon as possible.
    - Monitor breath sounds, SaO_2, ABGs, pulmonary artery pressures, cardiac output, and urine output, and obtain a chest x-ray as indicated.
- Client Education
    - Encourage coughing, deep breathing, and use of an incentive spirometer. Explain to the client that increasing activity reduces postoperative complications.

- Hypothermia
    - Hypothermia may cause vasoconstriction, metabolic acidosis and hypertension.
    - Nursing Actions
        - Monitor the client's temperature and provide warming measures, such as warm blankets and heat lamps.
        - Monitor the client's blood pressure.
        - Administer vasodilators if prescribed.
    - Client Education
        - Assure client that shivering is common following surgery.

- Decreased cardiac output
    - Decreased cardiac output can result from dysrhythmias, cardiac tamponade, hypovolemia, left ventricular failure, or MI.
        - Cardiac tamponade results from bleeding while chest tubes are occluded, causing fluid to build up in the pericardium. Increased pericardial fluid compresses the heart chambers and inhibits effective pumping.
            - Signs include a sudden decrease/cessation of chest-tube drainage following heavy drainage, jugular-venous distension with clear lung sounds, and equal pulmonary artery wedge pressure and central venous pressure values.
        - Hypovolemia may be the result of bleeding, decreased intravascular volume or vasodilation, and hypotension and decreased urine output are the results.
        - Left ventricular heart failure may occur with a MI or hypervolemia.
    - Nursing Actions
        - Monitor ECG, blood pressure, pulmonary artery pressures, cardiac output, urine output, and bleeding through the chest tube.
        - Administer inotropic medications and fluid and blood products as prescribed.
        - Treat dysrhythmias as prescribed.
            - Use pacemaker wires if heart block is present.

        □   Treatment of cardiac tamponade involves volume expansion (fluid administration) and an emergency sternotomy with drainage. Pericardiocentesis is avoided because blood may have clotted.

- ○ Electrolyte Disturbances

  - ▪ Potassium and magnesium depletion is common.

  - ▪ Nursing Actions

    - □ Always dilute potassium supplements in adequate fluid (40 to 80 mEq in 100 mL of IV solution).

    - □ Administer supplements with an infusion pump to control the rate of delivery.

    - □ Administer supplements through a central catheter.

    - □ Monitor ECG and electrolytes.

- ○ Neurologic deficits

  - ▪ Transient hypertension, hypotension, or a blood clot may cause an intraoperative cerebrovascular accident.

  - ▪ Nursing Actions

    - □ Assess the client's neurologic status, including pupils, level of consciousness, and sensory and motor function.

    - □ Maintain the client's blood pressure within prescribed parameters.

  - ▪ Client Education

    - □ Explain all procedures to the client.

    - □ Assure the client that memory loss and neuro deficits may be temporary.

Peripheral Bypass Grafts

- Bypass graft surgery aims to restore adequate blood flow to the areas affected by peripheral artery disease.

  - ○ A peripheral bypass graft involves suturing graft material or autogenous saphenous veins proximal and distal to an occluded area of an artery. This procedure improves blood supply to the area normally served by the blocked artery.

  - ○ If bypass surgery fails to restore circulation, the client may need to undergo amputation of the limb.

- Indications

  - ○ Acute circulatory compromise in limb

  - ○ Severe pain at rest that interferes with ability to work

○ Client Presentation

■ Subjective Data

    □ Numbness or burning pain to the lower extremity with exercise, and may stop with rest (intermittent claudication)

    □ Numbness or burning pain to the lower extremity at rest, and may wake client at night; pain may be relieved by lowering the extremity below heart

■ Objective Data

    □ Decreased or absent pulses to feet. Dry, hairless, shiny skin on calves. Muscles may atrophy with advanced disease. Skin may be cold and dark colored. Feet and toes may be mottled and dusky, and toenails may be thick. Skin may become reddened (rubor) when extremity is dropped to a dependent position. Ulcers or lesions may be noted on toes (arterial ulcers) or ankles (venous ulcers).

- Client Outcomes

○ The client will have increased circulation in the extremity/foot.

○ The client will be pain free, and the foot will be intact without ulcerations or lesions.

○ The client will follow a recommended diet, exercise, and maintain foot care.

- Preprocedure

○ Nursing Actions

■ Assess the client/family's understanding of the procedure.

■ Verify that that the client has signed the informed consent form.

■ Assess the client for allergies.

■ Document the client's baseline vital signs and peripheral pulses.

■ Administer prophylactic antibiotic therapy to the client as prescribed.

■ Instruct the client to maintain NPO status for at least 8 hr prior to surgery.

○ Client Education

■ Include information about postoperative pain management and teach the client deep breathing/ incentive spirometer exercises.

■ Advise the client not to cross his legs.

■ The client may have an arterial line inserted for blood work and blood pressure monitoring.

■ Explain to the client that pedal pulses will be checked frequently.

- Intraprocedure

○ Nursing Actions

■ Provide padding to bony prominences to provide comfort and to prevent skin breakdown.

- Communicate surgical progress to family members, if appropriate.

- Assist in monitoring urine output and blood loss.

- Document appropriate surgical events.

- Communicate client postoperative needs to postanesthesia care unit.

- Postprocedure

  o Nursing Actions

    - Assess and monitor the client's vital signs every 15 min for 1 hr and then hourly after the first hour (or per facility policy).

    - Follow standing orders to maintain blood pressure within the prescribed range. Hypotension may reduce blood flow to graft, and hypertension may cause bleeding.

    - Assess and monitor the client's the operative limb every 15 min for 1 hr and then hourly after that, paying particular attention to the following:

      □ Incision site for bleeding.

      □ Peripheral pulses and skin color/temperature for signs of bypass graft occlusion.

      □ That the site is marked with an indelible marker.

    - Administer IV fluids as prescribed.

    - Assess the type of pain experienced by the client.

      □ Throbbing pain is experienced due to an increase in blood flow to the extremity.

      □ Ischemic pain is often difficult to relieve with opioid administration.

    - Administer analgesics, such as morphine sulfate and fentanyl (Sublimaze), to provide pain relief.

    - Administer antibiotics as prescribed.

    - Use surgical aseptic technique for dressing changes.

    - Monitor the client's incision sites for signs of infection, such as erythema, tenderness, and drainage.

    - Administer anticoagulant therapy, such as warfarin (Coumadin), heparin, and enoxaparin (Lovenox), to prevent reocclusion.

    - Administer antiplatelet therapy, such as clopidogrel (Plavix), tirofiban (Aggrastat), and aspirin.

    - Help the client turn, cough, and deep breathe every 2 hr.

    - Maintain bed rest for 18 to 24 hr. The leg should be kept straight during this time.

    - Assist the client to get out of bed and ambulate. Encourage the use of a walker initially.

- Discourage the client from sitting for long periods of time.

- Apply support stockings to promote venous return.

- Set up a progressive exercise program that includes walking. Consider a physical therapy consult.

  o Client Education

    - Advise the client to completely abstain from smoking. Suggest community services that help smokers abstain.

    - Reinforce activity restrictions.

    - Remind the client to avoid crossing his legs.

    - Advise the client to avoid risk factors for atherosclerosis (smoking, sedentary life style, uncontrolled diabetes mellitus).

    - Teach the client techniques of foot inspection and care. Encourage the client to:

      □ Keep feet dry and clean.

      □ Avoid extreme temperatures.

      □ Use lotion.

      □ Avoid constraining garments.

      □ Wear clean, white, cotton socks and always wear shoes.

- Complications

  o Graft occlusion

    - The graft may occlude due to reduced blood flow and clot formation.

    - Nursing Actions

      □ Notify the provider immediately for any noted changes in pedal pulse, extremity color, or temperature.

      □ Prepare the client for thrombectomy or thrombolytic therapy.

      □ Monitor for bleeding with thrombolytics.

      □ Monitor coagulation studies.

      □ Monitor for anaphylaxis.

  o Compartment syndrome

    - Pressure from tissue swelling or bleeding within a compartment or a restricted space causes reduced blood flow to the area. Untreated, the affected tissue will become necrotic and die.

    - Nursing Actions

      □ Assess for worsening pain, swelling, and tense or taut skin.

      □ Report abnormal findings to the provider immediately.

      □ Prepare the client for a fasciotomy to relieve compartmental pressure.

○ Infection

- Infection of the surgical site may result in the loss of the graft and increased ischemia.

- Nursing Actions

  □ Assess the wound for increased redness, swelling, and drainage.

  □ Monitor WBC count and temperature.

  □ Collect specimens (wound or blood cultures).

  □ Administer antibiotic therapy.

- Client Education

  □ Advise the client to notify the provider of decreased sensation, increased ischemic pain, redness, or swelling at the incisional site or in the affected limb.

CHAPTER 34: INVASIVE CARDIOVASCULAR PROCEDURES

 Application Exercises

1. A nurse is caring for a client who is in the immediate postoperative period following CABG surgery. The client is 4 hr postextubation. He has refused to cough because he is tired and it hurts too much. He is only able to inspire 200 mL with the incentive spirometer. Which of the following is an appropriate nursing intervention?

    A. Let the client rest for now and return in 1 hr to try again.

    B. Administer morphine sulfate 4 mg IV bolus, and return in 10 to 15 min to try again.

    C. Document the 200 mL as an appropriate volume.

    D. Tell the client that he will have to learn to breathe through the pain if he does not want to get pneumonia.

Scenario: A nurse is caring for a client in the immediate postoperative period following peripheral bypass graft surgery.

2. Provide rationales for the following interventions.

NURSING INTERVENTION	RATIONALE
Assess the incision for bleeding.	
Assess distal pulse.	
Place an "X" on the site of the pulse.	
Discourage sitting for prolonged periods of time.	
Encourage participation in a walking program.	

3. Which of the following client findings pose an immediate concern? (Select all that apply.)

    _____ Trace of bloody drainage on the first dressing change

    _____ Capillary refill of affected limb of 6 seconds

    _____ Mottled appearance of the limb

    _____ Throbbing pain of affected limb that is decreased with morphine sulfate

    _____ Pulse of 2+ in the affected limb

4. List important topics for discharge teaching. Provide rationales for your choices.

TOPIC	RATIONALE

5. A nurse is caring for a client following an angioplasty that was inserted through the femoral artery. While turning the client, the nurse discovers blood underneath the client's lower back. The nurse should suspect

    A. retroperitoneal bleeding.

    B. cardiac tamponade.

    C. bleeding from the incisional site.

    D. heart failure.

CHAPTER 34: INVASIVE CARDIOVASCULAR PROCEDURES

 Application Exercises Answer Key

1. A nurse is caring for a client who is in the immediate postoperative period following CABG surgery. The client is 4 hr postextubation. He has refused to cough because he is tired and it hurts too much. He is only able to inspire 200 mL with the incentive spirometer. Which of the following is an appropriate nursing intervention?

A. Let the client rest for now and return in 1 hr to try again.

B. Administer morphine sulfate 4 mg IV bolus, and return in 10 to 15 min to try again.

C. Document the 200 mL as an appropriate volume.

D. Tell the client that he will have to learn to breathe through the pain if he does not want to get pneumonia.

It is important for the client to deep breathe and cough frequently. Pain medication should be administered to aid the client with deep breathing and coughing. Returning in 1 hr may result in a poor outcome. Two hundred milliliters is not an appropriate volume, and telling the client to breathe through the pain is not a therapeutic response.

 NCLEX® Connection: Reduction of Risk Potential, Potential for Complications from Surgical Procedures and Health Alterations

---

Scenario: A nurse is caring for a client in the immediate postoperative period following peripheral bypass graft surgery.

---

2. Provide rationales for the following interventions.

NURSING INTERVENTION	RATIONALE
Assess the incision for bleeding.	Arteries were involved in the bypass graft. An arterial bleed is life-threatening.
Assess distal pulse.	Distal pulse is an indicator of adequate circulation.
Place an "X" on the site of the pulse.	This allows for easier assessment of distal pulse.
Discourage sitting for prolonged periods of time.	Sitting puts pressure on vessels and increases the risk of venous stasis and edema.
Encourage participation in a walking program.	Exercise improves blood circulation.

 NCLEX® Connection: Reduction of Risk Potential, Potential for Complications from Surgical Procedures and Health Alterations

3. Which of the following client findings pose an immediate concern? (Select all that apply.)

_____   Trace of bloody drainage on the first dressing change

__X__   **Capillary refill of affected limb of 6 seconds**

__X__   **Mottled appearance of the limb**

_____   Throbbing pain of affected limb that is decreased with morphine sulfate

_____   Pulse of 2+ in the affected limb

Capillary refill greater than 3 seconds and a limb that appears mottled indicates decreased circulation and may indicate graft occlusion. The surgeon should be notified immediately. The other findings are expected and do not require immediate attention.

 NCLEX® Connection: Reduction of Risk Potential, System Specific Assessment

4. List important topics for discharge teaching. Provide rationales for your choices.

TOPIC	RATIONALE
Smoking cessation	Nicotine causes vasoconstriction, which will decrease perfusion and delay healing. Smoking will also increase progression of atherosclerosis.
Following medication regimen	Medications will increase circulation, prevent reocclusion, and prevent or treat infection.
Activity restrictions	This will prevent disruption of sutures.
Foot inspection	Skin remains fragile. Wounds will not heal well if circulation is compromised.
Dietary modification	An appropriate diet will slow the progression of atherosclerosis.

 NCLEX® Connection: Reduction of Risk Potential, Potential for Complications from Surgical Procedures and Health Alterations

5. A nurse is caring for a client following an angioplasty that was inserted through the femoral artery. While turning the client, the nurse discovers blood underneath the client's lower back. The nurse should suspect

    A. retroperitoneal bleeding.

    B. cardiac tamponade.

    C. bleeding from the incisional site.

    D. heart failure.

The incisional site is most likely leaking blood that is seeping under the client. The nurse should assess the incision for drainage, apply pressure, monitor blood pressure and heart rate, and notify the surgeon. Retroperitoneal bleeding, cardiac tamponade, and heart failure would not be indicative of these findings.

(N) NCLEX® Connection: Reduction of Risk Potential, Potential for Complications from Surgical Procedures and Health Alterations

UNIT 4	NURSING CARE OF CLIENTS WITH CARDIOVASCULAR DISORDERS
Section	Cardiac Disorders
Chapter 35	Angina and Myocardial Infarction

 Overview

- The continuum from angina to myocardial infarction (MI) is termed acute coronary syndrome. Symptoms of acute coronary syndrome are due to an imbalance between myocardial oxygen supply and demand.

 View Media Supplement: Myocardial Infarction (Image)

- Angina pectoris is a warning sign of an impending acute MI.

- Women and older adults do not always experience symptoms typically associated with angina or MI.

- The majority of deaths from an MI occur within 1 hr of symptom onset. The average time for a person seeking treatment is 4 hr. Early recognition and treatment of an acute MI is essential to prevent death.

- Research shows improved outcomes following an MI in clients treated with aspirin, beta-blockers, and angiotensin-converting enzyme (ACE) inhibitors.

- When blood flow to the heart is compromised, ischemia causes chest pain. Anginal pain is often described as a tight squeezing, heavy pressure, or constricting feeling in the chest. The pain can radiate to the jaw, neck, or arm.

- There are three types of angina:

  o Stable angina (exertional angina) occurs with exercise or emotional stress and is relieved by rest or nitroglycerin (Nitrostat).

  o Unstable angina (preinfarction angina) occurs with exercise or emotional stress, but it increases in occurrence, severity, and duration over time.

  o Variant angina (Prinzmetal's angina) is due to a coronary artery spasm, often occurring during periods of rest.

- Pain unrelieved by rest or nitroglycerin and lasting for more than 15 min differentiates an MI from angina.

- An abrupt interruption of oxygen to the heart muscle produces myocardial ischemia. Ischemia can lead to tissue necrosis (infarction) if blood supply and oxygen are not restored. Ischemia is reversible while an infarction results in permanent damage.

- When the cardiac muscle suffers ischemic injury, cardiac enzymes are released into the bloodstream, providing specific markers of MI.

- MIs are classified based on:

  ○ The affected area of the heart (anterior, anterolateral).

  ○ The depth of involvement (transmural versus nontransmural).

  ○ The EKG changes produced (Q wave, non-Q wave). Non-Q-wave MIs are more common in older adults, women, and clients who have diabetes mellitus.

ANGINA	MYOCARDIAL INFARCTION
Precipitated by exertion or stress	Can occur without cause, often in the morning after rest
Relieved by rest or nitroglycerin	Relieved only by opioids
Symptoms last < 15 min	Symptoms last > 30 min
Not associated with nausea, epigastric distress, dyspnea, anxiety, diaphoresis	Associated with nausea, epigastric distress, dyspnea, anxiety, diaphoresis

Health Promotion and Disease Prevention

- Encourage the client to maintain an exercise routine to remain physically active. The client should consult with a provider before starting any exercise regimen.

- The client should have her cholesterol level and blood pressure checked regularly.

- The client should consume a diet low in saturated fats and sodium. The client should also consult with a provider regarding diet restrictions.

- If the client is a smoker promote smoking cessation.

Assessment

- Risk Factors

  ○ Male gender or postmenopausal women

  ○ Hypertension

  ○ Tobacco use

  ○ Advanced age

  ○ Hyperlipidemia

  ○ Metabolic disorders (diabetes mellitus, hyperthyroidism)

  ○ Methamphetamine or cocaine use

- ○ Stress (occupational, physical exercise, and sexual activity)

(G)
- ○ An increased risk of coronary artery disease exists for older adult clients who are physically inactive, have one or more chronic diseases (hypertension, heart failure, and diabetes mellitus), or have lifestyle (smoking and diet) habits that contribute to atherosclerosis.

(G)
- ○ The incidence of cardiac disease increases with age, especially in the presence of hypertension, diabetes mellitus, hypercholesterolemia, elevated homocystine, and highly sensitive C-reactive protein (HS-CRP).

- ○ Atherosclerotic changes related to aging predispose the heart to poor blood perfusion and oxygen delivery.

- Subjective Data

(G)
- ○ Women and older adults may not experience typical symptoms associated with angina or an MI.

- ○ Anxiety, feeling of impending doom

- ○ Chest pain (substernal or precordial)

  - Pain can radiate down the shoulder or arm or may present in the form of jaw pain.

  - Pain may be described as a crushing or aching pressure.

- ○ Nausea

- ○ Dizziness

- Objective Data

- ○ Physical Assessment Findings

  - Pallor and cool, clammy skin

  - Tachycardia and/or heart palpitations

  - Diaphoresis

  - Vomiting

  - Decreased level of consciousness

- ○ Laboratory Tests

  - Cardiac enzymes released with cardiac muscle injury:

    - □ Myoglobin – Levels no longer evident after 24 hr

    - □ Creatine kinase-MB – Levels no longer evident after 3 days

    - □ Troponin I – Levels no longer evident after 7 days

    - □ Troponin T – Levels no longer evident after 14 to 21 days

- ○ Diagnostic Procedures
  - Electrocardiograms (ECG)
    - □ Electrocardiography uses an electrocardiograph to record the electrical activity of the heart over time. The electrocardiograph is connected by wires (leads) to skin electrodes placed on various areas of the body.
    - □ Nursing Actions
      - ‣ Position the client in a supine position with the chest exposed.
      - ‣ Wash the client's skin to remove oils.
      - ‣ Attach one electrode to each extremity by applying electrodes to flat surfaces above the wrists and ankles and the other six electrodes to the chest, avoiding chest hair. (On male clients, chest hair may need to be shaved.)
      - ‣ Check for changes on serial ECGs.
      - ‣ Angina – ST depression and/or T-wave inversion (ischemia)
      - ‣ MI – T-wave inversion (ischemia), ST-segment elevation (injury), and an abnormal Q wave (necrosis)
  - Thallium scans
    - □ Assess for ischemia or necrosis. Radioisotopes cannot reach areas with decreased or absent perfusion and they appear as "cold spots."
    - □ Nursing Actions
      - ‣ Instruct the client to avoid smoking and consuming caffeinated beverages 4 hr prior to the procedure. These can affect the test.
  - Cardiac catheterization
    - □ A coronary angiogram, also called a cardiac catheterization, is an invasive diagnostic procedure used to evaluate the presence and degree of coronary artery blockage.
    - □ Angiography involves the insertion of a catheter into a femoral (sometimes a brachial) vessel and threading it into the right or left side of the heart. Coronary artery narrowing and occlusions are identified by the injection of contrast media under fluoroscopy.
    - □ Nursing Actions
      - ‣ Ensure the client understands the procedure prior to signing the consent form.
      - ‣ Ensure that the client is kept NPO 8 hr prior to the procedure.
      - ‣ Assess that the client and family understand the procedure.
      - ‣ Assess for iodine/shellfish allergy (contrast media).

Collaborative Care

- Nursing Care
    - Monitor:
        - Vital signs every 15 min until stable, then every hour
        - Serial ECG, continuous cardiac monitoring
        - Location, severity, quality, and duration of pain
        - Hourly urine output – greater than 30 mL/hr indicates renal perfusion
        - Laboratory data (cardiac enzymes, electrolytes, ABGs)
    - Administer oxygen (2 to 4 L)
    - Obtain and maintain IV access.
    - Promote energy conservation (cluster nursing interventions).
- Medications
    - Vasodilators
        - Nitroglycerin (Nitrostat) prevents coronary artery vasospasm and reduces preload and afterload, decreasing myocardial oxygen demand.
        - Nursing Considerations
            - It is given to treat angina and help control blood pressure.
            - It should be used cautiously with other antihypertensive medications.
            - Vasodilators can cause orthostatic hypotension.
        - Client Education
            - Client education regarding response to chest pain:
                - Stop activity and rest.
                - Place nitroglycerin tablet under tongue to dissolve (quick absorption).
                - If pain is unrelieved in 5 min, the client should call 911 or be driven to an emergency department.
                - The client can take up to two more doses of nitroglycerin at 5-min intervals.
            - Remind the client that a headache is a common side effect of this medication.
            - Encourage the client to sit and lie down slowly.
    - Analgesics
        - Morphine sulfate is an opioid analgesic used to treat moderate to severe pain. Analgesics act on the mu and kappa receptors that help alleviate pain.
        - Activation of these receptors produces analgesia (pain relief), respiratory depression, euphoria, sedation, and a decrease in GI motility.

- Use cautiously with clients who have asthma or emphysema due to the risk of respiratory depression.

- Nursing Considerations

  □ For the client having chest pain, assess the client's pain every 5 to 15 min.

  □ Watch the client for signs of respiratory depression, especially older adults. If the respirations are 12/min or less, stop the medication and notify the provider immediately.

  □ Monitor the client's vital signs closely for signs of hypotension and decreased respirations.

  □ Observe the client for nausea and vomiting.

- Client Education

  □ If nausea and vomiting persist, advise the client to notify a nurse.

  □ Teach the client to use the PCA pump, if applicable.

    ▸ The client is the only person who should push the medication administration button. Reassure the client that the safety lockout mechanism on the PCA pump prevents overdosing of the medication.

○ Beta-blockers

- Metoprolol tartrate (Lopressor) has antidysrhythmic and antihypertensive properties that decrease the imbalance between myocardial oxygen supply and demand by reducing afterload.

- In an acute MI, beta-blockers decrease infarct size and improve short- and long-term survival rates.

- Nursing Considerations

  □ Beta-blockers can cause bradycardia and hypotension. Hold the medication if the client's apical pulse is less than 60/min and notify the provider.

  □ Avoid giving to clients who have asthma.

  □ Use with caution in clients who have heart failure.

- Client Education

  □ Encourage the client to sit and lie down slowly.

  □ Remind the client to notify the provider immediately if shortness of breath, edema, weight gain, or cough occur.

○ Thrombolytic agents

- Streptokinase (Streptase) and alteplase (Activase) are used to break up blood clots.

- Thrombolytic agents have similar side effects and contraindications as anticoagulants.

- For best results give within 6 hr of infarction.

- Nursing Considerations
  - Assess for contraindications (active bleeding, peptic ulcer disease, history of CVA, or recent trauma).
  - Monitor bleeding times – PT, aPTT, INR, fibrinogen levels, and CBC.
  - Monitor for the same side effects as anticoagulants (thrombocytopenia, anemia, or hemorrhage).
  - Administer streptokinase slowly to prevent hypotension.
- Client Education
  - Remind the client of the risk for bruising and bleeding while on this medication.

- Antiplatelet agents
  - Aspirin (Ecotrin) and clopidogrel (Plavix) prevent platelets from forming together, which can produce arterial clotting.
  - Nursing Considerations
    - Antiplatelet agents can cause gastrointestinal (GI) upset.
    - Use cautiously with clients who have a history of GI ulcers.
    - Tinnitus, ringing in the ears, can be a sign of aspirin toxicity.
  - Client Education
    - Remind the client of the risk for bruising and bleeding while on this medication.
    - Encourage the client to use aspirin tablets with enteric coating and to take with food.
    - Ask the client if she is experiencing ringing in the ears.

- Anticoagulants
  - Heparin and enoxaparin (Lovenox) are used to prevent clots from becoming larger or other clots from forming.
  - Nursing Considerations
    - Assess for contraindications (active bleeding, peptic ulcer disease, history of CVA, or recent trauma).
    - Monitor bleeding times – PT, aPTT, INR, and CBC.
    - Monitor for side effects of anticoagulants (thrombocytopenia, anemia, and hemorrhage).
  - Client Education
    - Remind the client of the risk for bruising and bleeding while on this medication.

- o Glycoprotein IIB/IIIA inhibitors

    - ■ Eptifibatide (Integrilin) is used to prevent the binding of fibrogen, in turn blocking platelet aggregation. In combination with aspirin therapy, IIB/IIA inhibitors are standard therapy.

    - ■ Nursing Considerations

        - □ This medication can cause active bleeding.

    - ■ Client Education

        - □ Instruct the client to report signs of bleeding during medication therapy.

- • Interdisciplinary Care

    - o Pain management services can be consulted if pain persists and/or is uncontrolled.

    - o Cardiac rehabilitation care can be consulted if the client has prolonged weakness and needs assistance with increasing level of activity.

    - o Nutritional services can be consulted for diet modification to promote low-sodium and low-saturated fat food choices.

- • Surgical Interventions

    - o Angioplasty (also known as PTCA)

        - ■ Percutaneous transluminal coronary angioplasty (PTCA) involves inflating a balloon to dilate the arterial lumen and the adhering plaque, thus widening the arterial lumen. A stent (mesh-wire device) is often placed to prevent restenosis of the artery.

        - ■ Nursing Actions

            - □ Ensure that the consent form is signed.

            - □ Ensure that the client is kept NPO 8 hr prior to the procedure.

            - □ Assess that the client and family understand the procedure.

            - □ Assess for iodine/shellfish allergy (contrast media).

    - o Bypass graft (also known as CABG)

        - ■ Coronary artery bypass graft (CABG) surgery restores myocardial tissue perfusion by the addition of grafts bypassing the obstructed coronary arteries. It is the most common form of cardiac surgery.

        - ■ Nursing Actions

            - □ A CABG can be an elective procedure or done in an emergency. When planned, preparation begins before the client comes to the hospital for the procedure.

            - □ Verify that the informed consent is signed.

            - □ Confirm recent chest x-ray, ECG, and blood work results are available or needed.

- Care after Discharge

  o Cardiac rehabilitation should be consulted for a specific exercise program related to the heart.

  o Nutritional services, such as a dietitian, can be consulted for diet modification or weight management.

  o Client Education

    ▪ Instruct the client to monitor and report signs of infection, such as fever, incisional drainage, and redness.

    ▪ Teach the client to avoid straining, strenuous exercise, or emotional stress, when possible.

    ▪ Client education regarding response to chest pain:

      □ Stop activity and rest.

      □ Place nitroglycerin tablet under tongue to dissolve (quick absorption).

      □ If pain is unrelieved in 5 min, the client should call 911 or be driven to an emergency department.

      □ The client can take up to two more doses of nitroglycerin at 5-min intervals.

    ▪ If the client is a smoker encourage smoking cessation.

    ▪ Encourage the client to remain active and to exercise regularly.

- Client Outcomes

  o The client will be free of pain.

  o The client will be able to maintain exercise routine.

  o The client will maintain medication regimen.

  o The client will remain free of infection.

Complications

- Acute MI

  o This is a complication of angina not relieved by rest or nitroglycerin.

  o Nursing Actions

    ▪ Administer oxygen to the client.

    ▪ Notify the provider immediately.

- Heart failure/cardiogenic shock

  o Injury to the left ventricle can lead to decreased cardiac output and heart failure.

  o Progressive heart failure can lead to cardiogenic shock.

    - This is a serious complication of pump failure, commonly following an MI of 40% blockage.

    - Symptoms include tachycardia, hypotension, inadequate urinary output, altered level of consciousness, respiratory distress (crackles and tachypnea) cool, clammy skin, decreased peripheral pulses, and chest pain.

  o Nursing Actions

    - Administration of oxygen; possible intubation and ventilation may be required.

    - IV administration of morphine, diuretics, and/or nitroglycerin to decrease preload; and IV administration of vasopressors and/or positive inotropes to increase cardiac output and to maintain organ perfusion.

    - Maintain continuous hemodynamic monitoring.

- Ischemic mitral regurgitation

  o Ischemia can be evidenced by the development of a new cardiac murmur.

  o Nursing Actions

    - Administer oxygen to the client.

    - Notify the provider immediately.

- Ventricular aneurysms/rupture

  o Necrosis due to an MI, can present as sudden chest pain, dysrhythmias, and severe hypotension.

  o Nursing Actions

    - Administer oxygen to the client.

    - Notify the provider immediately.

- Dysrhythmias

  o An inferior wall MI may lead to an injury to the AV node resulting in bradycardia and second-degree AV heart block.

  o An anterior wall MI may lead to an injury to the ventricle resulting in premature ventricular contractions, bundle branch, or a complete heart block.

  o Nursing Actions

    - Monitor ECG and vital signs.

    - Administer oxygen.

    - Administer antidysrhythmic medications as indicated.

    - Prepare for cardiac pacemaker if needed.

CHAPTER 35: ANGINA AND MYOCARDIAL INFARCTION

(A) Application Exercises

1. Which of the following findings will help a nurse distinguish angina from an MI?

    A. Angina can be relieved with rest and nitroglycerin.

    B. An MI will be relieved with nitroglycerin.

    C. An MI will have cardiac enzyme levels within the expected reference range.

    D. Angina can occur for longer than 30 min.

2. Match the following interventions with the correct rationale.

_____ Oxygen	A.	Increases myocardial oxygen supply
_____ Beta-blocker	B.	Removes a clot that is causing ischemia/infarction
_____ ACE inhibitor	C.	Reduces preload and afterload, dilates coronary arteries, increases myocardial oxygen supply, and reduces oxygen consumption
_____ Stool softener	D.	Reduces preload by venous vasodilation decreasing myocardial oxygen consumption, relieves pain, and decreases sympathetic nervous system stimulation
_____ Nitroglycerin	E.	Reduces straining, which could precipitate an MI and vasovagal effect
_____ Morphine	F.	It is an antidysrhythmic and antihypertensive; reduces afterload to decrease myocardial oxygen consumption, decreases infarct size, and improves survival rates
_____ Thrombolytic agent	G.	Decreases afterload and myocardial oxygen consumption

3. A client who has a diagnosis of an MI reports that dyspnea began 2 weeks ago. Which of the following cardiac enzymes should the nurse assess to determine if the infarction occurred 14 days ago?

    A. CK-MB

    B. Troponin I

    C. Troponin T

    D. Myoglobin

4. A client asks a nurse why her provider prescribed 1 aspirin per day. Which of the following responses should the nurse give?

    A. "Aspirin reduces the formation of blood clots that could cause a heart attack."

    B. "Aspirin decreases any pain due to myocardial ischemia."

    C. "Aspirin dissolves any clots that are forming in your coronary arteries."

    D. "Aspirin relieves any headaches that are caused by other medications."

5. A client who has angina reports that he is not able to make all of the lifestyle changes recommended. Which of the following changes should the nurse suggest that the client work on first?

    A. Diet modification

    B. Relaxation exercises

    C. Smoking cessation

    D. Taking omega-3 capsules

CHAPTER 35: ANGINA AND MYOCARDIAL INFARCTION

 Application Exercises Answer Key

1. Which of the following findings will help a nurse distinguish angina from an MI?

A. Angina can be relieved by rest and nitroglycerin.

B. An MI will with relieved with nitroglycerin.

C. An MI will have cardiac enzyme levels within the expected reference range.

D. Angina can occur for longer than 30 min.

Angina can be relieved with rest and nitroglycerin. An MI will need to be relieved using opioids. Cardiac enzymes are abnormal with an MI. Angina usually occurs for 15 min or less.

 NCLEX® Connection: Reduction of Risk Potential, System Specific Assessment

2. Match the following interventions with the correct rationale.

A	Oxygen	A. Increases myocardial oxygen supply
F	Beta-blocker	B. Removes a clot that is causing ischemia/infarction
G	ACE inhibitor	C. Reduces preload and afterload, dilates coronary arteries, increases myocardial oxygen supply, and reduces oxygen consumption
E	Stool softener	D. Reduces preload by venous vasodilation decreasing myocardial oxygen consumption, relieves pain, and decreases sympathetic nervous system stimulation
C	Nitroglycerin	E. Reduces straining, which could precipitate an MI and vasovagal effect
D	Morphine	F. It is an antidysrhythmic and antihypertensive; reduces afterload to decrease myocardial oxygen consumption, decreases infarct size, and improves survival rates
B	Thrombolytic agent	G. Decreases afterload and myocardial oxygen consumption

 NCLEX® Connection: Pharmacological and Parenteral Therapies, Expected Actions/ Outcomes

3. A client who has a diagnosis of an MI reports that dyspnea began 2 weeks ago. Which of the following cardiac enzymes should the nurse assess to determine if the infarction occurred 14 days ago?

    A. CK-MB

    B. Troponin I

    C. Troponin T

    D. Myoglobin

The Troponin T level will still be evident 14 to 21 days following an MI. Troponin I levels are no longer evident after 7 days, myoglobin levels are no longer evident after 24 hr, and creatine kinase-MB levels are no longer evident after 3 days.

 NCLEX® Connection: Reduction of Risk Potential, Laboratory Values

4. A client asks a nurse why her provider prescribed 1 aspirin per day. Which of the following responses should the nurse give??

    A. "Aspirin reduces the formation of blood clots that could cause a heart attack."

    B. "Aspirin decreases any pain due to myocardial ischemia."

    C. "Aspirin dissolves any clots that are forming in your coronary arteries."

    D. "Aspirin relieves any headaches that are caused by other medications."

Aspirin decreases platelet aggregation. One aspirin a day is not sufficient to alleviate ischemic pain. Aspirin does not dissolve clots. Other medications can cause headaches, but one aspirin per day is not administered as an analgesic.

 NCLEX® Connection: Pharmacological and Parenteral Therapies, Expected Actions/ Outcomes

5. A client who has angina reports that he is not able to make all of the lifestyle changes recommended. Which of the following changes should the nurse suggest that the client work on first?

    A. Diet modification

    B. Relaxation exercises

    C. Smoking cessation

    D. Taking omega-3 capsules

According to the airway, breathing, and circulation (ABC) priority setting framework, ensuring that the client has adequate oxygen should be the nurse's first priority. Nicotine causes vasoconstriction, elevates blood pressure, and narrows coronary arteries; therefore, the nurse should suggest that the client first work on a smoking cessation program.

 NCLEX® Connection: Physiological Adaptation, Illness Management

UNIT 4	NURSING CARE OF CLIENTS WITH CARDIOVASCULAR DISORDERS
Section	Cardiac Disorders
Chapter 36	Heart Failure and Pulmonary Edema

Overview

- Heart failure occurs when the heart muscle is unable to pump effectively, resulting in inadequate cardiac output, myocardial hypertrophy, and pulmonary/systemic congestion. The heart is unable to maintain adequate circulation to meet tissue needs.

- Heart failure is the result of an acute or chronic cardiopulmonary problem, such as systemic hypertension, myocardial infarction (MI), pulmonary hypertension, dysrhythmias, valvular heart disease, pericarditis, and cardiomyopathy.

- Pulmonary edema is a severe, life-threatening accumulation of fluid in the alveoli and interstitial spaces of the lung that can result from severe heart failure.

HEART FAILURE

Overview

- The severity of heart failure is graded on the New York Heart Association's functional classification scale indicating how little, or how much activity it takes to make the client symptomatic (chest pain, or shortness of breath).

  - Class I: Client exhibits no symptoms with activity.

  - Class II: Client has symptoms with ordinary exertion.

  - Class III: Client displays symptoms with minimal exertion.

  - Class IV: Client has symptoms at rest.

- Low-output heart failure can initially occur on either the left or right side of the heart.

  - Left-sided heart (ventricular) failure results in inadequate left ventricle (cardiac) output and consequently in inadequate tissue perfusion. Forms include:

    - Systolic heart (ventricular) failure (ejection fraction below 40%, pulmonary and systemic congestion).

    - Diastolic heart (ventricular) failure (inadequate relaxation or "stiffening" prevents ventricular filling).

  - Right-sided heart (ventricular) failure results in inadequate right ventricle output and systemic venous congestion (peripheral edema).

- An uncommon form of heart failure is high-output failure, in which cardiac output is normal or above normal.

Health Promotion and Disease Prevention

- Maintain an exercise routine to remain physically active and consult with the provider before starting any exercise regimen.

- Consume a diet low in sodium, along with fluid restrictions and consult with the provider regarding diet specifications.

- Refrain from smoking.

- Follow medication regimen and follow up with the provider as needed.

Assessment

- Risk Factors

  ○ Left-sided heart (ventricular) failure

    ▪ Hypertension

    ▪ Coronary artery disease, angina, MI

    ▪ Valvular disease (mitral and aortic)

  ○ Right-sided heart (ventricular) failure

    ▪ Left-sided heart (ventricular) failure

    ▪ Right ventricular MI

    ▪ Pulmonary problems (COPD, ARDS)

  ○ High-output heart failure

    ▪ Increased metabolic needs

    ▪ Septicemia (fever)

    ▪ Anemia

    ▪ Hyperthyroidism

  ○ Cardiomyopathy

    ▪ Coronary artery disease

    ▪ Infection or inflammation of the heart muscle

    ▪ Various cancer treatments

    ▪ Prolonged alcohol abuse

    ▪ Heredity

  ○ Systolic blood pressure is elevated in older adults, putting them at risk for coronary artery disease and heart failure.

- Subjective and Objective Data
  - Left-sided failure
    - Dyspnea, orthopnea (shortness of breath while lying down), nocturnal dyspnea
    - Fatigue
    - Displaced apical pulse (hypertrophy)
    - S_3 heart sound (gallop)
    - Pulmonary congestion (dyspnea, cough, bibasilar crackles)
    - Frothy sputum (can be blood-tinged)
    - Altered mental status
    - Symptoms of organ failure, such as oliguria (decrease in urine output)
  - Right-sided failure
    - Jugular vein distention
    - Ascending dependent edema (legs, ankles, sacrum)
    - Abdominal distention, ascites
    - Fatigue, weakness
    - Nausea and anorexia
    - Polyuria at rest (nocturnal)
    - Liver enlargement (hepatomegaly) and tenderness
    - Weight gain
  - Cardiomyopathy

    (M) View Media Supplement: Cardiomyopathy (Image)

    - Fatigue, weakness
    - Heart failure (left with dilated type, right with restrictive type)
    - Dysrhythmias (heart block)
    - S_3 gallop
    - Cardiomegaly (enlarged heart)
  - The presence of other chronic illnesses can mask the presence of heart failure in older adult clients.

- ○ Laboratory Tests

  - ▪ Human B-type natriuretic peptides (hBNP): Elevated in heart failure. Used to differentiate dyspnea related to heart failure versus respiratory problem and to monitor the need for and the effectiveness of aggressive heart failure intervention.

    - ▫ A level below 100 pg/mL indicates no heart failure.
    - ▫ Levels between 100 to 300 pg/mL suggest heart failure is present.
    - ▫ A level above 300 pg/mL indicates mild heart failure.
    - ▫ A level above 600 pg/mL indicates moderate heart failure.
    - ▫ A level above 900 pg/mL indicates severe heart failure.

- ○ Diagnostic Procedures

  - ▪ Hemodynamic monitoring

    - ▫ Heart failure generally results in increased central venous pressure (CVP), increased right arterial pressure, increased pulmonary wedge pressure (PAWP), increased pulmonary artery pressure (PAP), and decreased cardiac output (CO).

    - ▫ Left-sided failure findings:
      - ▸ CVP/right atrial pressure (normal = 1 to 8 mm Hg): Normal or elevated
      - ▸ PAP (normal = 15 to 26 mm Hg/5 to 15 mm Hg): Elevated
      - ▸ PAWP (normal = 4 to 12 mm Hg): Elevated
      - ▸ CO (normal = 4 to 7 L/min): Decreased

    - ▫ Right-sided failure findings:
      - ▸ CVP/right atrial pressure (normal = 1 to 8 mm Hg): Elevated

  - ▪ Ultrasound

    - ▫ An ultrasound (also called cardiac ultrasound or echocardiogram), 2-D (2-dimensional) or 3-D (3-dimensional), is used to measure both systolic and diastolic function of the heart.

      - ▸ Left ventricular ejection fraction (LVEF): The volume of blood pumped from the left ventricle into the arteries upon each beat. Normal is 55% to 70%.

      - ▸ Right ventricular ejection fraction (RVEF): The volume of blood pumped from the right ventricle to the lungs upon each beat. Normal is 45% to 60%.

  - ▪ A chest x-ray can reveal cardiomegaly and pleural effusions.

  - ▪ Electrocardiogram (ECG), cardiac enzymes, electrolytes, and ABGs are used to assess factors contributing to heart failure and/or the impact of heart failure.

Collaborative Care

- Nursing Care

    - Monitor daily weight and I&O.

    - Monitor for shortness of breath and dyspnea on exertion.

    - Administer oxygen as prescribed.

    - Monitor vital signs and hemodynamic pressures.

    - Position the client to maximize ventilation (high-Fowler's).

    - Check ABGs, electrolytes (especially potassium if on diuretics), SaO_2, and chest x-ray results.

    - Assess for signs of medication toxicity (digoxin toxicity)

    - Encourage bed rest until the client is stable.

    - Encourage energy conservation by assisting with care and ADLs.

    - Maintain dietary restrictions as prescribed (restricted fluid intake, restricted sodium intake).

    - Provide emotional support to the client and family.

- Medications

    - Diuretics

        - Diuretics are used to decrease preload.

            - Loop diuretics, such as furosemide (Lasix), bumetanide (Bumex)

            - Thiazide diuretics, such as hydrochlorothiazide (Hydrodiuril)

            - Potassium-sparing diuretics, such as spironolactone (Aldactone)

        - Nursing Considerations

            - Administer furosemide IV no faster than 20 mg/min.

            - Loop and thiazide diuretics can cause hypokalemia, and potassium supplementation may be required.

        - Client Education

            - Teach clients taking loop or thiazide diuretics to ingest foods and drinks that are high in potassium to counter the effects of hypokalemia.

    - Afterload-reducing agents

        - Afterload-reducing agents help the heart pump more easily by altering the resistance to contraction. These include:

            - Angiotensin-converting enzyme (ACE) inhibitors, such as enalapril (Vasotec), captopril (Capoten)

            - Angiotensin receptor II blockers, such as losartan (Cozaar)

- These are contraindicated for clients who have renal deficiency.
- Nursing Considerations
  - Monitor clients taking ACE inhibitors for hypotension following the initial dose.
    - ▸ ACE inhibitors can cause angioedema (swelling of the tongue and throat).
    - ▸ Monitor for increased levels in potassium.
    - ▸ ACE inhibitors can cause a decreased sense of taste or rash on the skin.
- Client Education
  - Inform the client that this medication can cause a dry cough.
  - Notify the provider if the client observes a rash or has a decreased sense of taste.
  - Notify the provider if swelling of the face or extremities occurs.
  - Remind the client that blood pressure needs to be monitored for 2 hr after the initial dose to detect hypotension.

○ Inotropic agents

- Inotropic agents, such as digoxin (Lanoxin), dopamine, dobutamine (Dobutrex), and milrinone (Primacor), are used to increase contractility and thereby improve cardiac output.
- Nursing Considerations
  - For a client taking digoxin, take the apical heart rate for 1 min. Hold the medication if apical pulse is less than 60/min and notify the provider.
  - Observe the client for nausea and vomiting.
  - Dopamine, dobutamine, and milrinone are administered via IV. The ECG, blood pressure, and urine output must be closely monitored.
- Client Education
  - Teach clients who are self-administering digoxin to:
    - ▸ Count pulse for 1 min before taking the medication. If the pulse rate is irregular or the pulse rate is outside of the limitations set by the provider (usually less than 60/min or greater than 100/min), instruct the client to hold the dose and to contact the provider.
    - ▸ Take the digoxin dose at the same time each day.
    - ▸ Do not take digoxin at the same time as antacids. Separate the two medications by at least 2 hr.
    - ▸ Report signs of toxicity, including fatigue, muscle weakness, confusion, and loss of appetite.
    - ▸ Regularly have digoxin and potassium levels checked.

- ○ Vasodilators
  - ■ Nitroglycerine (Nitrostat) and isosorbide mononitrate (Imdur) prevent coronary artery vasospasm and reduce preload and afterload, decreasing myocardial oxygen demand.
  - ■ Nursing Considerations
    - □ Vasodilators are given to treat angina and help control blood pressure.
    - □ Use cautiously with other antihypertensive mediations.
    - □ Vasodilators can cause orthostatic hypotension.
  - ■ Client Education
    - □ Remind the client that a headache is a common side effect of this medication.
    - □ Encourage the client to sit and lie down slowly.
- ○ Human B-type natriuretic peptides (hBNP)
  - ■ hBNPs, such as nesiritide (Natrecor), are used to treat acute heart failure by causing natriuresis (loss of sodium and vasodilation).
  - ■ Nursing Considerations
    - □ hBNPs can cause hypotension, as well as a number of cardiac effects that include, ventricular tachycardia and bradycardia.
    - □ BNP levels will increase while on this medication.
    - □ ECG, blood pressure, and other parameters must be closely monitored.
  - ■ Client Education
    - □ The client can be asymptomatic with a low blood pressure.
    - □ Remind the client to sit and lie down slowly.
- ○ Anticoagulants
  - ■ Anticoagulants, such as warfarin (Coumadin), can be prescribed if the client has a history of thrombus formation.
  - ■ Nursing Considerations
    - □ Assess for contraindications (active bleeding, peptic ulcer disease, history of cerebrovascular accident, recent trauma).
    - □ Monitor bleeding times – PT, aPTT, INR, and CBC.
  - ■ Client Education
    - □ Remind the client of the risk for bruising and bleeding while on this medication.
    - □ Remind the client to have blood monitored routinely to check bleeding times.

- Interdisciplinary Care

  o Cardiology and pulmonary services should be consulted to manage heart failure.

  o Respiratory services should be consulted for inhalers, breathing treatments, and suctioning for airway management.

  o Cardiac rehabilitation services can be consulted if the client has prolonged weakness and needs assistance with increasing level of activity.

  o Nutritional services can be consulted for diet modification to promote low sodium, and low-saturated fat food choices.

- Surgical Interventions

  o Ventricular assist device (VAD)

    □ A VAD is a mechanical pump that assists a heart that is too weak to pump blood through the body. A VAD is used in clients who are eligible for heart transplants or who have severe end-stage heart failure and are not candidates for heart transplants. Heart transplantation is the treatment of choice for clients who have severe dilated cardiomyopathy.

    ■ Nursing Actions

      □ Prepare the client for the procedure (NPO status and informed consent).

      □ Monitor postoperatively (vital signs, SaO_2, incision drainage, and pain management).

  o Heart Transplantation

    ■ Heart transplantation is a possible option for clients who have end-stage heart failure. Immunosuppressant therapy is required posttransplantation to prevent rejection.

    ■ Nursing Actions

      □ Prepare the client for the procedure (NPO status and informed consent).

      □ Monitor postoperatively (vital signs, SaO_2, incision drainage, and pain management).

    ■ Client Education

      □ Take medications as prescribed.

      □ Take diuretics in the early morning and early afternoon.

      □ Maintain fluid and sodium restriction – a dietary consult can be useful.

      □ Increase dietary intake of potassium (cantaloupe or bananas) if the client is taking potassium-losing diuretics, such as loop and thiazide diuretics.

      □ Check weight daily at the same time and notify the provider for a weight gain of 2 lb in 24 hr or 5 lb in 1 week.

      □ Schedule regular follow-up visits with the provider.

      □ Get vaccinations (pneumococcal and yearly influenza vaccines).

- Client Outcomes

  o The client will have adequate gas exchange.

  o The client will have a decrease in anxiety.

  o The client will maintain fluid balance.

  o The client will improve tolerance to activity.

  o The client will have an increase in cardiac output.

PULMONARY EDEMA

Overview

- Cardiogenic factors are the most common cause of pulmonary edema. It is a complication of various heart and lung diseases and usually occurs from increased pulmonary vascular pressure secondary to severe cardiac dysfunction.

- Noncardiac pulmonary edema can occur due to barbiturate or opiate overdose, inhalation of irritating gases, rapid administration of IV fluids, and after a pneumonectomy evacuation of pleural effusion.

- Neurogenic pulmonary edema develops following a head injury.

- For older adults, increased risk for pulmonary edema occurs related to decreased cardiac output and congestive heart failure (CHF).

- Increased risk for fluid and electrolyte imbalances occurs when the older adult client receives treatment with diuretics.

- For older adults, IV infusions must be administered at a slower rate to prevent circulatory overload.

Health Promotion and Disease Prevention

- Maintain an exercise routine to remain physically active and consult with the provider before starting any exercise regimen.

- Consume a diet low in sodium along with fluid restrictions and consult with the provider regarding diet specifications.

- Refrain from smoking.

- Follow medication regimen and follow up with the provider as needed.

Assessment

- Risk Factors

  o Acute MI

  o Fluid volume overload

- o Hypertension
- o Valvular heart disease
- o Postpneumonectomy
- o Postevacuation of pleural effusion
- o Acute respiratory failure
- o Left-sided heart failure
- o High altitude exposure or deep sea diving
- o Trauma
- o Sepsis
- o Drug overdose
- Subjective Data
  - o Anxiety
  - o Inability to sleep
- Objective Data
  - o Persistent cough with pink, frothy sputum (cardinal sign)
  - o Tachypnea, dyspnea, and orthopnea
  - o Hypoxemia (expected reference range > 95%)
  - o Cyanosis (later stage)
  - o Crackles
  - o Tachycardia
  - o Reduced urine output
  - o Confusion, stupor
  - o S_3 heart sound (gallop)
  - o Increased pulmonary artery occlusion pressure

Collaborative Care

- Nursing Care
  - o Monitor vital signs every 15 min until stable.
  - o Monitor intake and output.
  - o Monitor hemodynamic status (pulmonary wedge pressures, cardiac output).
  - o Check ABGs, electrolytes (especially potassium if on diuretics), SaO_2, and chest x-ray results.

○ Maintain a patent airway. Suction as needed.

○ Position the client in high-Fowler's position with feet and legs dependent or sitting on the side of the bed to decrease preload.

○ Administer oxygen using a high-flow rebreather mask. BiPAP or intubation/ventilation can become necessary. Be prepared to intervene quickly.

○ Restrict fluid intake (slow or discontinue infusing IV fluids).

○ Monitor hourly urine output. Watch for intake greater than output or hourly urine less than 30 mL/hr.

- Medications

  ○ Rapid-acting diuretics, such as furosemide (Lasix) and bumetanide (Bumex), promote fluid excretion.

  ○ Morphine decreases sympathetic nervous system response and anxiety and promotes mild vasodilation.

  ○ Vasodilators (nitroglycerin, sodium nitroprusside) decrease preload and afterload.

  ○ Inotropic agents, such as digoxin (Lanoxin) and dobutamine (Dobutrex), improve cardiac output.

  ○ Antihypertensives, such as ACE inhibitors and beta-blockers

- Care after Discharge

  ○ Client Education

    ▪ Provide emotional support for the client and family.

    ▪ Instruct the client on effective breathing techniques.

    ▪ Instruct the client on medications.

    ▪ Stress the importance of continuing to take medications even if the client is feeling better.

    ▪ Teach common side effects and reasons to contact the provider.

    ▪ Instruct the client on a low-sodium diet and fluid restriction.

    ▪ The client should measure weight daily at the same time. Notify the provider of a gain of more than 2 lb in 1 day or 5 lb in 1 week.

    ▪ Instruct the client to report swelling of feet or ankles or any shortness of breath or angina.

- Client Outcomes

  ○ The client will have adequate gas exchange.

  ○ The client will have a decrease in anxiety.

  ○ The client will maintain fluid balance.

  ○ The client will improve tolerance to activity.

  ○ The client will have an increase in cardiac output.

Complications

- Cardiomyopathy

  o Cardiomyopathy is an impaired cardiac function leading to heart failure. Blood circulation is impaired to the lungs or body when the cardiac pump is compromised. Of the three types (dilated cardiomyopathy, hypertrophic cardiomyopathy, and restrictive cardiomyopathy), dilated cardiomyopathy is the most common.

    ▪ Dilated – decreased contractility and increased ventricular filling pressures

    ▪ This can be a result of:

      □ Coronary artery disease

      □ Infection or inflammation of the heart muscle

      □ Various cancer treatments

      □ Prolonged alcohol abuse

- Acute pulmonary edema

  o Acute pulmonary edema is a life-threatening medical emergency.

  o Nursing Actions

    ▪ Administer prescribed medications to improve cardiac output.

    ▪ Teach the client about measures to improve tolerance to activity, such as alternating periods of activity with periods of rest.

    ▪ Symptoms include anxiety, tachycardia, acute respiratory distress, dyspnea at rest, change in level of consciousness, and an ascending fluid level within the lungs (crackles, cough productive of frothy, blood-tinged sputum).

    ▪ Prompt response to this emergency includes:

      □ Positioning the client in high-Fowler's position.

      □ Administration of oxygen, positive airway pressure, and/or intubation and mechanical ventilation.

      □ IV morphine (to decrease anxiety, respiratory distress, and decrease venous return).

      □ IV administration of rapid-acting loop diuretics, such as furosemide (Lasix).

      □ Effective intervention should result in diuresis (carefully monitor output), reduction in respiratory distress, improved lung sounds, and adequate oxygenation.

- Cardiogenic shock

  o This is a serious complication of pump failure that occurs commonly following an MI and injury to greater than 40% of the left ventricle.

  o Symptoms include tachycardia, hypotension, inadequate urinary output, altered level of consciousness, respiratory distress (crackles, tachypnea) cool, clammy skin, decreased peripheral pulses, and chest pain.

- o Nursing Actions

  - Monitor breath sounds. Assess for crackles or wheezing.

  - Monitor heart sounds.

  - Administration of oxygen; possible intubation and ventilation may be required.

  - IV administration of morphine, diuretics, and/or nitroglycerin to decrease preload; and IV administration of vasopressors and/or positive inotropes to increase cardiac output and to maintain organ perfusion.

  - Continuous hemodynamic monitoring.

- Pericardial tamponade

  - o Cardiac tamponade can result from fluid accumulation in the pericardial sac.

  - o Signs include hypotension, jugular venous distention, muffled heart sounds, and paradoxical pulse (variance of 10 mm Hg or more in systolic blood pressure between expiration and inspiration).

  - o Hemodynamic monitoring will reveal intracardiac and pulmonary artery pressures similar and elevated (plateau pressures).

  - o Nursing Actions

    - Notify the provider immediately.

    - Administer IV fluids to combat hypotension as prescribed.

    - Obtain a chest x-ray or echocardiogram to confirm diagnosis.

    - Prepare the client for pericardiocentesis (informed consent, gather materials, administer medications as appropriate).

    - Monitor hemodynamic pressures as they normalize.

    - Monitor heart rhythm; changes indicate improper positioning of the needle.

    - Monitor for reoccurrence of signs after the procedure.

CHAPTER 36: HEART FAILURE AND PULMONARY EDEMA

Ⓐ Application Exercises

1. Which of the following actions should a nurse include when planning discharge teaching for a client who has heart failure? (Select all that apply.)

_____ Conserve energy; the client should schedule rest periods between activities.

_____ Adhere to medication regimen.

_____ Weigh self weekly and notify the provider if there is a weight gain of 5 lb in 2 weeks.

_____ Get influenza vaccine yearly.

_____ If prescribed digoxin (Lanoxin), take pulse for 1 min, and notify the provider if the pulse is below the set limit.

_____ Take diuretics in the early morning and early afternoon (if prescribed twice daily) to allow for uninterrupted sleep.

_____ Notify the provider of increased dyspnea, orthopnea, and inability to wear rings or shoes.

2. A nurse is caring for a client who has heart failure and reports increased shortness of breath. The nurse increases the oxygen per protocol. Which of the following actions should the nurse take first?

A. Notify the primary care provider.

B. Assist the client into high-Fowler's position.

C. Auscultate the lungs, listening for increased crackles.

D. Check oxygen saturation with pulse oximeter.

3. A nurse is caring for a client who has a diagnosis of heart failure and asks how to limit fluid intake to 2,000 mL/day. Which of the following responses should the nurse give to the client?

A. "Pour the amount of fluid you drink into an empty 2 liter bottle to keep track of how much you drink."

B. "Each glass contains 8 ounces. There are 30 milliliters per ounce, so you can have a total of 8 glasses or cups of fluid each day."

C. "This is the same as 2 quarts, or about the same as two pots of coffee."

D. "Take sips of water or ice chips so you will not take in too much fluid."

4. Which of the following client findings suggests digitalis toxicity or a risk for developing digitalis toxicity? (Select all that apply.)

_____ Serum potassium level of 3.2 mEq/L

_____ Apical heart rate of 54/min

_____ Blurred vision

_____ Dysrhythmia

_____ Weight gain of 2 lb in 1 day

_____ Leg cramps

_____ Slurred speech

_____ Shortness of breath

_____ Anorexia

_____ Altered mental status

5. Identify which of the following food selections are high in sodium (mark with an S) and which are high in potassium (mark with a P).

_____ Cheese (cheddar and cottage cheese)

_____ Cantaloupe

_____ Milk

_____ Soy sauce

_____ Cured meats (pork)

_____ White potatoes

_____ Avocado

_____ Banana

_____ Raisins

_____ Meats (beef, pork, chicken, and veal)

_____ Codfish, salmon, and tuna

CHAPTER 36: HEART FAILURE AND PULMONARY EDEMA

 Application Exercises Answer Key

1. Which of the following actions should a nurse include when planning discharge teaching for a client who has heart failure? (Select all that apply.)

__X__	**Conserve energy; the client should schedule rest periods between activities.**
__X__	**Adhere to medication regimen.**
_____	Weigh self weekly and notify the provider if there is a weight gain of 5 lb in 2 weeks.
__X__	**Get influenza vaccine yearly.**
__X__	**If prescribed digoxin (Lanoxin), take pulse for 1 min, and notify the primary care provider if the pulse is below the set limit.**
__X__	**Take diuretics in the early morning and early afternoon (if prescribed twice daily) to allow for uninterrupted sleep.**
__X__	**Notify the primary care provider of increased dyspnea, orthopnea, and inability to wear rings or shoes.**

The client who has heart failure should take medications as prescribed. If prescribed digoxin, the client should take her pulse for 1 min, and notify the provider if her pulse rate is below the set limit. The client should take diuretics early in the morning and early in the afternoon to prevent interruptions in sleep. The client should also get vaccinations (pneumococcal and yearly influenza vaccines), maintain fluid and sodium restrictions (a dietary consult can be useful), weigh herself at the same time daily, and notify the provider of a weight gain of 2 lb in 24 hr or 5 lb in 1 week.

NCLEX® Connection: Physiological Adaptation, Illness Management

2. A nurse is caring for a client who has heart failure and reports increased shortness of breath. The nurse increases the oxygen per protocol. Which of the following actions should the nurse take first?

A. Notify the primary care provider.

B. Assist the client into high-Fowler's position.

C. Auscultate the lungs, listening for increased crackles.

D. Check oxygen saturation with pulse oximeter.

Using the airway, breathing, and circulation (ABC) priority setting framework, the first action is to assist the client into high-Fowler's position. Assisting the client into a high-Fowler's position will decrease venous return to the heart (preload) and will help relieve lung congestion. The other actions are appropriate but are not the priority, nor will they directly improve the client's oxygenation or relieve symptoms.

NCLEX® Connection: Physiological Adaptation, Illness Management

3. A nurse is caring for a client who has a diagnosis of heart failure and asks how to limit fluid intake to 2,000 mL/day. Which of the following responses should the nurse give to the client?

> **A. "Pour the amount of fluid you drink into an empty 2 liter bottle to keep track of how much you drink."**
>
> B. "Each glass contains 8 ounces. There are 30 milliliters per ounce, so you can have a total of 8 glasses or cups of fluid each day."
>
> C. "This is the same as 2 quarts, or about the same as two pots of coffee."
>
> D. "Take sips of water or ice chips so you will not take in too much fluid."

Pouring the amount of fluid consumed into an empty 2 L bottle will give the client a visual guide to how much fluid is consumed and how much is left. Glasses and cups vary in size. Providing frames of reference for the amount of fluid in 2 L or suggesting that the client take sips of water or ice chips are not concrete methods to determine intake.

 NCLEX® Connection: Physiological Adaptation, Fluid and Electrolyte Imbalances

4. Which of the following client findings suggests digitalis toxicity or a risk for developing digitalis toxicity? (Select all that apply.)

X	**Serum potassium level of 3.2 mEq/L**
X	**Apical heart rate of 54/min**
X	**Blurred vision**
X	**Dysrhythmia**
_____	Weight gain of 2 lb in 1 day
X	**Leg cramps**
_____	Slurred speech
_____	Shortness of breath
X	**Anorexia**
X	**Altered mental status**

Hypokalemia increases the risk of digitalis toxicity. Leg cramps are a possible sign of hypokalemia. Slowed pulse, blurred vision, dysrhythmias, anorexia, and altered mental status are signs of digitalis toxicity. Weight gain and shortness of breath are signs of heart failure. Slurred speech could be a sign of a cerebrovascular accident.

 NCLEX® Connection: Pharmacological and Parenteral Therapies, Adverse Effects/ Contraindications/Side Effects/Interactions

5. Identify which of the following food selections are high in sodium (mark with an S) and which are high in potassium (mark with a P).

S	Cheese (cheddar and cottage cheese)
P	Cantaloupe
S	Milk
S	Soy sauce
SP	Cured meats (pork)
P	White potatoes
P	Avocado
P	Banana
P	Raisins
P	Meats (beef, pork, chicken, and veal)
P	Codfish, salmon, and tuna

NCLEX® Connection: Basic Care and Comfort, Nutrition and Oral Hydration

UNIT 4	NURSING CARE OF CLIENTS WITH CARDIOVASCULAR DISORDERS
Section	Cardiac Disorders

Chapter 37   Valvular Heart Disease

 Overview

- Valvular heart disease describes an abnormality or dysfunction of any of the heart's four valves: the mitral and aortic valves (left side) and the tricuspid and pulmonic valves (right side).

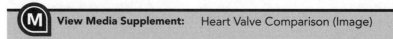
View Media Supplement: Heart Blood Flow (Image)

- Valvular heart disease is classified as:

  o   Stenosis – narrowed opening that impedes blood moving forward.

  o   Insufficiency – improper closure – some blood flows backward (regurgitation).

- Valvular heart disease can have congenital or acquired causes.

  o   Congenital valvular heart disease can affect all four valves and cause either stenosis or insufficiency.

  o   Acquired valvular heart disease is classified as one of three types:

  ▪   Degenerative disease – due to damage over time from mechanical stress. The most common cause is hypertension.

  ▪   Rheumatic disease – gradual fibrotic changes, calcification of valve cusps. The mitral valve is most commonly affected.

  ▪   Infective endocarditis – infectious organisms destroy the valve. Streptococcal infections are a common cause.

View Media Supplement: Heart Valve Comparison (Image)

- Valves on the left side are most commonly affected due to higher pressures.

- With age, fibrotic thickening occurs in the mitral and aortic valves. The aorta is stiffer in older adult clients, increasing systolic blood pressure and stress on the mitral valve.

Health Promotion and Disease Prevention

- Early detection and prevention of rheumatic fever helps prevent valvular disease.

- Encourage clients to consume a diet low in sodium and follow fluid restrictions prescribed by provider to prevent heart failure.

Assessment

- Risk Factors

    o Hypertension

    o Rheumatic fever (mitral stenosis and insufficiency)

    o Infective endocarditis

    o Congenital malformations

    o Marfan syndrome (connective tissue disorder that affects the heart and other areas of the body)

    o In older adult clients, the predominant causes of valvular heart disease are degenerative calcification, papillary muscle dysfunction, and infective endocarditis.

    o A murmur is heard with turbulent blood flow. The location of the murmur and timing (diastolic versus systolic) help determine the valve involved. Murmurs are graded on a scale of I (very faint) to VI (extremely loud).

- Subjective and Objective Data

LEFT-SIDED VALVE DAMAGE RESULTS IN DYSPNEA, FATIGUE, INCREASED PULMONARY ARTERY PRESSURE, AND DECREASED CARDIAC OUTPUT.			
MITRAL STENOSIS	MITRAL INSUFFICIENCY	AORTIC STENOSIS	AORTIC INSUFFICIENCY
<ul><li>Palpitations</li><li>Hemoptysis</li><li>Hoarseness</li><li>Dysphagia</li><li>Jugular vein distention</li><li>Orthopnea</li><li>Cough</li><li>Diastolic murmur</li><li>Atrial fibrillation</li></ul>	<ul><li>Proximal nocturnal</li><li>Dyspnea</li><li>Orthopnea</li><li>Palpitations</li><li>S_3 and/or S_4 sounds</li><li>Crackles in lungs</li><li>Possible diminished lung sounds</li><li>Systolic murmur</li><li>Atrial fibrillation</li></ul>	<ul><li>Angina</li><li>Syncope</li><li>Decreased SVR</li><li>S_3 and/or S_4 sounds</li><li>Systolic murmur</li><li>Narrowed pulse pressure</li></ul>	<ul><li>Angina</li><li>S_3 sounds</li><li>Diastolic murmur</li><li>Widened pulse pressure</li></ul>

RIGHT-SIDED VALVE DAMAGE RESULTS IN DYSPNEA, FATIGUE, INCREASED RIGHT ATRIAL PRESSURE, PERIPHERAL EDEMA, JUGULAR VEIN DISTENTION, AND HEPATOMEGALY.			
TRICUSPID STENOSIS	**TRICUSPID INSUFFICIENCY**	**PULMONIC STENOSIS**	**PULMONIC INSUFFICIENCY**
• Atrial dysrhythmias • Diastolic murmur • Decreased cardiac output	• Conduction delays • Supraventricular tachycardia • Systolic murmur	• Cyanosis • Systolic murmur	• Diastolic murmur

- o Diagnostic Procedures
    - ▪ Chest x-ray
        - □ A chest x-ray shows chamber enlargement, pulmonary congestion, and valve calcification.
    - ▪ 12-lead electrocardiogram (ECG)
        - □ An ECG shows chamber hypertrophy.
    - ▪ Echocardiogram
        - □ An echocardiogram shows chamber size, hypertrophy, specific valve dysfunction, ejection function, and amount of regurgitant flow.
    - ▪ Exercise tolerance testing/stress echocardiography
        - □ A stress echocardiography is used to assess the impact of the valve problem on cardiac functioning during stress.
    - ▪ Radionuclide studies
        - □ Radionuclide studies determine ejection fraction during activity and rest.
    - ▪ Angiography
        - □ Angiography reveals chamber pressures, ejection fraction, regurgitation, and pressure gradients.

Collaborative Care

- • Nursing Care
    - o Monitor current weight and note any recent changes.
    - o Assess heart rhythm (can be irregular or bradycardic, assess for murmur).
    - o Administer oxygen and medications as prescribed.
    - o Assess hemodynamic monitoring.
    - o Maintain fluid and sodium restriction.
    - o Assist the client to conserve energy.

- Medications
  - Diuretics
    - Diuretics are used to decrease preload.
      - Loop diuretics, such as furosemide (Lasix), bumetanide (Bumex)
      - Thiazide diuretics, such as hydrochlorothiazide (Hydrodiuril)
      - Potassium-sparing diuretics, such as spironolactone (Aldactone)
    - Nursing Considerations
      - Administer furosemide (Lasix) IV no faster than 20 mg/min.
      - Loop and thiazide diuretics can cause hypokalemia and a potassium supplement may be required.
    - Client Education
      - Teach clients who are taking loop or thiazide diuretics to ingest foods and drinks that are high in potassium to counter hypokalemia effect.
  - Afterload-reducing agents
    - Afterload-reducing agents help the heart pump more easily by altering the resistance to contraction.
      - Angiotensin-converting enzyme (ACE) inhibitors, such as enalapril (Vasotec), captopril (Capoten)
      - Beta-blockers
      - Calcium-channel blockers
    - Nursing Considerations
      - Monitor clients taking ACE inhibitors for initial dose hypotension.
  - Inotropic agents
    - Inotropic agents, such as digoxin (Lanoxin), dopamine, dobutamine (Dobutrex), and milrinone (Primacor), are used to increase contractility and thereby improve cardiac output.
    - Client Education
      - Teach clients who are self-administering digoxin to:
        - Count pulse for 1 min before taking the medication. If the pulse rate is irregular or the pulse rate is outside of the limitations set by the provider (usually less than 60/min or greater than 100/min), the client should hold the dose and contact the provider.
        - Take the dose of digoxin at the same time every day.
        - Do not take digoxin at the same time as antacids. Separate the two medications by at least 2 hr.
        - Report signs of toxicity, including fatigue, muscle weakness, confusion, visual changes, and loss of appetite.

- o Anticoagulants

  - Anticoagulation therapy is used for clients who have a mechanical valve replacement, atrial fibrillation, or severe left ventricle dysfunction.

- Interdisciplinary Care

  - o Respiratory services should be consulted for inhalers, breathing treatments, and suctioning for airway management.

  - o Cardiology can be consulted for cardiac management.

  - o Nutritional services can be contacted for weight loss or gain of this client related to medications or diagnosis.

  - o Rehabilitative care may need to be consulted if the client has prolonged weakness and needs assistance with increasing level of activity.

- Surgical Interventions

  - o Percutaneous balloon valvuloplasty

    - This procedure can open aortic or mitral valves affected by stenosis. A catheter is inserted through the femoral artery and advanced to the heart. A balloon is inflated at the stenotic lesion to open the fused commissures and improve leaflet mobility.

  - o Miscellaneous surgical management

    - Surgeries used in the treatment of valvular disorders include valve repair, chordae tendineae reconstruction, commissurotomy (relieve stenosis on leaflets), annuloplasty ring insertion (correct dilatation of valve annulus), and prosthetic valve replacement.

      - □ Prosthetic valves can be mechanical or tissue. Mechanical valves last longer but require anticoagulation. Tissue valves last 10 to 15 years.

    - Medical management is appropriate for many older adult clients; surgery is indicated when symptoms interfere with daily activities. The goal of surgery can be to improve the quality of life rather than to prolong life.

    - Nursing Actions

      - □ Postsurgery care is similar to coronary artery bypass surgery (care for sternal incision, activity limited for 6 weeks, report fever).

- Care after Discharge

  - o Nutritional services can be contacted for weight loss or weight gain related to medications or diagnosis.

  - o Rehabilitative care may need to be consulted if the client has prolonged weakness and needs assistance with increasing level of activity.

  - o Client Education

    - Prophylactic antibiotics are recommended prior to dental work, surgery, or other invasive procedures.

- Encourage the client to follow the prescribed exercise program.

- Encourage adherence to dietary restrictions; consider nutritional consultation.

- Teach the client energy conservation.

- Client Outcomes

  o The client will maintain the prescribed medication treatment regimen.

  o The client will maintain an unrestricted activity level without shortness of breath or chest pain.

  o The client will be free from anxiety.

  o The client will remain free from infection.

  o The client will be able to maintain within 10% of the ideal body weight.

Complications

- Heart Failure

  o Heart failure is the inability of the heart to maintain adequate circulation to meet tissue needs for oxygen and nutrients. Ineffective valves result in heart failure.

  o Nursing Actions

    - Monitoring a client's heart failure class (I to IV) is often the gauge for surgical intervention for valvular problems.

CHAPTER 37: VALVULAR HEART DISEASE

Ⓐ Application Exercises

1. Identify which specific valve problems can cause each of the following client findings.

CLIENT FINDING	ASSOCIATED VALVE PROBLEM
Atrial dysrhythmias (e.g., atrial fibrillation)	
Pulmonary edema	
Systolic murmurs	
Diastolic murmurs	
Angina	

2. Which of the following assessments are priorities for a client who is 2 hr postoperative following a mitral valve replacement? (Select all that apply.)

_____ Vital signs

_____ Cardiac rhythm

_____ Oxygen saturation

_____ Bowel sounds

_____ Heart and lung sounds

_____ Hemodynamics

3. Which of the following discharge teachings should a nurse provide to a client who had a mechanical valve replacement?

_____ Recommend that prophylactic antibiotics be taken before dental work, surgery, or other invasive procedures.

_____ Stress the importance of follow-up appointments.

_____ Inform the client of support groups in the area.

_____ Instruct the client to follow the prescribed medication regimen.

_____ Encourage the client to follow the prescribed exercise regimen.

_____ Encourage adherence to a diet high in sodium.

_____ Inform the client of findings that they should notify their provider of.

4. A nurse notes that a client has a history of mitral insufficiency. Which of the following is a sign of mitral valve insufficiency?

A. Ventricular arrhythmias

B. Petechiae

C. Crackles in lung bases

D. Splenomegaly

CHAPTER 37: VALVULAR HEART DISEASE

(A) Application Exercises Answer Key

1. Identify which specific valve problems can cause each of the following client findings.

CLIENT FINDING	ASSOCIATED VALVE PROBLEMS
Atrial dysrhythmias (e.g., atrial fibrillation)	Mitral stenosis, mitral insufficiency, tricuspid stenosis, or tricuspid insufficiency
Pulmonary edema	Mitral stenosis or mitral insufficiency
Systolic murmurs	Tricuspid insufficiency, pulmonic stenosis, mitral insufficiency, or aortic stenosis
Diastolic murmurs	Tricuspid stenosis, pulmonic insufficiency, mitral stenosis, or aortic insufficiency
Angina	Aortic stenosis or aortic insufficiency

(N) NCLEX® Connection: Reduction of Risk Potential, System Specific Assessment

2. Which of the following assessments are priorities for a client who is 2 hr postoperative following a mitral valve replacement? (Select all that apply.)

  X   **Vital signs**

  X   **Cardiac rhythm**

  X   **Oxygen saturation**

  _____ Bowel sounds

  X   **Heart and lung sounds**

  X   **Hemodynamics**

Auscultations for bowel sounds is not indicated at this time, since the client is postoperative and has been NPO. Vital signs, cardia rhythm, oxygen saturation, heart and lung sounds, and hemodynamics are all indicated for immediate assessment.

(N) NCLEX® Connection: Reduction of Risk Potential, Therapeutic Procedures

3. Which of the following discharge teachings should a nurse provide to a client who had a mechanical valve replacement?

   X   **Recommend prophylactic antibiotics be taken before dental work, surgery, or other invasive procedures.**

   X   **Stress the importance of follow-up appointments.**

   X   **Inform the client of support groups in the area.**

   X   **Instruct the client to follow the prescribed medication regimen.**

   X   **Encourage the client to follow the prescribed exercise regimen.**

          Encourage adherence to a diet high in sodium.

   X   **Inform the client of findings that they should notify the provider of.**

All the above findings are correct, except a diet high in sodium. A client who has a mechanical valve replacement should consume a diet low in sodium.

Ⓝ NCLEX® Connection: Reduction of Risk Potential, Therapeutic Procedures

4. A nurse notes that a client has a history of mitral insufficiency. Which of the following is a sign of mitral valve insufficiency?

A. Ventricular arrhythmias

B. Petechiae

C. Crackles in lung bases

D. Splenomegaly

Mitral insufficiency initially results in dyspnea, orthopnea, and pulmonary congestion. Angina, bilateral ankle edema, and jugular vein distention can occur with left ventricular failure due to progressive mitral insufficiency. Ventricular arrhythmias may be associated with tricuspid valve abnormalities. Petechiae can occur with endocarditis. Hepatomegaly, not splenomegaly, can occur with heart failure associated with mitral insufficiency.

Ⓝ NCLEX® Connection: Reduction of Risk Potential, System Specific Assessment

UNIT 4	NURSING CARE OF CLIENTS WITH CARDIOVASCULAR DISORDERS
Section	Cardiac Disorders
Chapter 38	**Inflammatory Disorders**

Overview

- Inflammation related to the heart is an extended inflammatory response that often leads to the destruction of healthy tissue. This primarily includes the layers of the heart.

- Inflammatory disorders related to the cardiovascular system that nurses should be familiar with include:

  o Pericarditis.

  o Myocarditis.

  o Rheumatic endocarditis.

  o Infective endocarditis.

Health Promotion and Disease Prevention

- Early treatment of streptococcal infections can prevent rheumatic fever.

- Prophylactic treatments (including antibiotics for clients who have cardiac defects) can prevent infective endocarditis.

- Influenza and pneumonia vaccinations are important for all clients in order to decrease the incidence of myocarditis, especially in older adults.

Assessment

- Risk Factors

  o Congenital heart defect/cardiac anomalies

  o Immunosuppression

  o Rheumatic endocarditis

  o School-age children who have long duration of streptococcus infection

  o Malnutrition

  o Overcrowding

  o Lower socioeconomic status

● Subjective and Objective Data

INFLAMMATORY DISORDER	DESCRIPTION OF DISEASE PROCESS	RELEVANT INFORMATION
Pericarditis	This is an inflammation of the pericardium.	<ul><li>This commonly follows a respiratory infection.</li><li>Pericarditis can be due to a myocardial infarction.</li><li>Findings include chest pressure/pain, friction rub auscultated in the lungs, shortness of breath, and pain relieved when sitting and leaning forward.</li></ul>
Myocarditis	This is an inflammation of the myocardium.	<ul><li>This can be due to a viral or fungal infection.</li><li>Myocarditis can be due to a systemic disease (Crohn's disease).</li><li>Findings include tachycardia, murmur, friction rub auscultated in the lungs, cardiomegaly, and dysrhythmias.</li></ul>
Rheumatic endocarditis	This is an infection of the endocardium due to streptococcal bacteria.	<ul><li>This is followed by an upper respiratory infection.</li><li>Rheumatic endocarditis produces lesions in the heart.</li><li>This occurs with half of the clients who have rheumatic fever.</li><li>Findings include fever, chest pain, joint pain, tachycardia, shortness of breath, rash on trunk and extremities, friction rub, murmur, and muscle spasms.</li></ul>
Infective endocarditis	This is also known as bacterial endocarditis, and is an infection of the endocardium due to streptococcal or staphylococcal bacteria.	<ul><li>This is most common in IV drug users or clients who have cardiac malformations.</li><li>Findings include fever, flu-like symptoms, murmur, petechiae (on the trunk and mucous membranes), positive blood cultures, and splinter hemorrhages (red streaks under the nail beds).</li></ul>

- o Laboratory Tests
  - Blood cultures can be drawn to detect a bacterial infection.
  - An elevated WBC count can be indicative of a bacterial infection.
  - Cardiac enzymes can be elevated with pericarditis.
  - Throat cultures can be taken to detect a streptococcal infection, which can lead to rheumatic fever.
- o Diagnostic Procedures
  - ECG can detect a murmur or heart block, which is indicative of rheumatic fever.

Collaborative Care

- Nursing Care
  - o Auscultate heart sounds (listen for murmur).
  - o Assess breath sounds in all lung fields (listen for friction rub).
  - o Check ABGs, SaO_2, and chest x-ray results.
  - o Administer oxygen as prescribed.
  - o Monitor vital signs (watch for fever).
  - o Monitor ECG and notify the provider of changes.
  - o Obtain throat cultures to identify bacteria to treat with antibiotics.
  - o Administer antibiotics as prescribed.
  - o Administer antipyretics as prescribed.
  - o Assess onset, quality, duration, and severity of the pain.
  - o Administer pain medication as prescribed.
  - o Encourage bed rest.
  - o Provide emotional support to the client and family, and encourage the verbalization of feelings regarding the illness.

- Medications

TYPE	PURPOSE	NURSING CONSIDERATIONS	CLIENT EDUCATION
Medication: Penicillin			
Antibiotic	This is given to treat an infection.	• Monitor for skin rash and hives. • Monitor electrolyte and kidney levels.	• Instruct the client to report signs of skin rash or hives. • Inform the client that the medication may cause GI distress.
Medication: Ibuprofen (Advil)			
NSAID (non-steroidal anti-inflammatory drug)	This is given to treat fever and inflammation.	• Do not use in clients with peptic ulcer disease. • Watch for signs of GI distress. • Monitor platelets, and liver and kidney levels.	• Instruct the client to take the medication with food. • Inform the client that the medication may cause GI distress. • Instruct the client to avoid alcohol consumption while taking the medication.
Medication: Prednisone (Deltasone)			
Glucocorticosteroid	This is given to treat inflammation.	• Use in low doses. • Monitor blood pressure. • Monitor electrolytes and blood sugar levels. • The client may heal slowly on this medication.	• Instruct the client to take the medication with food. • Instruct the client to avoid stopping the medication abruptly. • Instruct the client to report signs of an unexpected weight gain.
Medication: Amphotericin B (Amphocin)			
Antifungal	This is given to treat fungus.	• Monitor liver and kidney levels.	• Inform the client that the medication may cause GI distress.

TYPE	PURPOSE	NURSING CONSIDERATIONS	CLIENT EDUCATION
Medication: Diazepam (Valium)			
Benzodiazepine	This is given to treat anxiety.	• Start in low doses, and monitor for sleepiness and lightheadedness. • Monitor the client's liver function.	• Instruct the client to take the medication as prescribed. • Instruct the client to avoid alcohol consumption while taking the medication. • Instruct the client to avoid stopping the medication abruptly.

- Interdisciplinary Care

    o Cardiology services may be consulted to manage cardiac dysfunction.

    o Infectious disease services may be consulted to manage infection.

    o Physical therapy may be consulted to increase the client's level of activity once prescribed.

- Surgical Interventions

    o Pericarditis

        □ Pericardiocentesis

            ▸ A needle is inserted into the pericardium to aspirate pericardial fluid. This can be done in the emergency department or a procedure room.

        ■ Nursing Actions

            □ Pericardial fluid can be sent to the laboratory for culture and sensitivity.

            □ Monitor for reoccurrence of cardiac tamponade.

    o Infective endocarditis

        □ Valve debridement, draining of abscess, and repairing congenital shunts are procedures involved with infective endocarditis.

        ■ Nursing Actions

            □ Monitor for signs of bleeding, infection, and cardiac output.

- Care after Discharge

    ■ Home health services may be indicated if the client had surgery.

    ■ Intravenous antibiotics may be given by the home health service.

    ■ Pharmaceutical services may be indicated for IV supplies and medications.

    ■ Rehabilitation services may be indicated to help the client increase the level of activity.

- ○ Client Education
  - ■ Encourage the client to take rest periods as needed.
  - ■ Encourage the client to wash hands to prevent infection.
  - ■ Encourage the client to avoid crowded areas to reduce the risk of infection.
  - ■ Educate the client about the importance of good oral hygiene and the prevention of infection.
  - ■ Educate the client about the importance of taking medications as prescribed.
  - ■ Ask the client to demonstrate the administration of intravenous antibiotics and management before discharge.
  - ■ Encourage the client to quit smoking (if the client is a smoker).
  - ■ Educate the client and family about the illness and encourage expressing their feelings.
- • Client Outcomes
  - ○ The client will be free from infection.
  - ○ The client will be free from pain.
  - ○ The client will take medications as prescribed.

Complications

- • Cardiac tamponade
  - ○ Pericardial tamponade
    - ■ Cardiac tamponade can result from fluid accumulation in the pericardial sac.
      - □ Signs include hypotension, muffled heart sounds, jugular venous distention, and paradoxical pulse (variance of 10 mm Hg or more in systolic blood pressure between expiration and inspiration).
      - □ Hemodynamic monitoring will reveal intracardiac and pulmonary artery pressures similar and elevated (plateau pressures).
    - ■ Nursing Actions
      - □ Notify the provider immediately.
      - □ Administer IV fluids to combat hypotension as ordered.
      - □ Obtain a chest x-ray or echocardiogram to confirm the diagnosis.
    - ■ Prepare the client for pericardiocentesis (informed consent, gather materials, administer medications as appropriate).
      - □ Monitor hemodynamic pressures as they normalize.
      - □ Monitor heart rhythm as changes indicate improper positioning of the needle.
      - □ Monitor for reoccurrence of signs after the procedure.

CHAPTER 38: INFLAMMATORY DISORDERS

 Application Exercises

1. A nurse is caring for a client with pericarditis. Which of the following findings should the nurse anticipate?

    A. Petechiae

    B. Murmur

    C. Abdominal pain

    D. Friction rub

2. Which of the following clients has the greatest risk of acquiring rheumatic endocarditis?

    A. An older adult with chronic obstructive pulmonary disease

    B. A child with an upper respiratory streptococcus infection

    C. A middle age adult with Lupus

    D. A young adult who is 6 months pregnant

3. A nurse is assessing a client who has splinter hemorrhages in her nail beds and reports a fever. The client states that she recently had valve replacement surgery. Which of the following inflammatory disorders do the findings indicate?

    A. Infective endocarditis

    B. Pericarditis

    C. Myocarditis

    D. Rheumatic endocarditis

CHAPTER 38: INFLAMMATORY DISORDERS

 Application Exercises Answer Key

1. A nurse is caring for a client with pericarditis. Which of the following findings should the nurse anticipate?

    A. Petechiae

    B. Murmur

    C. Abdominal pain

    D. Friction rub

    A friction rub can be heard when listening to the lungs. Petechiae and a murmur are indicated for endocarditis. Abdominal pain is indicated for clients with endocarditis who are experiencing complications.

    NCLEX® Connection: Reduction of Risk Potential, System Specific Assessment

2. Which of the following clients has the greatest risk of acquiring rheumatic endocarditis?

    A. An older adult with chronic obstructive pulmonary disease

    B. A child with an upper respiratory streptococcus infection

    C. A middle age adult with Lupus

    D. A young adult who is 6 months pregnant

    A child with an upper respiratory streptococcus infection is at the greatest risk for acquiring rheumatic endocarditis. Rheumatic endocarditis develops due to an upper respiratory infection most commonly caused by the bacteria streptococcus. An older adult with chronic obstructive pulmonary disease, a middle age adult with Lupus, and a young adult who is 6 months pregnant are all at risk, but not the highest.

    NCLEX® Connection: Physiological Adaptation, Infectious Disease

3. A nurse is assessing a client who has splinter hemorrhages in her nail beds and reports a fever. The client states that she recently had valve replacement surgery. Which of the following inflammatory disorders do the findings indicate?

    A. Infective endocarditis

    B. Pericarditis

    C. Myocarditis

    D. Rheumatic endocarditis

    Splinter hemorrhages in nail beds and reports of fever are consistent with infective endocarditis. These findings do not indicate pericarditis, myocarditis, or rheumatic endocarditis.

    NCLEX® Connection: Reduction of Risk Potential, System Specific Assessment

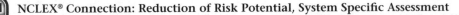

UNIT 4	NURSING CARE OF CLIENTS WITH CARDIOVASCULAR DISORDERS
Section	Vascular Disorders
Chapter 39	Peripheral Vascular Diseases

Overview

- Peripheral vascular diseases include peripheral arterial disease (PAD) and peripheral venous disorders, both of which interfere with normal blood flow.

- PAD affects the arteries (the blood vessels that carry blood away from the heart), and peripheral venous disease affects the veins (the blood vessels that carry blood toward the heart).

PERIPHERAL ARTERIAL DISEASE (PAD)

Overview

- PAD results from atherosclerosis that usually occurs in the arteries of the lower extremities and is characterized by inadequate flow of blood.

- Atherosclerosis is caused by a gradual thickening of the intima and media of the arteries, ultimately resulting in the progressive narrowing of the vessel lumen. Plaques may form on the walls of the arteries making them rough and fragile.

- Progressive stiffening of the arteries and narrowing of the lumen decreases the blood supply to affected tissues and increases resistance to blood flow.

- Atherosclerosis is actually a type of arteriosclerosis, which means "hardening of the arteries," and alludes to the loss of elasticity of arteries over time due to thickening of their walls.

- PAD is classified as inflow (distal aorta and iliac arteries) or outflow (femoral, popliteal, and tibial artery) and may range from mild to severe. Tissue damage occurs below the arterial obstruction.

- Buerger's disease, subclavian steal syndrome, thoracic outlet syndrome, Raynaud's disease and Raynaud's phenomenon, and popliteal entrapment are examples of PADs.

Assessment

- Risk Factors

  - Hypertension

  - Hyperlipidemia

- o Diabetes mellitus
- o Cigarette smoking
- o Obesity
- o Sedentary lifestyle
- o Familial predisposition
- o Age
  - Older adult clients have a higher incidence of PAD (rate of occurrence is increased in men over 45 and in women who are postmenopausal) and have a higher mortality rate from complications than younger individuals.
- Subjective Data
  - o Burning, cramping, and pain in the legs during exercise (intermittent claudication)
  - o Numbness or burning pain primarily in the feet when in bed
  - o Pain is relieved by placing legs at rest in a dependent position
- Objective Data
  - o Physical Assessment Findings
    - Bruit over femoral and aortic arteries

      View Media Supplement: Bruit (Audio)

    - Decreased capillary refill of toes (greater than 3 seconds)
    - Decreased or nonpalpable pulses
    - Loss of hair on lower calf, ankle, and foot
    - Dry, scaly, mottled skin
    - Thick toenails
    - Cold and cyanotic extremity
    - Pallor of extremity with elevation
    - Dependent rubor

      View Media Supplement: Rubor (Image)

    - Muscle atrophy
    - Ulcers and possible gangrene of toes

- o Diagnostic Procedures
  - Arteriography
    - ▸ Arteriography of the lower extremities involves arterial injection of contrast medium to visualize areas of decreased arterial flow on an x-ray.
    - ▸ It is usually done only to determine isolated areas of occlusion that can be treated during the procedure with percutaneous transluminal angioplasty and possible stent placement.
    - □ Nursing Actions
      - ▸ The nurse should observe for bleeding and hemorrhage.
      - ▸ Palpation of pedal pulses should also be done to assess for postprocedure occlusions.
  - Exercise tolerance testing
    - □ A stress test is done with or without the use of a treadmill (medications such as dipyridamole (Persantine) and adenosine (Adenocard) may be given to mimic the effects of exercise in clients who cannot tolerate a treadmill) with measurement of pulse volumes and blood pressures prior to and following the onset of symptoms or 5 min of exercise. Delays in return to normal pressures and pulse waveforms indicate arterial disease. It is used to evaluate claudication during exercise.
  - Plethysmography
    - □ Plethysmography is used to determine the variations of blood passing through an artery, thus identifying abnormal arterial flow in the affected limb.
    - □ Blood pressure cuffs are attached to the client's upper extremities and a lower extremity and attached to the plethysmograph machine. Variations in peripheral pulses between the upper and lower extremity are recorded.
    - □ A decrease in pulse pressure of the lower extremity indicates a possible blockage in the leg.
  - Segmental systolic blood pressure measurements
    - □ A Doppler probe is used to take various blood pressure measurements (thigh, calf, ankle, brachial) for comparison. In the absence of peripheral arterial disease, pressures in the lower extremities are higher than those of the upper extremities.
    - □ With arterial disease, the pressures in the thigh, calf, and ankle are lower.

Collaborative Care

- Nursing Care
  - o Encourage the client to exercise to build up collateral circulation – Initiate exercise gradually and increase slowly. Instruct the client to walk until the point of pain, stop and rest, and then walk a little farther.

- o Positioning
  - Instruct the client to avoid crossing her legs.
  - Tell the client to refrain from wearing restrictive garments.
  - Tell the client to elevate her legs to reduce swelling, but not to elevate them above the level of her heart because extreme elevation slows arterial blood flow to the feet.
- o Promote vasodilation and avoid vasoconstriction.
  - Provide a warm environment for the client.
  - Have the client wear insulated socks.
  - Tell the client to never apply direct heat to the affected extremity, as sensitivity is decreased and she may inadvertently burn herself.
  - Instruct the client to avoid exposure to cold (causes vasoconstriction and decreased arterial flow).
  - Instruct the client to avoid stress, caffeine, and nicotine, which also cause vasoconstriction. Complete abstinence from smoking or chewing tobacco is the most effective method of preventing vasoconstriction (vasoconstrictive effects last up to 1 hr after each cigarette smoked).
- Medications
  - o Antiplatelet medications – aspirin (acetylsalicylic acid), clopidogrel (Plavix), Pentoxifylline (Trental)
    - □ Antiplatelet medications reduce blood viscosity by decreasing blood fibrinogen levels, enhancing erythrocyte flexibility, and increasing blood flow in the extremities. Medications, such as aspirin (acetylsalicylic acid) and clopidogrel (Plavix), may be prescribed. Pentoxifylline (Trental), sometimes referred to as a hemorheologic medication, was one of the first to be used and is still used today, but less commonly than the other medications. It may be given to specifically treat intermittent claudication experienced by clients who have PAD.
    - Nursing Considerations
      - □ Give medication with meals.
    - Client Education
      - □ Inform the client that the medication's effects might not be apparent for several weeks.
      - □ Advise the client to monitor for signs of bleeding such as abdominal pain, coffee ground emesis, or black, tarry stools.

- Surgical Interventions

  o Surgical procedures for PAD

    - Percutaneous transluminal angioplasty

      □ Invasive intra-arterial procedure use a balloon and stent to open and help maintain the patency of the vessel.

      □ It is used for candidates who are not suitable for surgery or in cases where amputation is inevitable.

    - Laser-assisted angioplasty

      □ Laser-assisted angioplasty is an invasive procedure where a laser probe is advanced through a cannula to the site of stenosis.

      □ The laser is used to vaporize atherosclerotic plaque and open the artery.

    - Nursing Actions

      □ The priority for postoperative care is observing for bleeding at the puncture site.

      □ Closely monitor the client's vital signs, peripheral pulses, and capillary refill.

      □ If prescribed, keep the client on bed rest with his limb straight for 6 to 8 hr before ambulation.

      □ Anticoagulant therapy is used during the operative procedure, followed by antiplatelet therapy for 1 to 3 months.

    - Arterial revascularization surgery is used with clients who have severe claudication and/or limb pain at rest, or with clients who are at risk for losing a limb due to poor arterial circulation.

      □ Bypass grafts are used to reroute the circulation around the arterial occlusion.

      □ Grafts can be harvested from the client (autologous) or made from synthetic materials.

    - Nursing Actions

      □ The priority for postoperative care is to maintain adequate circulation in the repaired artery. The location of the pedal or dorsalis pulse should be marked and its pulsatile strength compared with the contralateral leg on a scheduled basis using a Doppler.

      □ Color, temperature, and capillary refill should also be compared with the contralateral extremity on a scheduled basis.

      □ Warmth, redness, and possibly edema of the affected limb should be present as a result of increased blood flow.

      □ Monitor the client for pain. Pain may be severe due to the reestablishment of blood flow to the extremity.

□ Monitor the client's blood pressure for hypotension or hypertension. Hypotension may result in an increased risk of clotting or graft collapse, while hypertension increases the risk for bleeding from sutures.

□ Instruct the client to limit bending of the hip and knee to decrease the risk of clot formation.

- Client Education

□ Instruct the client to avoid crossing his legs or raising his legs above the level of the heart.

□ Instruct the client to wear loose clothing.

□ Instruct the client on wound care if revascularization surgery was done.

□ Discourage smoking and cold temperatures with the client.

□ Instruct the client about foot care (keep feet clean and dry, wear good-fitting shoes, never go barefoot, cut toenails straight across or have the podiatrist cut nails).

- Client Outcomes

  ○ The client's extremity distal to the repaired occlusion will be warm, pink, and have a 2+ pulse.

  ○ The client will report being able to walk without pain in the affected leg.

Complications

- Graft Occlusion

  - Graft occlusion is a serious complication of arterial revascularization and often occurs within the first 24 hr following surgery.

  ○ Nursing Actions

    - Promptly notify the surgeon of signs and symptoms of occlusion, such as absent or reduced pedal pulses, increased pain, change in extremity color, or temperature.

    - Be prepared to assist with treatment, which may include an emergency thrombectomy (removal of a clot), local intraarterial thrombolytic therapy with an agent such as tissue plasminogen activator, infusion of a platelet inhibitor, or a combination of the above. With these treatments, closely assess the client for manifestations of bleeding.

- Compartment Syndrome

  - Compartment syndrome is considered a medical emergency. Tissue pressure within a confined body space can restrict blood flow and the resulting ischemia can lead to irreversible tissue damage.

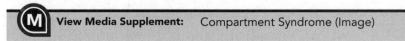

View Media Supplement: Compartment Syndrome (Image)

- ○ Nursing Actions

  - ■ Symptoms of compartment syndrome include tingling, numbness, worsening pain, edema, pain on passive movement, and unequal pulses. Immediately report symptoms to the provider.

  - ■ Loosen dressings.

  - ■ Prepare to assist with fasciotomy (surgical opening into the tissues), which may be necessary to prevent further injury and to save the limb.

PERIPHERAL VENOUS DISORDERS

Overview

- Peripheral venous disorders are problems with the veins that interfere with adequate return of blood flow from the extremities.

- There are superficial and deep veins in the lower extremities that have valves that prevent backflow of blood as it returns to the heart. The action of the skeletal muscles of the lower extremities during walking and other activities also promotes venous return.

- Three peripheral venous disorders that nurses should be familiar with are venous thromboembolism (VTE), venous insufficiency, and varicose veins.

  - ○ A VTE is a blood clot believed to form as a result of venous stasis, endothelial injury, or hypercoagulability Thrombus formation can lead to a pulmonary embolism, a life-threatening complication.

  - ○ Thrombophlebitis refers to a thrombus that is associated with inflammation.

  - ○ Venous insufficiency occurs secondary to incompetent valves in the deeper veins of the lower extremities, which allows pooling of blood and dilation of the veins. The veins' inability to carry fluid and wastes from the lower extremities precipitates the development of swelling, venous stasis ulcers, and in advanced cases, cellulitis.

  - ○ Varicose veins are enlarged, twisted and superficial veins that may occur in any part of the body; however, they are commonly observed in the lower extremities and in the esophagus.

Assessment

- Risk Factors

  - ○ Venous thromboembolism

    - ■ Hip surgery, total-knee replacement, open prostate surgery

    - ■ Heart failure

    - ■ Immobility

    - ■ Pregnancy

    - ■ Oral contraceptives

- Venous insufficiency
  - Sitting or standing in one position for a long period of time
  - Obesity
  - Pregnancy
  - Thrombophlebitis
- Varicose veins
  - Older than 30 years with an occupation requiring prolonged standing
  - Pregnancy
  - Obesity
  - Systemic diseases (heart disease)
  - Family history
- Subjective Data
  - Limb pain
    - Aching pain and feeling of fullness or heaviness in the legs after standing
- Objective Data
  - Physical Assessment Findings
    - Deep vein thrombosis (DVT) and thrombophlebitis
      - In DVT and thrombophlebitis, the client can become asymptomatic.
      - Classic signs of DVT and thrombophlebitis are calf or groin pain, or tenderness and a sudden onset of swelling of the legs.
      - Palpate the site for warmth, edema, and induration and hardness over the involved blood vessel.
      - Examine the area and compare it to the contralateral limb. Measure, record, and compare the right and left calf and thigh circumferences for changes over time; observe for localized edema.
      - Monitor the client for shortness of breath and chest pain, which can indicate that the embolus has moved to the lungs (pulmonary embolism).
    - Venous insufficiency
      - Stasis dermatitis is a brown discoloration along the ankles that extends up the calf relative to the level of insufficiency
      - Edema
      - Stasis ulcers (typically found around ankles)
    - Varicose veins
      - Distended, superficial veins that are visible just below the skin and are tortuous in nature

- ○ Laboratory Tests

  - ▪ A D-dimer test measures fibrin degradation products present in the blood produced from fibrinolysis. A positive D-dimer test indicates the presence of these products in a client's body, which indicates that thrombus formation has possibly occurred.

- ○ Diagnostic Procedures

  - ▪ DVT and thrombophlebitis

    - □ Venous duplex ultrasonography uses high-frequency sound waves to provide a real-time picture of the blood flow through a blood vessel.

    - □ Impedance plethysmography can be used to determine the variations of blood passing through a vein, thus identifying abnormal venous flow in the affected limb.

    - □ If the above tests are negative for a DVT, but one is still suspected, a venogram, which uses contrast material, may be needed for accurate diagnosis.

  - ▪ Varicose veins – the Trendelenburg test

    - ‣ The Trendelenburg test assists with a diagnosis of varicose veins.

    - □ Nursing Actions

      - ‣ Place the client in a supine position with legs elevated.

      - ‣ When the client sits up, the veins will fill from the proximal end if varicosities are present (veins normally fill from the distal end).

Collaborative Care

- • Nursing Care

  - ○ DVT and thrombophlebitis

    - ▪ Encourage the client to rest.

      - □ Facilitate bed rest in the client and elevation of the extremity above the level of the heart as prescribed (avoid using a knee gatch or pillow under knees).

      - □ Administer intermittent or continuous warm moist compresses to the client as prescribed.

      - □ To prevent thrombus from dislodging and becoming an embolus, do not massage the affected limb.

      - □ Provide thigh-high compression or antiembolism stockings as prescribed to reduce venous stasis and to assist in venous return of blood to the heart.

    - ▪ Prepare the client for an inferior vena cava interruption surgery (a filter traps emboli and prevents them from reaching the heart) as indicated.

- ○ Venous insufficiency

  - ▪ Ensure that the client elevates his legs several times a day for at least 15 to 30 min.

  - ▪ The client should elevate his feet approximately 6 inches at night.

  - ▪ The client should avoid crossing his legs and wearing constrictive clothing or stockings.

  - ▪ The client should wear elastic compression stockings and apply them after he has elevated his legs and when swelling is at a minimum.

- • Medications

  - ○ DVT and thrombophlebitis – anticoagulants

    - ▪ Unfractionated heparin is given IV to prevent formation of other clots and to prevent enlargement of the existing clot. It is has significant side effects and must be given in the facility. Prior to discharge, the client will be converted over to oral anticoagulation therapy with warfarin (Coumadin).

      - ☐ Nursing Actions

        - ▸ Monitor aPTT to allow for adjustments of heparin dosage.

        - ▸ Monitor platelet counts for heparin-induced thrombocytopenia.

        - ▸ Ensure that protamine sulfate, the antidote for heparin, is available if needed for excessive bleeding.

        - ▸ Monitor for hazards and side effects associated with anticoagulant therapy.

    - ▪ Low-molecular weight heparin is given subcutaneously and is based on a client's weight. Enoxaparin (Lovenox) is used for the prevention and treatment of DVT. It is usually given in the facility, but the twice daily injections can be given in the home setting if adequate medical support is available.

      - ☐ Nursing Actions

        - ▸ Ensure that protamine sulfate, the antidote for heparin, is available if needed for excessive bleeding.

        - ▸ Instruct the client to observe for signs of bleeding.

        - ▸ Instruct the client on bleeding precautions that should be taken (use electric instead of bladed razor and brush teeth with a soft toothbrush).

    - ▪ Warfarin inhibits synthesis of the four vitamin K-dependent clotting factors. The therapeutic effect takes 3 to 4 days to develop, so it is usually begun while the client is still on heparin.

      - ☐ Nursing Actions

        - ▸ Monitor the client for bleeding.

        - ▸ Monitor the client's PT and INR.

▸ Ensure that vitamin K (the antidote for warfarin) is available in case of excessive bleeding.

▸ Instruct the client about which signs of bleeding to look for.

▸ Instruct the client on bleeding precautions that should be taken (use electric instead of bladed razor and brush teeth with soft toothbrush).

○ DVT and thrombophlebitis – thrombolytic therapy

■ Thrombolytic therapy dissolves clots that have already developed. Therapy must be started within 5 days after the development of the clot for the therapy to be effective. Tissue plasminogen activator, a thrombolytic agent, and platelet inhibitors such as abciximab (ReoPro), and eptifibatide (Integrilin) can be effective in dissolving a clot or preventing new clots during the first 24 hr. Giving the medication in a manner that provides direct contact with the thrombus can be more effective and lessen the chance of bleeding.

□ Nursing Actions

▸ Monitor the client for bleeding (intracerebral bleeding).

▸ Instruct the client about bleeding precautions that should be taken (use electric instead of bladed razor and brush teeth with a soft toothbrush).

● Interdisciplinary Care

○ Venous insufficiency

■ Care of venous stasis ulcers requires long-term management.

■ Consultation with a dietitian and wound care specialist will facilitate the healing process.

● Therapeutic Procedures

○ Varicose veins – sclerotherapy

□ A sclerosing irritating chemical solution is injected into the varicose vein to produce localized inflammation, which will, over time, close the lumen of the vessel. For larger vessels, an incision and drainage of the trapped blood in a sclerosed vein may need to be performed 2 to 3 weeks after the injection. Pressure dressings are applied for approximately 1 week after each procedure to keep the vessel free of blood.

■ Client Education

□ Instruct the client to wear elastic stockings for prescribed time.

□ Mild analgesics such as Tylenol can be taken for discomfort.

● Surgical Interventions

○ Varicose veins – vein stripping

□ Vein stripping is the removal of large varicose veins that cannot be treated with less-invasive procedures.

- Nursing Actions
  - Preoperatively
    - Assist the provider with vein marking.
    - Evaluate the client's pulses as baseline for postoperative comparison.
  - Postoperatively
    - Maintain elastic bandages on the client's legs.
    - Monitor the client's groin and leg for bleeding through the elastic bandages.
    - Monitor the client's extremity for edema, warmth, color, and pulses.
    - Elevate the client's legs above the level of his heart.
    - Encourage the client to engage in range-of-motion exercises of the legs.
    - Instruct the client to elevate his legs when sitting, and avoid dangling them over the side of the bed.
- Client Education
  - Emphasize the importance of wearing elastic stockings after bandage removal.
  - Varicose veins – endovenous laser treatment
    - This type of treatment uses a laser fiber that is inserted into the vessel proximal to the area to be treated and then threaded to the involved area where heat from the laser is used to close the dilated vein.
  - Varicose veins – application of radiofrequency energy
    - This type of treatment uses a small catheter with a radiofrequency electrode, instead of a laser, that is inserted into the vessel proximal to the area to be treated that scars and closes a dilated vein.
- Client Outcomes
  - The client's lower extremities will be warm, pink, and free of pain.

Complications

- Ulcer Formation
  - Venous stasis ulcers often form over the medial malleolus. Venous ulcers are chronic, hard to heal, and often recur. They can lead to amputation and/or death.

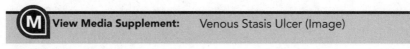
View Media Supplement: Venous Stasis Ulcer (Image)

  - Clients who also have neuropathy may not feel as much discomfort from the ulcer as its appearance may warrant.

- o Nursing Actions

  - Apply oxygen-permeable polyethylene films to superficial ulcers.

  - Apply occlusive, hydrocolloid dressings on deeper ulcers to promote granulation tissue and reepithelialization.

  - Leave a dressing on for 3 to 5 days.

  - If a wound needs chemical debridement, apply prescribed topical enzymatic agents to debride the ulcer, eliminate necrotic tissue, and promote healing.

  - Administer systemic antibiotics as prescribed.

- o Client Education

  - Recommend to the client a diet high in zinc, protein, and vitamins A and C.

- • Pulmonary Embolism

  - A pulmonary embolism occurs when a thrombus is dislodged, becomes an embolus, and lodges in a pulmonary vessel. This can lead to obstruction of pulmonary blood flow, decreased systemic oxygenation, pulmonary tissue hypoxia, and possible death.

- o Nursing Actions

  - Symptoms include sudden onset dyspnea, pleuritic chest pain, restlessness and apprehension, feelings of impending doom, cough and hemoptysis.

  - Signs include tachypnea, crackles, pleural friction rub, tachycardia, S_3 or S_4 heart sounds, diaphoresis, a low-grade fever, petechiae over chest and axillae, and decreased arterial oxygen saturation.

  - Notify the provider immediately, reassure the client, and assist him to a position of comfort with the head of the bed elevated.

  - Prepare for oxygen therapy and blood gas analysis while continuing to monitor and assess the client for other manifestations.

CHAPTER 39: PERIPHERAL VASCULAR DISEASES

 Application Exercises

1. A nurse is performing an assessment on a client who has chronic peripheral arterial disease (PAD). The nurse should expect to find

    A. edema around the client's ankles and feet.

    B. ulceration around the client's medial malleoli.

    C. scaling eczema of the client's lower legs with stasis dermatitis.

    D. pallor on elevation of the client's limbs and rubor when his limbs are dependent.

2. A nurse is caring for a client who has severe peripheral arterial disease (PAD). The nurse should expect that the client will sleep most comfortably in which of the following positions?

    A. With the affected limb hanging from the bed

    B. With the affected limb elevated on pillows

    C. With the head of the bed raised

    D. In a side-lying, recumbent position

3. A nurse is caring for a client who has chronic venous insufficiency. The provider prescribed thigh-high compression stockings. The nurse should instruct the client to

    A. massage both legs firmly with lotion prior to applying the stockings.

    B. apply the stockings in the morning upon awakening and before getting out of bed.

    C. roll the stockings down to the knees if they will not stay up on the thighs.

    D. remove the stocking while out of bed for 1 hr, four times a day to allow the legs to rest.

4. A nurse is caring for a client who has a deep vein thrombosis and has been taking unfractionated heparin (UFH) for 1 week. The client's condition is improving. Two days ago, the primary care provider also prescribed warfarin (Coumadin). The client questions the nurse about receiving both heparin and warfarin at the same time. Which of the following responses is appropriate for the nurse to give to the client?

    A. "Your provider must have forgotten that you were already taking heparin. I will remind her."

    B. "Your blood was so thick that two anticoagulants were needed."

    C. "Warfarin takes three to four days to achieve therapeutic anticoagulant effects. Heparin will be discontinued soon."

    D. "Only one of these medications is being given to treat your deep vein thrombosis."

CHAPTER 39: PERIPHERAL VASCULAR DISEASES

 Application Exercises Answer Key

1. A nurse performing an assessment with a client who has chronic peripheral arterial disease (PAD) should expect to find

   A. edema around the ankles and feet.

   B. ulceration around the medial malleoli.

   C. scaling eczema of the lower legs with stasis dermatitis.

   D. pallor on elevation of limbs and rubor when limbs are dependent.

   Findings depend on the severity of PAD. Observe the client for loss of hair on his lower calf, ankle, and foot; dry, if his skin is scaly, dusky, pale, or mottled; and whether his toenails are thickened. If the disease is severe, the client's extremity will be cold and gray-blue (cyanotic) or darkened. In chronic disease, pallor may occur when the client's extremity is elevated; dependent rubor may occur when the extremity is lowered. Muscle atrophy can accompany prolonged chronic arterial disease. Edema around the ankles and feet, ulceration around the medial malleoli, and scaling eczema of the lower legs with stasis dermatitis are seen with venous stasis.

 NCLEX® Connection: Reduction of Risk Potential, System-Specific Assessment

2. A nurse is caring for a client who has severe peripheral arterial disease (PAD). The nurse should expect that the client will sleep most comfortably in which of the following positions?

   A. With the affected limb hanging from the bed

   B. With the affected limb elevated on pillows

   C. With the head of the bed raised

   D. In a side-lying, recumbent position

   Clients who have severe PAD may find comfort with the affected limb in a dependent position. The other positions will not promote circulation in the lower extremities.

 NCLEX® Connection: Physiological Adaptation, Illness Management

3. A nurse is caring for a client who has chronic venous insufficiency. The provider prescribed thigh-high compression stockings. The nurse should instruct the client to

   A. massage both legs firmly with lotion prior to applying the stockings.

   B. apply the stockings in the morning upon awakening and before getting out of bed.

   C. roll the stockings down to the knees if they will not stay up on the thighs.

   D. remove the stocking while out of bed for 1 hr, four times a day to allow the legs to rest.

   Applying stockings in the morning upon awakening and before getting out of bed reduces venous stasis and assists in the venous return of blood to the heart. Legs are less edematous at this time. Massaging the affected area can dislodge a clot and cause embolism. Rolling stockings down can restrict circulation and cause edema. Stockings should be removed at night, before going to bed.

   Ⓝ NCLEX® Connection: Reduction of Risk Potential, Therapeutic Procedures

4. A nurse is caring for a client who has a deep vein thrombosis and has been taking unfractionated heparin for 1 week. The client's condition is improving. Two days ago, the primary care provider also prescribed warfarin (Coumadin). The client questions the nurse about receiving both heparin and warfarin at the same time. Which of the following responses is appropriate for the nurse to give to the client?

   A. "Your provider must have forgotten that you were already taking heparin. I will remind her."

   B. "Your blood was so thick that two anticoagulants were needed."

   C. "Warfarin takes three to four days to achieve therapeutic anticoagulant effects. Heparin will be discontinued soon."

   D. "Only one of these medications is being given to treat your deep vein thrombosis"

   Warfarin takes 3 to 4 days to achieve therapeutic anticoagulant effects because it depresses synthesis of clotting factors, but does not have any effect on clotting factors that are already present. Effects are delayed until the clotting factors that are present decay.

   Ⓝ NCLEX® Connection: Pharmacological and Parenteral Therapies, Expected Actions/ Outcomes

UNIT 4	NURSING CARE OF CLIENTS WITH CARDIOVASCULAR DISORDERS
Section	Vascular Disorders

Chapter 40	Hypertension

Ⓐ Overview

- Hypertension occurs when systolic blood pressure is at or above 140 mm Hg or diastolic blood pressure is at or above 90 mm Hg. Normal adult blood pressure is less than 120 mm Hg systolic and 80 mm Hg diastolic.

- Essential hypertension, also called primary hypertension, accounts for most cases of hypertension. There is no known cause. Secondary hypertension can be caused by certain disease states, such as renal disease, or as a side effect of some medications. Secondary hypertension can be treated by removing the cause (adrenal tumor, medication).

- Blood pressure is regulated by four bodily mechanisms.

  o Arterial baroreceptors

    ▪ Baroreceptors are located in the carotid sinus, aorta, and left ventricle.

    ▪ They control blood pressure by altering the heart rate and/or causing vasoconstriction or vasodilation.

  o Regulation of body-fluid volume

    ▪ Properly functioning kidneys either retain fluid when the client is hypotensive or excrete fluid when the client is hypertensive.

  o Renin-angiotensin system

    ▪ Angiotensin II vasoconstricts and controls aldosterone release, which causes the kidneys to reabsorb sodium and inhibit fluid loss.

  o Vascular autoregulation

    ▪ This maintains consistent levels of tissue perfusion.

- Clients who have a systolic blood pressure of 120 to 139 mm Hg or a diastolic blood pressure of 80 to 89 mm Hg are considered prehypertensive. Lifestyle changes are needed for these clients to help prevent cardiovascular disease.

- Prolonged, untreated, or poorly controlled hypertension can cause peripheral vascular disease, especially affecting the heart, brain, eyes, and kidneys. The risk of developing complications increases as blood pressure increases.

- Hypertrophy of the left ventricle can develop as the heart pumps against resistance caused by the hypertension.

Health Promotion and Disease Prevention

- The client should maintain a body mass index of less than 30.

- Clients who have diabetes mellitus should keep blood glucose within a recommended reference range.

- The client should limit caffeine and alcohol intake.

- The client should use stress-management techniques during times of stress.

- The client should stop smoking. Nicotine patches or engaging in a smoking cessation class may be indicated.

- The client should engage in exercise that provides aerobic benefits at least 3 times a week.

Assessment

- Risk Factors

  - Essential hypertension

    - Positive family history
    - Excessive sodium intake
    - Physical inactivity
    - Obesity
    - High alcohol consumption
    - African American
    - Smoking
    - Hyperlipidemia
    - Stress

  - Secondary hypertension

    - Renal disease
    - Cushing's disease (excessive glucocorticoid secretion)
    - Primary aldosteronism (causes hypertension and hypokalemia)
    - Pheochromocytoma (excessive catecholamine release)
    - Brain tumors, encephalitis
    - Medications such as estrogen, steroids, sympathomimetics

- Subjective Data

  - Clients who have hypertension can experience few or no symptoms. The nurse should monitor for:

    - Headaches, particularly in the morning.

- Dizziness.

- Fainting.

- Retinal changes, visual disturbances.

- Nocturia.

- Objective Data

  - Physical Assessment Findings

    - When a blood pressure reading is elevated, it should be taken in both arms and with the client sitting and standing.

    - There are several levels of hypertension, as defined by the Joint National Committee on Prevention, Detection, Evaluation, and Treatment of High Blood Pressure.

      - Prehypertension – systolic 120 to 139; diastolic 80 to 89

      - Stage I hypertension – systolic 140 to 159; diastolic 90 to 99

      - Stage II hypertension – systolic greater than or equal to 160; diastolic greater than or equal to 100

  - Laboratory Tests

    - No laboratory tests exist to diagnose hypertension; however, several laboratory tests can identify the causes of secondary hypertension and target organ damage.

      - BUN, creatinine – elevation indicative of renal disease

      - Elevated serum corticoids to detect Cushing's disease

      - Blood glucose and cholesterol studies can identify contributing factors related to blood vessel changes.

  - Diagnostic Procedures

    - An ECG is used to evaluate cardiac function.

      - Tall R-waves are often seen with left-ventricular hypertrophy.

    - A chest x-ray may show cardiomegaly.

Collaborative Care

- Nursing Care

  - Discuss factors with the client that increase the risk of hypertension and how they can be managed.

- Medications

  - Medications that are added to treat hypertension are not responsive to lifestyle changes alone. Diuretics are often used as the first-line medications. However, clients can require a combination of medications to control hypertension.

- Clients who are taking antihypertensives should be instructed to change positions slowly, be careful when getting out of bed, driving, and climbing stairs until the medication's effects are fully known.

○ Diuretics

□ Thiazide diuretics, such as hydrochlorothiazide (Hydrodiuril), inhibit water and sodium reabsorption, and increase potassium excretion.

□ Other diuretics may be used to treat hypertension not responsive to the thiazide diuretics.

▸ Loop diuretics, such as furosemide (Lasix), decrease sodium reabsorption and increase potassium excretion. Monitor the client closely for hypokalemia.

▸ Potassium-sparing diuretics, such as spironolactone (Aldactone), affect the distal tubule and prevent reabsorption of sodium in exchange for potassium. Monitor the client closely for hyperkalemia.

- Nursing Considerations

□ Monitor the client's potassium levels and watch for muscle weakness, irregular pulse, and dehydration. Thiazide and loop diuretics can cause hypokalemia, and potassium-sparing diuretics can cause hyperkalemia.

- Client Education

□ Encourage the client to keep all appointments with the provider to monitor efficacy of pharmacologic treatment and possible electrolyte imbalance (hyponatremia, hyperkalemia).

□ If the client is taking a potassium-depleting diuretic, encourage consumption of potassium-rich foods, such as bananas.

○ Calcium-channel blockers

□ Verapamil hydrochloride (Calan), amlodipine (Norvasc), and diltiazem (Cardizem) alter the movement of calcium ions through the cell membrane, causing vasodilation and lowering blood pressure.

- Nursing Considerations

□ Monitor the client's blood pressure and pulse, and change the client's position slowly. Hypotension is a common side effect.

□ Calcium-channel blockers should be used cautiously with clients who have heart failure.

- Client Education

□ Constipation can occur with verapamil hydrochloride, so encourage intake of foods that are high in fiber

□ Decreased or increased heart rate and atrioventricular (AV) block can occur, so teach the client how to take her pulse and call the provider if the pulse is irregular or lower than the established rate.

□ Instruct the client to avoid grapefruit juice, which potentiates the medication's effects, increases hypotensive effects, and increases the risk of medication toxicity.

○ Angiotensin-converting enzyme (ACE) inhibitors

▪ ACE inhibitors prevent the conversion of angiotensin I to angiotensin II, which prevents vasoconstriction.

▪ Nursing Considerations

□ Monitor the client's blood pressure and pulse. Hypotension is a common side effect.

□ Monitor the client for signs of heart failure, such as edema. This medication may cause heart and renal complications.

▪ Client Education

□ Teach the client to report a cough, which is a side effect of ACE inhibitors. The client should notify the provider of this side effect, as the medication can be discontinued due to its persistent nature and occasional relationship to angioedema (swelling of the tissues in the throat that can progress to a life-threatening obstruction).

□ Teach the client to reports signs of heart failure (edema).

○ Angiotensin-II receptor antagonists

□ Also called angiotensin-receptor blockers (ARBs), these medications, such as candesartan (Atacand), losartan (Cozaar), and telmisartan (Micardis), are a good option for clients taking ACE inhibitors who report cough and those who have hyperkalemia. Also, ARBs do not require a dosage adjustment for older adult clients.

▪ Nursing Considerations

□ Monitor the client for signs of angioedema or of heart failure. Angioedema is a serious, but uncommon adverse effect, and heart failure can result from taking this medication.

▪ Client Education

□ Teach the client to change positions slowly.

□ Teach the client to report signs of angioedema (swollen lips or face) or heart failure (edema).

○ Aldosterone-receptor antagonists

□ Aldosterone-receptor antagonists, such as eplerenone (Inspra), block aldosterone action. The blocking effect of eplerenone on aldosterone receptors promotes the retention of potassium and excretion of sodium and water.

- Nursing Considerations
  - Monitor the client's renal function, triglycerides, sodium, and potassium levels. The risk of adverse effects increases with deteriorating renal function. Hypertriglyceridemia, hyponatremia, and hyperkalemia can occur as the dose increases.
    - Monitor the client's potassium levels every 2 weeks for the first few months and every 2 months thereafter. Do not give the client potassium supplements or potassium-sparing diuretics.
- Client Education
  - Teach the client about potential medication and herbal interactions. Grapefruit juice and St. John's wort can increase adverse effects.
  - Instruct the client not to take salt substitutes with potassium or other foods that are rich in potassium.

○ Beta blockers
  - Beta blockers, such as metoprolol (Lopressor) and atenolol (Tenormin), are indicated for clients who have unstable angina or MI. They decrease cardiac output and block the release of renin, subsequently decreasing vasoconstriction of the peripheral vasculature.
- Nursing Considerations
  - Monitor the client's blood pressure and pulse.
  - These medications can mask hypoglycemia in clients who have diabetes mellitus.
- Client Education
  - Teach the client that these medications may cause fatigue, weakness, depression, and sexual dysfunction.
  - Advise the client not to suddenly stop taking the medication without consulting with the provider. Stopping suddenly can cause rebound hypertension.
  - Teach the client symptoms of hypoglycemia that do not include tachycardia, which is suppressed with beta blockers.

○ Central-alpha agonists
  - Central-alpha agonists, such as clonidine (Catapres), reduce peripheral vascular resistance and decrease blood pressure by inhibiting the reuptake of norepinephrine.
- Nursing Considerations
  - Monitor the client's blood pressure and pulse.
  - This medication is not indicated for first-line management of hypertension.

- Client Education
  - Teach the client that side effects include sedation, orthostatic hypotension, and impotence.
- Alpha-adrenergic Antagonists
  - Alpha-adrenergic antagonists, such as prazosin (Minipress), reduce blood pressure by causing vasodilation.
- Nursing Considerations
  - Start treatment with a low dose of the medication.
  - Give the client the first dose at night and monitor her blood pressure for 2 hr after initiation of treatment.
- Client Education
  - Advise the client to rise slowly to prevent postural hypotension. Tell the client to use caution when driving until the effects of the medication are known.

- Care After Discharge
  - Express to the client and family the importance of adhering to the medication regimen, even if the client is asymptomatic.
  - Provide verbal and written education to the client regarding medications and their side effects.
  - Ensure that the client has the resources necessary to pay for and obtain prescribed antihypertensive medication.
  - Encourage the client to schedule regular provider appointments to monitor hypertension and cardiovascular status.
  - If the client has blood pressure that is difficult to manage, teach the client or a significant other how to take their blood pressure.
  - Encourage the client to report symptoms or side effects, as they may be indicative of additional problems. Medications can often be changed to alleviate side effects.
    - Older adult clients are more likely to experience medication interactions.
    - Older adult clients are more likely to experience orthostatic hypotension.
  - Treatment involves the client making lifestyle changes.
    - Sodium restriction
      - Monitor potassium with salt substitute use.
      - Consume less than 2.3 g/day of sodium.
    - Weight reduction
      - Consume a diet low in fat, saturated fat, and cholesterol.
      - Control alcohol intake (2 oz of liquor, 8 oz of wine, 24 oz of beer per day).

- Exercise
  - Begin slowly and gradually advance the program with the guidance of the primary care provider and physical therapist.
  - Exercise at least three times a week in a manner that provides aerobic benefits.
- Smoking cessation
  - Smoking is not directly linked to hypertension, but it should be avoided due to its high association with the development of cardiovascular diseases.
- Stress reduction
  - Encourage the client to try yoga, massage, hypnosis, or other forms of relaxation.

- Client Outcomes
  - The client's blood pressure will be maintained with a systolic pressure less than 140 and a diastolic pressure less than 90.
  - The client will be able to verbalize proper administration of medications and side effects that should be reported to the provider.
  - The client will not report side effects such as postural hypotension, dizziness, weakness or fatigue.

Complications

- Hypertensive Crisis
  - Hypertensive crisis often occurs when clients do not follow the medication therapy regimen.
  - Nursing Actions
    - Recognize signs and symptoms
      - Severe headache
      - Extremely high blood pressure (generally, systolic blood pressure greater than 240 mm Hg, diastolic greater than 120 mm Hg)
      - Blurred vision, dizziness, and disorientation
      - Epistaxis
    - Administer IV antihypertensive therapies, such as nitroprusside (Nipride), nicardipine (Cardene IV), and labetalol (Normodyne).
    - Before, during, and after administration of IV antihypertensive, closely monitor blood pressure every 5 to 15 min as prescribed.
    - Assess the client's neurological status such as pupils, level of consciousness, and muscle strength, frequently to monitor for cerebrovascular change.
    - Monitor the ECG to assess the client's cardiac status.

CHAPTER 40: HYPERTENSION

(A) Application Exercises

1. Which of the following practices should be avoided by clients who are predisposed to or who have hypertension? (Select all that apply.)

_____ Drinking 8 oz of nonfat milk daily

_____ Eating popcorn at the movie theater

_____ Walking 1 mile daily at 12 min/mile pace

_____ Consuming 36 oz of beer daily

_____ Smoking a pipe

2. A nurse is caring for a client who is diagnosed with hypertension and is prescribed spironolactone (Aldactone) 25 mg/day. Which of the following statements by the client indicates a need for further teaching?

A. "I should eat a lot of fruits and vegetables, especially bananas and potatoes."

B. "I will report any changes in heart rate or rhythm."

C. "I should use a salt substitute that is low in potassium."

D. "I will continue to take this medication even if I am feeling better."

3. A nurse is caring for a client who is admitted to the emergency department with a blood pressure of 266/147 mm Hg. The client reports a headache and states that she is seeing double. The client states that she ran out of her diltiazem (Cardizem) 3 days ago, and she has not been able to purchase more. Which of the following nursing interventions should the nurse expect to perform first?

A. Administer acetaminophen for headache.

B. Provide teaching in regard to the importance of not abruptly stopping an antihypertensive.

C. Obtain IV access and prepare to administer an IV antihypertensive.

D. Call social services for a referral for financial assistance in obtaining prescribed medication.

4. A nurse is providing discharge teaching for a client who has a prescription for furosemide (Lasix) 40 mg by mouth daily. What time of day should the client be encouraged to take this medication?

A. Morning

B. Immediately after lunch

C. Immediately before dinner

D. Bedtime

CHAPTER 40: HYPERTENSION

 Application Exercises Answer Key

1. Which of the following practices should be avoided by clients who are predisposed to or who have hypertension? (Select all that apply.)

_____	Drinking 8 oz of nonfat milk daily
X	**Eating popcorn at the movie theater**
_____	Walking 1 mile daily at 12 min/mile pace
X	**Consuming 36 oz of beer daily**
X	**Smoking a pipe**

Popcorn at a movie theater contains a large amount of sodium and fat, which should be limited for a client who has hypertension. Consuming more than 24 oz of beer per day can contribute to weight gain. Smoking causes vasoconstriction, which can increase a client's blood pressure. Clients should consume low-fat foods and beverages, and engage in regular exercise.

 NCLEX® Connection: Physiological Adaptation, Hemodynamics

2. A nurse is caring for a client who is diagnosed with hypertension and is prescribed spironolactone (Aldactone) 25 mg/day. Which of the following statements by the client indicates a need for further teaching?

A. "I should eat a lot of fruits and vegetables, especially bananas and potatoes."
B. "I will report any changes in heart rate or rhythm."
C. "I should use a salt substitute that is low in potassium."
D. "I will continue to take this medication even if I am feeling better."

Potatoes and bananas are high in potassium, and spironolactone is a potassium-sparing diuretic. Consuming these foods can lead to hyperkalemia. The client should report any changes in heart rate or rhythm, use salt substitutes that are low in potassium to prevent hyperkalemia, and know to continue taking the medication even if he is symptom free.

 NCLEX® Connection: Pharmacological and Parenteral Therapies, Adverse Effects/ Contraindications/Side Effects/Interactions

3. A nurse is caring for a client who is admitted to the emergency department with a blood pressure of 266/147 mm Hg. The client reports a headache and states that she is seeing double. The client states that she ran out of her diltiazem (Cardizem) 3 days ago, and she has not been able to purchase more. Which of the following nursing interventions should the nurse expect to perform first?

    A. Administer acetaminophen for headache.

    B. Provide teaching in regard to the importance of not abruptly stopping an antihypertensive.

    C. Obtain IV access and prepare to administer an IV antihypertensive.

    D. Call social services for a referral for financial assistance in obtaining prescribed medication.

The greatest risk to the client is injury due to a blood pressure of 266/147 mm Hg, which can be life-threatening. The highest priority is to decrease the client's blood pressure as quickly as possible. An IV should be started for IV access. Medications given by the IV route will be absorbed and distributed much faster than by the oral route. Administering acetaminophen for headache, providing teaching regarding medication administration, and obtaining financial assistance is important, but not the priority at this time.

 NCLEX® Connection: Physiological Adaptation, Medical Emergencies

4. A nurse is providing discharge teaching for a client who has a prescription for furosemide (Lasix) 40 mg by mouth daily. What time of day should the client be encouraged to take this medication?

    A. Morning

    B. Immediately after lunch

    C. Immediately before dinner

    D. Bedtime

The client should take the furosemide in the morning so that the peak action and duration of the medication occurs during waking hours. All other times may increase the likelihood of interrupting the client's sleep with the need to urinate.

 NCLEX® Connection: Pharmacological and Parenteral Therapies, Adverse Effects/ Contraindications/Side Effects/Interactions

UNIT 4   NURSING CARE OF CLIENTS WITH CARDIOVASCULAR DISORDERS

Section   Vascular Disorders

Chapter 41   Hemodynamic Shock

Overview

- Shock is a state of inadequate tissue perfusion that impairs cellular function and may lead to organ failure. Any condition that compromises the delivery of oxygen delivery to organs and tissues can lead to shock.

- Shock is a rapidly progressing, life-threatening process. Early detection with rapid response is necessary to improve client outcome.

- Older adult clients can have reduced compensatory mechanisms and rapidly progress through the stages of shock. Decreased baroreceptor response to catecholamine secretions may not improve cardiac contractibility or cause vasoconstriction as in younger adults. Decreased ability to compensate can cause sustained low cardiac output and blood pressure.

- Shock is identified by its underlying cause

  o   Cardiogenic – pump failure or heart failure

  o   Hypovolemic – a decrease in intravascular volume of 10 to 15% or more

  o   Obstructive – mechanical blockage in the heart or great vessels

  o   Distributive – widespread vasodilation and increased capillary permeability

- All types of shock progress through the same stages and produce similar effects on body systems.

  o   Initial – no visible changes in client parameters; only changes on the cellular level

  o   Compensatory – measures to increase cardiac output to restore tissue perfusion and oxygenation.

  o   Progressive – compensatory mechanisms begin to fail

  o   Refractory – irreversible shock and total body failure

- The cause of shock, category of shock, and the stage of shock (initial, compensatory, progressive, or refractory) direct treatment.

Health Promotion and Disease Prevention

- Client Education

TYPE OF SHOCK	CLIENT EDUCATION
Cardiogenic	• Educate the client about ways to reduce the risk of an MI, such as exercise, diet, stress reduction and smoking cessation.
Hypovolemic	• Advise the client to drink plenty of fluids when exercising or when in hot weather. • Advise the client to obtain early medical attention with illness or trauma and with any signs of dehydration or bleeding. • Educate the client about the signs of dehydration, including thirst, decreased urine output, and dizziness.
Obstructive/distributive/hypovolemic	• Educate the client about wearing seatbelts, helmets, and the use of caution with dangerous equipment, machinery, or activities.
Septic shock	• Advise the client to obtain early medical attention with any sign of an infection, such as localized redness, swelling, drainage, fever, and urinary frequency and burning. • Advise the client to complete the entire course of antibiotics as directed.
Anaphylactic	• Advise the client to wear a medical identification wristband, avoid allergens, and to have an epinephrine pen available at all times. • Teach the client and family how to use the epinephrine pen and to be alert to early signs of an allergic reaction.

Assessment

- Risk Factors

  - Cardiogenic – cardiac pump failure due to MI, heart failure, cardiomyopathy, dysrhythmias, and valvular rupture or stenosis

    - Older adult clients are more at risk for MI and cardiomyopathy.

  - Hypovolemic – excessive fluid loss from diuresis or vomiting/diarrhea, or blood loss secondary to surgery, trauma, gynecologic/obstetric causes, burns, and diabetic ketoacidosis.

    - Older adult clients are more prone to dehydration due to decreased fluid and protein intake and the use of medications, such as diuretics. It will not take as much in the way of fluid losses through vomiting/diarrhea for older adult clients to become dehydrated.

- o Obstructive – blockage of great vessels, pulmonary artery stenosis, pulmonary embolism, cardiac tamponade, tension pneumothorax, and aortic dissection are among the causes

- o Distributive is divided into three types

  - Septic – endotoxins and other mediators causing massive vasodilation; most common cause is gram-negative bacteria

    - □ Urosepsis is more frequent in older adult clients. This may be due to an inability to recognize early symptoms of a urinary tract infection due to decreased sensation of urethral burning and awareness of urinary urgency. Many older adult clients live in extended care facilities where urinary catheters are used, increasing the likelihood of urosepsis.

  - Neurogenic – loss of sympathetic tone causing massive vasodilation; trauma, spinal shock, and epidural anesthesia are among the causes

  - Anaphylactic – antigen-antibody reaction causing massive vasodilation; allergens inhaled, swallowed, contacted, or introduced IV are causes

- Subjective Data

  - o Symptoms can include chest pain, lethargy, somnolence, restlessness, anxiousness, dyspnea, diaphoresis, thirst, muscle weakness, nausea, and constipation

- Objective Data

  - o Physical Assessment Findings

    - Hypoxia, tachypnea progressing to greater than 40/min, hypocarbia

    - Skin may be pale, mottled or dusky in color, cool, diaphoretic, warm, flushed with fever (distributive shock), and exhibit a rash (anaphylactic and septic shock)

    - Angioedema (anaphylactic)

    - Wheezing

    - Blood pressure may be within the expected reference range during the initial stage, but can increase during the progressive stage and then drop to less than 50 to 60 mm Hg

    - Tachycardia progressing to greater than 140/min

    - Pulse that is weak, thready, or bound with distributive shock

    - Decreased cardiac output

    - Central venous pressure is decreased in hypovolemic shock

    - Central venous pressure is increased with increased systemic vascular resistance in cardiogenic shock

    - Decreased urine output

    - Seizures

- o Laboratory Tests

  - ABGs – decreased tissue oxygenation (decreased pH, decreased PaO_2, increased $PaCO_2$)

  - Serum lactic acid – increases due to anaerobic metabolism

  - Serum glucose and electrolytes – serum glucose can increase during shock

  - Cardiogenic shock

    - □ Cardiac enzymes – creatine phosphokinase, troponin

  - Hypovolemic shock

    - □ Hgb and Hct – decreased with hemorrhage, increased with dehydration

  - Septic shock

    - □ Cultures – blood, urine, wound

    - □ Coagulation tests – PT, INR, aPTT

- o Diagnostic Procedures

  - Hemodynamic monitoring

    - □ Arterial line insertion

      - ▸ Needed for continuous blood pressure monitoring and access to withdraw ABG sample and other blood work

    - □ Pulmonary artery catheter insertion

      - ▸ A pulmonary artery catheter is inserted to measure cerebrovascular pressure, pulmonary artery pressures, and cardiac output. Continuous hemodynamic monitoring is important to manage fluids and dosage of inotropic medications

    - □ Nursing Actions

      - ▸ Monitor ECG during catheter insertion.

      - ▸ Have resuscitation medications and equipment ready.

      - ▸ Monitor hemodynamic waveforms and readings.

      - ▸ Confirm catheter placement using a chest x-ray.

    - □ Client Education

      - ▸ Explain all procedures to the client. The client may be anxious and scared.

  - Cardiogenic and obstructive shock

    - □ ECG

      - ▸ Assess for ECG changes associated with MI and dysrhythmias.

- Echocardiogram
  - Diagnostic procedure used for cardiomegaly, cardiomyopathy, the evaluation of cardiac contractility and function, ejection fraction, and valve function
- Computerized tomography (CT)
  - Diagnostic procedure used for cardiomegaly, cardiac tamponade, pulmonary emboli, cardiomyopathy, aortic dissection or aneurysm, and pericardial effusion
- Cardiac catheterization
  - Diagnostic procedure used to identify cardiac artery blockage
- Chest x-ray
  - Diagnostic procedure used to diagnose cardiomegaly, pneumothorax, and to evaluate lungs

- **Hypovolemic shock – miscellaneous diagnostic procedures**
  - Investigate possible sources of bleeding
    - Blood in nasogastric drainage or stools
    - Esophagogastroduodenoscopy
    - CT scan of abdomen
  - Nursing Actions
    - Continuously monitor the client's airway and vital signs.
    - Provide hemodynamic support through fluids and medications.
    - The client with suspected shock may be hemodynamically unstable.
    - Have resuscitation equipment available when transporting the client to and from procedures.
  - Client Education
    - Explain all procedures to the client.

Collaborative Care

- Nursing Care
  - Monitor
    - Oxygenation status (priority)
    - Vital signs
    - Cardiac rhythm with continuous cardiac monitoring
    - Urine output – hourly, report if less than 30 mL/hr
    - Level of consciousness
    - Skin color, temperature, moisture, capillary refill, turgor

- o Explain procedures and findings to the client and family while providing reassurance.
- o Place the client on high-flow oxygen, such as a 100% nonrebreather face mask.
  - ■ If the client has COPD, insert a 2 L/min nasal cannula and increase the oxygen flow as needed.
- o Be prepared to intubate the client. Have emergency resuscitation equipment ready.
- o Maintain patent IV access.
- o For hypotension, place the client flat with his legs elevated to increase venous return.
- o If change in status occurs, notify the primary care provider of the findings.
- o Initiate orders to intervene during shock, including transfer to the intensive care unit, surgery, other specialty unit, or diagnostic area.
- o Prepare for and carry out hemodynamic monitoring.
  - ■ Monitor cerebrovascular pressure, pulmonary artery pressures, cardiac output, and pulse pressure.
  - ■ Titrate continuous IV drips to maintain hemodynamic parameters as prescribed.
- • Medications

PHARMACOLOGICAL AGENTS	ACTIONS	NURSING CONSIDERATIONS
Inotropic agents • Milrinone lactate (Primacor)	Strengthens cardiac contraction and increases cardiac output	• Give through a continuous IV drip with constant hemodynamic monitoring. • Can titrate agent to maintain prescribed hemodynamic parameters. • Agent can cause vasodilation in some clients. • Agents are often given in combination with a vasopressor.
Vasopressors • Dobutamine (Dobutrex) • Dopamine hydrochloride (Intropin) • Norepinephrine (Levophed)	• Strengthens cardiac contraction and increases cardiac output • Increases renal perfusion at low doses • Decreases renal perfusion at high doses	• Give through a continuous IV drip with constant hemodynamic monitoring. • Can titrate vasopressor to maintain prescribed hemodynamic parameters. • Monitor urine output. • Give through a central line to prevent extravasation. Rapid onset occurs in 5 min, and short duration occurs in 10 min.
Pituitary Hormone • Vasopressin (Pitressin Synthetic)	• Strengthens cardiac contraction • Causes vasoconstriction, increases systemic vascular resistance blood pressure, and increases cardiac output	

 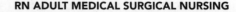

PHARMACOLOGICAL AGENTS	ACTIONS	NURSING CONSIDERATIONS
Opioid analgesics • Morphine sulfate • Fentanyl (Sublimaze)	Pain management	• Monitor respirations on clients who are nonventilated. • Monitor the client's blood pressure, heart rate, and SaO$_2$. • Monitor the client's ABGs. • Use opioid analgesics cautiously in conjunction with hypnotic sedatives. • Assess and document the client's pain level and response to medication. • Use cautiously due to risk of increased vasodilation and hypotension. • Have naloxone (Narcan) and resuscitation equipment available for severe respiratory depression in a client who is nonventilated.
Proton-pump inhibitors • Pantoprazole (Protonix)	Protects against stress ulcer development	• Do not mix with other medications.
Anticoagulant • Low-molecular weight heparin, enoxaparin sodium (Lovenox)	Deep vein thrombosis prophylaxis	• Give subcutaneously, usually in abdomen. • Do not rub injection site.
Isotonic crystalloids or colloids (including blood products) • 0.9% sodium chloride in water) or lactated Ringer's solution	Hypovolemic shock – volume replacement	• ALERT – During hypovolemic shock, replace volume first. • Use vasopressors only if the client's blood pressure remains low after volume is replaced.
Vasodilator • Sodium nitroprusside (Nipride)	• Used to treat cardiogenic shock • Reduces afterload and preload • Causes vasodilation • Decreases cardiac output and afterload	• Assess the client's blood pressure every 15 min. • Use medication with caution because it is a potent vasodilator. • Protect the solution from light.
Antihistamines • Diphenhydramine (Benadryl)	• Used to treat anaphylactic shock • Blocks histamine at receptor sites	• Diphenhydramine can cause drowsiness, hypotension, and tachycardia.

PHARMACOLOGICAL AGENTS	ACTIONS	NURSING CONSIDERATIONS
Sympathomimetics • Epinephrine (Adrenaline)	• Rapid-acting bronchodilator • Increases heart rate and cardiac output	• Monitor the client's blood pressure, pulse, and cardiac output. • Epinephrine can cause sloughing if infiltrates tissue.
Corticosteroids • Hydrocortisone (Solu-Cortef) • Methylprednisolone (Solu-Medrol)	• Reduces WBC migration and decrease inflammation	• Hydrocortisone can cause hypertension. • Discontinue medication gradually. • Give hydrocortisone with an antiulcer medication to prevent peptic ulcer formation. • Monitor the client's weight and blood pressure. • Monitor the client's glucose and electrolytes.
Antibiotics sensitive to cultured organism(s) • Vancomycin (Vancocin)	• Used to treat septic shock • Inhibits cell growth or reproduction of undesired organism	• Monitor the client for hypersensitivity reaction. • Give IV dosages of vancomycin slowly. • Culture infected area prior to administration of the first dose of vancomycin. • Monitor the IV site for infiltration. • Do not give vancomycin with other medications. • Monitor coagulopathy and renal function.
Activated protein C • Drotrecogin alfa (activated) (Xigris)	Anti-inflammatory, anticoagulant, fibrinolysis properties	• Use drotrecogin alfa only in severe shock. • Drotrecogin alfa can cause bleeding. • Do not mix with other medications. • Do not use in clients who are experiencing active bleeding. • Monitor the client for signs of hemorrhage. • Monitor the client's coagulation studies and CBC.

- Interdisciplinary Care

  ○ Respiratory therapy

    ■ The respiratory therapist typically manages the ventilator, adjusts the settings, and provides chest physical therapy to improve ventilation and chest expansion. The respiratory therapist may also suction the endotracheal tube and administer inhalation medications such as bronchodilators.

- Therapeutic Procedures

  ○ Intubation and mechanical ventilation

    ■ An artificial airway is inserted, and the client's respirations are controlled by mechanical ventilation.

    ■ Nursing Actions

      □ Preintubation:

        ‣ Monitor the client's ECG, SaO_2, breath sounds, and color.

        ‣ Sedate the client as needed.

        ‣ Preoxygenate the client with 100% oxygen.

        ‣ Assist the client with ventilation with a manual resuscitation bag and a face mask.

        ‣ Have suction equipment, manual emergency resuscitation, and a face mask readily available.

        ‣ Suction the client's secretions as needed.

        ‣ Provide reassurance to calm client.

      □ Postintubation:

        ‣ Assess bilateral breath sounds, symmetrical chest movement, and a chest x-ray to confirm placement of the endotracheal tube.

        ‣ Secure the endotracheal tube per facility guidelines.

        ‣ Assess the balloon cuff for air leak periodically.

      □ Positive end expiratory pressure (PEEP)

        ‣ Positive pressure is applied at the end of expiration to keep the alveoli expanded.

        ‣ PEEP is added to the ventilator setting to increase oxygenation and improve lung expansion.

    ■ Client Education

      □ Explain all procedures to the client.

      □ Provide reassurance to calm the client.

      □ Explain to the client and family that the client will be unable to talk with the endotracheal tube in place.

- ○ Needle decompression and chest tube insertion

  - ▪ Used to relieve pressure from a tension pneumothorax that may be causing obstructive shock

  - ▪ Nursing Actions

    - □ Monitor the client's ECG, SaO_2, breath sounds, and color.

    - □ Sedate the client as needed.

    - □ Set up a water seal chest-drainage system and attach it to suction.

    - □ Apply a dressing.

    - □ Assess the chest tube for air leaks.

    - □ Monitor and document the drainage.

    - □ Obtain a chest x-ray postprocedure.

  - ▪ Client Education

    - □ Explain all procedures to the client.

    - □ Reassure and calm the client.

- ○ Pericardiocentesis

  - ▪ Drainage of pericardial fluid that is causing cardiac tamponade and obstructive shock

  - ▪ Nursing Actions

    - □ Monitor the client's ECG, SaO_2, breath sounds, and color.

    - □ Sedate the client as needed.

    - □ Obtain a postprocedure chest x-ray.

  - ▪ Client Education

    - □ Explain all procedures to the client.

    - □ Reassure and calm the client.

- • Surgical Interventions

  - ○ Surgical intervention may be needed to correct the cause of shock, such as a hemorrhaging ulcer, wound, artery or vein.

    - ▪ Nursing Actions

      - □ Preprocedure

        - ‣ Manage the client's airway and provide supplemental oxygen and intubation if needed.

        - ‣ Provide hemodynamic support with fluids and medications to stabilize the client prior to surgical intervention, if possible.

       □ Postprocedure

          ▸ Continue to monitor the client's blood pressure, ECG, pulmonary artery pressures, cardiac output, central venous pressure, and urine output.

          ▸ Titrate and administer medications as prescribed.

          ▸ Assess the surgical site for bleeding.

          ▸ Monitor the client's airway, breath sounds, and ABGs.

          ▸ Monitor the client's CBC.

- Client Education

       □ Explain all procedures to the client.

       □ Be aware that the client may be awake and frightened.

- Client Outcomes

  o The client should use caution and wear a helmet and seatbelt to avoid serious injury.

  o The client should seek early medical attention with any sign of an infection as well as complete the course of antibiotics as prescribed.

  o The client should prevent dehydration by drinking plenty of fluids and seek early medical attention with any sign of dehydration.

  o The client who has severe allergies should wear a medical identification wristband, carry an epinephrine pen, and avoid allergens.

Complications

- Multiple organ dysfunction syndrome (MODS)

  o MODS may develop from severe hypotension and reperfusion of ischemic cells causing further tissue injury. Inadequate tissue perfusion may cause organ failure in the lungs (adult respiratory distress syndrome), kidneys (renal failure), heart (decreased coronary artery perfusion, decreased cardiac contractibility), and the gastrointestinal tract (necrosis).

  o Nursing Actions

    - Assess organ function and provide support measures that can increase tissue perfusion and improve organ function (ventilatory support, inotropic medications).

    - Take interventions to compensate for dysfunction (administration of clotting factors, dialysis).

- Disseminated Intravascular Coagulation (DIC)

  o DIC is a complication of septic shock. Thousands of small clots form within organ capillaries (liver, kidney, heart, brain), creating hypoxia and anaerobic metabolism. As a result of massive, multiple clot formation, platelets and other clotting factors such as fibrinogen are depleted and the client is at increased risk for hemorrhage. The client can develop diffuse petechiae and ecchymoses, and blood can leak from membranes and puncture sites.

  o Nursing Actions

    ▪ Administer platelets and clotting factors and other blood products as prescribed.

    ▪ Monitor the client's hemodynamic levels.

    ▪ Assess the client for further signs of bleeding.

    ▪ Apply pressure to leaking IV/central line/arterial line sites.

  o Client Education

    ▪ Explain procedures and care to the client and family.

CHAPTER 41: HEMODYNAMIC SHOCK

(A) Application Exercises

Scenario: A client is admitted following a colon resection. The client is receiving oxygen at 3 L/min per nasal cannula and has a right forearm IV with lactated Ringer's infusing at 125 mL/hr, a saline lock in the left forearm, an indwelling urinary catheter, and an epidural catheter for pain management. The abdominal dressing is dry and intact. Provider prescriptions include:

Cefotaxime sodium (Claforan) 1 g IV every 12 hr

Metronidazole (Flagyl) 1 g IV every 12 hr

Dextrose 5% in 0.45% sodium chloride IV at 125 mL/hr

1. What types of shock is the client at risk for developing?

2. What should the nurse monitor to determine if each type of shock is developing?

3. A nurse should anticipate the use of afterload-reducing agents in which of the following types of shock?

    A. Cardiogenic

    B. Obstructive

    C. Hypovolemic

    D. Distributive

4. Which of the following is the highest priority of collaborative management for septic shock?

    A. Maintaining adequate fluid volume with IV infusions

    B. Treating the cause of the infection

    C. Monitoring hemodynamic status

    D. Administering dopamine (Intropin) at low does to increase renal perfusion

5. A client is brought to the emergency department with an allergic reaction to a bee sting. The client is experiencing wheezing and swelling of the tongue. Which of the following medications should the nurse expect to administer first?

    A. Methylprednisolone (Solu-Medrol) IVP

    B. Diphenhydramine (Benadryl) subcutaneously

    C. Epinephrine (Adrenaline) IV

    D. Albuterol (Proventil) inhaler

6. A nurse is assessing a client who in shock. Which of the following findings should the nurse expect? (Select all that apply.)

_____ Heart rate 60/min

_____ Seizure activity

_____ Respiratory rate 42/min

_____ Increased urine output

_____ Weak, thready pulse

CHAPTER 41: HEMODYNAMIC SHOCK

(A) Application Exercises Answer Key

Scenario: A client is admitted following a colon resection. The client is receiving oxygen at 3 L/min per nasal cannula and has a right forearm IV with lactated Ringer's infusing at 125 mL/hr, a saline lock in the left forearm, an indwelling urinary catheter, and an epidural catheter for pain management. The abdominal dressing is dry and intact. Provider prescriptions include:

Cefotaxime sodium (Claforan) 1 g IV every 12 hr

Metronidazole (Flagyl) 1 g IV every 12 hr

Dextrose 5% in 0.45% sodium chloride IV at 125 mL/hr

1. What types of shock is the client at risk for developing?

Hypovolemic – due to bleeding and fluid collection in peritoneal cavity

Obstructive – due to pulmonary emboli if deep vein thrombosis develops

Septic – due to colon surgery

Neurogenic – due to epidural analgesia

Anaphylactic – due to antibiotics

(N) **NCLEX® Connection: Physiological Adaptation, Hemodynamics**

2. What should the nurse monitor to determine if each type of shock is developing?

Hypovolemic – vital signs, I&O, skin turgor, abdominal girth

Obstructive – for deep vein thrombosis

Septic – vital signs, temperature, wound

Neurogenic – vital signs, movement and sensation of legs, peripheral pulses

Anaphylactic – vital signs, lung sounds

(N) **NCLEX® Connection: Reduction of Risk Potential, System-Specific Assessment**

3. A nurse should anticipate the use of afterload-reducing agents in which of the following types of shock?

   A. Cardiogenic

   B. Obstructive

   C. Hypovolemic

   D. Distributive

   Reducing afterload will allow the heart to pump more effectively. The high afterload is due to obstruction of blood flow, and afterload-reducing agents will not remove the obstruction. Fluid replacement and reduction of further fluid loss are the focus of management of hypovolemic shock. All three forms of distributive shock result in decreased afterload from vasodilation.

    NCLEX® Connection: Pharmacological and Parenteral Therapies, Pharmacological Agents/ Actions

4. Which of the following is the highest priority of collaborative management for septic shock?

   A. Maintaining adequate fluid volume with IV infusions

   B. Treating the cause of the infection

   C. Monitoring hemodynamic status

   D. Administering dopamine (Intropin) at low does to increase renal perfusion

   The highest priority for management of septic shock is to determine and treat the cause of the infection to halt the infection process. Other important actions include administering large amounts of IV fluid to fill the increased vascular space caused by the vasodilation, monitoring hemodynamic status to determine effectiveness of therapy and, administering dopamine to increase renal perfusion.

    NCLEX® Connection: Physiological Adaptation, Hemodynamics

5. A client is brought to the emergency department with an allergic reaction to a bee sting. The client is experiencing wheezing and swelling of the tongue. Which of the following medications should the nurse expect to administer first?

   A. Methylprednisolone (Solu-Medrol) IV

   B. Diphenhydramine (Benadryl) subcutaneously

   C. Epinephrine (Adrenaline) IV

   D. Albuterol (Proventil) inhaler

   Epinephrine will treat both symptoms. Clients who are experiencing allergic reactions are given prescriptions for epinephrine pens that they should carry with them at all times. Methylprednisolone, diphenhydramine, and albuterol may all be administered, but will not be administered first.

    NCLEX® Connection: Pharmacological and Parenteral Therapies, Expected Actions/ Outcomes

6. A nurse is assessing a client who in shock. Which of the following findings should the nurse expect? (Select all that apply.)

_____	Heart rate 60/min
__X__	**Seizure activity**
__X__	**Respiratory rate 42/min**
_____	Increased urine output
__X__	**Weak, thready pulse**

A client in shock may exhibit seizure activity, a respiratory rate of 42/min, and a weak thready pulse. A heart rate of 60/min, and increased urine output would not be present in a client who is in shock.

Ⓝ NCLEX® Connection: Physiological Adaptation, Hemodynamics

UNIT 4	NURSING CARE OF CLIENTS WITH CARDIOVASCULAR DISORDERS
Section	Vascular Disorders
Chapter 42	Aneurysms

 Overview

- A weakness in a section of a dilated artery that causes a widening or ballooning in the wall of the blood vessel is called an aneurysm.

- Aneurysms can occur in two forms. They can be saccular (only affecting one side of the artery), or they can be fusiform (involving the complete circumference of the artery).

- Seventy-five percent of aneurysms are abdominal aortic aneurysms.

> **View Media Supplement:** Common Aneurysm Sites (Image)

- Aortic dissection can occur when blood accumulates within the aortic wall (hematoma) following a tear in the lining of the aorta (usually due to hypertension).

Health Promotion and Disease Prevention

- Promote smoking cessation.

- Maintain appropriate weight for height and body frame.

- Encourage a healthy diet and physical activity.

- Control blood pressure with regular monitoring and medication if needed.

Assessment

- Risk Factors

  - Atherosclerosis

  - Uncontrolled hypertension

  - Tobacco use

  - With age, arterial stiffening caused by loss of elastin in arterial walls, thickening of intima of arteries, and progressive fibrosis of media occurs; therefore, older adult clients are more prone to aneurysms and have a higher mortality rate from aneurysms than younger individuals

- Subjective Data and Objective Data

  ○ Initially, clients are often asymptomatic.

  ○ Abdominal aortic aneurysm (most common related to atherosclerosis)

    ■ Constant gnawing feeling in abdomen; flank or back pain

    ■ Pulsating abdominal mass

    ■ Bruit

    ■ Elevated blood pressure (unless in cardiac tamponade or rupture of aneurysm)

  ○ Aortic dissections (often associated with Marfan's syndrome)

    ■ Sudden onset of "tearing," "ripping," and "stabbing" abdominal or back pain

    ■ Hypovolemic shock

      □ Diaphoresis, nausea, vomiting, faintness, apprehension

      □ Decreased or absent peripheral pulses

      □ Neurological deficits

      □ Hypotension and tachycardia (initial)

  ○ Thoracic aortic aneurysm

    ■ Coolness and/or cyanosis of extremities below graft

    ■ Hoarseness, shortness of breath, and difficulty swallowing

    ■ Severe back pain

    ■ Decrease in urinary output

  ○ Diagnostic procedures

    ■ X-ray

      □ X-rays can reveal the classic "eggshell" appearance of an aneurysm. Aneurysms are often discovered when examining the client for some other clinical possibility.

    ■ Computed tomography (CT) and ultrasonography

      □ CT scans and ultrasonography are used to assess the size and location of aneurysms and are often repeated at periodic intervals to monitor the progression of an aneurysm.

Collaborative Care

- Nursing Care

  ○ Take the client's vital signs every 15 min until stable, then every hour (Watch for increased blood pressure.).

  ○ Assess the onset, quality, duration, and severity of the client's pain.

  ○ Assess the client's temperature, circulation, and function of all extremities.

- Continuously monitor the client's cardiac rhythm.

- Monitor the client's hemodynamic values.

- Monitor ABGs, SaO$_2$, electrolytes, and CBC laboratory values.

- Monitor the client's hourly urine output – greater than 30 mL/hr indicates adequate renal perfusion.

- Administer oxygen as prescribed.

- Obtain and maintain IV access.

- Administer medications as prescribed.

  - Note – All aneurysms can be life-threatening and need medical attention.

- Medications

  - The priority intervention is to reduce systolic blood pressure between 100 and 120 mm Hg during an emergency and to maintain a systolic blood pressure at or less than 130 to 140 mm Hg.

    - Administer antihypertensive agents as prescribed. Often more than one is prescribed (beta blockers and calcium blockers).

- Interdisciplinary Care

  - Cardiology services may be consulted to manage and treat hypertension.

  - Radiology should be consulted for diagnostic studies to determine an aneurysm.

  - Vascular services may be consulted for surgical intervention.

- Surgical Interventions

  - Abdominal aortic aneurysm (AAA) resection

    - An AAA resection involves the excision of the aneurysm and the placement of a synthetic graft. Surgical management may be either elective or emergency. A rupturing aneurysm requires prompt emergency surgery. AAA of 6 cm or greater in diameter may be managed with elective surgery. Mortality rates are 2 to 5% for elective AAA resections and 50% when rupture has occurred. Risks include significant blood loss and the consequences of reduced cardiac output and tissue ischemia (MI, renal failure, respiratory distress, paralytic ileus).

    - Nursing Actions
      - Priority interventions include monitoring the client's arterial pressure, heart rhythm, and hemodynamic values as well as monitoring for signs of graft occlusion or rupture postoperatively.

      - Monitor the client's vital signs and circulation (pulses distal to graft) every 15 min. Listen to breath sounds.

      - Avoid flexion of the graft (keep the head of the bed below 45°).

- Monitor and maintain normal blood pressure on the client. Prolonged hypotension can cause thrombi to form within the graft, and severe hypertension can cause leakage or rupture at the arterial anastomosis suture line.

- Administer IV fluids to the client at prescribed rates to ensure adequate hydration and renal perfusion.

- Maintain a warm environment to prevent temperature-induced vasoconstriction.

- Monitor the client's urinary output (report less than 50 mL/hr), daily weights, BUN, and serum creatinine to detect for signs of altered renal perfusion and renal failure (secondary to surgical clamping of aorta).

- Encourage the client to cough and deep breathe every 2 hr. Encourage splinting with coughing.

- Assess onset, quality, duration, and severity of the client's pain.

  ▸ Administer pain medication as prescribed.

- Monitor the client's bowel sounds and observe for abdominal distention. Maintain nasogastric suction as prescribed.

- Take measures to reduce the risk of thromboembolism (sequential compression devices, early ambulation, administer prescribed antiplatelet or anticoagulant medications).

- Monitor the client for signs of infection such as elevated body temperature, WBC count, heart rate, and respiratory rate; decreased blood pressure; erythema and warmth along the incision line; persistent drainage from incisions as well as at sites of invasive lines; and separation of wound edges.

- Administer antibiotics to the client as prescribed to maintain adequate blood levels of the medication.

- Any signs of graft occlusion or rupture should be reported immediately (changes in pulses, coolness of extremity below graft, white or blue extremities or flanks, severe pain, abdominal distention, decreased urine output).

- Client Education

  - Provide client teaching regarding postoperative activity restrictions (avoid lifting more than 15 lb, strenuous activity).

  - Ensure adequate nutrition – specifically a diet high in protein, vitamin C, vitamin A, and zinc – to promote healing.

○ Percutaneous aneurysm repair

- Percutaneous insertion of endothelial stent grafts for aneurysm repair avoids abdominal incision and shortens the postoperative period (can be used to repair a thoracic aortic aneurysm).

- Nursing Actions
  - Nursing care after the procedure is similar to care following an arteriogram or cardiac catheterization (pedal pulse checks).
- Client Education
  - Provide client teaching regarding postoperative activity restrictions (avoidance of lifting more than 15 lb, strenuous activity).
  - Ensure adequate nutrition – specifically a diet high in protein, vitamin C, vitamin A, and zinc – to promote healing. Refer to Chapter 34: Invasive Cardiac Procedures.

○ Thoracic aortic aneurysm repair

- Procedure similar to thoracic surgery, such as open heart. The course of action depends on the location of the aneurysm. Cardiopulmonary bypass is commonly used for this procedure.
- Nursing Actions
  - Nursing care after the procedure is similar to care following coronary artery bypass graft surgery (monitor respiratory status; respiratory distress is common after this type of procedure).
- Client Education
  - Provide client teaching regarding postoperative activity restrictions (avoid lifting more than 15 lb, strenuous activity) and introduce cardiac rehabilitation information.
  - Ensure adequate nutrition – specifically a diet high in protein, vitamin C, vitamin A, and zinc – to promote healing.
- Care After Discharge
  - Cardiac rehabilitation services may be consulted for prolonged weakness and assistance in increasing the client's level of activity.
  - Nutritional services may be consulted for food choices that are low in fat and cholesterol.

○ Client Education

- Emphasize with the client the importance of monitoring and controlling blood pressure.
- Emphasize with the client the importance of following through on scheduled tests to monitor size (nonsurgical client).
- Promote smoking cessation if the client smokes.
- Instruct the client to wash her hands to prevent infection.
- Encourage the client to consume a low-fat, low-cholesterol diet.
- Explain symptoms of aneurysm rupture to the client that need to be promptly reported (abdominal fullness or pain, chest or back pain, shortness of breath, difficulty swallowing, hoarseness).

- Inform the client about weight restrictions and activities that should be avoided, how to take care for the incision, and the signs and symptoms of infection. (surgical client).

- Client Outcomes

  o The client will be free of pain.

  o The client will have blood pressure within the expected reference range.

  o The client will be free from infection.

Complications

- Rupture

  o Aneurysm rupture is a life-threatening emergency. A ruptured aneurysm may result in massive hemorrhage causing shock and death.

  o It requires simultaneous resuscitation and immediate surgical repair.

    - Aneurysms greater than 6 cm (2.4 in) in diameter have a 50% chance of rupture within 1 year.

- Thrombus formation

  o A thrombus may form inside the aneurysm. Emboli may be dislodged, blocking arteries distal to the aneurysm, which causes ischemia and shuts down other body systems.

  o Assess circulation distal to aneurysm, including pulses and color and temperature of the lower extremities. Monitor the client's urine output.

CHAPTER 42: ANEURYSMS

(A) Application Exercises

Scenario: A middle adult client presents with reports of a persistent, chronic cough unrelieved by sinus and cold medications. On assessment, the nurse notes that the client's voice sounds hoarse, blood pressure is 164/98 mm Hg, heart rate is 96/min, and respirations are 22/min. The client confirms episodes of epigastric discomfort unrelieved by antacids. Chest x-ray results indicate a 5-cm enlargement of the ascending aorta.

1. What do these findings indicate?

2. Identify appropriate nursing interventions for the care of this client.

3. Four months later, the client experiences a change in her condition and calls 911. The client arrives by ambulance into the emergency department with a blood pressure of 86/30 mm Hg, diaphoresis, mental obtundation, an irregular heart rhythm, severe back pain, and bilateral bruising in the flanks. List the findings that indicate that this client is experiencing a medical emergency?

4. Which of the following is the priority intervention?

    A. Give pain medication.

    B. Obtain blood specimen.

    C. Administer IV fluids.

    D. Initiate a 12-lead ECG.

5. Which of the following are priority nursing interventions postoperatively? (Select all that apply.)

    _____ Assess temperature, circulation, and function of extremities.

    _____ Monitor and report increased pain below the graft site.

    _____ Maintain a cold environment.

    _____ Restrict fluids due to the risk of pulmonary congestion.

    _____ Administer anticoagulants and/or antiplatelet agents.

CHAPTER 42: ANEURYSMS

 Application Exercises Answer Key

Scenario: A middle adult client presents with reports of a persistent, chronic cough unrelieved by sinus and cold medications. On assessment, the nurse notes that the client's voice sounds hoarse, blood pressure is 164/98 mm Hg, heart rate is 96/min, and respirations are 22/min. The client confirms episodes of epigastric discomfort unrelieved by antacids. Chest x-ray results indicate a 5-cm enlargement of the ascending aorta.

1. What do these findings indicate?

> **This client is experiencing symptoms related to pressure from the 5-cm aneurysm on surrounding structures. The client is probably experiencing hoarseness as a result of pressure on the laryngeal nerve. Pressure on pulmonary structures can result in coughing, dyspnea, and airway obstruction. Epigastric discomfort is probably a result of pressure on the esophagus and stomach. Pressure on the esophagus can cause dysphagia. Pressure on the superior vena cava can result in decreased venous drainage resulting in distended neck veins and edema of the head and arms. Elevated blood pressure may be a contributing factor.**

 NCLEX® Connection: Physiological Adaptation, Pathophysiology

2. Identify appropriate nursing interventions for the care of this client.

> **Emphasize the importance of following through on scheduled CT scans, which are used to monitor the growth of the aneurysm.**
>
> **Explain manifestations of the aneurysm to the client that need to be promptly reported.**
>
> **Assess the client for indications of rupture (paleness; weakness; tachycardia; hypotension; abdominal, back, or groin pain; changes in sensorium; or a pulsating abdominal mass).**
>
> **Assess the client for normal tissue perfusion and intact motor and sensory function.**
>
> **Provide the client with education about how to control hypertension, the medication regimen, smoking cessation, and a low-fat, low-cholesterol diet.**

 NCLEX® Connection: Physiological Adaptation, Illness Management

3. Four months later, the client experiences a change in her condition and calls 911. The client arrives by ambulance into the emergency department with a blood pressure of 86/30 mm Hg, diaphoresis, mental obtundation, an irregular heart rhythm, severe back pain, and bilateral bruising in the flanks. List the findings that indicate that this client is experiencing a medical emergency?

> **Symptoms of shock (blood pressure of 86/30 mm Hg, diaphoresis, mental obtundation, dysrhythmia) and rupture of the aneurysm (severe back pain, bilateral bruising in the flanks) are indicative of a critical, immediate, life-threatening situation.**

 NCLEX® Connection: Physiological Adaptation, Pathophysiology

4. Which of the following is the priority intervention?

> A. Give pain medication.
>
> B. Obtain blood specimen.
>
> **C. Administer IV fluids.**
>
> D. Initiate a 12-lead ECG.

Using the ABC priority setting framework, the greatest risk to the client is inadequate circulatory volume. Therefore, the highest priority intervention is to administer IV fluids. Giving pain medication, obtaining a blood specimen, and initiating a 12-lead ECG are important actions, but not the priority.

Ⓝ NCLEX® Connection: Physiological Adaptation, Pathophysiology

5. Which of the following are priority nursing interventions postoperatively? (Select all that apply.)

> __X__ **Assess temperature, circulation, and function of extremities.**
>
> __X__ **Monitor and report increased pain below the graft site.**
>
> _____ Maintain a cold environment.
>
> _____ Restrict fluids due to the risk of pulmonary congestion.
>
> __X__ **Administer anticoagulants and/or antiplatelet agents.**
>
> _____ Report an hourly urine output of 60 mL.

The client's extremities should be assessed for signs of complications, such as occlusion of the graft. Pain can be an indicator of graft occlusion or rupture. IV fluids are given (not restricted) to maintain renal perfusion. Anticoagulants and or antiplatelet agents are used to prevent thrombus formation. A warm environment is maintained to prevent temperature-induced thrombus formation. An hourly urine output of 60 mL/hr is an expected finding.

Ⓝ NCLEX® Connection: Physiological Adaptation, Alterations in Body Systems=

UNIT 5: NURSING CARE OF CLIENTS WITH HEMATOLOGIC DISORDERS

- Diagnostic and Therapeutic Procedures
- Hematologic Disorders

NCLEX® CONNECTIONS

When reviewing the chapters
in this unit, keep in mind
the relevant sections of the
NCLEX® outline, in particular:

CLIENT NEEDS: PHARMACOLOGICAL AND PARENTERAL THERAPIES

Relevant topics/tasks include:
- Blood and Blood Products
  - Identify the client according to facility policy prior to administration of red blood cells/blood products.
  - Check the client for appropriate venous access for red blood cell/blood product administration .
  - Administer blood products and evaluate the client's response.

CLIENT NEEDS: REDUCTION OF RISK POTENTIAL

Relevant topics/tasks include:
- Laboratory Values
  - Recognize deviations from normal for values of albumin (blood), ALT (SGPT), AST (SGOT), ammonia, bilirubin, bleeding time, calcium (total), cholesterol (HDL and LDL), digoxin, ESR, lithium, magnesium, phosphorous/ phosphate, protein (total), urine (specific gravity, albumin, pH, WBC).
  - Educate the client about the purpose and procedure of prescribed laboratory tests.

CLIENT NEEDS: PHYSIOLOGICAL ADAPTATION

Relevant topics/tasks include:
- Alterations in Body Systems
  - Assess the adaptation of the client to health alteration, illness and/ or disease.
- Fluid and Electrolyte Imbalances
  - Manage the care of the client with a fluid and electrolyte imbalance.
- Hemodynamics
  - Intervene to improve the client's cardiovascular status.

UNIT 5	NURSING CARE OF CLIENTS WITH HEMATOLOGIC DISORDERS
Section	Diagnostic and Therapeutic Procedures
Chapter 43	Hematologic Diagnostic Procedures

Overview

- Hematologic assessment and diagnostic procedures are used to evaluate blood function by testing indicators such as erythrocytes (RBC), leukocytes (WBC), platelets, and coagulation times.

- By testing the blood, diagnosis of a disease and efficacy of treatment can be determined.

- Bone marrow is responsible for the production of many blood cells including RBCs, WBCs, and platelets. A bone marrow biopsy provides diagnostic information about how the bone marrow is functioning.

Blood Collection/Testing

- Blood diagnostic procedures that nurses should be knowledgeable about:

  - Serum RBC count

  - Serum WBC count

  - Mean corpuscular volume (MCV)

  - Mean corpuscular Hgb (MCH)

  - Total iron-binding count (TIBC)

  - Iron

  - Platelets

  - Hgb

  - Hct

  - Coagulation studies

    - Prothrombin time (PT)

    - Partial thromboplastin time (aPTT)

    - International normalized ratio (INR)

      - D-dimer

      - Fibrinogen levels

      - Fibrin degradation products

- CBC is a series of tests which include RBC, WBC, MCV, MCH, Hgb, and Hct.

- Indications/interpretation of findings

TEST	EXPECTED REFERENCE RANGE	PURPOSE FOR TEST
RBC	Females: 4.2 to 5.4 million/uL Males: 4.7 to 6.1 million/uL	• Decreased level of RBCs can be evidence of anemia.
WBC	5,000 to 10,000/uL	• Elevated level of WBCs can be evidence of infection. • Decreased level of WBCs can be evidence of immunosuppression.
MCV	80 to 95 mm^3	• Elevated level can be evidence of macrocytic (large) cells, possible anemia. • Decreased level can be evidence of microcytic (small) cells, possible iron deficiency anemia.
MCH	27 to 31 pg/cell	• Same as above for MCV, but measure the amount of Hgb by weight per RBC.
TIBC	250 to 460 mcg/dL	• Elevated level can be evidence of iron deficiency. • Decreased level can be evidence of anemia, hemolysis, or hemorrhage.
Iron	Females: 60 to 160 mcg/dL Males: 80 to 180 mcg/dL	• Elevated level can be evidence of hemochromatosis, iron excess, liver disorder, or megaloblastic anemia. • Decreased level can be evidence of iron deficiency anemia, or hemorrhage.
Platelets	150,000 to 400,000 mm^3	• Increased level can be evidence of malignancy or polycythemia vera. • Decreased level can be evidence of autoimmune disease, bone marrow suppression, or enlarged spleen.
Hgb	Females: 12 to 16 g/dL Males: 14 to 18 g/dL	• Same as above for RBC
Hct	Females: 37 to 47% Males: 42 to 52%	• Same as above for RBC
PT	11 to 12.5 seconds, 85 to 100%, or 1:1 client-control ratio	• Increased time can be evidence of deficiency or clotting. • Decreased time can be evidence of vitamin K excess.
aPTT	1.5 to 2 times normal range of 30 to 40 seconds (desired range for anticoagulation)	• Measures the intrinsic clotting factors. • Monitored for heparin therapy. • Increased time can be evidence of hemophilia, disseminated intravascular coagulation (DIC), or liver disease.

TEST	EXPECTED REFERENCE RANGE	PURPOSE FOR TEST
INR	2 to 3 on warfarin therapy	Measures the mean of PT. Client's PT divided by average mean PT. Monitored for warfarin (Coumadin) therapy.
D-dimer	0.43 to 2.33 mcg/mL 0 to 250 ng/mL	Measures hypercoagulability of the blood. Elevated D-dimer indicates clot formation has occurred.
Fibrinogen levels	170 to 340 mg/dL	Reflects available fibrinogen for clotting. Decreased levels may indicate decreased ability to clot.
Fibrin degradation products	Less than 10 mcg/mL	Increases when clot dissolving activity (fibrinolysis) is occurring. Monitors efficacy of medications for DIC.

- Preprocedure

  - Nursing Actions

    - Use standard precautions in collecting and handling blood for specimen collection.

- Intraprocedure

  - Nursing Actions

    - Vials are usually labeled according to laboratory value that will be tested.

    - A sufficient quantity of a blood should be collected and placed in a vial and filled to the black line indicated on the vial tube.

    - The specimen must be properly labeled and delivered to the laboratory promptly for appropriate storage and analysis. Check facility protocol regarding timeframe within which the specimen must be delivered to the laboratory.

    - For coagulation studies, blood will be required to be drawn at specific times and sent to the laboratory immediately so that the nurse can adjust the dose of anticoagulant therapy based on the results.

- Postprocedure

  - Nursing Actions

    - Results of hematologic tests are usually available preliminarily within 24 to 48 hr, with final results in 72 hr.

    - If results are out of expected reference range, it is the nurse's responsibility to report the results to the provider for further intervention.

Bone Marrow Aspiration/Biopsy

- A biopsy is the extraction of a very small amount of tissue, such as bone marrow, to definitively diagnose cell type and to confirm or rule out malignancy. A bone marrow tissue sample is removed by needle aspiration for cytological (histological) examination.

  ○ Biopsies can be performed with local anesthesia or conscious sedation in an ambulatory setting, intraoperatively, and/or during scope procedures.

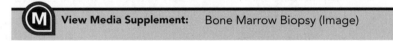

View Media Supplement: Bone Marrow Biopsy (Image)

- Indications

  ○ A bone marrow biopsy is commonly performed to diagnose causes of blood disorders, such as anemia or thrombocytopenia, or to rule-out diseases, such as leukemia and other cancers.

- Interpretation of Findings

  ○ After a procedure is completed, the tissue sample is sent to pathology for interpretation.

- Preprocedure

  ○ Nursing Actions

    ▪ Ensure that the client has signed the informed consent form.

    ▪ Position the client in a prone or side lying position to expose the ileac crest for the procedure.

  ○ Client Education

    ▪ Explain the procedure to the client. The biopsy site will be anesthetized with a local anesthetic, and the client may feel pressure during the aspiration.

- Intraprocedure

  ○ Nursing Actions

    ▪ Medicate the client with a sedative if prescribed.

      □ Older adult clients are at greater risk for complications associated with sedation for biopsy procedures due to chronic illnesses.

      □ An older adult's renal clearance also needs to be considered when using any analgesics for sedation.

    ▪ Assist the provider with the test/procedure as needed.

    ▪ As appropriate, apply pressure to the biopsy site to control bleeding.

    ▪ As appropriate, place a sterile dressing over the biopsy site.

- Postprocedure

  - Nursing Actions

    - Monitor the client for evidence of infection (fever, increased WBCs, pain, and swelling at the site) and bleeding.

    - Apply ice to the incision site if prescribed.

    - Postprocedure discomfort is usually relieved by mild analgesics.

    - Avoid aspirin and other medications that affect clotting.

  - Client Education

    - Teach the client to report excessive bleeding and/or signs of infection to the provider.

    - Teach the client to check the incision daily. The incision should be clean, dry, and intact.

    - If sutures are in place, remind the client to return in 7 to 10 days to have them removed.

- Complications

  - Infection

    - Infection can occur at the aspiration site.

    - Nursing Actions

      - Monitor the site and keep it clean and dry.

  - Bleeding

    - Bleeding can occur from the site.

    - Nursing Actions

      - Report bleeding to the primary care provider immediately.

CHAPTER 43: HEMATOLOGIC DIAGNOSTIC PROCEDURES

Ⓐ Application Exercises

1. A nurse is admitting a client in the emergency department who reports thirst, tiredness, and difficulty concentrating. Upon assessment, the nurse notices that the client is pale and has heart palpitations. The nurse suspects that the client may be anemic. Which of the following tests should the nurse anticipate to be ordered?

    A. International normalized ratio (INR)

    B. Platelet count

    C. WBC count

    D. Hgb

2. A nurse is caring for a client who has hemophilia. Which of the following tests should the nurse anticipate to be ordered to check for this diagnosis?

    A. RBC

    B. WBC

    C. aPTT

    D. INR

3. A nurse is providing teaching for a client who needs to have a bone marrow aspiration of the iliac crest. Which of the following statements made by the client indicates a need for further teaching?

    A. "Cancer can be detected in the fluid being tested."

    B. "I will feel a heavy pressure sensation in my hip bone."

    C. "The need for antibiotics can be determined with this test."

    D. "I will be awake during the procedure."

CHAPTER 43: HEMATOLOGIC DIAGNOSTIC PROCEDURES

 Application Exercises Answer Key

1. A nurse is admitting a client in the emergency department who reports thirst, tiredness, and difficulty concentrating. Upon assessment, the nurse notices that the client is pale and has heart palpitations. The nurse suspects that the client may be anemic. Which of the following tests should the nurse anticipate to be ordered?

    A. International normalized ratio (INR)

    B. Platelet count

    C. WBC count

    D. Hemoglobin

    An Hgb test is ordered to check for anemia. INR, platelet count, and WBC count are not indicated for anemia.

 NCLEX® Connection: Reduction of Risk Potential, Diagnostic Tests

2. A nurse is caring for a client who has hemophilia. Which of the following tests should the nurse anticipate to be ordered to check for this diagnosis?

    A. RBC

    B. WBC

    C. aPTT

    D. INR

    PTT checks the clotting factors and is indicated for a client who has hemophilia. RBC, WBC, and INR are not indicated for this client.

 NCLEX® Connection: Reduction of Risk Potential, Diagnostic Tests

3. A nurse is providing teaching for a client who needs to have a bone marrow aspiration of the iliac crest. Which of the following statements made by the client indicates a need for further teaching?

    A. "Cancer can be detected in the fluid being tested."

    B. "I will feel a heavy pressure sensation in my hip bone."

    C. "The need for antibiotics can be determined with this test."

    D. "I will be awake during the procedure."

    The fluid from a bone marrow aspiration is not being tested for the presence of an infection and the need for antibiotics. Cancer can be detected in the fluid; the client will feel a heavy pressure in the hip bone; and the client will be awake during the procedure.

 NCLEX® Connection: Reduction of Risk Potential, Diagnostic Tests

UNIT 5	NURSING CARE OF CLIENTS WITH HEMATOLOGIC DISORDERS
Section	Diagnostic and Therapeutic Procedures
Chapter 44	Blood and Blood Product Transfusions

Overview

- Whole blood or components of whole blood can be transfused for clients who require replacement due to blood loss or blood disease.

- Blood components:

  - Packed RBCs

  - Plasma

  - Albumin

  - Clotting factors

  - Prothrombin complex

  - Cryoprecipitate

  - Platelets

Transfusions

- Blood and blood products must be administered intravenously through a cannula of large caliber (usually a 20-gauge needle).

  - Transfusion Types

    - Homologous transfusions – blood from donors is used

    - Autologous transfusions – the client's own blood is collected in anticipation of future transfusions (elective surgery); this blood is designated for and can be used only by the client

      - Intraoperative blood salvage – blood loss during certain surgeries can be recycled through a cell-saver machine and transfused intraoperatively or postoperatively (orthopedic surgeries, CABG)

- Indications

  - Diagnoses

    - Excessive blood loss (Hgb 6 to 10 g/dL, depending on symptoms) – whole blood

    - Anemia (Hgb 6 to 10 g/dL, depending on symptoms) – packed RBCs

- Chronic renal failure – packed RBCs
- Coagulation factor deficiencies such as hemophilia – fresh frozen plasma
- Thrombocytopenia/platelet dysfunction (platelets < 20,000 or < 80,000 and actively bleeding) – platelets

- Preprocedure

  - Incompatibility is a major concern when administering blood or blood products, and preventing incompatibility requires strict adherence to blood transfusion protocols.

    - Blood is typed based on the presence of antigens.

BLOOD TYPE	ANTIGEN	ANTIBODIES AGAINST	COMPATIBLE WITH
A	A	B	A, O
B	B	A	B, O
AB	AB	None	A, B, AB, O
O	None	A, B	O

    - Another consideration is the Rh-factor – blood that contains D antigen makes the Rh factor positive. Rh-positive blood given to an Rh-negative person will cause hemolysis.

  - Nursing Actions

    - Assess laboratory values, such as Hgb and Hct. Packed RBCs are usually prescribed for clients with an Hgb of less than 8 g/dL.
    - Verify the prescription for a specific blood product.
    - Obtain blood samples for compatibility determination, such as type and crossmatch.
    - Initiate large-bore IV access. A 20-gauge needle is standard for administering blood products.
      - For older adult clients, venous access for blood transfusions may be limited due to age-related vascular and skin changes.
    - Assess the client for a history of blood-transfusion reactions.
    - Obtain blood products from the blood bank. Inspect the blood for discoloration, excessive bubbles, or cloudiness.
    - Following specific institution protocol: confirm the client's identity, blood compatibility, and expiration time of the blood product with another nurse.
    - Prime the blood administration set with normal saline (NS). Blood products are only infused with 0.9% sodium chloride. Never add medications to blood products.
    - Ascertain whether or not a filter should be used.
    - Obtain the client's baseline vital signs.

- Begin the transfusion and use a blood warmer if indicated.
  - o Client Education
    - Explain to the client the reason for the blood transfusion.
- Intraprocedure
  - o Nursing Actions
    - Remain with the client for the first 15 to 30 min of the infusion (reactions occur most often during first 15 min) and monitor:
      - □ Vital signs (then every hour afterward).
      - □ Rate of infusion.
      - □ Respiratory status.
      - □ Sudden increase in anxiety.
      - □ Breath sounds.
      - □ Neck-vein distention.
    - For older adult clients, assess vital signs more frequently because changes in pulse, blood pressure, and respiratory rate may indicate fluid overload or may be the sole indicators of a transfusion reaction. Older adult clients with cardiac or renal dysfunction are at an increased risk for heart failure and fluid-volume excess when receiving a blood transfusion.
    - Notify the primary health care provider immediately if any signs of a reaction occur.
    - Complete the transfusion within a 2 to 4 hr time frame to avoid bacterial growth.
- Postprocedure
  - o Nursing Actions
    - Obtain the client's vital signs upon completion of the transfusion.
    - Dispose of the blood-administration set appropriately (biohazard bags).
    - Monitor blood values as prescribed (CBC, Hgb, Hct).
      - □ Hgb levels should rise by approximately 1 g/dL with each unit transfused.
    - Complete paperwork and file in the appropriate places.
    - Document the client's response.
- Complications
  - o Transfusion Reactions

TYPE OF REACTION	ONSET	SIGNS AND SYMPTOMS
Acute hemolytic	Immediate	This reaction may be mild or life-threatening. Symptoms include: chills, fever, low back pain, tachycardia, flushing, hypotension, chest tightening or pain, tachypnea, nausea, anxiety, and hemoglobinuria. This reaction may cause cardiovascular collapse, acute renal failure, disseminated intravascular coagulation, shock, and death.
Febrile	30 min to 6 hr after transfusion	Symptoms include: chills, fever, flushing, headache, and anxiety. Use WBC filter. Administer antipyretics.
Mild allergic	During or up to 24 hr after transfusion	Symptoms include: itching, urticaria, and flushing. Administer antihistamines, such as diphenhydramine (Benadryl).
Anaphylactic	Immediate	Symptoms include: wheezing, dyspnea, chest tightness, cyanosis, and hypotension. Maintain airway; administer oxygen, IV fluids, antihistamines, corticosteroids, and vasopressors.

- Nursing Actions

  □ Stop the transfusion immediately if a reaction is suspected.

  □ Initiate an infusion of 0.9% sodium chloride. The infusion should be initiated with a separate line, so as not to infuse more blood from the transfusion tubing.

  □ Save the blood bag with the remaining blood and the blood tubing for testing at the laboratory following agency protocol.

- Client Education

  □ Explain to client the reason that the blood is being discontinued.

○ Circulatory overload

- Clients with impaired cardiac function can experience circulatory overload as a result of a transfusion.

  □ Signs and symptoms include – dyspnea, chest tightness, tachycardia, tachypnea, headache, hypertension, jugular-vein distention, peripheral edema, orthopnea, sudden anxiety, and crackles in the base of the lungs.

- Nursing Actions

  □ Administer oxygen, monitor vital signs, slow the infusion rate, and administer diuretics as prescribed.

  □ Notify the primary health care provider immediately.

- ○ Sepsis and septic shock
  - ■ Symptoms include – fever, nausea, vomiting, abdominal pain, chills, and hypotension.
  - ■ Nursing Actions
    - □ Maintain patent airway and administer oxygen.
    - □ Administer antibiotic therapy as prescribed.
    - □ Obtain samples for blood cultures.
    - □ Administer vasopressors, such as dopamine, to combat vasodilation in the late phase.
    - □ Elevate the client's feet.
    - □ If disseminated intravascular coagulation (DIC) occurs:
      - ▸ Administer anticoagulants, such as heparin, in the early phase.
      - ▸ Administer clotting factors and blood products during the late phase (clotting factors are used up in the early stage).
      - ▸ Administer activated protein C (Xigris) to control inflammatory response.

CHAPTER 44: BLOOD AND BLOOD PRODUCT TRANSFUSIONS

(A) Application Exercises

1. Fill in the types of blood that each of the following clients may receive.

CLIENT'S BLOOD TYPE	COMPATIBLE BLOOD TYPES
A⁺	
A⁻	
B⁺	
B⁻	
AB⁺	
AB⁻	
O⁺	
O⁻	

2. A nurse should remain with a client during the first 15 min of a blood transfusion to

    A. verify the blood is being transfused.

    B. assess for an adverse reaction.

    C. explain the procedure to the client.

    D. obtain consent for the blood transfusion.

3. What actions should a nurse take if there is a possible transfusion reaction? (Select all that apply.)

    _____ Stop the transfusion.

    _____ Send the blood bag and IV tubing to the blood bank for analysis.

    _____ Maintain an IV infusion with 0.9% sodium chloride.

    _____ Notify the primary care provider.

    _____ Obtain blood cultures.

4. A nurse is monitoring a client who began receiving a unit of blood 10 min ago. Which of the following should pose an immediate concern for the nurse? (Select all that apply.)

    _____ Temperature change from 37° C (98.6° F) pretransfusion to 37.2° C (99.0° F) posttransfusion

    _____ Dyspnea

    _____ Restlessness

    _____ Heart rate increase: 74/min pretransfusion, 81/min posttransfusion

    _____ Client report of itching

    _____ Client appears flushed

CHAPTER 44: BLOOD AND BLOOD PRODUCT TRANSFUSIONS

 Application Exercises Answer Key

1. Fill in the types of blood that each of the following clients may receive.

CLIENT'S BLOOD TYPE	COMPATIBLE BLOOD TYPES
A⁺	A⁺, A⁻, O⁺, O⁻
A⁻	A⁻, O⁻
B⁺	B⁺, B⁻, O⁺, O⁻
B⁻	B⁻, O⁻
AB⁺	AB⁺, AB⁻, A⁺, A⁻, B⁺, B⁻, O⁺, O⁻
AB⁻	AB⁻, A⁻, B⁻, O⁻
O⁺	O⁺, O⁻
O⁻	O⁻

 NCLEX® Connection: Pharmacological and Parenteral Therapies, Blood and Blood Products

2. The nurse should remain with the client during the first 15 min of a blood transfusion to

    A. verify the blood being transfused.

    B. assess for an adverse reaction.

    C. explain the procedure to the client.

    D. obtain consent for the blood transfusion.

Assessing for a blood reaction typically occurs within the first 15 min of the transfusion. Verifying the blood, explaining the procedure, and obtaining consent should all be done prior to administrating the blood.

 NCLEX® Connection: Pharmacological and Parenteral Therapies, Blood and Blood Products

3. What actions should a nurse take if there is a possible transfusion reaction? (Select all that apply.)

    __X__ **Stop the transfusion.**

    __X__ **Send the blood bag and IV tubing to the blood bank for analysis.**

    __X__ **Maintain an IV infusion with 0.9% sodium chloride.**

    __X__ **Notify the primary care provider.**

    _____ Obtain blood cultures.

When a possible transfusion reaction is suspected, the nurse should stop the infusion, send the blood bag and IV tubing to the blood bank for analysis, maintain an IV infusion with 0.9% sodium chloride, and notify the provider. Blood and urine specimens are usually obtained to determine hemolysis, but blood cultures are not routinely done unless sepsis is suspected.

 NCLEX® Connection: Pharmacological and Parenteral Therapies, Blood and Blood Products

4. A nurse is monitoring a client who began receiving a unit of blood 10 min ago. Which of the following should pose an immediate concern for a nurse? (Select all that apply.)

_____ Temperature change from 37° C (98.6° F) pretransfusion to 37.2° C (99.0° F) posttransfusion

__X__ **Dyspnea**

__X__ **Restlessness**

_____ Heart rate increase: 74/min pretransfusion, 81/min post-transfusion

__X__ **Client report of itching**

__X__ **Flushed appearance**

Dyspnea, restlessness, report of itching and a flushed appearance may indicate a transfusion reaction. A slight increase in heart rate and temperature is an expected finding.

Ⓝ NCLEX® Connection: Pharmacological and Parenteral Therapies, Blood and Blood Products

UNIT 5	NURSING CARE OF CLIENTS WITH HEMATOLOGIC DISORDERS
Section	Hematologic Disorders
Chapter 45	Anemias

 Overview

- Anemia is an abnormally low amount of circulating RBCs, Hgb concentration, or both.

- Anemia results in diminished oxygen-carrying capacity and delivery to tissues and organs. The goal of treatment is to restore and maintain adequate tissue oxygenation.

- Anemias are due to:

    o   Blood loss.

    o   Inadequate RBC production (hypoproliferative).

    o   Increased RBC destruction (hemolytic).

    o   Deficiency of necessary components such as folic acid, iron, and/or vitamin B_{12}.

- Iron-deficiency anemia due to inadequate intake is the most common cause of anemia in children, adolescents, and pregnant women.

- Iron-deficiency anemia due to blood loss (such as from a gastrointestinal ulcer) is the most common cause of anemia in men and women who are post menopausal. Women who are menstruating can develop anemia secondary to menorrhagia.

Health Promotion and Disease Prevention

- Women who are pregnant or menstruating should ensure that their diet contains adequate amounts of iron-rich foods. Otherwise, they should take an iron supplement.

    o   Women who are pregnant should plan to take an adequate amount of folic acid to prevent neural tube defects (spina bifida) in the newborn.

- Individuals who are iron deficient, but have elevated cholesterol levels, should integrate iron-rich foods that are not red or organ meats into their diets (iron-fortified cereal and breads, fish and poultry, and dried peas and beans).

Assessment

- Risk Factors

    - Acute or chronic blood loss

        - Menorrhagia

        - Gastrointestinal bleed (ulcers, tumor)

        - Intra or postsurgical blood loss or hemorrhage

    - Increased hemolysis

        - Defective Hgb (sickle-cell disease) – RBCs become malformed during periods of hypoxia and obstruct capillaries in joints and organs

        - Impaired glycolysis – Glucose-6-phosphate-dehydrogenase (G6PD) deficiency anemia

        - Immune disorder or destruction (transfusion reactions, autoimmune diseases)

        - Mechanical trauma to RBCs (mechanical heart valve, cardiopulmonary bypass)

    - Inadequate dietary intake

        - Iron deficiency

        - Vitamin B_{12} deficiency – Pernicious anemia due to deficiency of intrinsic factor produced by gastric mucosa, which is necessary for absorption of vitamin B_{12}

        - Folic-acid deficiency

        - Pica, or a persistent eating of substances not normally considered food (non nutritive substances), such as soil or chalk, for at least 1 month, may limit the amount of healthy food choices a client makes

    - Bone-marrow suppression

        - Exposure to radiation or chemicals (such as insecticides or solvents)

        - Aplastic anemia results in a decreased number of RBCs as well as decreased platelets and WBCs.

    - Older adult clients are at risk for nutrition-deficient anemias (iron, vitamin B_{12}, folate).

    - Anemia may be misdiagnosed as depression or debilitation in older adult clients.

    - Gastrointestinal bleeding is a common cause of anemia in older adult clients.

- Subjective Data

    - May be asymptomatic in mild cases

    - Pallor

    - Fatigue

    - Irritability

    - Numbness and tingling of extremities

- o Dyspnea on exertion
- o Sensitivity to cold
- o Pain and hypoxia with sickle-cell crisis
- Objective Data
  - o Physical Assessment Findings
    - Shortness of breath/fatigue, especially upon exertion
    - Tachycardia and palpitations
    - Dizziness or fainting upon standing or with exertion
    - Pallor with pale nail beds and mucous membranes
    - Nail bed deformities
    - Smooth, sore, bright red tongue (vitamin B_{12} deficiency)
  - o Laboratory Tests
    - CBC count
      - □ RBCs are the major carriers of hemoglobin in the blood.
      - □ Hgb transports oxygen and carbon dioxide to and from the cells and can be used as an index of the oxygen-carrying capacity of the blood.
      - □ Hct is the percentage of RBCs in relation to the total blood volume.
    - RBC indices are used to determine the type and cause of most anemias
      - □ Mean corpuscular volume (MCV) – Size of red blood cells
        - ‣ Normocytic – Normal size
        - ‣ Microcytic – Small cells
        - ‣ Macrocytic – Large cells
    - Mean corpuscular Hgb (MCH): to determine the amount of Hgb per RBC
      - □ Normochromic – normal amount of Hgb per cell
      - □ Hypochromic – decreased Hgb per cell
    - Mean corpuscular Hgb concentration (MCHC) – To indicate Hgb amount relative to the size of the cell

RBC INDICES	CLASSIFICATION	POSSIBLE CAUSES
Normal MCV, MCH, MCHC	Normocytic, normochromic anemia	• Acute blood loss • Sickle-cell disease
Decreased MCV, MCH, MCHC	Microcytic, hypochromic anemia	• Iron-deficiency anemia • Anemia of chronic illness • Chronic blood loss
Increased MCV	Macrocytic anemia	• Vitamin B_{12} deficiency • Folic-acid deficiency

- Iron studies
  - Total iron-binding capacity (TIBC) reflects an indirect measurement of serum transferrin, a protein that binds with iron and transports it for storage.
  - Serum ferritin is an indicator of total iron stores in the body.
  - Serum iron measures the amount of iron in the blood. Low serum iron and elevated TIBC indicates iron-deficiency anemia.
- Hgb electrophoresis separates normal Hgb from abnormal. It is used to detect thalassemia and sickle-cell disease.
- A sickle-cell test evaluates the sickling of RBCs in the presence of decreased oxygen tension.

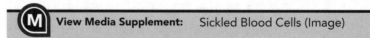

View Media Supplement: Sickled Blood Cells (Image)

- A Schilling test measures vitamin B_{12} absorption with and without intrinsic factor. It is used to differentiate between malabsorption and pernicious anemia.
  - Diagnostic Procedures
    - Bone-marrow examination
      - It is used to diagnose aplastic anemia (failure of bone marrow to produce RBCs as well as platelets and WBCs).

Collaborative Care

- Nursing Care
  - Encourage the client to increase her dietary intake of the deficient nutrient (iron, vitamin B_{12}, folic acid).
  - Administer medications to the client, as prescribed, at the proper time for optimal absorption, and using an appropriate technique.
  - Teach the client and family about energy conservation in the client and the risk of the client experiencing dizziness upon standing.
  - Teach the client about the time frame for resolution.

- Medications

    o Iron supplements - ferrous sulfate (Feosol), ferrous fumarate (Feostat), ferrous gluconate (Fergon)

        ■ Oral iron supplements are used to replenish the client's serum iron and iron stores. Iron is an essential component of Hgb, and subsequently, oxygen transport.

        ■ Parenteral iron supplements (iron dextran) are only given for severe anemia.

        ■ Nursing Considerations

            □ Administer parenteral iron to a client using the Z-track method.

        ■ Client Education

            □ Instruct to have hemoglobin checked in 4 to 6 weeks to determine efficacy.

            □ Vitamin C may increase oral iron absorption.

            □ Instruct the client to take iron supplements between meals to increase absorption, if tolerated.

    o Erythropoietin – Epoetin alfa (Epogen, Procrit)

        ■ A hematopoietic growth factor used to increase production of RBCs

        ■ Nursing Considerations

            □ Observe the client for an increase in blood pressure.

            □ Monitor Hgb and Hct twice a week.

            □ Monitor the client for cardiovascular event if Hgb increases too rapidly (>1 gm/dL in 2 weeks).

        ■ Client Education

            □ Reinforce the importance of having Hgb and Hct evaluated on a twice-a-week basis.

    o Vitamin B_{12} supplementation (cyanocobalamin)

        ■ Vitamin B_{12} is necessary to convert folic acid from its inactive form to its active form. All cells rely on folic acid for DNA production.

        ■ Vitamin B_{12} supplementation can be given orally if the deficit is due to inadequate dietary intake. However, if deficiency is due to lack of intrinsic factor being produced by the parietal cells of the stomach or malabsorption syndrome, it must be given parenterally or intranasally to be absorbed.

        ■ Nursing Considerations

            □ Give vitamin B_{12} according to appropriate route related to cause of Vitamin B_{12} anemia (parenteral versus oral).

            □ Administer parenteral forms of vitamin B_{12} intramuscularly or deep subcutaneous to decrease irritation. Do not mix other medications in the syringe.

- Client Education

  □ Clients who lack intrinsic factor or have an irreversible-malabsorption syndrome should be informed that this therapy must be continued for the rest of their life.

  □ A client should receive vitamin B_{12} injections on a monthly basis.

  o Folic acid supplements

  - Folic-acid is a water-soluble, B-complex vitamin. It is necessary for the production of new RBCs.

  - Nursing Considerations

    □ Folic acid can be given orally or parenterally.

  - Client Education

    □ Large doses of folic acid will turn the client's urine dark yellow.

- Therapeutic Procedures

  o Blood transfusions – lead to an immediate improvement in blood-cell counts and client signs and symptoms.

  - Typically only used when the client has significant symptoms of anemia, because of the risk of blood-borne infections.

- Client Outcomes

  o The client's Hgb and Hct will return to a value within the normal reference range

  o The client will report less fatigue

Complications

- Heart failure

  o Heart failure can develop due to the increased demand on the heart to increase oxygen to tissues.

  o A low Hct decreases the amount of oxygen carried to tissues in the body, which makes the heart work harder and beat faster (tachycardia, palpitations).

  o Nursing Actions

  - Administer oxygen and monitor the client's pulse oximetry.

  - Monitor the client's cardiac rhythm.

  - Obtain the client's daily weight.

  - Administer a blood transfusion to the client as prescribed.

  - Give the client cardiac medications as prescribed (diuretics, antidysrhythmics).

  - Give the client antianemia medications as prescribed.

CHAPTER 45: ANEMIAS

 Application Exercises

1. Provide assessment findings for each of the following body systems that indicate anemia.

BODY SYSTEM	ASSESSMENT FINDINGS
Integumentary	
Gastrointestinal	
Cardiovascular	
Respiratory	
Musculoskeletal	
Neurologic	

2. A nurse is caring for a client who was admitted with an Hgb of 7.5 and an Hct of 21.5. Which of the following should the nurse include in the client's plan of care? (Select all that apply.)

_____ Provide assistance when ambulating to the restroom.

_____ Monitor pulse rate.

_____ Weigh the client daily.

_____ Test stools for occult blood.

_____ Schedule a time for rest periods.

_____ Encourage intake of potato products.

3. A nurse is teaching a client about how to take an oral iron supplement. Which of the following is appropriate information to include?

A. Stools will be dark red in color.

B. Iron may be taken with a glass of milk if gastrointestinal distress occurs.

C. Foods high in vitamin C will increase iron absorption.

D. Iron therapy will only be needed for 2 consecutive weeks.

4. A nurse is instructing a client who is in the first trimester of her pregnancy about prenatal vitamins. Which of the following must be taken in adequate amounts to prevent spina bifida in the fetus?

    A. Vitamin B_{12}

    B. Folic acid

    C. Calcium

    D. Iron

5. A nurse is providing education to a client who has just had a gastrectomy for stomach cancer. Which of the following information is appropriate to include? (Select all that apply.)

    _____ You must receive a monthly vitamin B_{12} injection for the rest of your life.

    _____ Taking vitamin B_{12} on a daily basis in the form of cyanocobalamin (CaloMist) nasal spray may be an option.

    _____ A vitamin B_{12} oral supplement must be taken on a daily basis.

    _____ You should increase the amount of vitamin B_{12} in your diet by eating more animal protein, legumes, and dairy products.

    _____ You can drink soy milk fortified with vitamin B_{12} to decrease your risk of pernicious anemia.

CHAPTER 45: ANEMIAS

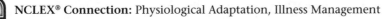 Application Exercises Answer Key

1. Provide assessment findings for each of the following body systems that indicate anemia.

BODY SYSTEM	ASSESSMENT FINDINGS
Integumentary	Pallor of skin, mucous membranes, conjunctiva and nail beds; petechiae, purpura, cheilosis, spoon-shaped nail, sore beefy red tongue
Gastrointestinal	Anorexia, diarrhea, nausea, abdominal pain
Cardiovascular	Tachycardia, palpitations
Respiratory	Tachypnea, dyspnea on exertion
Musculoskeletal	Fatigue, weakness, night cramps, joint pain
Neurologic	Paresthesias, headache, dizziness, forgetfulness, pain, pica

NCLEX® Connection: Reduction of Risk Potential, Potential for Alterations in Body Systems

2. A nurse is caring for a client who was admitted with an Hgb of 7.5 and an Hct of 21.5. Which of the following should the nurse include in the client's plan of care? (Select all that apply.)

   X   **Provide assistance when ambulating to the restroom.**
   X   **Monitor pulse rate.**
   X   **Weigh the client daily.**
   X   **Test stools for occult blood.**
   X   **Schedule a time for rest periods.**
          Encourage intake of potato products.

Clients who have anemia and an Hgb of 7.5 and an Hct of 21.5 will experience fatigue, dizziness, fainting, and tachycardia. Heart failure can also develop due to the heart working harder to adequately oxygenate tissues. Thus, the nurse should ensure that the client is assisted to the bathroom to prevent falls, his pulse rate and rhythm be monitored, his daily weight gain reported to the provider, stools be evaluated as a possible source of bleeding, and rest periods should be scheduled for him to prevent undue fatigue. Potato products are not high in iron and will not help alleviate the anemia.

NCLEX® Connection: Physiological Adaptation, Illness Management

3. A nurse is teaching a client about how to take an oral iron supplement. Which of the following is appropriate information to include?

    A. Stools will be dark red in color.

    B. Iron may be taken with a glass of milk if gastrointestinal distress occurs.

    C. Foods high in vitamin C will increase iron absorption.

    D. Iron therapy will only be needed for 2 consecutive weeks.

Vitamin C will increase the amount of iron absorbed by the intestinal tract. Stools will be green to black in color, milk will bind to the iron and decrease the absorption, and iron therapy usually takes 4 to 6 weeks for the Hgb and Hct to return its normal reference range.

 NCLEX® Connection: Physiological Adaptation, Illness Management

4. A nurse is instructing a client who is in the first trimester of her pregnancy about prenatal vitamins. Which of the following must be taken in adequate amounts to prevent spina bifida in the fetus?

    A. Vitamin B_{12}

    B. Folic acid

    C. Calcium

    D. Iron

Folic acid must be taken in adequate amounts to prevent neural tube defects in the fetus. While it is important to ingest adequate amounts of vitamin B_{12}, calcium, and iron, inadequate intake of these vitamins or minerals will not cause neural tube defects.

 NCLEX® Connection: Basic Care and Comfort, Nutrition, and Oral Hydration

5. A nurse is providing education to a client who has just had a gastrectomy for stomach cancer. Which of the following information is appropriate to include? (Select all that apply.)

    __X__ You must receive a monthly vitamin B_{12} injection for the rest of your life.

    __X__ Taking vitamin B_{12} on a daily basis in the form of cyanocobalamin (CaloMist) nasal spray may be an option.

    _____ A vitamin B_{12} oral supplement must be taken on a daily basis.

    _____ You should increase the amount of Vitamin B_{12} in your diet by eating more animal protein, legumes, and dairy products.

    _____ You can drink soy milk fortified with vitamin B_{12} to decrease your risk of pernicious anemia.

A client who has had a gastrectomy will need to receive monthly injections of vitamin B_{12} for the rest of his life or be placed on daily inhalations of CaloMist, a nasal form of cyanocobalamin. Oral preparations and food containing vitamin B_{12} will no longer be absorbed due to the lack of intrinsic factor normally produced by the stomach.

 NCLEX® Connection: Pharmacological and Parenteral Therapies, Expected Actions/Outcomes

UNIT 5	NURSING CARE OF CLIENTS WITH HEMATOLOGIC DISORDERS
Section	Hematologic Disorders
Chapter 46	Leukemia and Lymphoma

Overview

- Leukemias are cancers of white blood cells or of cells that will develop into white blood cells.

    o In leukemia, the white blood cells are not functional. They invade and destroy bone marrow, and they can metastasize to the liver, spleen, lymph nodes, testes, and brain.

    o Leukemias are divided into acute (acute lymphocytic leukemia and acute myelogenous leukemia) and chronic (chronic lymphocytic leukemia and chronic myelogenous leukemia) and are further classified by the type of white blood cells primarily affected.

    o Clients with leukemia are vulnerable to infection and can develop anemia secondary to bone marrow destruction.

    o The goal of treatment is to eliminate all leukemia cells.

- Lymphomas are cancers of lymphocytes (a type of white blood cell) and lymph nodes (which produce antibodies and fight infection).

    o There are two types of lymphomas – Hodgkin's lymphoma (HL) and non-Hodgkin's lymphoma (NHL).

    o Lymphomas can metastasize to almost any organ.

- The exact cause of leukemia is not known.

- Incidence and Cure Rates

    o Acute lymphocytic leukemia (ALL) – Various factors influence the prognosis for children but 5 year survival rate is approximately 85% (age at diagnosis, gender, cell type involved); less than 50% of adults can be cured.

    o Acute myelogenous leukemia (AML) – Most common leukemia among adults; prognosis is poor.

    o Chronic lymphocytic leukemia (CLL) – Most cases involve people older than 60. This disease does not occur in children – disease progresses slowly in three phases over time.

    o Chronic myelogenous leukemia (CML) – Most cases involve adults. The disease is uncommon in children; prognosis is less than two years of survival from time of diagnosis.

- Lymphoma
  - Hodgkin's Lymphoma (HL)
    - Most cases involve adults.
    - Possible causes include viral infections and exposure to chemical agents.
  - Non-Hodgkin's Lymphoma (NHL)
    - More common in clients older than 50 years.
    - Possible causes include gene damage, viral infections, autoimmune disease, and exposure to radiation or to toxic chemicals.

Health Promotion and Disease Prevention

- Use protective equipment such as a mask and ensure proper ventilation while working in environments that contain carcinogens or particles in the air.
- Influenza and pneumonia vaccinations are important for all clients who are immunosuppressed.

Assessment

- Risk Factors
  - Immunologic factors (immunosuppression)
  - Exposure to some chemicals and medications (chemotherapy agents and drugs that suppress bone marrow)
  - Genetic factors (hereditary conditions)
  - Ionizing radiation (radiation therapy, environmental)
    - Older adult clients often have diminished immune function and decreased bone marrow function, which increases their risk of complications of leukemia and lymphoma.
    - Older adult clients also have decreased energy reserves and will tire more easily during treatment. Safety is a concern with ambulation.
- Subjective and Objective Data
  - Acute leukemia
    - Bone pain
    - Joint swelling
    - Enlarged liver and spleen
    - Weight loss

- Fever

- Poor wound healing (infected lesions)

- Signs of anemia (fatigue, pallor, tachycardia, dyspnea on exertion)

- Signs of bleeding (ecchymoses, hematuria, bleeding gums)

○ HL and NHL:

- Some clients may only experience an enlarged lymph node (usually in the neck with HL).

- Other possible findings include fever, fatigue, and infections.

○ Laboratory Tests

- White blood cell (WBC) – Count Often elevated (20,000 to 100,000/mm^3) with immature WBCs in leukemia prior to treatment; decreased with treatment

- Hemoglobin, hematocrit, and platelets Decreased

- Bleeding times – Increased

○ Diagnostic Procedures

- Bone marrow aspiration and biopsy

    □ Identification of prolific quantities of immature leukemic blast cells and protein markers indicates the specific type of leukemia – lymphoid or myeloid.

    □ Nursing Actions

        ▸ Apply pressure to the site for 5 to 10 min.

        ▸ Assess vital signs frequently.

        ▸ Apply pressure dressing.

        ▸ Monitor for signs of bleeding and infection for 24 hr.

- Lymph node biopsy

    □ This biopsy involves a tissue sample to diagnose disease. Dye can sometimes be used with this type of biopsy.

    □ Hodgkin's lymphoma (HL) – The presence of Reed-Sternberg cells (B-lymphocytes that have become cancerous) is diagnostic for Hodgkin's disease.

Collaborative Care

- Nursing Care

    ○ Monitor for any signs of infection or bleeding and report immediately.

    ○ Prevent infection.

        - Frequent, thorough hand hygiene is a priority intervention.

        - Place the client in a private room.

- - Screen visitors carefully.

  - Encourage good nutrition (low-bacteria diet-Avoid salads, raw fruits, and vegetables) and fluid intake.

  - Monitor WBC counts.

  - Encourage good personal hygiene.

  - Avoid crowds if possible.

  - These interventions are especially important during chemotherapy induction and for clients who have received a bone marrow transplant.

  - Prevent injury.

    - Monitor platelet counts.

    - Assess the client frequently for obvious and occult signs of bleeding.

    - Protect the client from trauma (avoid injections and venipunctures, apply firm pressure, increase vitamin K intake).

    - Teach the client how to avoid trauma (use electric shaver, soft bristled toothbrush, avoid contact sports).

  - Conserve the client's energy.

    - Encourage rest, good nutrition, and fluid intake.

    - Ensure the client gets adequate sleep.

    - Assess the client's energy resources/capability.

    - Plan activities as appropriate.

- Medications

  - Chemotherapy

    - Chemotherapy is used to treat leukemia and lymphoma. Treatment may also include radiation of the brain and spinal cord.

PHASE	GOAL	PROCEDURE	LENGTH OF TIME
Induction therapy – Places client at high risk for infection and hemorrhage following this phase	To induce remission – defined as absence of all signs of leukemia including less than 5% blasts in bone marrow	CNS prophylaxis administered as chemotherapy to the CSF (intrathecal) or as radiation to the brain and spinal cord	Lasts 4 to 6 weeks
Consolidation or intensification therapy	To eradicate any residual leukemic cells	High doses of chemotherapy frequently administered	Lasts about 6 months
Maintenance therapy	Prevention of relapse	Use of oral chemotherapy	Lasts 2 to 3 years

PHASE	GOAL	PROCEDURE	LENGTH OF TIME
Reinduction therapy – for the client who relapses	Primary purpose is to place the client back in remission	Combinations of chemotherapy used to achieve remission	Probability of relapse occurring decreases over time

- Client Education
    - Inform client of potential side effects of medications and other treatments and actions to take
    - Encourage client to inform nurse if nausea and vomiting persist. Nutritional consult may be helpful if adequate intake is difficult to assume.
    - Instruct client to use frequent oral hygiene and use a soft toothbrush. Avoid alcohol-based mouthwash.
    - Report signs and symptoms of infection or illness immediately to provider.
    - Inform client that hair loss (alopecia) occurs 7 to 10 days after treatment begins. Encourage client to select hairpiece before treatment starts.
- Colony-stimulating medications such as filgrastim (Neupogen)
    - Stimulate the production of leukocytes
    - Nursing Considerations
        - Monitor for signs of bone pain. Monitor CBC twice weekly to check leukocyte level. Use cautiously with clients who have bone marrow cancer.
    - Client Education
        - Encourage clients to inform nurse if bone discomfort occurs.
- Interdisciplinary Care
    - Oncology services may be consulted for chemotherapy.
    - Nutritional services may be contacted for weight loss or gain of client related to medications or diagnosis.
    - Rehabilitation team may be consulted if client has prolonged weakness and needs assistance with increasing level of activity.
    - Bone marrow transplantation
        - Bone marrow is destroyed or "ablated" using radiation or chemotherapy.
        - Closely matched donor stem cells are infused to replace destroyed cells.
            - Autologous cells are the client's own cells that are collected before chemotherapy.
            - Syngeneic cells are donated from the client's identical twin.
            - Allogeneic cells are obtained from an HLA-matched donor, such as a relative or from umbilical cord blood.
        - Following transplantation, the client is at high risk for infection and bleeding until the transfused stem cells begin producing white blood cells again.

- ○ Care after Discharge
  - Home health services may be consulted if client is going to receive infusions at home or on an outpatient basis.
  - Nutritional services may be consulted to meet the client's dietary needs.
- ○ Client Education
  - Teach the client/family to recognize signs of infection, skin breakdown, and nutritional deficiency.
  - Encourage the client to maintain good hygiene.
  - Teach the client to avoid individuals with colds/infections/viruses.
  - Instruct the client/family to administer medications and nutritional support at home.
  - Instruct the client/family in the proper use of vascular access devices.
  - Instruct the client/family about bleeding precautions and management of active bleeding.
- Client Outcomes
  - ○ Client will be free from infection.
  - ○ Client will have no signs of bleeding.
  - ○ Client will have increased level of activity.

Complications

- Pancytopenia – Decrease in white and red blood cells and platelets
  - ○ Neutropenia secondary to disease and/or treatment, which greatly increases the client's risk for infection
    - Nursing Actions
      - □ Maintain a hygienic environment and encourage the client to do the same.
      - □ Monitor the client closely for signs of infection (cough, alterations in breath sounds, urine, or feces). Report temperature greater than 37.8° C (100° F).
      - □ Administer antimicrobial, antiviral, and antifungal medications as prescribed.
      - □ An absolute neutrophil count (ANC) less than 2,000/mm^3 suggests an increased risk of infection. An ANC of less than 500/mm^3 indicates a severe risk of infection.
      - □ Administer blood products (granulocytes) as needed.

- o Thrombocytopenia secondary to disease and/or treatment, which greatly increases the client's risk for bleeding
  - ■ Nursing Actions
    - □ Minimize the risk of trauma (safe environment).
    - □ The greatest risk is at platelet counts less than 50,000/mm^3, and spontaneous bleeds can occur at less than 20,000/mm^3.
    - □ Administer blood products (platelets) as needed.
- o Anemia secondary to disease and/or treatment, which greatly increases the client's risk for hypoxemia
  - ■ Nursing Actions
    - □ Maintain an environment that does not overly tax the client's energy resources/capability.
    - □ Monitor red blood cell counts.
    - □ Provide a diet high in protein and carbohydrates.
    - □ Administer colony-stimulating factors, such as epoetin alfa (Procrit), as prescribed.
    - □ Administer blood products (packed red blood cells) as needed.
- • Bone Marrow Transplant Complications
  - o Failure of stem cells to engraft
    - ■ Stem cells fail to grow. Bone marrow transplant must be repeated.
  - o Graft-versus-host disease
    - ■ Graft rejection
    - ■ Nursing Actions
      - □ Administer immunosuppressants as prescribed.
  - o Phlebitis
    - ■ May occur in the blood vessels of the liver
      - □ May occur up to one month after bone marrow transplant
    - ■ Nursing Actions
      - □ Monitor for jaundice, abdominal pain, and liver enlargement.
      - □ Monitor daily weights and abdominal girth to assess for fluid retention.

CHAPTER 46: LEUKEMIA AND LYMPHOMA

Ⓐ Application Exercises

1. A client who has leukemia develops thrombocytopenia following chemotherapy. Based on this specific finding, which of the following nursing interventions is the priority?

    A. Encourage the client to turn, cough, and deep breathe every 2 hr.

    B. Monitor the client's temperature every 4 hr.

    C. Monitor the client's platelet counts.

    D. Encourage the client to take frequent rest periods throughout the day.

2. Which of the following nursing interventions and client instructions are appropriate in caring for a client who has pancytopenia? (Select all that apply and identify the rationale for each chosen option.)

    _____ Restrict fresh fruits and vegetables in the diet.

    _____ Restrict all visitors.

    _____ Insert a Foley catheter to monitor intake and output.

    _____ Restrict fluids.

    _____ Report low-grade temperature.

    _____ Hold firm pressure for 5 min following necessary venipunctures.

    _____ Report an ANC of 2,500/mm³.

    _____ Administer epoetin alfa (Procrit) as prescribed.

3. A client's platelet count is 10,000/mm³. Based on this laboratory value, which of the following is the priority nursing assessment?

    A. Level of consciousness

    B. Skin turgor

    C. Bowel sounds

    D. Breath sounds

4. Match the following.

    _____ Hodgkin's lymphoma   A. Most common leukemia in adults

    _____ Acute myelogenous leukemia (AML)   B. Most cases are in adults over the age of 60

    _____ Chronic lymphocytic leukemia (CLL)   C. Reed-Sternberg cells

    _____ Non-Hodgkin's lymphoma   D. Can be caused by radiation

CHAPTER 46: LEUKEMIA AND LYMPHOMA

 Application Exercises Answer Key

1. A client who has leukemia develops thrombocytopenia following chemotherapy. Based on this specific finding, which of the following nursing interventions is the priority?

    A. Encourage the client to turn, cough, and deep breathe every 2 hr.

    B. Monitor the client's temperature every 4 hr.

    C. Monitor the client's platelet counts.

    D. Encourage the client to take frequent rest periods throughout the day.

The greatest risk to the client who has thrombocytopenia is bleeding. Bleeding precautions are generally implemented for platelet counts less than 50,000/mm³. Encouraging the client to turn, cough, and deep breath, monitoring the client's temperature, and encouraging frequent rest periods are important, but none of them is the priority at this time.

 NCLEX® Connection: Reduction of Risk Potential, Potential for Alterations in Body Systems

2. Which of the following nursing interventions and client instructions are appropriate in caring for a client who has pancytopenia? (Select all that apply and identify the rationale for each chosen option.)

    __X__   **Restrict fresh fruits and vegetables in the diet.**

    _____   Restrict visitors.

    _____   Insert a Foley urinary catheter to monitor intake and output.

    _____   Restrict fluids.

    __X__   **Report low-grade temperature.**

    __X__   **Hold firm pressure for 5 min following necessary venipunctures.**

    _____   Report an ANC of 2,500/mm³.

    __X__   **Administer epoetin alfa (Procrit) as prescribed.**

Fresh fruits and vegetables pose a risk for introduction of bacteria into the gastrointestinal systems. A low-grade temperature may represent an immune response to an infection for clients who are immunosuppressed. Clients are at greater risk for bleeding due to low platelet counts. Firm pressure for longer periods of time is indicated following invasive procedures. Anemia is a probable consequence of the disease and/or treatment. Administration of a colony stimulating factor, such as epoetin alfa, can be vital in RBC production to counter disease/treatment-induced anemia. An absolute neutrophil count (ANC) less than 2,000/mm³ increases the risk of infection. Visitors should wear a protective mask and practice good hand hygiene. Only individuals who have a communicable disease should be restricted. There is no reason to insert an indwelling urinary catheter or restrict fluids.

 NCLEX® Connection: Reduction of Risk Potential, Potential for Complications of Diagnostic Tests/Treatments/Procedures

3. A client's platelet count is 10,000/mm³. Based on this laboratory value, which of the following is the priority nursing assessment?

   A. level of consciousness

   B. Skin turgor

   C. Bowel sounds

   D. Breath sounds

   The greatest risk to the client is spontaneous bleeding, including the risk for a fatal cerebral bleed, due to a platelet count less than 20,000/mm³. A change in level of consciousness can be an early sign of cerebral hemorrhage. Assessing skin turgor, bowel sounds, and breath sounds are not priority actions.

   Ⓝ NCLEX® Connection: Reduction of Risk Potential, System Specific Assessment

4. Match the following.

__C__	Hodgkin's lymphoma	A. Most common leukemia in adults
__A__	Acute myelogenous leukemia (AML)	B. Most cases are in adults over the age of 60
__B__	Chronic lymphocytic leukemia (CLL)	C. Reed-Sternberg cells
__D__	Non-Hodgkin's lymphoma	D. Can be caused by radiation

   Reed-Sternberg cells are significant for Hodgkin's lymphoma. The most common leukemia in adults is AML. Chronic lymphocytic leukemia is an uncommon form of leukemia that may develop in adults over age 60. Non-Hodgkin's lymphoma can be caused by radiation.

   Ⓝ NCLEX® Connection: Physiological Adaptation, Pathophysiology

UNIT 5	NURSING CARE OF CLIENTS WITH HEMATOLOGIC DISORDERS
Section	Hematologic Disorders
Chapter 47	Coagulation Disorders

Overview

- Coagulation disorders occur secondary to an alteration in platelets, clotting factors, or both. Coagulopathy is the term for any condition that affects an individual's ability to coagulate. Coagulopathies are suspected when the usual measures used to stop bleeding fail.

- Coagulopathy may occur secondary to an autoimmune disorder or extensive blood loss in which platelets and clotting factors are lost. In some cases, the development of microemboli in the circulatory system paradoxically "uses up" the clotting factors that cause hemorrhages to occur at the same time intravascular clotting occurs.

- Coagulation disorders include:

  o Idiopathic thrombocytopenic purpura (ITP) – A coagulopathy that is an autoimmune disorder in which the life span of platelets is decreased by antiplatelet antibodies. This can result in severe hemorrhage following a cesarean birth or lacerations.

  o Disseminated intravascular coagulation (DIC) – A coagulopathy in which clotting and anticlotting mechanisms occur at the same time.

    ▪ The client with DIC is at risk for both internal and external bleeding, as well as damage to organs resulting from ischemia caused by microclots.

Risk Factors

- Risk factors for ITP

  o Female

  o Autoimmune disorder

  o Recent virus (children only)

- Risk factors for DIC that occur secondary to other complications include:

  o Septicemia

  o Cardiopulmonary arrest

  o Hemorrhage

Assessment

- Objective Data
  - ○ Physical Assessment Findings
    - ■ Unusual spontaneous bleeding from the client's gums and nose (epistaxis)
    - ■ Oozing, trickling, or flow of blood from incisions or lacerations
    - ■ Petechiae and ecchymoses
    - ■ Excessive bleeding from venipuncture, injection sites, or slight traumas
    - ■ Tachycardia, hypotension, and diaphoresis
    - ■ Organ failure secondary to microemboli
  - ○ Laboratory Tests
    - ■ Platelet levels (thrombocytopenia) decreased with DIC and ITP
    - ■ Fibrinogen levels (decreased with DIC)
    - ■ Prothrombin time (increased with DIC)
    - ■ Partial thromboplastin (increased with DIC)
    - ■ Fibrin split product levels/fibrin degradation products (increased with DIC)
    - ■ D-dimer (increased with DIC)
    - ■ Blood typing and crossmatch

Collaborative Care

- Nursing Care
  - ○ DIC
    - ■ Nursing interventions for DIC initially focus on assessing for and correcting the underlying cause (sepsis, hemorrhage). The focus then turns to preventing organ damage secondary to microemboli and replacing the blood's clotting components.
    - ■ Monitor for signs of microemboli (cyanotic nail beds, pain).
  - ○ DIC and ITP
    - ■ Regularly take vital signs and assess hemodynamic status.
    - ■ Monitor for signs of organ failure or intracranial bleed (oliguria, decreased level of consciousness).
    - ■ Monitor laboratory values for clotting factors.
    - ■ Administer fluid volume replacement.
    - ■ Transfuse blood, platelets, and other clotting products.
    - ■ Monitor for complications from the administration of blood and blood products.
    - ■ Avoid use of NSAIDs.

- ■ Administer supplemental oxygen.

- ■ Provide protection from injury.

- ■ Instruct client to avoid Valsalva maneuver (could cause cerebral hemorrhage).

- ■ Implement bleeding precautions (avoid use of needles).

- Medications

  - ○ ITP – Corticosteroids and immunosuppressants

  - ○ DIC – Anticoagulants (heparin)

    - ■ May be used to decrease microclots from forming and using up clotting factors

- Surgical Interventions

  - ○ ITP – Splenectomy may be performed by the provider if client does not respond to medical management.

- Desired Client Outcomes

  - ○ Client's bleeding stops and is free from recurrence of bleeding incidences.

CHAPTER 47: COAGULATION DISORDERS

 Application Exercises

1. A nurse is caring for a client who has disseminated intravascular coagulation (DIC) secondary to hemorrhage that occurred during a motor vehicle crash. Which of the following indicates that the client's clotting factors are becoming depleted? (Select all that apply.)

    _____ Platelets 100,000/mm³

    _____ Fibrinogen levels 97 mg/dL

    _____ Fibrin degradation products 4.3 mcg/mL

    _____ D-dimer 179 ng/mL

    _____ Sedimentation rate 38 mm/hr

2. A nurse is caring for a client who is demonstrating uncontrollable bleeding after a cardiac bypass and is prescribed heparin by the provider. Identify why low-dose heparin is indicated in this situation.

3. A nurse is caring for a client who has idiopathic thrombocytopenic purpura (ITP). The nurse should call the provider and report possible small vessel clotting when which of the following is found during assessment?

    A. Petechiae on the upper chest

    B. Hypotension

    C. Cyanotic nail beds

    D. Severe headache

CHAPTER 47: COAGULATION DISORDERS

 Application Exercises Answer Key

1. A nurse is caring for a client who has disseminated intravascular coagulation (DIC) secondary to hemorrhage that occurred during a motor vehicle crash. Which of the following indicates that the client's clotting factors are becoming depleted? (Select all that apply.)

      X   **Platelets 100,000/mm³**

      X   **Fibrinogen levels 97 mg/dL**

   _____ Fibrin degradation products 4.3 mcg/mL

   _____ D-dimer 179 ng/mL

   _____ Sedimentation rate 38 mm/hr

   During DIC, clotting factors are depleted and clotting times are increased significantly, raising the risk of fatal hemorrhage. The platelet and fibrinogen levels indicate this is occurring. The fibrin degradation products and D-dimer are within the expected reference range. While the sedimentation rate is elevated, it is not an indicator of coagulation.

    NCLEX® Connection: Reduction of Risk Potential, Laboratory Values

2. A nurse is caring for a client who is demonstrating uncontrollable bleeding after a cardiac bypass and is prescribed heparin by the provider. Identify why low-dose heparin is indicated in this situation.

   The client is likely in DIC. Low-dose heparin may be used to treat DIC to stop microclotting from occurring, which may be contributing to the depletion of clotting factors and bleeding.

   NCLEX® Connection: Pharmacological and Parenteral Therapies, Expected Actions/ Outcomes

3. A nurse is caring for a client who has idiopathic thrombocytopenic purpura (ITP). The nurse should call the provider and report possible small vessel clotting when which of the following is found during assessment?

   A. Petechiae on the upper chest

   B. Hypotension

   C. Cyanotic nail beds

   D. Severe headache

   Cyanotic nail beds indicate microvascular clotting is occurring and should be immediately reported to avoid ischemic loss of the fingers or toes. Petechiae and hypotension indicate impaired clotting and a severe headache may indicate a cerebral bleed.

   NCLEX® Connection: Reduction of Risk Potential, System Specific Assessment

UNIT 6: NURSING CARE OF CLIENTS WITH FLUID/ELECTROLYTE/ACID-BASE IMBALANCES

- Fluid Imbalances

- Electrolyte Imbalances

- Acid-Base Imbalances

NCLEX® CONNECTIONS

When reviewing the chapters in this unit, keep in mind the relevant sections of the NCLEX® outline, in particular:

CLIENT NEEDS: PHYSIOLOGICAL ADAPTATION

Relevant topics/tasks include:
- Fluid and Electrolyte Imbalances
  - Evaluate the client's response to interventions to correct fluid or electrolyte imbalance.
- Hemodynamics
  - Apply knowledge of pathophysiology to interventions in response to the client's abnormal hemodynamics.
- Medical Emergencies
  - Evaluate and document the client's response to emergency interventions.

UNIT 6	NURSING CARE OF CLIENTS WITH FLUID/ELECTROLYTE/ ACID-BASE IMBALANCES
Chapter 48	Fluid Imbalances

Overview

- Body fluids are distributed between intracellular (ICF) and extracellular (ECF) fluid compartments.

- Fluid can move between compartments (through selectively permeable membranes) by a variety of methods (diffusion, active transport, filtration, osmosis) to maintain homeostasis.

- Fluid imbalances that nurses should be familiar with are:

  o Fluid Volume Deficits

  o Fluid Volume Excess

FLUID VOLUME DEFICITS

Overview

- Fluid volume deficits (FVDs) include hypovolemia-isotonic (loss of water and electrolytes from the ECF) and dehydration-osmolar (loss of water with no loss of electrolytes).

- Hemoconcentration occurs with dehydration, resulting in increases in Hct, serum electrolytes, and urine specific gravity.

- Note – Compensatory mechanisms include sympathetic nervous system responses of increased thirst, antidiuretic hormone (ADH) release, and aldosterone release.

- Hypovolemia can lead to hypovolemic shock.

Health Promotion and Disease Prevention

- Increase fluid intake with vigorous exercise.

- Increase fluid intake in high altitudes and dry climates to promote hydration.

- Avoid drinking fluids that contain alcohol or caffeine. This increases fluid excretion.

- Older adults have an increased risk for dehydration due to a decrease in total body mass, which includes total body water content.

Assessment

- Risk Factors
  - Causes of Hypovolemia
    - Abnormal gastrointestinal (GI) losses – Vomiting, nasogastric suctioning, diarrhea
    - Abnormal skin losses – Diaphoresis
    - Abnormal renal losses – Diuretic therapy, diabetes insipidus, renal disease, adrenal insufficiency, osmotic diuresis
    - Third spacing – Peritonitis, intestinal obstruction, ascites, burns
    - Hemorrhage
    - Altered intake, such as nothing by mouth (NPO)
  - Causes of Dehydration
    - Hyperventilation
    - Diabetic ketoacidosis
    - Enteral feeding without sufficient water intake
- Subjective Data and Objective Data
  - Vital signs – Hyperthermia, tachycardia, thready pulse, hypotension, orthostatic hypotension, decreased central venous pressure, tachypneic (increased respirations), hypoxia
  - Neuromusculoskeletal – Dizziness, syncope, confusion, weakness, fatigue
  - Gastrointestinal – Thirst, dry furrowed tongue, nausea/vomiting, anorexia, acute weight loss
  - Renal – Oliguria (decreased production of urine)
  - Other signs – Diminished capillary refill, cool clammy skin, diaphoresis, sunken eyeballs, flattened neck veins
  - Laboratory Tests
    - Hematocrit (Hct)
      - Hypovolemia – Increased Hct
    - Serum osmolarity
      - Dehydration – Increased (hemoconcentration) osmolarity (> 300 mOsm/L), — increased protein, blood urea nitrogen (BUN), electrolytes, glucose
    - Urine specific gravity and osmolarity
      - Dehydration – Increased (concentration)
    - Serum sodium
      - Dehydration – Increased (hemoconcentration)

Collaborative Care

- Nursing Care

  - Check urinalysis, oxygen saturation (SaO_2, and CBC and electrolytes.

  - Administer supplemental oxygen as prescribed.

  - Monitor vital signs and heart rhythm.

  - Auscultate lung sounds.

  - Initiate and maintain IV access.

  - Place the client in shock position (on back with legs elevated).

  - Fluid replacement – Administer IV fluids as prescribed (isotonic solutions, such as lactated Ringer's, normal saline, blood transfusions).

  - Monitor intake and output. Alert the provider for urine output less than 30 cc/hr.

  - Monitor level of consciousness and maintain client safety.

  - Assess level of gait stability. Encourage client to use call light and ask for assistance.

  - Encourage the client to change positions, slowly rolling from side to side, or standing up.

- Interdisciplinary Care

  - Respiratory services may be consulted for oxygen management.

- Care After Discharge

  - Client Education

    - Encourage the client to drink plenty of liquids to promote hydration.

    - Educate the client regarding causes of dehydration, such as nausea/vomiting.

- Client Outcomes

  - The client will maintain adequate oxygen level.

  - The client will be able to maintain adequate hydration.

  - The client will be able to tolerate food and liquids.

  - The client will be free from anxiety.

  - The client will be free from falls/injury.

Complications

- Hypovolemic Shock

  - Vital organ hypoxia/anoxia – Decreased hemoglobin oxygen saturation and pulse pressure (systolic-diastolic blood pressure)

- Nursing Actions
  - Administer oxygen.
  - Provide fluid replacement with:
    - Colloids (whole blood, packed RBCs, plasma, synthetic plasma expanders)
    - Crystalloids (Ringer's lactate, normal saline)
  - Administer vasoconstrictors, such as dopamine (Intropin) and norepinephrine (Levophed); coronary vasodilators, such as sodium nitroprusside (Nipride); and/or positive inotropic medications, such as dobutamine (Dobutrex).
  - Perform hemodynamic monitoring.

FLUID VOLUME EXCESSES

Overview

- Fluid volume excesses (FVEs) include hypervolemia-isotonic (water and sodium are retained in abnormally high proportions) and overhydration-osmolar (more water is gained than electrolytes).

- Note – Severe hypervolemia can lead to pulmonary edema and heart failure.

- Note – Compensatory mechanisms include increased release of natriuretic peptides, resulting in increased loss of sodium and water by the kidneys and the decrease in the release of aldosterone.

Health Promotion and Disease Prevention

- Consume a diet low in sodium. Consult with provider regarding diet restrictions.

- Promote fluid restriction intake. Consult with provider regarding prescribed restrictions.

Assessment

- Risk Factors
  - Causes of Hypervolemia
    - Chronic stimulus to the kidney to conserve sodium and water (heart failure, cirrhosis, increased glucocorticosteroids)
    - Abnormal renal function with reduced excretion of sodium and water (renal failure)
    - Interstitial to plasma fluid shifts (hypertonic fluids, burns)
    - Age-related changes in cardiovascular and renal function
    - Excessive sodium intake
  - Causes of Overhydration
    - Water replacement without electrolyte replacement (strenuous exercise with profuse diaphoresis)

- Subjective Data and Objective Data

  - Vital signs – Tachycardia, bounding pulse, hypertension, tachypnea, increased central venous pressure

  - Neuromusculoskeletal – Confusion, muscle weakness

  - Gastrointestinal – Weight gain, ascites

  - Respiratory – Dyspnea, orthopnea, crackles, diminished breath sounds

  - Other signs – Edema, distended neck veins

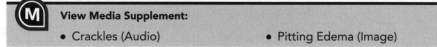

View Media Supplement:
- Crackles (Audio)
- Pitting Edema (Image)

  - Laboratory Findings

    - Hematocrit

      - Hypervolemia – Decreased hematocrit (Hct)

    - Serum osmolarity

      - Overhydration – Decreased (hemodilution) osmolarity (< 270 mOsm/L)

    - Serum sodium

      - Hypervolemia – Sodium within expected reference range

    - Electrolytes, BUN, and creatinine

      - Overhydration/hypervolemia – Decreased electrolytes, BUN, and creatinine

    - Arterial Blood Gases

    - Respiratory alkalosis – Decreased $PaCO_2$ (< 35 mm Hg), increased PH (>7.45)

  - Diagnostic Procedures

    - Chest x-ray – Reveals possible pulmonary congestion.

Collaborative Care

- Nursing Care

  - Check ABGs, SaO_2, CBC, and chest x-ray results.

  - Position the client in a semi-Fowler's position.

  - Obtain daily weight.

  - Monitor intake and output.

  - Administer supplemental oxygen as prescribed.

  - Reduce IV flow rates.

  - Administer diuretics (osmotic, loop) as prescribed.

- ○ Limit fluid and sodium intake as ordered.

- ○ Monitor and document presence of edema (pretibial, sacral, periorbital).

- ○ Reposition the client at least every 2 hr.

- ○ Support arms and legs to decrease dependent edema as appropriate.

- ○ Monitor vital signs and heart rhythm.

- ○ Auscultate lung sounds (listen for crackles).

- • Interdisciplinary Care

  - ○ Respiratory services may be consulted for oxygen management.

  - ○ Pulmonology may be consulted if fluid moves into lungs.

- • Care After Discharge

  - ○ Client Education

    - ▪ Encourage client to weigh themselves daily. Notify provider if 1 to 2-pound gain in 24 hr, or a 3-pound gain in a week.

    - ▪ Consume a low-sodium diet. Read food labels to check sodium content and keep record of daily sodium intake.

    - ▪ Promote fluid restriction intake. Consult with provider regarding prescribed restrictions.

- • Client Outcomes

  - ○ The client will maintain adequate oxygen level.

  - ○ The client will be free from anxiety.

  - ○ The client will be compliant with fluid restriction intake.

  - ○ The client will consume a low-sodium diet.

Complications

- • Pulmonary Edema

  - ○ Pulmonary edema can be caused by severe fluid overload.

    - ▪ Symptoms include anxiety, tachycardia, acute respiratory distress, increased vein distention, dyspnea at rest, change in level of consciousness, and ascending crackles (fluid level within lungs) and cough, productive of frothy pink-tinged sputum.

  - ○ Nursing Actions

    - ▪ Position the client in high-Fowler's position to maximize ventilation.

    - ▪ Administer oxygen, positive airway pressure, and/or possible intubation and mechanical ventilation.

    - ▪ Administer morphine and diuretic as prescribed.

CHAPTER 48: FLUID IMBALANCES

 Application Exercises

1. A middle adult male client is seen in the emergency department with reports of nausea, vomiting, dizziness, and weakness. History reveals that he had just completed a 10-mile run when the onset of symptoms occurred. Physical assessment reveals dry oral mucous membranes, temperature 38.5° C (101.3° F), pulse 92 beats/min and thready, respirations 20/min, skin cool and tenting present, and blood pressure 102/64 mm Hg. His urine is concentrated with a high specific gravity. Which of the following are consistent with the presence of fluid volume deficit? (Select all that apply.)

_____ Decreased skin turgor

_____ Concentrated urine

_____ Tachycardia

_____ Low-grade fever

_____ Tachypnea

_____ Hypertension

Scenario: An older adult female client is admitted to an acute care facility with dyspnea, weakness, weight gain of 2 lb, 1+ pitting edema of both lower extremities to mid calf, and bilateral crackles in lung bases. Assessment findings include – Temperature 37.2° C (99° F), pulse 96/min and bounding, respirations 26/min, oxygen saturation 94% on 3 L oxygen via nasal cannula, and blood pressure 152/96 mm Hg. She is diagnosed with heart failure and fluid volume excess. IV furosemide (Lasix) is prescribed.

---

2. Which of the following present fluid volume excess? (Select all that apply.)

_____ Dyspnea

_____ Edema

_____ Bradycardia

_____ Hypertension

_____ Weakness

3. Why is fluid volume excess a common complication of heart failure?

4. Which electrolyte should the nurse carefully monitor in this client and why?

Scenario: An older adult male client living in an assisted living facility has become weak and confused. Usually a good eater, today he has eaten only 40% of his breakfast and lunch. He has required constant encouragement to drink. Assessment findings include – Temperature 38.3° C (100.9° F), pulse rate 92/min, respirations 20/min, and blood pressure 108/60 mm Hg. He has lost ¾ lb and he reports dizziness when assisted to the bathroom. He also has a non-productive cough with diminished breath sounds in the right lower lobe. His urine is dark yellow.

5. Which of the above data supports fluid volume deficit?

6. Which of the following interventions should the nurse take?

    A. Initiate fluid restrictions to limit intake and output.

    B. Observe for signs of hypertension.

    C. Encourage client to ambulate to promote oxygenation.

    D. Monitor respirations for shortness of breath.

7. Which of the following should the nurse look for when assessing for fluid volume deficit?

    A. Moist skin

    B. Distended neck veins

    C. Increased urinary output

    D. Hypotension

8. A client receiving 0.9% sodium chloride should be monitored for signs of

    A. fluid overload.

    B. fluid deficit.

CHAPTER 48: FLUID IMBALANCES

 Application Exercises Answer Key

1. A middle adult male client is seen in the emergency department with reports of nausea, vomiting, dizziness, and weakness. History reveals that he had just completed a 10-mile run when the onset of symptoms occurred. Physical assessment reveals dry oral mucous membranes, temperature 38.5° C (101.3° F), pulse 92 beats/min and thready, respirations 20/min, skin cool and tenting present, and blood pressure 102/64 mm Hg. His urine is concentrated with a high specific gravity. Which of the following are consistent with the presence of fluid volume deficit? (Select all that apply.)

__X__	**Decreased skin turgor**
__X__	**Concentrated urine**
__X__	**Tachycardia**
__X__	**Low-grade fever**
__X__	**Tachypnea**
_____	Hypertension

Decreased skin turgor, concentrated urine, tachycardia, low-grade fever, and tachypnea are all findings related to fluid volume deficit. Hypertension would be a finding related to fluid volume excess.

 NCLEX® Connection: Physiological Adaptation, Fluid and Electrolyte Imbalances

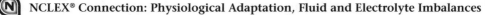

Scenario: An older adult female client is admitted to an acute care facility with dyspnea, weakness, weight gain of 2 lb, 1+ pitting edema of both lower extremities to mid calf, and bilateral crackles in lung bases. Assessment findings include – Temperature 37.2° C (99° F), pulse 96/min and bounding, respirations 26/min, oxygen saturation 94% on 3 L oxygen via nasal cannula, and blood pressure 152/96 mm Hg. She is diagnosed with heart failure and fluid volume excess. IV furosemide (Lasix) is prescribed.

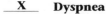

2. Which of the following present fluid volume excess? (Select all that apply.)

__X__	**Dyspnea**
__X__	**Edema**
_____	Bradycardia
__X__	**Hypertension**
__X__	**Weakness**

Dyspnea, edema, hypertension, and weakness are all symptoms related to fluid volume excess. Bradycardia would not be a finding related to this diagnosis.

NCLEX® Connection: Physiological Adaptation, Fluid and Electrolyte Imbalances

3. Why is fluid volume excess a common complication of heart failure?

Heart failure occurs when the cardiac muscle is too weak to maintain adequate cardiac output. This results in decreased renal blood flow and renal perfusion. This prompts the retention of sodium and water. Poor myocardial contraction also results in insufficient ventricle emptying resulting in pulmonary and/or peripheral edema.

 NCLEX® Connection: Physiological Adaptation, Fluid and Electrolyte Imbalances

4. Which electrolyte should the nurse carefully monitor in this client and why?

Potassium, because furosemide (Lasix) administration may result in hypokalemia.

 NCLEX® Connection: Physiological Adaptation, Fluid and Electrolyte Imbalances

Scenario: An older adult male client living in an assisted living facility has become weak and confused. Usually a good eater, today he has eaten only 40% of his breakfast and lunch. He has required constant encouragement to drink. Assessment findings include – Temperature 38.3° C (100.9° F), pulse rate 92/min, respirations 20/min, and blood pressure 108/60 mm Hg. He has lost ¾ lb and he reports dizziness when assisted to the bathroom. He also has a non-productive cough with diminished breath sounds in the right lower lobe. His urine is dark yellow.

5. Which of the above data supports fluid volume deficit?

Weak and confused, ate only 40% of his breakfast and lunch, requires encouragement to drink, temperature 38.3° C (100.9° F), pulse rate 92 beats/min, respirations 20/min, blood pressure 108/60 mm Hg, ¾ lb weight loss, dizziness, non-productive cough with diminished breath sounds in the right lower lobe, dark yellow urine

 NCLEX® Connection: Physiological Adaptation, Fluid and Electrolyte Imbalances

6. Which of the following interventions should the nurse take?

A. Initiate fluid restrictions to limit intake and output.

B. Observe for signs of hypertension.

C. Encourage client to ambulate to promote oxygenation.

D. Monitor respirations for shortness of breath.

Monitoring respirations for shortness of breath is an intervention that the nurse should take when caring for a client with a fluid volume deficit. The other interventions are for fluid volume excess.

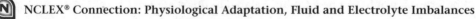 **NCLEX® Connection: Physiological Adaptation, Fluid and Electrolyte Imbalances**

7. Which of the following should the nurse look for when assessing for fluid volume deficit?

    A. Moist skin

    B. Distended neck veins

    C. Increased urinary output

    D. Hypotension

    Hypotension is a sign of fluid volume deficit. The other findings are symptoms related to fluid volume excess.

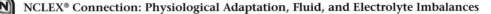 NCLEX® Connection: Physiological Adaptation, Fluid, and Electrolyte Imbalances

8. A client receiving 0.9% sodium chloride should be monitored for signs of

    A. fluid overload.

    B. fluid deficit.

    0.9% NS is an isotonic solution given for dehydration. Extracellular fluid is lost during dehydration and this isotonic fluid helps replace this fluid. Hypertonic fluids pose a risk for fluid volume deficits due to their level of osmosis and that they pull fluid from the isotonic spaces.

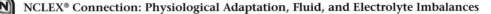 NCLEX® Connection: Physiological Adaptation, Fluid, and Electrolyte Imbalances

UNIT 6	NURSING CARE OF CLIENTS WITH FLUID/ELECTROLYTE/ ACID-BASE IMBALANCES
Chapter 49	Electrolyte Imbalances

Overview

- Electrolytes are minerals (sometimes called salts) that are present in all body fluids. They regulate fluid balance and hormone production, strengthen skeletal structures, and act as catalysts in nerve response, muscle contraction, and the metabolism of nutrients.

- When dissolved in water or other solvent, electrolytes separate into ions and conduct either a positive (cations – magnesium, potassium, sodium, calcium) or negative (anions – phosphate, sulfate, chloride, bicarbonate) electrical current.

- Electrolytes are distributed between intracellular (ICF) and extracellular (ECF) fluid compartments. While laboratory tests can accurately reflect the electrolyte concentrations in plasma, it is not possible to directly measure electrolyte concentrations within cells.

ELECTROLYTE	EXPECTED REFERENCE RANGE
Sodium	136 to 145 mEq/L
Potassium	3.5 to 5.0 mEq/L
Chloride	98 to 106 mEq/L
Calcium	9.0 to 10.5 mg/dL
Magnesium	1.3 to 2.1 mEq/L
Phosphorus	3.5 to 4.5 mg/dL

SODIUM IMBALANCES

Overview

- Sodium (Na^+) is the major electrolyte found in extracellular fluid.

- Sodium is essential for maintaining acid-base balance, active and passive transport mechanisms, and maintaining irritability and conduction of nerve and muscle tissue.

- Normal serum sodium levels are between 136 to 145 mEq/L.

  o Decreased sodium levels are referred to as hyponatremia.

  o Elevated sodium levels are referred to as hypernatremia.

Hyponatremia

- Hyponatremia is a net gain of water or loss of sodium-rich fluids that results in sodium levels less than 136 mEq/L.

    o Hyponatremia delays and slows the depolarization of membranes.

    o Water moves from the ECF into the ICF causing cells to swell (cerebral edema).

    o Compensatory mechanisms include the renal excretion of sodium-free water.

- Assessment

    o Risk Factors

        ■ Causes of hyponatremia include:

            □ Deficient ECF volume

                ▸ Abnormal gastrointestinal (GI) losses: Vomiting, nasogastric suctioning, diarrhea, tap water enemas, gastrointestinal obstructions

                ▸ Renal losses: Diuretics, kidney disease, adrenal insufficiency

                ▸ Skin losses: Excessive sweating, burns, wound drainage, ascites (as it relates to cirrhosis)

            □ Increased or normal ECF volume

                ▸ Excessive oral water intake

                ▸ Syndrome of inappropriate antidiuretic hormone (SIADH) – excess secretion of antidiuretic hormone (ADH)

            □ Edematous states: Heart failure, cirrhosis, nephrotic syndrome

            □ Excessive hypotonic IV fluids

            □ Inadequate sodium intake (nothing by mouth status {NPO})

        ■ Older adult clients are at a greater risk due to the increased incidence of chronic illnesses, use of diuretic medications, and risk for insufficient sodium intake.

    o Subjective Data and Objective Data

        ■ Clinical indicators depend on whether it is associated with a normal (euvolemic), decreased (hypovolemic), or increased ECF (hypervolemic) volume.

        ■ Vital signs: hypothermia, tachycardia, rapid thready pulse, hypotension, orthostatic hypotension (vital signs can vary based on state of ECF volume)

        ■ Neuromusculoskeletal: headache, confusion, lethargy, muscle weakness to the point of possible respiratory compromise, fatigue, decreased deep tendon reflexes, seizures

- Gastrointestinal: increased motility, hyperactive bowel sounds, abdominal cramping, nausea
- Laboratory Tests
  - Serum sodium
    - ▸ Decreased: < 136 mEq/L
  - Serum osmolarity
    - ▸ Decreased: < 270 mOsm/L
- Collaborative Care
  - Nursing Care
    - Report abnormal laboratory findings to the provider.
    - Fluid overload: Restrict water intake as prescribed by the provider.
    - For clients with heart failure and hyponatremia, provide loop diuretics and ACE inhibitors, as prescribed.
    - Acute hyponatremia:
      - Administer hypertonic oral and IV fluids as prescribed.
      - Administer 3% sodium chloride slowly and monitor sodium levels frequently.
      - Encourage foods and fluids high in sodium (cheeses, milk, condiments).
    - Restoration of normal ECF volume: Administer isotonic IV therapy (0.9% sodium chloride, Ringer's lactate).
    - Monitor intake and output, and daily weight.
    - Monitor vital signs and level of consciousness, report abnormal findings to the provider.
    - Encourage the client to change positions slowly.
  - Interdisciplinary Care
    - Nephrology may be consulted for electrolyte and fluid replacement.
    - Respiratory services may be consulted for oxygen management.
    - Nutritional services may be consulted for food choices high in sodium and restricting fluid intake.
  - Care After Discharge
    - Client Education
      - Encourage the client to weigh daily and to notify the provider of a 1 to 2 lb gain in 24 hr, or 3 lb gain in a week.
      - Instruct the client to consume a high-sodium diet, including reading food labels to check sodium content, and keeping a daily record of sodium intake.

- Client Outcomes

  - The client will maintain normal fluid balance as indicated by urinary output, vital signs, and cognitive functioning.

  - The client will identify three ways to maintain the fluid restriction.

  - The client will consume a high-sodium diet.

- Complications

  - Acute Hyponatremia

    - Complications (coma, seizures, respiratory arrest) can result from acute hyponatremia if not treated immediately.

    - Nursing Actions

      - Maintain an open airway and monitor client's vital signs.

      - Implement seizure precautions and take appropriate action if seizures occur.

      - Monitor the client's level of consciousness.

Hypernatremia

- Increased sodium causes hypertonicity of the serum. This causes a shift of water out of the cells, resulting in dehydrated cells.

  - Hypernatremia is a serum sodium level greater than 145 mEq/L.

  - Hypernatremia is a serious electrolyte imbalance. It can cause significant neurological, endocrine, and/or cardiac disturbances.

Assessment

  - Risk Factors

    - Causes of hypernatremia (loss of water) include:

      - Water deprivation (NPO)

      - Excessive sodium intake: Dietary sodium intake, hypertonic IV fluids, bicarbonate intake

      - Excessive sodium retention: Renal failure, Cushing's syndrome, aldosteronism, some medications (glucocorticosteroids)

      - Fluid losses: Fever, diaphoresis, burns, respiratory infection, diabetes insipidus, hyperglycemia, watery diarrhea

      - Age-related changes, specifically decreased total body water content and inadequate fluid intake related to an altered thirst mechanism

      - Compensatory mechanisms include increased thirst and production of ADH.

- ○ Subjective Data and Objective Data
  - ■ Vital signs: hyperthermia, tachycardia, orthostatic hypotension
  - ■ Neuromusculoskeletal: restlessness, irritability, muscle twitching to the point of muscle weakness including respiratory compromise, decreased deep tendon reflexes (DTR) to the point of absent DTRs, seizures, coma
  - ■ Gastrointestinal: thirst, dry mucous membranes, increased motility, hyperactive bowel sounds, abdominal cramping, nausea
  - ■ Other signs: edema, warm flushed skin, oliguria (decreased production of urine)
  - ■ Laboratory Tests
    - □ Serum sodium: increased: > 145 mEq/L
    - □ Serum osmolarity: increased: > 300 mOsm/L
- • Collaborative Care
  - ○ Nursing Care
    - ■ Report abnormal laboratory findings to the provider.
    - ■ Fluid loss:
      - □ Based on serum osmolarity and hemodynamic stability:
        - ▸ Administer hypotonic IV fluids (0.45% sodium chloride).
        - ▸ Administer isotonic IV fluids (0.9% sodium chloride).
    - ■ Excess sodium
      - □ Encourage water intake and discourage sodium intake.
      - □ Administer diuretics (loop diuretics) for clients with poor renal excretion.
    - ■ Monitor level of consciousness and ensure safety.
    - ■ Monitor the client's vital signs and heart rhythm.
    - ■ Auscultate lung sounds.
    - ■ Provide oral hygiene and other comfort measures to decrease thirst.
    - ■ Monitor intake and output, and alert the provider of inadequate renal output.
  - ○ Interdisciplinary Care
    - ■ Nephrology may be consulted for electrolyte and fluid management.
    - ■ Respiratory services may be consulted for oxygen management.
    - ■ Nutritional services may be consulted for food choices low in sodium and to restrict fluid intake.

- o Care After Discharge
  - Client Education
    - □ Encourage the client to weigh daily. Notify the provider of a 1 to 2 lb gain in 24 hr, or 3 lb gain in a week.
    - □ Encourage the client to consume a low-sodium diet, read food labels to check sodium content, and keep a record of daily sodium intake.
    - □ Encourage fluids as prescribed by the provider.
  - o Client Outcomes
    - The client will be free from injury.
    - The client will maintain a normal fluid balance as indicated by urinary output, vital signs, and cognitive functioning.
    - The client will maintain a serum sodium level within the expected reference range.
- Complications
  - o Acute Hypernatremia
    - Complications (seizures, convulsion, death) can result from acute hypernatremia if not treated immediately.
    - Nursing Actions
      - □ Maintain open airway and monitor the client's vital signs.
      - □ Implement seizure precautions and take appropriate action if seizures occur.
      - □ Monitor the client's level of consciousness.

POTASSIUM IMBALANCES

Overview

- Potassium (K^+) is the major cation in the intracellular fluid (ICF).
- Potassium plays a vital role in cell metabolism, transmission of nerve impulses, functioning of cardiac, lung, and muscle tissues, and acid-base balance.
- Potassium has a reciprocal action with sodium.
- Normal serum potassium levels are between 3.5 and 5.0 mEq/L.
  - o Decreased potassium levels are referred to as hypokalemia.
  - o Elevated potassium levels are referred to as hyperkalemia.

Hypokalemia

- Hypokalemia is the result of an increased loss of potassium from the body or movement of potassium into the cells, resulting in a serum potassium less than 3.5 mEq/L.

- Assessment

  - Risk Factors

    - Causes of hypokalemia include:

      - Decreased total body potassium

        ‣ Abnormal GI losses: Vomiting, nasogastric suctioning, diarrhea, inappropriate laxative use

        ‣ Renal losses: Excessive use of diuretics (furosemide [Lasix], corticosteroids)

        ‣ Skin losses: Diaphoresis, wound losses

      - Insufficient potassium

        ‣ Inadequate dietary intake (rare)

        ‣ Prolonged administration of non-electrolyte containing IV solutions (D_5W)

      - Intracellular shift: Metabolic alkalosis, after correction of acidosis, during periods of tissue repair (burns, trauma, starvation), total parenteral nutrition

    - Older adult clients are at greater risk due to increased use of diuretics and laxatives.

  - Subjective Data and Objective Data

    - Vital signs: weak, irregular pulse, hypotension, respiratory distress

    - Neuromusculoskeletal: weakness to the point of respiratory collapse and paralysis, muscle cramping, decreased muscle tone and hypoactive reflexes, paresthesias, mental confusion

    - ECG: premature ventricular contractions (PVCs), bradycardia, blocks, ventricular tachycardia, inverted T waves, and ST depression

    - Gastrointestinal: decreased motility, abdominal distention, constipation, ileus, nausea, vomiting, anorexia

    - Other signs: polyuria (dilute urine)

- Laboratory Tests
  - Serum potassium: decreased (< 3.5 mEq/L)
  - Arterial blood gases: metabolic alkalosis (pH > 7.45)
- Diagnostic Procedures
  - Electrocardiogram (ECG)
    - ECG will show findings of dysrhythmias (premature ventricular contractions [PVCs], ventricular tachycardia, inverted T waves, ST depression).

- Collaborative Care
  - Nursing Care
    - Report abnormal findings to the provider.
    - Replacement of potassium:
      - Encourage foods high in potassium (avocados, broccoli, dairy products, dried fruit, cantaloupe, bananas).
      - Provide oral potassium supplementation.
    - IV potassium supplementation:
      - Never IV bolus (high risk of cardiac arrest).
      - The maximum recommended rate is 5 to 10 mEq/hr.
    - Assess for phlebitis (tissue irritant).
    - Monitor and maintain adequate urine output.
    - Observe for shallow ineffective respirations and diminished breath sounds.
    - Monitor the client's cardiac rhythm and intervene promptly as needed.
    - Monitor clients receiving digoxin (Lanoxin). Hypokalemia increases the risk for digoxin toxicity.
    - Monitor level of consciousness and maintain client safety.
    - Monitor bowel sounds and abdominal distention and intervene as needed.
    - Monitor kidney function (BUN, GFR, Creatinine).
    - Monitor magnesium, calcium, and phosphorus.
    - Provide assistance with ADLs (weakness is usually pronounced if the client has a K+ < 2.5).
  - Interdisciplinary Care
    - Nephrology may be consulted for electrolyte and fluid management.
    - Respiratory services may be consulted for oxygen management.
    - Nutritional services may be consulted for food choices and potassium-rich foods.
    - Cardiology may be consulted for dysrhythmias.

- o Care After Discharge
  - ■ Client Education
    - □ Educate the client regarding potassium-rich foods to consume.
    - □ Teach the client ways to prevent a decrease in potassium by excessive use of diuretics and laxatives.
- o Client Outcomes
  - ■ The client will maintain adequate gas exchange.
  - ■ The client will be free from injury.
  - ■ The client will have electrolyte lab values within the expected reference range.
- Complications
  - o Respiratory Failure
    - ■ Nursing Actions
      - □ Maintain an open airway and monitor the client's vital signs.
      - □ Monitor the client's level of consciousness.
      - □ Monitor for hypoxemia and hypercapnia.
      - □ Assist with intubation and mechanical ventilation if indicated.
  - o Cardiac Arrest
    - ■ Nursing Actions
      - □ Perform continuous cardiac monitoring.
      - □ Treat dysrhythmias.

Hyperkalemia

- Hyperkalemia is the result of an increased intake of potassium, movement of potassium out of the cells, or inadequate renal excretion resulting in a serum potassium level greater than 5.0 mEq/L.

- Assessment
  - o Risk Factors
    - ■ Causes of hyperkalemia include:
      - □ Increased total body potassium: IV potassium administration, salt substitute.
      - □ Extracellular shift: Decreased insulin, acidosis (diabetic ketoacidosis), tissue catabolism (sepsis, trauma, surgery, fever, myocardial infarction)

- ☐ Hypertonic states: Uncontrolled diabetes
- ☐ Decreased excretion of potassium: Renal failure, severe dehydration, potassium-sparing diuretics, angiotensin-converting enzyme inhibitors, NSAIDs, adrenal insufficiency

- ■ Older adult clients are at a greater risk due to the increased use of salt substitutes, ACE inhibitors, and potassium-sparing diuretics.
  - ○ Subjective Data and Objective Data
    - ■ Vital signs: slow, irregular pulse, hypotension
    - ■ Neuromusculoskeletal: restlessness, irritability, weakness to the point of ascending flaccid paralysis, paresthesias
    - ■ ECG: premature ventricular contractions, ventricular fibrillation, peaked T waves, and widened QRS
    - ■ Gastrointestinal: nausea, vomiting, increased motility, diarrhea, hyperactive bowel sounds
    - ■ Other signs: oliguria
    - ■ Laboratory Tests
      - ☐ Serum potassium: increased (> 5.0 mEq/L)
      - ☐ Arterial blood gases: metabolic acidosis (pH < 7.35)
    - ■ Diagnostic Procedures
      - ☐ Electrocardiogram
        - ► Will show dysrhythmias (ventricular fibrillation, peaked T waves, widened QRS)
- • Collaborative Care
  - ○ Nursing Care
    - ■ Report abnormal findings to the provider.
    - ■ Cardiac protection: Prepare to administer calcium gluconate or calcium chloride.
    - ■ Decrease potassium intake:
      - ☐ Stop the infusion of IV potassium.
      - ☐ Withhold oral potassium.
      - ☐ Provide a potassium-restricted diet (avoid foods high in potassium [avocados, broccoli, dairy products, dried fruit, cantaloupe, bananas]).
    - ■ Promote movement of potassium from ECF to ICF:
      - ☐ Administer IV fluids with dextrose and Regular insulin.
      - ☐ Administer sodium bicarbonate to reverse acidosis.
    - ■ Monitor the client's cardiac rhythm and intervene promptly as needed.

- ○ Medications (to increase potassium excretion)
  - ■ Administer loop diuretics (furosemide [Lasix]) if renal function is adequate.
    - □ Loop diuretics increase the depletion of potassium from the renal system.
    - □ Nursing Considerations
      - ‣ Maintain IV access.
    - □ Client Education
      - ‣ Educate the client on a potassium-restricted diet.
      - ‣ Instruct the client to hold oral potassium supplements until further advised by the provider.
  - ■ Administer cation exchange resins (sodium polystyrene sulfonate [Kayexalate]).
    - □ Works as a laxative and excretes excess potassium from the body. Can be used on clients with renal problems.
    - □ Nursing Considerations
      - ‣ If potassium levels are extremely high, dialysis may be required.
    - □ Client Education
      - ‣ Educate the client on a potassium-restricted diet.
      - ‣ Instruct the client to hold oral potassium supplements until further advised by the provider.
- ○ Interdisciplinary Care
  - ■ Nephrology may be consulted if dialysis is needed and for electrolyte and fluid management.
  - ■ Nutritional services may be consulted for food choices containing potassium-restricted foods.
  - ■ Cardiology may be consulted for dysrhythmias.
- Care After Discharge
  - ○ Client Education
    - ■ Educate the client about potassium-restricted foods to consume.
    - ■ Teach the client ways to prevent an increase in potassium by reading food labels and avoiding salt substitutes containing potassium.
- Client Outcomes
  - ○ The client will be free from injury.
  - ○ The client will maintain a potassium level within the expected reference range.
  - ○ The client will consume a low-potassium diet.

- Complications
  - Cardiac Arrest
    - Nursing Actions
      - Treat dysrhythmias.
      - Perform continuous cardiac monitoring.

OTHER ELECTROLYTE IMBALANCES

Overview

- Other electrolyte imbalances are:
  - Calcium
    - Hypocalcemia
    - Hypercalcemia
  - Chloride
    - Hypochloremia
    - Hyperchloremia
  - Magnesium
    - Hypomagnesemia
    - Hypermagnesemia
  - Phosphorus
    - Hypophosphatemia
    - Hyperphosphatemia
- In particular, nurses should be aware of the implications of hypocalcemia and hypomagnesemia.

Hypocalcemia

- Hypocalcemia is a serum calcium less than 9.0 mg/dL or ionized calcium less than 4.5 mg/dL.
- Assessment
  - Risk Factors
    - Malabsorption syndromes (Crohn's disease)
    - Hypoalbuminemia
    - End-stage kidney disease
    - Post thyroidectomy
    - Hypoparathyroidism

- Inadequate intake of calcium
- Vitamin D deficiency (becoming more common today) or lack of 25-hydroxy vitamin D related to ESKD
- Pancreatitis
- Hyperphosphatemia
- Medications that block parathyroid function, cause hyperphosphatemia, chelate calcium, or prevent absorption of calcium
- Sepsis
- Subjective Data and Objective Data
  - Paresthesia of the fingers and lips (early symptom)
  - Muscle twitches/tetany
  - Frequent, painful muscle spasms at rest
  - Hyperactive deep tendon reflexes
  - Positive Chvostek's sign (tapping on the facial nerve triggering facial twitching)
  - Positive Trousseau's sign (hand/finger spasms with sustained blood pressure cuff inflation)
  - Cardiovascular: decreased myocardial contractility (decreased heart rate and hypotension)
  - Gastrointestinal: hyperactive bowel sounds, diarrhea, abdominal cramping
  - Laboratory Tests
    - Calcium level less than 9.0 mg/dL
  - Diagnostic Procedures
    - Electrocardiogram
      - ECG changes: prolonged QT interval
- Collaborative Care
  - Nursing Care
    - Administer oral or IV calcium supplements.
    - Implement seizure precautions.
    - Have emergency equipment on standby.
    - Encourage foods high in calcium including dairy products and dark green vegetables.
  - Interdisciplinary Care
    - Endocrinology may be consulted for electrolyte and fluid management.
    - Respiratory services may be consulted for oxygen management.
    - Nutritional services may be consulted for food choices high in calcium.
    - Cardiology may be consulted for dysrhythmias.

- ○ Care After Discharge
  - ■ Client Education
    - □ Educate the client about consuming foods high in calcium (yogurt, milk).
    - □ Teach the client ways to increase in calcium by reading food labels.
- ○ Client Outcomes
  - ■ The client will maintain serum calcium levels within the normal range.
  - ■ The client will be free from injury.
  - ■ The client will be free from convulsions.

Hypomagnesemia

- Hypomagnesemia is a serum magnesium level less than 1.3 mg/dL.
- Assessment
  - ○ Risk Factors
    - ■ Causes of hypomagnesemia
      - □ Malnutrition (insufficient magnesium intake)
      - □ Alcohol ingestion (magnesium excretion)
    - ■ Subjective and Objective Data
      - □ Neuromuscular: increased nerve impulse transmission (hyperactive deep tendon reflexes, paresthesias, muscle tetany), positive Chvostek's and Trousseau's signs
      - □ Gastrointestinal: hypoactive bowel sounds, constipation, abdominal distention, paralytic ileus.
- Collaborative Care
  - ○ Nursing Care
    - ■ Discontinue magnesium-losing medications (e.g., loop diuretics).
    - ■ Administer oral or IV magnesium sulfate following safety protocols. IV route used as IM can cause pain and tissue damage. Oral magnesium can cause diarrhea and increase magnesium depletion. Monitor the client closely.
    - ■ Encourage foods high in magnesium, including dairy products and dark green vegetables.
    - ■ Oral magnesium can cause diarrhea and increase magnesium depletion. Monitor the client closely.
  - ○ Interdisciplinary Care
    - ■ Endocrinology may be consulted for electrolyte and fluid management.
    - ■ Respiratory services may be consulted for oxygen management.

- ■ Nutritional services may be consulted for food choices high in magnesium.
- ■ Cardiology may be consulted for dysrhythmias.
- ○ Care After Discharge
  - ■ Client Education
    - □ Educate the client regarding foods that are high in magnesium.
    - □ Teach the client ways to increase magnesium in diet by reading food labels.
- ○ Client Outcomes
  - ■ The client will be free from injury.
  - ■ The client will be free from seizures.

CHAPTER 49: ELECTROLYTE IMBALANCES

(A) Application Exercises

1. A nurse is caring for a client with the following electrolyte results: Na+ 133 mEq/L and K+ 3.4 mEq/L. Which of the following treatments likely caused these results?

   A. Three tap water enemas

   B. 0.9% sodium chloride 50 mL/hr

   C. D_5W with 20 K+ 80 mL/hr

   D. Administration of glucocorticoids

2. A nurse is caring for a client who has a potassium level of 5.4 mEq/L. The nurse should assess the client for

   A. ECG changes.

   B. constipation.

   C. polyuria.

   D. hypotension.

3. For which of the following electrolyte imbalances should the nurse monitor a client who has a nasogastric tube with suctioning?

   A. Hyperkalemia

   B. Hypernatremia

   C. Hypokalemia and hyponatremia

   D. Hypomagnesemia

4. Which of the following conditions might result in hyperkalemia?

   A. Diabetic ketoacidosis

   B. Heart failure

   C. Diabetes insipidus

   D. Thyroidectomy

5. When testing a client for Chvostek's sign, where should the nurse tap?

CHAPTER 49: ELECTROLYTE IMBALANCES

 Application Exercises Answer Key

1. A nurse is caring for a client with the following electrolyte results: Na+ 133 mEq/L and K+ 3.4 mEq/L. Which of the following treatments likely caused these results?

   A. Three tap water enemas

   B. 0.9% sodium chloride 50 mL/hr

   C. D_5W with 20 K+ 80 mL/hr

   D. Administration of glucocorticoids

   Tap water is hypotonic and gastrointestinal losses are isotonic. This creates an imbalance and solute dilution. Administering normal saline, D_5W with 20 K + 80mL/hr, or glucocorticoids should not cause these results.

   (N) NCLEX® Connection: Physiological Adaptation, Fluid and Electrolyte Imbalances

2. A nurse is caring for a client who has a potassium level of 5.4 mEq/L. The nurse should assess the client for

   A. ECG changes.

   B. constipation.

   C. polyuria.

   D. hypotension.

   Potassium levels can affect the heart resulting in arrhythmias. An ECG would indicate these findings. Constipation and polyuria are signs of hypokalemia and hypotension is a sign of hypokalemia.

   (N) NCLEX® Connection: Physiological Adaptation, Fluid and Electrolyte Imbalances

3. For which of the following electrolyte imbalances should the nurse monitor a client who has a nasogastric tube with suctioning?

   A. Hyperkalemia

   B. Hypernatremia

   C. Hypokalemia and hyponatremia

   D. Hypomagnesemia

   Nasogastric losses are isotonic, containing both sodium and potassium. Hyperkalemia, hypernatremia, and hypomagnesemia would not be indicated for the client.

   (N) NCLEX® Connection: Physiological Adaptation, Fluid and Electrolyte Imbalances

4. Which of the following conditions might result in hyperkalemia?

   A. Diabetic ketoacidosis
   B. Heart failure
   C. Diabetes insipidus
   D. Thyroidectomy

   Diabetic ketoacidosis might result in hyperkalemia. Heart failure, diabetes insipidus, and thyroidectomy would not result in hyperkalemia.

   (N) NCLEX® Connection: Physiological Adaptation, Fluid and Electrolyte Imbalances

5. When testing a client for Chvostek's sign, where should the nurse tap?

   The nurse should tap on the client's facial nerve just below and anterior to the ear. A positive response is facial twitching of the mouth, nose, and cheek on the side being tested.

   (N) NCLEX® Connection: Physiological Adaptation, Fluid and Electrolyte Imbalances

UNIT 6	NURSING CARE OF CLIENTS WITH FLUID/ELECTROLYTE/ ACID-BASE IMBALANCES
Chapter 50	Acid-Base Imbalances

Overview

- For cells to function optimally, metabolic processes must maintain a steady balance between the acids and bases found in the body.

  ○ Acid-base balance represents homeostasis of hydrogen (H^+) ion concentration in body fluids. Hydrogen shifts between the extracellular and intracellular compartments to compensate for acid-base imbalances.

  ○ Minor changes in hydrogen concentration have major effects on normal cellular function.

- Arterial pH is an indirect measurement of hydrogen ion concentration and is a result of respiratory and renal compensational function. Arterial blood gases (ABGs) are most commonly used to evaluate acid-base balance.

  ○ The pH is the expression of the balance between carbon dioxide (CO_2), which is regulated by the lungs, and bicarbonate (HCO_3^-), a base regulated by the kidneys.

    ■ The greater the concentration of hydrogen, the more acidic the body fluids and the lower the pH.

    ■ The lower the concentration of hydrogen, the more alkaline the body fluids and the higher the pH.

Maintenance of Acid-Base Balance

- Acid-base balance is maintained by chemical, respiratory, and renal processes.

  ○ Chemical and protein buffers:

    ■ Are the first line of defense.

    ■ Either bind or release hydrogen ions as needed.

    ■ Respond quickly to changes in pH.

  ○ Respiratory buffers:

    ■ Are the second line of defense.

    ■ Control the level of hydrogen ions in the blood through the control of CO_2 levels.

    ■ When a chemoreceptor senses a change in the level of CO_2, a signal is sent to the brain to alter the rate and depth of respirations.

      □ Hyperventilation = decrease in hydrogen ions

      □ Hypoventilation = increase in hydrogen ions

- ○ Renal buffers:
  - ■ The kidneys are the third line of defense.
  - ■ This buffering system is much slower to respond, but it is the most effective buffering system with the longest duration.
  - ■ The kidneys control the movement of bicarbonate in the urine. Bicarbonate can be reabsorbed into the bloodstream or excreted in the urine in response to blood levels of hydrogen.
  - ■ The kidneys may also produce more bicarbonate when needed.
    - ☐ High hydrogen ions = bicarbonate reabsorption and production
    - ☐ Low hydrogen ions = bicarbonate excretion
- Compensation refers to the process by which the body attempts to correct changes and imbalances in pH levels.
  - ○ Full compensation occurs when the pH level of the blood returns to normal (7.35 to 7.45).
  - ○ If the pH level is not able to normalize, then it is referred to as partial compensation.
- Metabolic alkalosis, metabolic acidosis, respiratory alkalosis, and respiratory acidosis are examples of acid-base imbalances.
- Acid-base imbalances are a result of insufficient compensation. Respiratory and renal function plays a large role in the body's ability to effectively compensate for acid-base alterations. Organ dysfunction negatively affects acid-base compensation.

Respiratory Compensation   Metabolic Compensation

$$H_2O + CO_2 \longleftrightarrow H_2CO_3 \longleftrightarrow H^+ + HCO_3^-$$

Water Carbon   Carbonic   Hydrogen Bicarbonate
       dioxide   acid   ion

Expelled   Expelled
by lungs   by kidneys

Health Promotion and Disease Prevention

- Encourage a healthy diet and physical activity.
- Limit the consumption of alcohol.
- Encourage drinking six to eight glasses of water daily.
- Maintain an appropriate weight for height and body frame.
- Promote smoking cessation.

Assessment

- Risk Factors/Causes of Acid-Base Imbalances

RESPIRATORY ACIDOSIS–HYPOVENTILATION	RESPIRATORY ALKALOSIS–HYPERVENTILATION
Respiratory acidosis results from: - Respiratory depression from poisons, anesthetics, trauma, or neurological diseases (myasthenia gravis, Guillain-Barré). - Inadequate chest expansion due to muscle weakness, pneumothorax/hemothorax, flail chest, obesity, tumors, or deformities. - Airway obstruction that occurs in laryngospasm, asthma, and some cancers. - Alveolar-capillary blockage secondary to a pulmonary embolus, thrombus, cancer, or pulmonary edema. - Inadequate mechanical ventilation. Respiratory acidosis results in: - Increased CO_2. - Increased H^+ concentration.	Respiratory alkalosis results from: - Hyperventilation due to fear, anxiety, intracerebral trauma, salicylate toxicity, or excessive mechanical ventilation. - Hypoxemia from asphyxiation, high altitudes, shock, or early-stage asthma or pneumonia. Respiratory alkalosis results in: - Decreased CO_2. - Decreased H^+ concentration.
METABOLIC ACIDOSIS	METABOLIC ALKALOSIS

Metabolic acidosis results from:
- Excess production of hydrogen ions
  o DKA
  o Lactic acidosis
  o Starvation
  o Heavy exercise
  o Seizure activity
  o Fever
  o Hypoxia
  o Intoxication with ethanol or salicylates
- Inadequate elimination of hydrogen ions
  o Renal failure
- Inadequate production of bicarbonate
  o Renal failure
  o Pancreatitis
  o Liver failure
  o Dehydration
- Excess elimination of bicarbonate
  o Diarrhea, ileostomy
Metabolic acidosis results in:
- Decreased HCO_3^-.
- Increased $H+$ concentration.
	Metabolic alkalosis results from:
	- Base excess
	  o Oral ingestion of bases (antacids)
	  o Venous administration of bases (blood transfusions, TPN, or sodium bicarbonate)
	- Acid deficit
	  o Loss of gastric secretions (through prolonged vomiting, NG suction)
	  o Potassium depletion (due to thiazide diuretics, laxative abuse, Cushing's syndrome)
	Metabolic alkalosis results in:
	- Increased HCO_3^-.
	- Decreased $H+$ concentration.

- Subjective and Objective Data

RESPIRATORY ACIDOSIS–HYPOVENTILATION	RESPIRATORY ALKALOSIS–HYPERVENTILATION
- Vital signs: Tachycardia (severe acidosis may lead to bradycardia), tachypnea - Dysrhythmias - Neurological: Anxiety, irritability, confusion, coma - Respiratory: Ineffective, shallow, rapid breathing - Skin: Pale or cyanotic	- Vital Signs: Tachypnea - Neurological: Anxiety, tetany, convulsions, tingling, numbness - CV: Palpitations, chest pain, dysrhythmias - Respiratory: Rapid, deep respirations
METABOLIC ACIDOSIS	**METABOLIC ALKALOSIS**
- Vital Signs: Bradycardia, weak peripheral pulses, hypotension, tachypnea - Dysrhythmias - Neurological: Muscle weakness, hyporeflexia, flaccid paralysis, fatigue, confusion - Respiratory: Rapid, deep respirations (Kussmaul respirations) - Skin: Warm, dry, flushed	- Vital Signs: Tachycardia, normotensive or hypotensive - Dysrhythmias - Neurological: Numbness, tingling, tetany, muscle weakness, hyperreflexia, confusion, convulsion - Respiratory: Depressed skeletal muscles resulting in ineffective breathing

- Laboratory Tests and Diagnostic Procedures

  - To determine the type of imbalance, follow these steps:

Step 1: Look at pH.

If < 7.35, diagnose as acidosis.
If > 7.45, diagnose as alkalosis.

Step 2: Look at $PaCO_2$ and HCO_3^- simultaneously.

Determine which is in the normal range.

Conclude that the other is the indicator of imbalance.

Diagnose < 35 or > 45 $PaCO_2$ as respiratory in origin.

Diagnose < 22 or > 26 HCO_3^- as metabolic in origin.

Step 3: Combine diagnoses of Steps 1 and 2 to name the type of imbalance

Step 4: Evaluate the PaO_2 and the SaO_2.

If the results are below the normal range, the client is hypoxic.

Step 5: Determine compensation as follows:

Uncompensated: The pH will be abnormal and either the HCO_3^- or the $PaCO_2$ will be abnormal.

Partially compensated: The pH, HCO_3^-, and $PaCO_2$ will be abnormal.

Fully compensated: The pH will be normal, but the $PaCO_2$ and HCO_3^- will both be abnormal. Looking back at the pH will provide a clue as to which system initiated the problem, respiratory or metabolic. If the pH is < 7.40, think "acidosis" and determine which system has the acidosis value. If the pH is > 7.40, think "alkalosis" and determine which system has the alkalosis value.

- The following are the five classic types of ABG results demonstrating balance and imbalance.

STEP 1	STEP 2		STEP 3
If	Determine which is in normal range		Combine names
pH	$PaCO_2$	HCO_3^-	Diagnosis
7.35-7.45	35-45	22-26	Homeostasis
< 7.35	> 45	22-26	Respiratory acidosis
< 7.35	35-45	< 22	Metabolic acidosis
> 7.45	< 35	22-26	Respiratory alkalosis
> 7.45	35-45	> 26	Metabolic alkalosis

Collaborative Care

- Nursing Care

  o For all acid-base imbalances, it is imperative to treat the underlying cause.

  o Respiratory acidosis: Oxygen therapy, maintain patent airway, and enhance gas exchange (positioning and breathing techniques, ventilatory support, bronchodilators, mucolytics).

  o Respiratory alkalosis: Oxygen therapy, anxiety reduction interventions, and rebreathing techniques.

  o Metabolic acidosis: Varies with causes (if DKA, administer insulin; if related to GI losses, administer antidiarrheals and provide rehydration; if serum bicarbonate is low, administer sodium bicarbonate [1 mEq/kg]).

  o Metabolic alkalosis: Varies with causes (if GI losses, administer antiemetics, fluids, and electrolyte replacements; if related to potassium depletion, discontinue causative agent).

- Interdisciplinary Care

  o Respiratory services can be consulted for oxygen therapy, breathing treatments, and ABGs.

  o Pulmonology services can be consulted for respiratory management.

- Care after Discharge
  - Client Education
    - Education may vary in relation to the client's condition.
    - Encourage adherence to the prescribed diet and dialysis regimen for clients who have kidney dysfunction.
    - Encourage the client to weigh self daily and notify the provider if there is a 1 to 2 lb gain in 24 hr or a 3 lb gain in 1 week.
    - Promote smoking cessation if the client is a smoker.
    - Teach the client to take medication as prescribed. Encourage adherence to the medication regimen for clients who have COPD.
  - Set up referral services (home oxygen).
- Client Outcomes
  - The client will be free from anxiety.
  - The client will maintain an adequate gas exchange.
  - The client will have arterial blood gas results within the expected reference range.

Complications

- Convulsions, Coma, and Respiratory Arrest
  - These are potential complications of acid-base imbalances.
  - Nursing Actions
    - Implement seizure precautions and perform management interventions if necessary.
    - Provide life-support interventions if necessary.

CHAPTER 50: ACID-BASE IMBALANCES

 Application Exercises

1. Interpret each of the following ABG results.

Possible interpretations: Respiratory acidosis, respiratory alkalosis, metabolic acidosis, metabolic alkalosis, partially compensated metabolic acidosis, partially compensated metabolic alkalosis, partially compensated respiratory acidosis, partially compensated respiratory alkalosis, normal.

pH 7.28 $PaCO_2$ 56 mm Hg HCO_3^- 25 mEq/L SaO_2 89% Interpretation: _____	pH 7.49 $PaCO_2$ 30 mm Hg HCO_3^- 23 mEq/L SaO_2 96% Interpretation: _____
pH 7.28 $PaCO_2$ 43 mm Hg HCO_3^- 18 mEq/L SaO_2 96% Interpretation: _____	pH 7.40 $PaCO_2$ 40 mm Hg HCO_3^- 24 mEq/L SaO_2 98% Interpretation: _____
pH 7.50 $PaCO_2$ 36 mm Hg HCO_3^- 27 mEq/L SaO_2 97% Interpretation: _____	pH 7.33 $PaCO_2$ 29 mm Hg HCO_3^- 16 mEq/L SaO_2 95% Interpretation: _____
pH 7.35 $PaCO_2$ 42 mm Hg HCO_3^- 26 mEq/L SaO_2 95% Interpretation: _____	pH 7.12 $PaCO_2$ 60 mm Hg HCO_3^- 29 mEq/ SaO_2 94% Interpretation: _____
pH 7.48 $PaCO_2$ 33 mm Hg HCO_3^- 24 mEq/L SaO_2 96% Interpretation: _____	pH 7.58 $PaCO_2$ 47 mm Hg HCO_3^- 30 mEq/L SaO_2 95% Interpretation: _____
pH 7.36 $PaCO_2$ 44 mm Hg HCO_3^- 24 mEq/L SaO_2 98% Interpretation: _____	pH 7.30 $PaCO_2$ 59 mm Hg HCO_3^- 38 mEq/L SaO_2 94% Interpretation: _____

2. A young adult female client who has a history of depression is admitted with confusion and lethargy. She was found at home with an empty bottle of aspirin next to her in the bed. Vital signs reveal a blood pressure of 104/72 mm Hg, pulse rate of 116 beats/min with a regular rhythm, and a respiratory rate of 42/min and deep. Which of the following arterial blood gas results should the nurse expect?

    A. pH 7.38, PaO_2 96 mm Hg, $PaCO_2$ 38 mm Hg, HCO_3^- 24 mEq/L

    B. pH 7.48, PaO_2 100 mm Hg, $PaCO_2$ 28 mm Hg, HCO_3^- 23 mEq/L

    C. pH 6.98, PaO_2 100 mm Hg, $PaCO_2$ 30 mm Hg, HCO_3^- 18 mEq/L

    D. pH 7.58, PaO_2 96 mm Hg, $PaCO_2$ 38 mm Hg, HCO_3^- 29 mEq/L

3. An adult male client was involved in a single-vehicle car crash. He is reporting chest pain and difficulty breathing, A chest x-ray reveals a pneumothorax and blood gas analysis is obtained. Which of the following results should the nurse expect?

    A. pH 7.06, PaO_2 86 mm Hg, $PaCO_2$ 52 mm Hg, HCO_3^- 24 mEq/L

    B. pH 7.42, PaO_2 100 mm Hg, $PaCO_2$ 38 mm Hg, HCO_3^- 23 mEq/L

    C. pH 6.98, PaO_2 100 mm Hg, $PaCO_2$ 30 mm Hg, HCO_3^- 18 mEq/L

    D. pH 7.58, PaO_2 96 mm Hg, $PaCO_2$ 38 mm Hg, HCO_3^- 29 mEq/L

4. A client is in the first trimester of pregnancy. She has experienced approximately 1 week of severe nausea with frequent vomiting. Which of the following conditions should the nurse expect to find if an arterial blood gas is analyzed?

    A. Respiratory acidosis

    B. Respiratory alkalosis

    C. Metabolic acidosis

    D. Metabolic alkalosis

CHAPTER 50: ACID-BASE IMBALANCES

 Application Exercises Answer Key

1. Interpret each of the following ABG results.

Possible interpretations: Respiratory acidosis, respiratory alkalosis, metabolic acidosis, metabolic alkalosis, partially compensated metabolic acidosis, partially compensated metabolic alkalosis, partially compensated respiratory acidosis, partially compensated respiratory alkalosis, normal.

pH 7.28 $PaCO_2$ 56 mm Hg HCO_3^- 25 mEq/L SaO_2 89% **Interpretation: Respiratory acidosis**	pH 7.49 $PaCO_2$ 30 mm Hg HCO_3^- 23 mEq/L SaO_2 96% **Interpretation: Respiratory alkalosis**
pH 7.28 $PaCO_2$ 43 mm Hg HCO_3^- 18 mEq/L SaO_2 96% **Interpretation: Metabolic acidosis**	pH 7.40 $PaCO_2$ 40 mm Hg HCO_3^- 24 mEq/L SaO_2 98% **Interpretation: Normal**
pH 7.50 $PaCO_2$ 36 mm Hg HCO_3^- 27 mEq/L SaO_2 97% **Interpretation: Metabolic alkalosis**	pH 7.33 $PaCO_2$ 29 mm Hg HCO_3^- 16 mEq/L SaO_2 95% **Interpretation: Partially compensated metabolic acidosis**
pH 7.35 $PaCO_2$ 42 mm Hg HCO_3^- 26 mEq/L SaO_2 95% **Interpretation: Normal**	pH 7.12 $PaCO_2$ 60 mm Hg HCO_3^- 29 mEq/L SaO_2 94% **Interpretation: Partially compensated respiratory acidosis**
pH 7.48 $PaCO_2$ 33 mm Hg HCO_3^- 24 mEq/L SaO_2 96% **Interpretation: Respiratory alkalosis**	pH 7.58 $PaCO_2$ 47 mm Hg HCO_3^- 30 mEq/L SaO_2 95% **Interpretation: Partially compensated metabolic alkalosis**
pH 7.36 $PaCO_2$ 44 mm Hg HCO_3^- 24 mEq/L SaO_2 98% **Interpretation: Normal**	pH 7.30 $PaCO_2$ 59 mm Hg HCO_3^- 38 mEq/L SaO_2 94% **Interpretation: Partially compensated respiratory acidosis**

Ⓝ NCLEX® Connection: Reduction of Risk Potential, Laboratory Values

2. A young adult female client who has a history of depression is admitted with confusion and lethargy. She was found at home with an empty bottle of aspirin next to her in the bed. Vital signs reveal a blood pressure of 104/72 mm Hg, pulse rate of 116 beats/min with a regular rhythm, and a respiratory rate of 42/min and deep. Which of the following arterial blood gas results should the nurse expect?

    A. pH 7.38, PaO_2 96 mm Hg, $PaCO_2$ 38 mm Hg, HCO_3^- 24 mEq/L

    B. pH 7.48, PaO_2 100 mm Hg, $PaCO_2$ 28 mm Hg, HCO_3^- 23 mEq/L

    C. pH 6.98, PaO_2 100 mm Hg, $PaCO_2$ 30 mm Hg, HCO_3^- 18 mEq/L

    D. pH 7.58, PaO_2 96 mm Hg, $PaCO_2$ 38 mm Hg, HCO_3^- 29 mEq/L

An aspirin overdose would result in metabolic acidosis. Metabolic alkalosis, respiratory acidosis, and respiratory alkalosis would not be indicated in the client.

 NCLEX® Connection: Reduction of Risk Potential, Laboratory Values

3. An adult male client was involved in a single-vehicle car crash. He is reporting chest pain and difficulty breathing, A chest x-ray reveals a pneumothorax and blood gas analysis is obtained. Which of the following results should the nurse expect?

    A. pH 7.06, PaO_2 86 mm Hg, $PaCO_2$ 52 mm Hg, HCO_3^- 24 mEq/L

    B. pH 7.42, PaO_2 100 mm Hg, $PaCO_2$ 38 mm Hg, HCO_3^- 23 mEq/L

    C. pH 6.98, PaO_2 100 mm Hg, $PaCO_2$ 30 mm Hg, HCO_3^- 18 mEq/L

    D. pH 7.58, PaO_2 96 mm Hg, $PaCO_2$ 38 mm Hg, HCO_3^- 29 mEq/L

Pneumothorax can cause alveolar hypoventilation and increased carbon dioxide levels, resulting in a state of respiratory acidosis. Respiratory alkalosis, metabolic alkalosis, and metabolic acidosis would not be indicated in the client.

 NCLEX® Connection: Reduction of Risk Potential, Laboratory Values

4. A client is in the first trimester of pregnancy. She has experienced approximately 1 week of severe nausea with frequent vomiting. Which of the following conditions should the nurse expect to find if an arterial blood gas is analyzed?

    A. Respiratory acidosis

    B. Respiratory alkalosis

    C. Metabolic acidosis

    D. Metabolic alkalosis

Excessive vomiting causes a loss of gastric acids and an accumulation of bicarbonate in the blood, resulting in metabolic alkalosis. Respiratory acidosis, respiratory alkalosis, and metabolic acidosis would not be indicated in the client.

 NCLEX® Connection: Reduction of Risk Potential, Laboratory Values

UNIT 7: NURSING CARE OF CLIENTS WITH GASTROINTESTINAL DISORDERS

- Diagnostic and Therapeutic Procedures
- Upper Gastrointestinal Disorders
- Lower Gastrointestinal Disorders
- Gallbladder and Pancreas Disorders
- Liver Disorders

NCLEX® CONNECTIONS

When reviewing the chapters in this unit, keep in mind the relevant sections of the NCLEX® outline, in particular:

CLIENT NEEDS: BASIC CARE AND COMFORT

Relevant topics/tasks include:
- Elimination
  - Assess and manage the client with an alteration in elimination.
  - Evaluate whether the client's elimination is restored/maintained.
- Nutrition and Oral Hydration
  - Provide/maintain special diets based on the client's diagnosis/nutritional needs and cultural considerations.

CLIENT NEEDS: PHARMACOLOGICAL AND PARENTERAL THERAPIES

Relevant topics/tasks include:
- Blood and Blood Products
  - Document necessary information on the administration of red blood cells/blood products.
- Pharmacological Pain Management
  - Assess the client's need for administration of a PRN pain medication.
- Total Parenteral Nutrition (TPN)
  - Administer parenteral nutrition and evaluate the client's response.

CLIENT NEEDS: REDUCTION OF RISK POTENTIAL

Relevant topics/tasks include:
- Diagnostic Tests
  - Perform diagnostic testing.
- Potential for Complications of Diagnostic Tests/Treatments/Procedures
  - Insert, maintain, and remove nasogastric tubes and/or urethral catheters.
- Therapeutic Procedures
  - Manage the client during and following a procedure with moderate sedation.

UNIT 7	NURSING CARE OF CLIENTS WITH GASTROINTESTINAL DISORDERS
Section	Diagnostic and Therapeutic Procedures
Chapter 51	Gastrointestinal Diagnostic Procedures

Overview

- Gastrointestinal diagnostic procedures involve the use of scopes and x-rays to visualize parts of the gastrointestinal system, as well as evaluate gastrointestinal fluid.

- Gastrointestinal diagnostic procedures that nurses should be knowledgeable about

    o Liver function tests and other blood tests

    o Urine bilinogen

    o Fecal occult blood test (FOBT) and stool samples

    o Endoscopy

    o Gastrointestinal (GI) series

Liver Function Tests and Other Blood Tests

- Liver function tests – Aspartate aminotransferase (AST), alanine aminotransferase (ALT), alkaline phosphatase (ALP), bilirubin, and albumin

- Other blood tests that provide information on the functioning of the gastrointestinal system include – Amylase, lipase, alpha-fetoprotein, and ammonia.

- Indications

    o Suspected liver, pancreatic, or biliary tract disorder

- Interpretation of Findings

BLOOD TEST	NORMAL VALUES	INTERPRETATION OF FINDINGS
Aspartate aminotransferase (AST)	5 to 40 units/L	Elevation occurs with hepatitis or cirrhosis
Alanine aminotransferase (ALT)	8 to 20 units/L 3 to 35 IU/L	Elevation occurs with hepatitis or cirrhosis
Alkaline phosphatase (ALP)	42 to 128 units/L 30 to 85 IU/L	Elevation indicates liver damage
Amylase	56 to 90 IU/L	Elevation occurs with pancreatitis
Lipase	0 to 110 units/L	Elevation occurs with pancreatitis
Total bilirubin	0 to 1.0 mg/dL	Elevations indicate altered liver functioning, bile duct obstruction, or other hepatobiliary disorder
Direct (conjugated) bilirubin	0 to 0.3 mg/dL	Elevations indicate altered liver functioning, bile duct obstruction, or other hepatobiliary disorder
Indirect (unconjugated) bilirubin	0.1 to 1.0 mg/dL	Elevations indicate altered liver functioning, bile duct obstruction, or other hepatobiliary disorder
Albumin	3.5 to 5.0 g/dL	Decrease may indicate hepatic disease
Alpha-fetoprotein	< 40 mcg/L	Elevated in liver cancer
Ammonia	15 to 110 mg/dL	Elevated in liver disease

- Preprocedure

  - Explain to the client how blood will be drawn and what information this will provide.

- Postprocedure

  - Let the client know when and how results will be provided.

Urine Bilirubin

- Also known as urobilinogen, this is a urine test done to determine the presence of bilirubin the in urine.

- Indications

  - Suspected liver or biliary tract disorder

- Interpretation of Findings

  - A positive or elevated finding indicates possible liver disorder (cirrhosis, hepatitis) or biliary obstruction.

- Preprocedure
  - Nursing Actions
    - The test may be performed by using a dipstick (urine bilirubin) or a 24-hr urine collection (urobilinogen).
  - Client Education
    - Teach the client how to collect urine and provide proper collection container.
- Postprocedure
  - Nursing Actions
    - Let the client know when and how results will be provided.

Fecal Occult Blood Test and Stool Samples

- A stool sample is collected and tested for blood, ova and parasites (Giardia), and bacteria (*Clostridium difficile*).
- Indications
  - Client Presentation
    - Gastrointestinal bleeding
    - Unexplained diarrhea
- Interpretation of Findings
  - A positive finding for blood is indicative of gastrointestinal bleeding (ulcer, colitis, cancer).
  - A positive finding for ova and parasites is indicative of a gastrointestinal parasitic infection.
  - A positive finding for *clostridium difficile* is indicative of this opportunistic infection, which usually becomes established secondary to use of broad-spectrum antibiotics.
- Preprocedure
  - Nursing Actions
    - Occult blood – Provide the client with cards impregnated with guaiac that can be mailed to provider or with a container for a specimen collection cup. If the cards are used, three samples are usually required.
    - Stool for ova and parasites and bacteria – Provide the client with a specimen collection cup.

- o Client Education

  - ▪ Occult blood – Instruct the client about proper collection of a stool sample using a card or sample collection cup. The client may also need to be instructed about dietary and medication restrictions to follow prior to obtaining samples (red meat, anticoagulants).

  - ▪ Stool for ova and parasites and bacteria – Instruct the client about proper collection technique (time frame for submission to laboratory, need for refrigeration).

- • Postprocedure

  - o Nursing Actions

    - ▪ Let the client know when and how the results will be provided.

Endoscopy

- • Endoscopic procedures allow direct visualization of body cavities, tissues, and organs through the use of a flexible, lighted tube (endoscope). They are performed for diagnostic and therapeutic purposes.

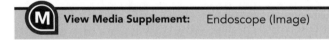

View Media Supplement: Endoscope (Image)

- o Endoscopic procedures can be performed in outpatient diagnostic centers, provider offices, and acute-care settings. Endoscopic procedures are primarily performed for diagnostic purposes. However, during an endoscopic procedure, the provider can perform biopsies, remove abnormal tissue, and perform minor surgery, such as cauterizing a bleeding ulcer.

- o During some endoscopic procedures a contrast medium is injected to allow visualization of structures beyond the capabilities of the scope.

- o Gastrointestinal scope procedures

  - ▪ Colonoscopy – Allows visualization of the anus, rectum, and colon

  - ▪ Esophagogastroduodenoscopy – Allows visualization of the oropharynx, esophagus, stomach, and duodenum.

  - ▪ Endoscopic retrograde cholangiopancreatography – Allows visualization of the liver, gallbladder, and bile ducts

  - ▪ Sigmoidoscopy – Allows visualization of the anus, rectum, and sigmoid colon

- • Indications

  - o Potential Diagnoses

    - ▪ Gastrointestinal bleeding, ulcerations or inflammation, polyps, malignant tumors

○ Client Presentation

- Anemia (secondary to bleeding)

- Abdominal discomfort

- Abdominal distention or mass

- Interpretation of Findings

  ○ Findings may indicate a need for medication or surgical removal of a lesion.

- General endoscopic procedures

  ○ Preprocedure

    - Nursing Actions

      □ Evaluate the client's understanding of the procedure.

      □ Verify that a consent form has been signed for the specific procedure.

      □ Assess vital signs and verify the client's allergies.

      □ Evaluate baseline laboratory tests and report unexpected or abnormal findings to the provider. Laboratory tests may include CBC, electrolyte panel, BUN, creatinine, PT, aPTT, and liver function studies. A chest x-ray and ECG may also be ordered. ABGs may be measured before and after the procedure to assess oxygenation.

      □ Evaluate if the client's medical history increases the risk for complications.

        ▸ Age can influence the client's ability to understand the procedures, tolerance of the positioning required for some of the procedures, and compliance with any pretest preparation required for a procedure.

          ▷ Current health status – Evaluate the client's medical history for conditions and medications that can affect the client's tolerance for and recovery from the procedure.

          ▷ Cognitive status – Assess the client's understanding of the procedure and establish a baseline mental status.

          ▷ Support system – Evaluate the client's support system to determine whether a support person will assist the client after the procedure.

        ▸ Recent food or fluid intake – The presence of food or fluid in the gastrointestinal tract may affect the provider's ability to visualize key structures and increase the client's risk for complications (aspiration). Notify the provider if dietary restrictions were not followed.

        ▸ Medications – Some medications could place the client at greater risks for complications (NSAIDs, warfarin, aspirin). Notify the provider if medication restrictions were not followed.

        ▸ Previous radiographic examinations – Any recent radiographic examinations using barium may affect the provider's ability to view key structures. Notify the provider if contrast has been recently used.

▸ Ensure that the client followed proper bowel preparation (laxatives, enemas). Inadequate bowel preparation prior to a lower gastrointestinal endoscopic examination can result in cancellation and delays in completing this diagnostic examination. This situation can also lead to the client experiencing extended periods of being NPO or on a liquid diet.

▸ Electrolyte and fluid imbalances secondary to repeated enemas may affect the client's ability to tolerate any bowel preparation orders.

▸ Ensure that the client is NPO for 6 to 8 hr prior to most endoscopic examinations.

■ Client Education

☐ Provide the client with instructions regarding medication and food restrictions.

☐ Provide prescriptions for medications used as a part of the bowel prep.

☐ Instruct the client about the number and type of enemas, if prescribed.

○ Postprocedure

■ Nursing Actions

☐ Monitor the client's vital signs.

☐ Assess the client for complications.

■ Client Education

☐ If a biopsy was done during the procedure, food restrictions may be prescribed.

● Specific Endoscopic Procedures

ANESTHESIA	POSITIONING	PREPARATION	POSTPROCEDURE
Colonoscopy – Involves the use of a flexible fiberoptic colonoscope to visualize the colon. After entering through the anus, the rectum, sigmoid, descending, transverse, and ascending colon can be visualized.			
● Moderate sedation – midazolam (Versed) usually given with an opiate analgesic	● Left side with knees to chest	● Bowel prep 　○ May include laxatives, such as bisacodyl (Dulcolax®) and polyethylene glycol (GoLYTELY®) 　○ Clear liquid diet; NPO after midnight ● Instruct the client to avoid medications per the provider's order.	● Monitor for rectal bleeding. ● Resume normal diet if ordered. ● Encourage plenty of fluids. ● Monitor vital signs and respiratory status. ● Instruct the client that there may be increased flatulence due to air instillation during procedure.

ANESTHESIA	POSITIONING	PREPARATION	POSTPROCEDURE
EGD – Involves insertion of an endoscope through the client's mouth and esophagus, stomach, and duodenum. Allows visualization of these structures.			
• Moderate sedation – topical anesthetic	• Left side-lying	• NPO 6 to 8 hr; remove dentures prior to procedure.	• Monitor vital signs and respiratory status. • Notify provider of bleeding, abdominal or chest pain, and any evidence of infection. • Withhold fluids until return of gag reflex.
ERCP – Involves insertion of an endoscope through the client's mouth and into the biliary tree via the duodenum. Allows visualization of the biliary ducts and gall bladder.			
• Conscious sedation – topical anesthetic	Initially semi-prone with repositioning throughout procedure	• NPO 6 to 8 hr; remove dentures prior to procedure • Explain procedure and need to change positions during procedure.	• Monitor vital signs and respiratory status. • Notify provider of bleeding, abdominal or chest pain, and any evidence of infection. • Withhold fluids until the client's gag reflex returns.
Sigmoidoscopy – Similar to colonoscopy, but scope is shorter, thus allowing visualization of only the anus, rectum, and sigmoid colon.			
• None required	• On left side	• Bowel prep, which may include laxatives such as, bisacodyl (Dulcolax®) and polyethylene glycol (GoLYTELY®) • Clear liquid diet • NPO after midnight • Instruct the client to avoid medications per the provider's prescription.	• Monitor for rectal bleeding. • Resume normal diet if prescribed. • Encourage plenty of fluids. • Monitor vital signs and respiratory status. • Instruct the client that there may be increased flatulence due to air instillation during procedure.

- Complications
  - Oversedation
    - Any endoscopic procedure using moderate sedation places the client at risk for oversedation.
      - Symptoms of oversedation – Difficulty arousing the client, poor respiratory effort, evidence of hypoxemia, tachycardia, and elevated or low blood pressure
    - Nursing Actions
      - The nurse should be prepared to administer antidotes to the sedatives administered prior to and during the procedure, maintain an open airway, administer oxygen, and monitor the client's vital signs.
      - If evidence of oversedation occurs, the provider should be informed immediately.
    - Client Education
      - Driving and major decision making should be restricted until the effects of the sedation has worn off and this varies with the type of agents used.
  - Hemorrhage
    - Bleeding can occur after any endoscopic procedure. The nurse should monitor the client for evidence of bleeding after these procedures.
      - Symptoms of hemorrhage include bleeding, cool clammy skin, hypotension, tachycardia, dizziness, and tachypnea.
    - Nursing Actions
      - The nurse should monitor the client's vital signs after the procedure, monitor diagnostic test results (particularly Hgb and Hct), and assess for evidence of bleeding from the site.
      - The primary care provider should be notified immediately if these symptoms occur.
    - Client Education
      - Report fever, pain, and bleeding.
  - Aspiration
    - Aspiration may occur after any procedure using moderate sedation or any procedure using topical anesthesia that affects the gag reflex.
      - Symptoms of aspiration include dyspnea, tachypnea, adventitious breath sounds, tachycardia, and fever.

- ■ Nursing Actions
  - □ The client should remain NPO until the gag reflex returns. The nurse should ensure that the client is awake and alert prior to the client consuming any food or fluid. In addition, the nurse should encourage the client to deep breathe and cough to keep his airway open.
  - □ The provider should be notified if these symptoms occur.
- ■ Client Education
  - □ Have the client report any respiratory congestion or compromise.
- ○ Perforation
  - ■ Perforation of the gastrointestinal tract can occur with many of these endoscopic procedures.
    - □ Symptoms include chest or abdominal pain, fever, nausea, vomiting, and abdominal distention.
  - ■ Nursing Actions
    - □ The nurse should monitor diagnostic tests for evidence of infection, including elevated WBC counts.
    - □ The provider should be notified if these symptoms occur.
  - ■ Client Education
    - □ Have the client report fever, pain, and bleeding.

Gastrointestinal Series

- • Gastrointestinal studies are radiographic studies, done with or without contrast, that help define anatomic or functional abnormalities.
  - ○ Gastrointestinal studies provide for imaging of the esophagus, stomach and entire intestinal tract.
  - ○ Upper gastrointestinal imaging is done by having the client drink a radiopaque liquid (barium).
  - ○ A barium enema is done by instilling a radiopaque liquid into the client's rectum and colon.
- • Indications
  - ○ Potential Diagnoses
    - ■ Gastric ulcers, peristaltic disorders, tumors, varices, and intestinal enlargements or constrictions
  - ○ Client Presentation
    - ■ The client may present with abdominal pain, altered elimination habits (constipation, diarrhea), or gastrointestinal bleeding.

- Interpretation of Findings
  - Abnormal findings are those that indicate abnormal bowel shape and size, increased motility or obstruction.
- Preprocedure
  - Nursing Actions
    - Inform the client about medications, food and fluid restrictions (clear liquid and/or low residue diet, NPO after midnight), and avoiding smoking or chewing gum (increases peristalsis).
    - Inform the client of bowel preparation (laxatives, enemas) so image will not be distorted by feces.
    - Barium enema studies must be scheduled prior to upper gastrointestinal studies.
    - Assess for contraindications to bowel preparation (possible bowel perforation or obstruction, inflammatory disease).
  - Client Education
    - Tell the client to restrict food and fluids for bowel preparation.
    - Inform the client if the small intestine is to be visualized, additional radiographs will be done over the next 24 hr.
- Postprocedure
  - Nursing Actions
    - Monitor the client's elimination of contrast material and administer a laxative if prescribed.
    - Force fluids to promote elimination of contrast material.
  - Client Education
    - Instruct the client to monitor elimination of contrast material and to report retention of contrast material (constipation) or diarrhea accompanied by weakness.
    - Discuss the possible need for an over-the-counter medication to prevent constipation resulting from the barium.

CHAPTER 51: GASTROINTESTINAL DIAGNOSTIC PROCEDURES

(A) Application Exercises

1. A client is scheduled for a colonoscopy this morning and the nurse notes the client is continuing to have stool in the last output after the prescribed phospho-soda enema. The appropriate action for the nurse to take is to

    A. continue to administer enemas until return is clear.

    B. cancel the procedure.

    C. notify the provider.

    D. document the findings.

2. A client is scheduled for a colonoscopy. The provider has ordered a bowel prep using polyethylene glycol (GoLYTELY®). The nurse should include which of the following in the instructions to the client?

    A. Medication taken with this prep will not be absorbed.

    B. Eat a normal diet until the bowel prep has begun.

    C. This solution will usually not begin acting until morning.

    D. You should consume at least half of this solution to get the best results.

3. After a scope procedure a client is difficult to arouse. The priority action for the nurse to perform at this time is to

    A. assess the client's airway.

    B. allow the client to sleep.

    C. increase rate of IV fluids.

    D. evaluate preprocedure laboratory tests for abnormalities.

4. A client is scheduled for both an upper gastrointestinal and barium enema. How should the nurse schedule these exams?

    A. The upper gastrointestinal should be scheduled the same day but before the barium enema.

    B. The barium enema should be scheduled the same day but before the upper gastrointestinal.

    C. The upper gastrointestinal should be scheduled the day before the barium enema.

    D. The barium enema should be scheduled when the client is not NPO.

CHAPTER 51: GASTROINTESTINAL DIAGNOSTIC PROCEDURES

 Application Exercises Answer Key

1. A client is scheduled for a colonoscopy this morning, and the nurse notes the client is continuing to have stool in the last output after the prescribed phospho-soda enema. The appropriate action for the nurse to take is to

    A. continue to administer enemas until return is clear.

    B. cancel the procedure.

    C. notify the provider.

    D. document the findings.

    Stool will impede visualization. Additional interventions may be necessary, including delay or cancellation of the procedure.

 NCLEX® Connection: Reduction of Risk Potential, Potential for Complications of Diagnostic Tests/Treatments/Procedures

2. A client is scheduled for a colonoscopy. The provider has ordered a bowel prep using polyethylene glycol (GoLYTELY®). The nurse should include which of the following in the instructions to the client?

    A. Medication taken with this prep will not be absorbed.

    B. Eat a normal diet until the bowel prep has begun.

    C. This solution will usually not begin acting until morning.

    D. You should consume at least half of this solution to get the best results.

    The client should be NPO for at least 4 hr prior to beginning the bowel prep. The client will need to consume the full prescribed amount of polyethylene glycol. Its effects should be observed within 1 hr. Motility will be increased with the effects of the polyethylene glycol, which would greatly reduce the likelihood of medication absorption.

 NCLEX® Connection: Reduction of Risk Potential, Potential for Complications of Diagnostic Tests/Treatments/Procedures

3. After a scope procedure a client is difficult to arouse. The priority action for the nurse to perform at this time is to

    A. assess the client's airway.

    B. allow the client to sleep.

    C. increase rate of IV fluids.

    D. evaluate preprocedure laboratory tests for abnormalities.

Following the airway, breathing and circulation (ABC) priority framework, the priority intervention is airway maintenance. The other interventions are important, but not the priority.

    NCLEX® Connection: Reduction of Risk Potential, Potential for Complications of Diagnostic Tests/Treatments/Procedures

4. A client is scheduled for both an upper gastrointestinal and barium enema. How should the nurse schedule these exams?

    A. The upper gastrointestinal should be scheduled the same day but before the barium enema.

    B. The barium enema should be scheduled the same day but before the upper gastrointestinal.

    C. The upper gastrointestinal should be scheduled the day before the barium enema.

    D. The barium enema should be scheduled when the client is not NPO.

The barium enema can be done on the same day as the upper gastrointestinal, but it needs to be done first to avoid barium entering the colon from the upper intestinal track. Both procedures are done with the client NPO.

    NCLEX® Connection: Reduction of Risk Potential, Potential for Complications of Diagnostic Tests/Treatments/Procedures

UNIT 7	NURSING CARE OF CLIENTS WITH GASTROINTESTINAL DISORDERS
Section	Diagnostic and Therapeutic Procedures
Chapter 52	**Gastrointestinal Therapeutic Procedures**

Overview

- Gastrointestinal therapeutic procedures are performed for reasons including treatment of obesity, treatment of gastrointestinal obstructions and other disorders, and the maintenance of nutritional intake.

- Gastrointestinal therapeutic procedures that nurses should be knowledgeable about

  o Bariatric surgeries

  o Nasogastric decompression

  o Ostomies

  o Enteral feedings

  o Total parenteral nutrition (TPN)

  o Paracentesis

Bariatric Surgeries

- Bariatric surgeries are done as a treatment for morbid obesity when other weight control methods have failed.

  o Bariatric surgeries reduce the functional size of the stomach.

  o There are several types of procedures that can be done.

    ▪ Stapling a portion of the stomach shut to decrease the functional size of it.

    ▪ Using a band that constricts the functional size of the stomach - can be done laparoscopically.

    ▪ Intestinal bypass that will decrease the length of the functional small intestine to decrease absorption of nutrients.

  o Some procedures combine more than one of these approaches.

  o Many clients will undergo body contouring to remove excess skin after weight is lost.

View Media Supplement:
- Stomach Stapling
- Gastric Band
- Intestinal Bypass (Images)

- Indications
  - Diagnoses
    - Long history of morbid obesity
  - Client Presentation
    - BMI > 40
    - BMI > 35 with comorbidities
- Client Outcome
  - The client will experience resolution of obesity-related problems.
- Preprocedure
  - Nursing Actions
    - Assess the client's psychosocial issues related to weight loss.
    - Ensure that the client understands dietary and lifestyle changes that will be required.
    - Prepare the client for postoperative course and potential complications.
    - Arrange for a bariatric bed to be available and mechanical lifting devices to prevent client/staff injury.
- Postprocedure
  - Nursing Actions
    - Provide postoperative care and prevent postoperative complications.
    - Monitor for the development of postoperative complications that are at increased risk due to obesity (atelectasis, thromboemboli, incisional hernia, peritonitis).
    - Assess the client's airway and oxygenation frequently. Keep the client in a semi-Fowler's position for better lung expansion.
    - Monitor the client's bowel sounds.
    - Apply an abdominal binder if the client has an abdominal incision to prevent dehiscence.
    - Ambulate the client as soon as possible after surgery.
    - Provide 6 small meals a day when the client can resume intake. Observe for signs of dumping syndrome (cramps, diarrhea, tachycardia, dizziness, and fatigue). The client's first feeding may only consist of 30 mL of liquid.
  - Client Education
    - The client should be limited to liquids or pureed foods for the first 6 weeks.
    - The client's meal size should not exceed 1 cup.
    - The client should walk daily for at least 30 min.

- Remind the client that overeating can dilate the surgically created pouch causing weight to be gained back.

- Instruct the client to take vitamin and mineral supplements.

- Complications

  ○ Warn the client that excessive thirst or concentrated urine may be a sign of dehydration and the surgeon should be notified.

  ○ Malabsorption/malnutrition

    - Since bariatric surgeries reduce the size of the stomach or length of the intestinal track, fewer nutrients will be able to be ingested and absorbed.

    - Nursing Actions

      □ Monitor the client's tolerance of increasing amounts of food and fluids.

      □ Refer the client for dietary management.

    - Client Education

      □ Tell the client to eat 2 servings of protein a day.

      □ Tell the client to eat only nutrition-dense foods. Avoid empty calories, such as colas and fruity juice drinks.

Nasogastric Decompression

- Nasogastric decompression is a procedure done for client's who have an intestinal obstruction. Decompression is accomplished by insertion of an NG tube with suction applied until obstruction is relieved. The obstruction can be mechanical (tumors, adhesions, fecal impaction) or functional (paralytic ileus).

- Indications

  ○ Diagnoses

    - Any disorder that causes a mechanical or functional intestinal obstruction

  ○ Client Presentation

    - Vomiting (begins with stomach contents and continues until fecal material is also being regurgitated)

    - Bowel sounds may be absent (paralytic ileus) or hyperactive and high pitched (obstruction)

    - Intermittent, colicky abdominal pain and distention; hiccups

- Client Outcome

  ○ The client will resume normal gastrointestinal function.

- Preprocedure

  ○ Nursing Actions

    - Gather necessary equipment and supplies.

- ○ Client Education

  - ■ Instruct the client on the purpose of the NG tube and the client's role in its placement.

- • Postprocedure

  - ○ Nursing Actions

    - ■ Assess and maintain proper functioning of the tube and suction equipment.

    - ■ Monitor the client for fluid and electrolyte imbalance (metabolic acidosis – low obstruction; alkalosis – high obstruction).

    - ■ Monitor the client's I&O observing for discrepancies.

    - ■ Assess the client's bowel sounds and abdominal girth; return of flatus.

  - ○ Client Education

    - ■ Instruct the client to maintain NPO status.

- • Complications

  - ○ Strangulated obstruction/intestinal infarction

    - ■ Occurs when a portion of the intestine is twisted or the blood supply is compromised, which may cause ischemia

      - □ Peritonitis and septicemia can result.

      - □ Gangrene of the affected bowel may necessitate removal of a section of bowel.

    - ■ Nursing Actions

      - □ Monitor the client for an increase in abdominal pain, abdominal rigidity, fever, tachycardia, and hypotension.

Ostomies

- • An ostomy is a surgical opening from the inside of the body to the outside. Ostomies can be permanent or temporary and are located in various parts of the body.

  - ○ A stoma is an artificial opening from the inside of the body to the outside created during the ostomy surgery.

  - ○ The main types of ostomies performed in the abdominal area

    - ■ Ileostomy – a surgical opening into the ileum to drain stool

    - ■ Colostomy – a surgical opening into the large intestine to drain stool

View Media Supplement:

- • Colostomy (Image)
- • Healthy Stoma (Image)

- Indications

  o Diagnoses

    ▪ Ileostomy is performed when the entire colon must be removed due to disease (Crohn's disease)

    ▪ Colostomy is performed when colon cancer necessitates removal of a portion of the bowel.

- Client Outcomes

  o The client will demonstrate ostomy care.

	ILEOSTOMY	TRANSVERSE COLOSTOMY	SIGMOID COLOSTOMY
Normal postoperative output	• Less than 1,000 mL/day • May be bile-colored and liquid	• Small semi-liquid with some mucus 2 to 3 days after surgery • Blood may be present in the first few days after surgery	• Small to moderate amount of mucus with semi-formed stool 4 to 5 days after surgery
Postoperative changes in output	• After several days to weeks, the output will decrease to approximately 500 to 1,000 mL/day • Becomes more paste-like as the small intestine assumes the absorptive function of the large intestine	• After several days to weeks, output will become more stool-like, semi-formed, or formed	• After several days to weeks, output will resemble semi-formed stool
Pattern of output	• Continuous output	• Resumes a pattern similar to the preoperative pattern	• Resumes a pattern similar to the preoperative pattern

- Preprocedure

  o Nursing Actions

    ▪ Determine the client's readiness for the procedure. Assess visual acuity, manual dexterity, cognitive status, cultural influences, and support systems.

  o Client Education

    ▪ Instruct the client and a support person regarding care and management of an ostomy before surgery.

- Postprocedure

  - Nursing Actions

    - Assess the type and fit of the ostomy appliance. Monitor for leakage (risk to skin integrity). Fit the ostomy appliance based on:

      □ Type of ostomy.

      □ Location of the ostomy.

      □ Visual acuity and manual dexterity of the client.

    - Assess peristomal skin integrity and the appearance of the stoma. The stoma should appear pink and moist.

    - Apply skin barriers and creams, such as stoma adhesive paste, when applying wafers to protect the peristomal skin. Let the skin sealants dry before applying a new appliance.

    - Evaluate output from the stoma. The higher up an ostomy is placed in the small intestine, the more liquid and acidic the output will be from the ostomy.

    - Empty the ostomy bag when it is ¼ to ½ full of drainage.

    - Assess for fluid and electrolyte imbalances, particularly with a new ileostomy.

  - Client Education

    - Educate the client regarding dietary changes and ostomy appliances that can help manage flatus and odor.

      □ Foods that can cause odor include fish, eggs, asparagus, garlic, beans, and dark green leafy vegetables.

      □ Foods that can cause gas include dark green leafy vegetables, beer, carbonated beverages, dairy products, and corn. Yogurt can be ingested to help decrease gas.

      □ After an ostomy is placed involving the small intestine, the client should be instructed to avoid high-fiber foods for the first 2 months after surgery, chew food well, drink plenty of fluids, and evaluate for any evidence of blockage when slowly adding high-fiber foods.

      □ Do not put anything in the bag to mask odor such as a mint. Keep appliance clean and empty frequently to decrease odor.

    - Provide opportunities for the client to discuss feelings about the ostomy and concerns about its impact on the client's life. Encourage the client to look at and touch the stoma.

    - Refer the client to a local ostomy support group.

- Complications

  - Stomal Ischemia/necrosis

    - The stomal appearance should normally be pink or red and moist.

- □ Signs of stomal ischemia are pale pink or bluish/purple in color and dry in appearance.

- □ If the stoma appears black or purple in color, this indicates a serious impairment of blood flow and requires immediate intervention.

- ■ Nursing Actions

- □ Obtain the client's vital signs, pulse oximetry, and current laboratory results. Notify the provider or surgeon of abnormal findings.

- ■ Client Education

- □ Teach the client to watch for signs of stomal ischemia/necrosis following discharge.

- ○ Intestinal obstruction

- ■ An obstruction can occur for a variety of reasons.

- ■ Nursing Actions

- □ Monitor and record output from the stoma.

- □ Assess the client for symptoms of obstruction including abdominal pain, hypoactive or absent bowel sounds, distention, nausea, and vomiting. Notify the surgeon of abnormal findings.

- ■ Client Education

- □ Teach client to watch for signs of an intestinal obstruction following discharge.

Enteral Feedings

- • Enteral feedings are instituted when a client can no longer take adequate nutrition orally.

- • Indications

- ○ Diagnoses

- ■ Clients who are intubated

- ■ Pathologies that cause difficulty swallowing and/or increase risk of aspiration (stroke, advanced Parkinson's disease, and multiple sclerosis)

- ■ Clients who cannot maintain adequate oral nutritional intake and need supplementation

- ○ Client Presentation

- ■ Malnutrition

- ■ Aspiration pneumonia

- • Client Outcomes

- ○ The client will maintain adequate caloric intake to meet nutritional needs and maintain or increase weight.

- Complications

  - Diarrhea

    - Diarrhea occurs secondary to concentration of feeding or its constituents.

    - Nursing Actions

      - Slow rate of feeding and notify the provider.

      - Confer with the dietitian.

      - Provide skin care and protection.

  - Aspiration pneumonia

    - Pneumonia can occur secondary to aspiration of feeding.

    - Nursing Actions

      - Stop the feeding.

      - Turn the client to his side and suction the airway. Provide oxygen if indicated.

      - Monitor the client's vital signs for an elevated temperature.

      - Auscultate breath sounds for increased congestion.

      - Notify the provider and obtain a chest x-ray if prescribed.

Total Parenteral Nutrition

- Total parenteral nutrition (TPN) is a hypertonic intravenous (IV) bolus solution that provides complete nutrition to a client who does not have a functioning gastrointestinal (GI) tract or needs additional nutritional supplementation (burns). The purpose of TPN administration is to prevent or correct nutritional deficiencies and minimize the adverse effects of malnourishment.

  - TPN administration is usually through a central line, such as a nontunneled triple lumen catheter or a single- or double-lumen peripherally inserted central line (PICC).

  - TPN contains complete nutrition, including calories (through a high concentration – 20 to 50% – of dextrose), lipids/essential fatty acids, protein, electrolytes, vitamins, and trace elements. Standard IV bolus therapy is typically ≤ 700 calories a day.

  - Partial parenteral nutrition or peripheral parenteral nutrition (PPN) is less hypertonic and intended for short-term use in a large peripheral vein. Usual dextrose concentration is 10% or less. Risks include phlebitis.

- Indications

  - Diagnoses

    - Potential indications for TPN include any condition that

      - Affects the ability to absorb nutrition.

      - Has a prolonged recovery.

- □ Creates a hypermetabolic state.
- □ Creates a chronic malnutrition.
  - ■ Specific conditions
    - □ Chronic pancreatitis
    - □ Diffuse peritonitis
    - □ Short bowel syndrome
    - □ Gastric paresis from diabetes mellitus
    - □ Severe burns
  - ○ Client Presentation
    - ■ Basic guidelines regarding when to initiate TPN
      - □ A weight loss of 7% body weight and NPO for 5 days or more
      - □ A hypermetabolic state
- Client Outcomes
  - ■ The client will maintain current weight.
  - ■ The client's laboratory values will be within normal ranges.
  - ■ The client will maintain a positive nitrogen balance.
- Nursing Actions
  - ○ Preparation of the Client
    - ■ Determine the client's readiness for TPN.
      - □ Obtain daily laboratory values, including electrolytes. Solutions are customized for each client according to daily laboratory results.
  - ○ Ongoing Care
    - ■ The flow rate is gradually increased and gradually decreased to allow body adjustment (usually no more than a 10% hourly increase in rate).
      - □ Never abruptly stop TPN. Speeding up/slowing down the rate is contraindicated. An abrupt rate changes can alter glucose levels significantly.
    - ■ Monitor the client's vital signs every 4 to 8 hr.
    - ■ Follow sterile procedures to minimize the risk of sepsis.
      - □ TPN solution is prepared by the pharmacy using aseptic technique with a laminar flow hood.
      - □ Change tubing and solution bag (even if not empty) every 24 hr.
      - □ A filter is used on the IV bolus line (to collect particles from the solution).
      - □ Do not use the line for other IV bolus solutions (prevents contamination and interruption of the flow).

▫ Do not add anything to the solution due to risks of contamination and incompatibility.

▫ Use sterile procedures, including a mask, when changing the central line dressing (per facility procedure).

○ Interventions

■ Check capillary glucose every 4 to 6 hr for at least the first 24 hr.

▫ Clients receiving TPN frequently need supplemental Regular insulin until the pancreas can increase its endogenous production of insulin.

▫ Keep dextrose 10% in water at the bedside in case the solution is unexpectedly ruined or the next bag is not available. This will minimize the risk of hypoglycemia with abrupt changes in dextrose concentrations.

▫ Older adult clients have an increased incidence of glucose intolerance.

Ⓖ

• Complications

○ Metabolic complications

■ Metabolic complications include hyperglycemia, hypoglycemia, and vitamin deficiencies.

■ Nursing Actions

▫ Daily laboratory work must be ordered and results obtained before a new solution is prepared.

▫ Fluid needs are typically replaced with a separate IV bolus to prevent fluid volume excess.

▫ Monitor the client for signs of hyperglycemia.

○ Air embolism

■ A pressure change during tubing changes can lead to an air embolism.

■ Nursing Actions

▫ Signs and symptoms of an air embolism (sudden onset of dyspnea, chest pain, anxiety, hypoxia) should be treated emergently by clamping the catheter and placing the client in a Trendelenburg position and on the left side to trap air. Administer oxygen and notify the provider stat so that trapped air can be aspirated.

○ Infection

■ Concentrated glucose is a medium for bacteria.

■ Nursing Actions

▫ Observe the central line insertion site frequently for local infection (erythema, tenderness, exudate).

▫ Change the sterile dressing on a central line per protocol (typically every 72 hr).

- Observe the client for signs of systemic infection (fever, increased WBC, chills, malaise).

- Do NOT use TPN line for other IV bolus fluids and medications (repeated access increases the risk for infection).

  ○ Fluid Imbalance

  - In particular, fluid volume excess is possible due to the hyperosmotic solution (three to six times the osmolarity of blood), which poses a risk for fluid shifts.

    - Older adult clients are more vulnerable to complications, particularly fluid and electrolyte imbalances. Clients who have a history of congestive heart failure may need a more concentrated solution to avoid fluid overload.

  - Nursing Actions

    - Assess the client's lungs for crackles and monitor him for evidence of respiratory distress.

    - Monitor the client's daily weights and I&O.

    - Use a controlled infusion pump to administer TPN at the prescribed rate.

    - Do not speed up the infusion to "catch up."

    - Gradually increase the flow rate until the prescribed infusion rate is achieved.

Paracentesis

- Therapeutically, a paracentesis is performed by inserting a needle or trocar through the abdominal wall into the peritoneal cavity and withdrawing ascitic fluid to relieve abdominal pressure from ascites buildup.

  ○ A paracentesis can be performed in the provider's office, an outpatient center, or in an acute care setting at the bedside.

- Indications

  ○ Diagnoses

    - Ascites is an abnormal accumulation of protein-rich fluid in the abdominal cavity most often caused by cirrhosis of the liver.

      - Respiratory distress is the determining factor in the use of a paracentesis in the treatment of ascites, and in the evaluation of treatment effectiveness.

  ○ Client Presentation

    - Compromised lung expansion

- Client Outcomes

  ○ The client will be free of respiratory distress as evidenced by regular, even respirations, and the absence of shortness of breath.

  ○ The client will be free of abdominal discomfort.

- Preprocedure

  - Nursing Actions

    - Determine the client's readiness for the procedure.

    - Variables such as the age of the client and chronic and acute diseases can influence the client's ability to tolerate and recover from this procedure.

    - Have the client void or insert a temporary indwelling urinary catheter.

    - Take the client's baseline vital signs, record weight, and measure abdominal girth.

    - Gather equipment for the procedure.

    - Verify that the client has signed the informed consent forms.

    - Position the client as tolerated. Clients with ascites are typically more comfortable sitting up.

    - Administer sedation prescribed by the provider.

    - Administer prescribed IV bolus fluids or albumin, prior to or after a paracentesis, to restore fluid balance.

  - Client Education

    - Explain the procedure and its purpose to the client.

    - Instruct the client that local anesthetics will be used at the needle-insertion site.

    - Explain that there may be pressure or pain with needle insertion.

    - Assess the client's knowledge of the procedure.

- Intraprocedure

  - Nursing Actions

    - Monitor the client's vital signs.

    - Adhere to standard precautions.

    - Label laboratory specimens and send to the laboratory.

    - Between 4 and 6 L of fluid is slowly drained from the abdomen by gravity. The nurse is responsible for monitoring the amount of drainage and notifying the primary care provider of any evidence of complications.

- Postprocedure

  - Nursing Actions

    - Maintain pressure at the insertion site for several minutes. Apply a dressing to the site.

    - If the needle-insertion site continues to leak after holding pressure for several minutes, dry sterile gauze dressings should be applied and changed as often as necessary.

    - Take the client's vital signs, record weight, and measure abdominal girth. Document and compare to preprocedure measurements.

- Continue to monitor the client's vital signs and insertion site per facility protocol.

- Monitor the client's temperature every 4 hr for a minimum of 48 hr.

- Assess I&O every 4 hr.

- Diuretics such as spironolactone (Aldactone) and furosemide (Lasix) may be prescribed to control fluid volume. Potassium supplements may be necessary when a loop diuretic such as furosemide has been administrated.

- Administer IV bolus fluids or albumin as prescribed by the provider.

- Assist the client into a position of comfort.

- Document color, odor, consistency, and amount of fluid removed; location of needle insertion; any evidence of leakage at the insertion site; signs and symptoms of hypovolemia; and changes in mental status.

- Prior to and after a paracentesis, the client's serum albumin, protein, glucose, amylase, BUN, and creatinine levels should be monitored.

- Complications

  - Hypovolemia

    - Albumin levels can drop dangerously low because the peritoneal fluid removed contains a large amount of protein. The removal of this protein-rich fluid can cause shifting of intravascular volume, resulting in hypovolemia.

    - Nursing Actions

      - Preventive measures include slow drainage of fluid and administration of plasma expanders, such as albumin, to counter albumin losses.

      - Monitor clients for evidence of hypovolemia, such as tachycardia, hypotension, pallor, diaphoresis, and dizziness.

      - Any abnormal symptoms should be reported to the provider.

  - Bladder perforation

    - Bladder perforation is a rare, but possible complication.

    - Symptoms of bladder perforation include hematuria, low or no urine output, suprapubic pain and/or distention, symptoms of cystitis, and fever.

    - Nursing Actions

      - If a bladder perforation is suspected, the nurse should notify the provider immediately.

    - Client Education

      - Inform the client to report symptoms of bladder perforation as described above.

○ Peritonitis

- Peritonitis can occur as the result of injury to the intestines during needle insertion.

  □ Symptoms of peritonitis include sharp, constant abdominal pain, fever, nausea, vomiting, and diminished or absent bowel sounds.

- Nursing Actions

  □ If the client exhibits symptoms of peritonitis, the nurse should notify the provider immediately.

- Client Education

  □ Inform the client to report symptoms listed above.

CHAPTER 52: GASTROINTESTINAL THERAPEUTIC PROCEDURES

Ⓐ Application Exercises

Scenario: A male client had a paracentesis completed 15 min ago with removal of 1750 mL of pale, straw-colored liquid due to ascites. Prior to the procedure, his vital signs were blood pressure 136/88 mm Hg, heart rate 96/min, respirations 24/min, and temperature 37.2° C (99.0° F). The client's weight is 100.4 kg (221 lb), and his abdominal girth is 121.9 cm (48 in). Currently, his vital signs are blood pressure 100/60 mm Hg, heart rate 124/min, respirations 24/min, and temperature 37.1° C (98.8° F). His weight is now 99.8 kg (219.5 lb), and his abdominal girth is 109.2 cm (43 in).

1. What are the implications of this assessment data?

2. What nursing interventions should be taken at this time?

3. What are the signs and symptoms a client may exhibit if the bowel is perforated during a paracentesis?

4. A nurse is providing care to a client who is 1 day postoperative paracentesis. The nurse notes that a clear, pale yellow fluid is leaking out of the needle puncture site. Which of the following is an appropriate nursing intervention?

    A. Notify the provider.

    B. Apply a dry, sterile gauze dressing.

    C. Attach an ostomy bag.

    D. Place the client in a supine position.

5. A nurse is assessing a client in the immediate postoperative period after having a colostomy established. The nurse notes that the stoma appears red and moist. The appropriate action by the nurse at this time is to

    A. notify the primary care provider.

    B. check the client's oxygenation.

    C. document the findings.

    D. encourage the client to cough and deep breathe.

6. A nurse is assigned at 0700 to care for a client who started receiving TPN yesterday for chronic pancreatitis. Which of the following should be included in the nurse's plan of care for this client? (Select all that apply.)

    _____ Obtain a capillary blood glucose four times daily.

    _____ Add the prescribed IV bolus potassium to the bag of TPN solution.

    _____ Take a set of vital signs three times during the 12-hr shift.

    _____ Contact the primary care provider for a specific gravity of 1.002.

    _____ Ensure a daily aPTT is obtained.

7. It has been 24 hr since the last bag of TPN was hung for a client. There is 400 mL of TPN solution remaining. Which of the following is the appropriate action for the nurse to take?

    A. Remove the old bag and hang a new bag.

    B. Let the remaining solution infuse at the current rate and hang a new bag when the current bag is empty.

    C. Increase the rate of the TPN infusion so as to administer the remaining solution within the next hour before starting a new bag.

    D. Clarify the procedure with the pharmacist.

CHAPTER 52: GASTROINTESTINAL THERAPEUTIC PROCEDURES

 Application Exercises Answer Key

Scenario: A male client had a paracentesis completed 15 min ago with removal of 1750 mL of pale, straw-colored liquid due to ascites. Prior to the procedure, his vital signs were blood pressure 136/88 mm Hg, heart rate 96/min, respirations 24/min, and temperature 37.2° C (99.0° F). The client's weight is 100.4 kg (221 lb), and his abdominal girth is 121.9 cm (48 in). Currently, his vital signs are blood pressure 100/60 mm Hg, heart rate 124/min, respirations 24/min, and temperature 37.1° C (98.8° F). His weight is now 99.8 kg (219.5 lb), and his abdominal girth is 109.2 cm (43 in).

1. What are the implications of this assessment data?

The client is exhibiting symptoms of hypovolemia.

 NCLEX® Connection: Reduction of Risk Potential, Changes/Abnormalities in Vital Signs

2. What nursing interventions should be taken at this time?

The response should include notifying the provider of the symptoms, preparing for interventions such as the administration of IV bolus fluids or albumin, and laboratory tests. Maintain the client in a position of comfort with the head of the bed elevated. Instruct the client about the purpose of the interventions being performed, and document all of the client's symptoms and all of the nursing interventions.

 NCLEX® Connection: Reduction of Risk Potential, Potential for Complications of Diagnostic Tests/Treatments/Procedures

3. What are the signs and symptoms a client may exhibit if the bowel is perforated during a paracentesis?

Symptoms may include abdominal pain and rigidity, low or diminished bowel sounds, fever, nausea, vomiting, anorexia, and rebound tenderness in the abdomen.

 NCLEX® Connection: Reduction of Risk Potential, System Specific Assessment

4. A nurse is providing care to a client who is 1 day postoperative paracentesis. The nurse notes that a clear, pale yellow fluid is leaking out of the needle puncture site. Which of the following is an appropriate nursing intervention?

    A. Notify the provider.

    B. Apply a dry, sterile gauze dressing.

    C. Attach an ostomy bag.

    D. Place the client in a supine position.

Drainage of clear, yellow fluid can occur after a paracentesis, as ascitic fluid continues to escape. Application of a sterile gauze dressing after the trocar is removed will contain the drainage and allow continuous assessment of color and quantity. Draining of ascitic fluid often occurs through the trocar wound after a paracentesis and does not require notification of the provider. It would not be appropriate to apply an ostomy bag to the puncture wound and the client should be maintained in a Fowler's position due to the respiratory compromise that occurs secondary to excess abdominal fluid.

 NCLEX® Connection: Reduction of Risk Potential, Potential for Complications of Diagnostic Tests/Treatments/Procedures

5. A nurse is assessing a client in the immediate postoperative period after having a colostomy established. The nurse notes that the stoma appears red and moist. The appropriate action by the nurse at this time is to

    A. notify the primary care provider.

    B. check the client's oxygenation.

    C. document the findings.

    D. encourage the client to cough and deep breathe.

These are expected findings for a healthy stoma. There is no indication to notify the provider, check the client's oxygen saturation, or encourage the client to cough and deep breathe.

 NCLEX® Connection: Reduction of Risk Potential, Potential for Complications of Diagnostic Tests/Treatments/Procedures

6. A nurse is assigned at 0700 to care for a client who started receiving TPN yesterday for chronic pancreatitis. Which of the following should be included in the nurse's plan of care for this client? (Select all that apply.)

    X   **Obtain a capillary blood glucose four times daily.**

    _____   Add the prescribed IV bolus potassium to the bag of TPN solution.

    X   **Take a set of vital signs three times during the 12-hr shift.**

    X   **Contact the primary care provider for a specific gravity of 1.002.**

    _____   Ensure a daily aPTT is obtained.

The client is at risk for hyperglycemia during the administration of TPN and may require supplemental insulin. Vital signs are recommended every 4 to 8 hr to assess for fluid volume excess and infection. No additional substances such as potassium should be added to the bag of TPN on the unit due to the risk of contamination and incompatibility. TPN candidates are at risk for osmotic diuresis, so specific gravity should be closely monitored. A specific gravity of 1.002 indicates osmotic diuresis may be occurring and dehydration could result; the provider should be notified. The aPTT measures the coagulability of the blood, which is unnecessary during the administration of TPN.

 NCLEX® Connection: Reduction of Risk Potential, Potential for Complications of Diagnostic Tests/Treatments/Procedures

7. It has been 24 hr since the last bag of TPN was hung for a client. There is 400 mL of TPN solution remaining. Which of the following is the appropriate action for the nurse to take?

A. Remove the old bag and hang a new bag.

B. Let the remaining solution infuse at the current rate and hang a new bag when the current bag is empty.

C. Increase the rate of the TPN infusion so as to administer the remaining solution within the next hour before starting a new bag.

D. Clarify the procedure with the pharmacist.

The current bag of TPN should not hang more than 24 hr due to the risk of infection. The TPN infusion rate should never be increased/decreased abruptly due to the risk of phlebitis and hyperglycemia. There is no reason to clarify the procedure with the pharmacist.

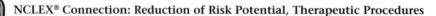

NCLEX® Connection: Reduction of Risk Potential, Therapeutic Procedures

UNIT 7	NURSING CARE OF CLIENTS WITH GASTROINTESTINAL DISORDERS
Section	Upper Gastrointestinal Disorders
Chapter 53	Esophageal Disorders

Overview

- The esophagus is a tube that consists of smooth muscle and leads from the throat to the stomach. Esophageal disorders can affect any part of the esophagus.

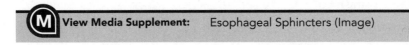
View Media Supplement: Esophageal Sphincters (Image)

- There are two sphincters (upper esophageal – UES; lower esophageal–LES) that prevent the reflux of food and fluids back into the mouth or esophagus.

- Contractions of the esophagus propel food and fluids toward the stomach, while the relaxation of the gastroesophageal sphincter allows them to pass into the stomach.

- Esophageal disorders that nurses should be knowledgeable about include:

  ○ Gastroesophageal Reflux Disease (GERD)

  ○ Esophageal Varices

  ○ Esophageal Cancer

GERD

Overview

- Gastroesophageal reflux disease, or GERD is a common condition characterized by gastric content and enzyme leakage into the esophagus. These corrosive fluids irritate the esophageal tissue and limit its ability to clear them from the esophagus.

- The primary treatment of GERD is diet and lifestyle changes, advancing into medication use (antacids, H_2 receptor antagonists, proton pump inhibitors), and surgery.

- Untreated GERD leads to inflammation, breakdown, and long-term complications including adenocarcinoma of the esophagus.

Health Promotion and Disease Prevention

- Maintain a weight below the BMI of 30.

- Stop smoking.

- Drink alcohol in moderation.

Assessment

- Risk Factors

  - Obesity

  - Older age

  - Sleep apnea

  - Nasogastric tube

  - Contributing factors

    - Diet: Excessive ingestion of foods that relax the LES include: fatty and fried foods, chocolate, caffeinated beverages (coffee, peppermint, spicy foods, tomatoes, citrus fruits, alcohol)

    - Distended abdomen from overeating or delayed emptying

    - Increased abdominal pressure resulting from obesity, pregnancy, bending at the waist, ascites or tight clothing at the waist

    - Drugs that relax the LES (theophylline, nitrates, calcium channel blockers, anticholinergics, and diazepam [Valium])

    - Drugs (NSAIDs), or events (stress) that increase gastric acid

    - Debilitation or age-related conditions resulting in weakened LES tone

    - Hiatal hernia (LES displacement into the thorax with delayed esophageal clearance)

    - Lying flat

- Subjective Data

  - The chief symptom of GERD is frequent and prolonged substernal heartburn (dyspepsia) and regurgitation (acid reflux) in relationship to eating activities or position.

  - Classic symptoms: Dyspepsia after eating an offending food or fluid, and regurgitation.

  - Other symptoms: Throat irritation (chronic cough, laryngitis), hypersalivation, eructation, flatulence, bitter taste in mouth, or atypical chest pain from esophageal spasm. Chronic GERD can lead to dysphagia.

  - GERD may mimic a heart attack due to the substernal pain that can radiate to the jaw and back.

- o Symptoms occurring four to five times per week on a consistent basis are considered diagnostic.

- o Symptoms may come from expected physiological changes (delayed gastric emptying) related to aging.

- Objective Data

  - o Physical Assessment Findings

    - Tooth erosion

    - Hoarseness

  - o Diagnostic Procedures

    - Esophagogastroduodenoscopy (EGD) allows visualization of the esophagus revealing esophagitis or Barrett's epithelium (premalignant cells). It is done using moderate sedation to observe for tissue damage (in 60% of clients with GERD) and possibly to dilate structures.

      - □ Nursing Actions: Verify gag response has returned prior to providing oral fluids or food following the procedure.

    - 24 hr ambulatory esophageal pH monitoring. A small catheter is placed through the client's nose and into the distal esophagus where pH readings are taken in relation to food, position, and activity.

    - Esophageal manometry records lower esophageal sphincter pressure.

      - □ Nursing Actions: Instruct the client to keep a diary of symptoms related to food, position, and activity throughout the day.

    - Barium swallow to identify a hiatal hernia, which would contribute to or cause GERD

Collaborative Care

- Medications

  - o Antacids

    - Antacids (aluminum hydroxide [Mylanta])) neutralize excess acid.

    - Nursing Considerations

      - □ Ensure aluminum is not contraindicated with other prescribed medications (levothyroxine).

    - Client Education

      - □ Instruct the client to take antacids when acid secretion is the highest (1 to 3 hr after eating and at bedtime), and to separate from other medications by at least 1 hr.

- ○ Histamine$_2$ Receptor Antagonists

  - ▪ Histamine$_2$ receptor antagonists (ranitidine [Zantac], famotidine [Pepcid], nizatidine [Axid]) reduce the secretion of acid. The onset is longer than antacids, but the effect has a longer duration.

    - □ Cimetidine (Tagamet) is no longer first-line as it has a higher risk profile in older adult clients and interacts with more than 60 other medications.

  - ▪ Nursing Considerations

    - □ Use cautiously in clients who are at a high risk for pneumonia (clients with chronic obstructive pulmonary disease [COPD]).

  - ▪ Client Education

    - □ Encourage adherence to the medication regimen.

- ○ Proton Pump Inhibitors (PPIs)

  - ▪ PPIs (pantoprazole [Protonix], omeprazole [Prilosec], esomeprazole [Nexium], and lansoprazole [Prevacid]) reduce gastric acid by inhibiting the cellular pump necessary for secretion.

  - ▪ Nursing Considerations

    - □ Use cautiously in clients at a high risk for pneumonia (clients with COPD).

  - ▪ Client Education

    - □ Suggest the client sprinkle the contents of the sustained-release capsule over food if experiencing difficulty swallowing.

- ○ Prokinetics

  - ▪ Prokinetic medications (metoclopramide hydrochloride [Reglan]) increase the motility of the esophagus and stomach.

  - ▪ Nursing Considerations

    - □ Monitor the client for extrapyramidal side effects.

  - ▪ Client Education

    - □ Instruct the client to report abnormal, involuntary movement.

- • Therapeutic Procedures

  - ○ Stretta Procedure

    - ▪ The Stretta procedure uses radiofrequency energy, applied by an endoscope, to the LES muscle. This causes the tissue to contract and tighten.

- • Surgical Interventions

  - ○ Fundoplication

    - ▪ This surgical option may be indicated for clients who fail to respond to other treatments. The fundus of the stomach is wrapped around and behind the esophagus through a laparoscope to create a physical barrier.

- ○ Client Education
  - ■ Diet
    - □ Avoid offending foods.
    - □ Avoid large meals.
    - □ Remain upright after eating.
    - □ Avoid eating before bed.
  - ■ Lifestyle
    - □ Avoid tight-fitting clothing around the middle.
    - □ Lose weight, if applicable.
    - □ Elevate the head of the bed 15.2 to 20.3 cm (6 to 8 in) with blocks. The use of pillows is not recommended as this rounds the back bringing the stomach contents up closer to the chest.
    - □ Sleep on the right side.
- Client Outcomes
  - ○ The client will report less epigastric pain.
  - ○ The client will not experience gastric reflux during sleeping hours.

Complications

- Aspiration of gastric secretion
  - ○ Causes
    - ■ Reflux of gastric fluids into the esophagus can be aspirated into the trachea.
    - ■ Risks associated with aspiration include:
      - □ Asthma exacerbations from inhaled aerosolized acid.
      - □ Frequent upper respiratory, sinus, or ear infections.
      - □ Aspiration pneumonia.
      - □ Barrett's epithelium (premalignant) and esophageal adenocarcinoma.
  - ○ Cause
    - ■ Reflux of gastric fluids can cause esophagitis. Chronic esophagitis requires the body to continuously heal inflamed tissue, eventually replacing normal esophageal epithelium with premalignant tissue (Barrett's epithelium) or malignant adenocarcinoma.
  - ○ Nursing Actions
    - ■ Determine the cause of GERD with the client and review lifestyle changes that can decrease gastric reflux.

ESOPHAGEAL VARICES

Overview

- Esophageal varices are swollen, fragile blood vessels in the esophagus. As a result of liver damage, blood flow through the liver is restricted and is diverted to other vessels (the vessels of the lower esophagus). The increased blood flow (portal hypertension) causes swelling, and varices result.

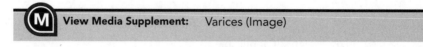

View Media Supplement: Varices (Image)

- When esophageal varices hemorrhage, it is often a medical emergency associated with a high mortality rate. Reoccurrence of esophageal bleeding is common.

Health Promotion and Disease Prevention

- Avoid alcohol consumption.

Assessment

- Risk Factors

    ○ Portal hypertension is the primary risk factor for the development of esophageal varices. Portal hypertension (elevated blood pressure in veins that carry blood from the intestines to the liver) is caused by impaired circulation of blood through the liver. Collateral circulation is subsequently developed creating varices in the upper stomach and esophagus. Varices are fragile and can bleed very easily.

    ○ Alcoholic cirrhosis.

    ○ Viral hepatitis.

    ○ Older adult clients frequently have depressed immune function, decreased liver function, and cardiac disorders that make them especially vulnerable to bleeding.

- Subjective Data

    ○ An endoscopy is indicated for clients who have cirrhosis to determine the presence of esophageal varices.

    ○ The client may experience no symptoms until the varices begin to bleed.

- Objective Data

  - Physical Assessment Findings (Bleeding Esophageal Varices)

    - Factors that precipitate bleeding are the Valsalva maneuver, lifting heavy objects, coughing, sneezing, and alcohol.

    - Hematemesis

    - Melena

    - Hypotension

    - Tachycardia

  - Laboratory Tests

    - Liver function tests indicate a liver disorder

    - Hemoglobin and hematocrit tests can indicate anemia secondary to occult bleeding or overt bleeding

  - Diagnostic Procedures

    - Endoscopy

      - Endoscopic evaluation is the first step in treatment of esophageal varices. Therapeutic interventions can be performed during the endoscopy.

      - Nursing Actions: Endoscopy requires a pre-procedure sedation. After the procedure, it is important to monitor the client's vital signs and to take measures to prevent aspiration.

Collaborative Care

- Nursing Care

  - If the client is bleeding, establish IV access with a large bore needle, monitor vital signs and hematocrit, type and crossmatch for possible blood transfusions, and monitor for overt and occult bleeding.

- Medications

  - Nonselective Beta-Blockers

    - Nonselective beta-blockers (propranolol [Inderal]) are prescribed to decrease heart rate and consequently reduce hepatic venous pressure.

    - Recommended for prophylactic use and not emergency treatment for hemorrhage.

  - Vasoconstrictors

    - Vasoconstrictors (vasopressin [Desmopressin], octreotide [Sandostatin]), are prescribed to decrease portal inflow.

    - Nursing Considerations

      - Vasopressin cannot be given to clients with coronary artery disease due to resultant coronary constriction.

- Interdisciplinary Care

  o Alcohol recovery program if varices due to alcohol abuse

- Therapeutic Procedures

  o Endoscopic injection sclerotherapy or variceal band ligation

    ▪ Ligating bands can be placed, and/or injection sclerotherapy can be performed through an endoscopic procedure. Used only for active bleeding and not prophylactically.

    ▪ Nursing Actions: Endoscopy requires a pre-procedure sedation. After the procedure, it is important to monitor the client's vital signs and to take measures to prevent aspiration.

    ▪ Sclerotherapy carries a greater risk of postoperative hemorrhage.

    ▪ Antacids and/or H2 receptor blockers are administered postoperatively.

  o Transjugular Intrahepatic Portal-Systemic Shunt (TIPS)

    ▪ While the client is under sedation or general anesthesia, a catheter is passed into the liver via the jugular vein in the neck. A stent is then placed between the portal and hepatic veins bypassing the liver. Portal hypertension is subsequently relieved.

    ▪ Nursing Actions

      □ Monitor the client's vital signs.

      □ Keep the head of the bed elevated.

  o Esophagogastric Balloon Tamponade

    ▪ An esophagogastric tube with esophageal and gastric balloons is used to compress blood vessels in the esophagus and stomach. Check balloons for leaks prior to insertion. Traction is applied after balloons are inflated to desired pressure. When the bleeding is stopped, the traction is released and the pressure in the balloons is reduced gradually. Reserved for clients who have unsuccessful TIPS procedures.

    ▪ Nursing Actions

      □ Irrigate the tube as prescribed and document color of return (clear versus bloody).

      □ Monitor placement of the tube and observe for possible obstruction of airway.

      □ Monitor for aspiration into the lungs and secretions or blood from the esophagus.

      □ Maintain balloon pressure at prescribed pressure for prescribed time to decrease risk of esophageal or gastric necrosis from ischemia.

      □ Provide oral suction as needed.

      □ Monitor the client with decreased mentation or confusion who may pull on the tube.

- Surgical Interventions

    ○ Surgery for esophageal varices is considered as a last resort.

    ○ Bypass procedures

        ■ Bypass procedures establish a venous shunt that bypasses the liver, decreasing portal hypertension.

        ■ Common shunts include splenorenal (splenic, left renal veins), mesocaval (mesenteric vein, vena cava), portacaval (portal vein, inferior vena cava).

        ■ Nursing Actions (pre, post)

            □ Monitor the client for an increase in liver dysfunction or encephalopathy.

- Client Outcomes

    ○ The client's esophageal varices will stop bleeding.

    ○ The client will not experience future variceal bleeds.

Complications

- Hypovolemic Shock

    ○ Hemorrhage from esophageal varices can lead to hypovolemic shock.

    ○ Nursing Actions

        ■ Observe the client carefully for signs of hemorrhage and shock.

        ■ Monitor vital signs, hemoglobin, and hematocrit.

        ■ Replace losses and support therapeutic procedures to stop and control bleeding.

ESOPHAGEAL CANCER

Overview

- Esophageal cancer is a fast-growing and metastasizing type of cancer.

- Cancers of the upper esophagus are typically squamous cell and cancers of the lower esophagus are typically adenomas.

- Early symptoms are often vague and the delay before medical attention is sought significantly affects the prognosis.

- Treatment often involves several weeks of chemotherapy and radiation therapy followed by surgery.

Health Promotion and Disease Prevention

- Avoid alcohol consumption.

- Smoking cessation.

- Avoid foods containing nitrites.

- Treat GERD with diet, positioning, and medications.

Assessment

- Risk Factors

  - Smoking

  - Alcohol abuse

  - Nitrites

  - GERD

  - Barrett's esophagus

- Subjective Data

  - Dysphagia

  - Odynophagia (painful swallowing)

  - Feeling of a lump in the throat

- Objective Data

  - Physical Assessment Findings

    - Weight loss

    - Halitosis

    - Regurgitation

    - Hiccups

  - Diagnostic Procedures

    - Barium swallow may be done initially to determine cause of dysphagia.

    - Esophagogastroduodenoscopy (EGD) is done to visualize tumors and take a biopsy of suspicious tissue.

    - CT or positron emission tomography (PET) scans of the chest and abdomen can assess for metastatic disease of the lungs and liver.

    - Esophageal ultrasound can determine presence of cancer in mediastinum and lymph nodes.

Collaborative Care

- Nursing Care

    o Weigh the client daily

    o Support nutrition with a high-caloric diet, semi-soft foods and thickened liquids, and supplements. Record calorie count.

    o Monitor for aspiration during meals. Enteral feedings through a gastrostomy tube may be needed.

    o Keep the client elevated at least 30 degrees at all times, and higher after meals.

- Medications

    o Chemotherapy

        ▪ Chemotherapy may be given prior to surgery to aid in shrinking the tumor, in place of surgery if the tumor is too extensive, or for palliation. Chemotherapy can make the tumor cells more susceptible to radiation.

        ▪ Traditional chemotherapy (5-fluorouracil, cisplatin) or more targeted medications (monoclonal antibodies [MABs]) may be used.

    o Targeted medication therapy – Monoclonal antibodies (MABs)

        ▫ Angiogenesis inhibitors (inhibits growth of new blood vessels to tumors): bevacizumab (Avastin)

        ▫ Tyrosine kinase inhibitors (decreases cell proliferation and increases cell death of certain cancers): cetuximab (Erbitux) and panitumumab (Vectibix)

- Interdisciplinary Care

    o Dietary consult for appropriate diet

    o Speech therapy consult for swallowing instruction

    o Home health nurse upon discharge from hospital

    o Cancer support groups

- Therapeutic Procedures

  - Radiation (Refer to Chapter 104: Cancer Treatment Options.)

    - Radiation is often given along with chemotherapy or may be given alone. It can be effective in reducing the size of the tumor making swallowing easier. Esophageal dilation may be needed after treatment in relation to esophageal strictures caused by scarring.

  - Photodynamic therapy (PDT)

    - Photodynamic therapy involves the injection of a photosensitizing agent that is absorbed by all the cells in the body. One to three days later when the agent remains in only the cancer cells, the tumor is exposed to a specific wavelength of light via an endoscope. Cells are subsequently destroyed and tumors are eliminated or reduced in size.

      - Nursing Actions

        - Treat chest pain with opioids.

        - Treat nausea with antiemetic.

        - Monitor for difficulty breathing or swallowing.

      - Client Education

        - Instruct the client to avoid sun exposure for at least 6 weeks.

        - Instruct the client to consume a liquid diet for several days until pain subsides.

- Surgical Interventions

  - Esophagectomy/esophagogastrostomy

    - Removal of all or part of the esophagus and stomach. Some of the intestine may be used as an anatomic graft for the missing length of the esophagus. A more minimally invasive procedure may be done using a laparoscope, but esophageal cancer is usually too extensive for this type of surgery.

    - Nursing Actions (pre, post)

      - Provide preoperative teaching and postoperative care

      - Due to the location of the surgical incision, preoperative radiation pulmonary complications are common. The client should be premedicated with an analgesic and encouraged to cough and deep breathe every 1 to 2 hr and use the inspirometer.

      - Maintain the client in a semi-Fowler's position or higher.

      - Monitor chest tube and drainage.

      - Maintain NG tube patency and monitor drainage – do not replace NG tube if it comes out.

      - Do not manipulate or irrigate NG tube unless prescribed by the provider.

      - Provide enteral feedings if jejunostomy tube was placed.

- ☐ Keep the client NPO until anastomosis has been determined to be patent (barium swallow).

- ☐ Monitor for anastomotic leak (fever, saliva seeping through incision).

- ☐ Provide the client with suction for oral secretions.

- ☐ Closely observe for aspiration when oral feedings are resumed. Keep the client upright for at least 2 hr after meals.

- ■ Client Education

  - ☐ Instruct the client to slowly progress diet beginning with thick liquids and moving to semisolid and well-chewed solid foods.

  - ☐ Instruct the client to weigh regularly and increase caloric intake as tolerated to maintain or increase weight.

  - ☐ Instruct the client to monitor the incision closely for signs of infection or abnormal drainage (saliva).

- Client Outcomes

  - ○ The client will be able to ingest a regular diet without aspiration or dysphagia.

  - ○ The client will maintain or gain weight.

  - ○ The client will not develop aspiration pneumonia.

Complications

- Vagotomy syndrome

  - ○ Causes

    - ■ Due to an interruption of the vagal nerve, a syndrome similar to "dumping syndrome" occurs after esophagectomy. This is related to the quick passage of food into the duodenum, which creates an osmotic gradient with large amounts of fluids entering the bowel and manifesting itself as watery diarrhea. It typically occurs 15 to 60 minutes after a meal.

  - ○ Nursing Actions

    - ■ Observe for postprandial symptoms (diaphoresis, diarrhea, tachycardia, abdominal pain).

    - ■ Refer the client to a dietician to determine what foods to avoid and develop a meal program (six small meals a day that are lactose free).

CHAPTER 53: ESOPHAGEAL DISORDERS

(A) Application Exercises

Scenario: A nurse is caring for a client diagnosed with gastroesophageal reflux disease (GERD). The client is overweight and has been experiencing dyspepsia, belching, bloating after meals, dysphagia, and chest pain.

1. What pathophysiologic problem is causing the client to experience chest pain?

2. What client education should be provided?

3. What classifications of medications will help to relieve the symptoms of GERD that result from the reflux of gastrointestinal contents containing acid? (Select all that apply.)

_____ Antacids

_____ Histamine$_2$ receptor antagonists

_____ Opioid analgesics

_____ Fiber laxatives

_____ Proton pump inhibitors

4. Identify which of the following factors contribute to decreased lower esophageal sphincter (LES) and the occurrence of GERD. (Select all that apply.)

_____ Cigarette smoking

_____ Decaffeinated coffee

_____ Ice cream with chocolate sauce

_____ Peppermint candy cane

_____ Diltiazem (Cardizem)

_____ Cheeseburger and french fries

_____ Low-fat milk

_____ Tomato salsa

_____ Alcohol

_____ Exercise

_____ Weight loss

5. A client has been admitted to the hospital with a diagnosis of bleeding esophageal varices. Which of the following medications should the nurse anticipate will be prescribed?

A. Propranolol (Inderal)

B. Metoclopramide (Reglan)

C. Cetuximab (Erbitux)

D. Vasopressin (Desmopressin)

CHAPTER 53: ESOPHAGEAL DISORDERS

 Application Exercises Answer Key

Scenario: A nurse is caring for a client diagnosed with gastroesophageal reflux disease (GERD). The client is overweight and has been experiencing dyspepsia, belching, bloating after meals, dysphagia, and chest pain.

1. What pathophysiologic problem is causing the client to experience chest pain?

Chest pain in clients with GERD is caused by spasms of the esophagus as a result of the reflux of acidic stomach contents and inflammatory response.

 NCLEX® Connection: Physiological Adaptation, Pathophysiology

2. What client education should be provided?

The nurse should instruct the client to eat small frequent meals; chew foods thoroughly; avoid evening snacks, fatty foods, chocolate, alcohol, coffee, and tea; and start a weight-loss program. The client should be instructed to avoid tight-fitting clothing. The client should elevate the head of the bed on blocks, and should avoid elevating her head with pillows. The client should keep a food diary to see what foods trigger symptoms. If the client smokes, she should seek assistance in quitting.

 NCLEX® Connection: Physiological Adaptation, Illness Management

3. What classifications of medications will help to relieve the symptoms of GERD that result from the reflux of gastrointestinal contents containing acid? (Select all that apply.)

X	**Antacids**
X	**Histamine₂ receptor antagonists**
_____	Opioid analgesics
_____	Fiber laxatives
X	**Proton pump inhibitors**

Antacids neutralize gastric acid, histamine$_2$ receptor antagonists decrease the secretion of gastric acid, and proton pump inhibitors decrease the production of gastric acid; these are all given to treat GERD. Opioid analgesics and fiber laxatives are not effective in the treatment of symptoms of GERD that result from the reflux of gastrointestinal contents containing acid.

 NCLEX® Connection: Physiological Adaptation, Illness Management

4. Identify which of the following factors contribute to decreased lower esophageal sphincter (LES) and the occurrence of GERD. (Select all that apply.)

   X   **Cigarette smoking**

          Decaffeinated coffee

   X   **Ice cream with chocolate sauce**

   X   **Peppermint candy cane**

   X   **Diltiazem (Cardizem)**

   X   **Cheeseburger and french fries**

          Low-fat milk

   X   **Tomato salsa**

   X   **Alcohol**

          Exercise

          Weight loss

Cigarette smoking, chocolate sauce, peppermint candy canes, diltiazem (Cardizem), cheeseburger and french fries, tomato salsa, and alcohol all relax the lower esophageal sphincter. Decaffeinated coffee, low-fat milk, exercise, and weight loss do not result in relaxation of the lower esophageal sphincter.

(N) **NCLEX® Connection: Physiological Adaptation, Pathophysiology**

5. A client has been admitted to the hospital with a diagnosis of bleeding esophageal varices. Which of the following medications should the nurse anticipate will be prescribed?

   A. Propranolol (Inderal)

   B. Metoclopramide (Reglan)

   C. Cetuximab (Erbitux)

   D. Vasopressin (Desmopressin)

Vasopressin is given for active esophageal bleeds due to its ability to constrict blood vessels. Propranolol is not appropriate to give for an active bleed; it may be given prophylactically to decrease portal hypertension. Metoclopramide (Reglan) increases the motility of the esophagus and stomach. Cetuximab (Erbitux) is used in the treatment of esophageal cancer.

(N) **NCLEX® Connection: Pharmacological and Parenteral Therapies, Expected Actions/ Outcomes**

UNIT 7	NURSING CARE OF CLIENTS WITH GASTROINTESTINAL DISORDERS
Section	Upper Gastrointestinal Disorders
Chapter 54	Peptic Ulcer Disease

 Overview

- A peptic ulcer is an erosion of the mucosal lining of the stomach or duodenum. The mucous membranes can become eroded to the point that the epithelium is exposed to gastric acid and pepsin, and can precipitate bleeding and perforation. Perforation that extends through all the layers of the stomach or duodenum can cause peritonitis. An individual with a peptic ulcer has peptic ulcer disease (PUD).

- There are gastric ulcers, duodenal ulcers, and stress ulcers (these occur after major stress or trauma).

Health Promotion and Disease Prevention

- Drink alcohol in moderation.

- Smoking cessation.

- Use stress management techniques.

- Avoid NSAIDS as indicated.

Assessment

- Risk Factors

  o Causes of peptic ulcers:

    ▪ *Helicobacter pylori (H. pylori)* infection.

    ▪ Nonsteroidal anti-inflammatory drug (NSAID) and corticosteroid use.

    ▪ Severe stress.

    ▪ Hypersecretory states.

    ▪ Type O blood.

    ▪ Excess alcohol ingestion.

    ▪ Chronic pulmonary or renal disease.

    ▪ Zollinger-Ellison syndrome (combination of peptic ulcers, hypersecretion of gastric acid, and gastrin secreting tumors).

- Subjective Data

    o Dyspepsia – heartburn, bloating, nausea, and vomiting. May be perceived as uncomfortable fullness or hunger.

    o Pain

GASTRIC ULCER	DUODENAL ULCER
30 to 60 min after a meal	1.5 to 3 hr after a meal
Rarely occurs at night	Often occurs at night
Pain exacerbated by ingestion of food	Pain may be relieved by ingestion of food or antacid.

- Objective Data

    o Physical Assessment Findings

        ■ Epigastric pain upon palpation. Pain that radiates to the back may indicate perforation is imminent.

        ■ Bloody emesis (hematemesis) or stools (melena)

        ■ Weight loss

    o Laboratory Tests

        ■ *H. pylori* testing:

            □ Gastric samples are collected via an endoscopy to test for *H. pylori*.

            □ C 13 Urea breath testing is when the client exhales into a collection container (baseline), drinks carbon-enriched urea solution, and is asked to exhale into a collection container. The client should take nothing by mouth (NPO) prior to the test. If *H. pylori* is present, the solution will break down and carbon dioxide will be released. The two collections are compared to confirm the presence of *H. pylori*.

            □ IgG serologic testing documents the presence of *H. pylori* based on antibody assays.

            □ Stool sample tests for the presence of the *H. pylori* antigen.

        ■ Hemoglobin and hematocrit (decreased values secondary to bleeding).

        ■ Stool sample for occult blood.

○ Diagnostic Procedures

- Esophagogastroduodenoscopy (EGD)

  □ An EGD is the most definitive diagnosis of peptic ulcers and may be repeated to evaluate the effectiveness of treatment. Gastric samples are taken to test for H. pylori.

  □ Nursing Actions

    ▸ Several medications (bismuth, misoprostol, sucralfate, histamine$_2$ antagonists) can interfere with testing for *H. pylori* (false negatives). Therefore, a complete medication history should be collected prior to testing.

  □ Client Education

    ▸ Avoid taking the medications listed above prior to the test.

Collaborative Care

- Nursing Care

  ○ Monitor for orthostatic changes in vital signs and tachycardia as these findings are suggestive of gastrointestinal bleeding.

  ○ Administer saline lavage via nasogastric tube, if prescribed.

  ○ Administer medication as prescribed.

  ○ Decrease environmental stress.

  ○ Encourage rest periods.

  ○ Encourage smoking cessation and avoid alcohol consumption.

- Medications

  ○ Antibiotics: Metronidazole (Flagyl), amoxicillin (Amoxil), bismuth (Pepto-Bismol), clarithromycin (Biaxin), tetracycline (Achromycin V)

    - Eliminate *H. pylori* infection

    - Nursing Considerations

      □ The client may require a combination of two to three different antibiotics.

    - Client Education

      □ Instruct the client to complete a full course of medication.

  ○ Histamine$_2$ receptor antagonists: Ranitidine hydrochloride (Zantac), famotidine (Pepcid)

    - Suppress the secretion of gastric acid by selectively blocking H_2 receptors in parietal cells lining the stomach.

    - Used in conjunction with antibiotics to treat ulcers caused by *H. pylori*.

- Used to prevent stress to individuals who are NPO after major surgery, have large areas of burns, are septic, or have increased intracranial pressure.
- Nursing Considerations
  - Ranitidine and famotidine can be administered IV for acute situations.
  - Ranitidine can be taken with or without food.
  - Treatment of peptic ulcer disease is usually started as an oral dose twice a day until the ulcer is healed, followed by a maintenance dose usually taken once a day at bedtime.
- Client Education
  - Instruct clients to notify the provider for any sign of obvious or occult GI bleeding (coffee-ground emesis).

- Proton pump inhibitors: Pantoprazole (Protonix), esomeprazole (Nexium)
  - Reduce gastric acid secretion by irreversibly inhibiting the enzyme that produces gastric acid.
  - Reduce basal and stimulated acid production.
  - Nursing Considerations
    - Insignificant side effects and adverse effects with short-term treatment.
  - Client Education
    - Instruct the client not to crush, chew, or break sustained-release capsules.
    - Instruct the client to take omeprazole once a day prior to eating in the morning.
    - Encourage the client to avoid alcohol and irritating medications (NSAIDs).

- Antacids: Aluminum carbonate, magnesium hydroxide (Milk of Magnesia)
  - Antacids are given 1 to 3 hr after meals to neutralize gastric acid, which occurs with food ingestion and at bedtime.
  - Nursing Considerations
    - Give 1 hr apart from other medications to avoid reducing the absorption of other medications.
  - Client Education
    - Encourage compliance by reinforcing the intended effect of the antacid (relief of pain, healing of ulcer).
    - Teach clients to take all medications at least 1 hr before or after taking an antacid.

- Mucosal protectant: Sucralfate (Carafate).
  - Nursing Considerations
    - Give 1 hr before meals and at bedtime.
    - Monitor for side effects of constipation.

- Interdisciplinary Care

  ○ Nutrition consult – diet that restricts acid-producing foods (milk products, caffeine, decaffeinated coffee, spicy foods, medications [NSAIDs]).

- Therapeutic Procedures

  ○ Endoscopic therapies

    ■ During an esophagogastroduodenoscopy (EGD), areas of bleeding may be treated with epinephrine or laser coagulation.

- Surgical Interventions

  ○ Gastric Surgery

    ■ Gastric surgeries include:

      □ Gastrectomy – All or part of the stomach is removed. This surgery may be performed with laparoscopic or open approach.

      □ Antrectomy – The antrum portion of the stomach is removed.

      □ Gastrojejunostomy (Billroth II procedure) – The lower portion of the stomach is excised and the remaining stomach is anastomosed to the jejunum, and the remaining duodenum is surgically closed.

      □ Vagotomy – The branches of the vagus nerve that supply the stomach are cut to disrupt acid production.

      □ Pyloroplasty – The opening between the stomach and small intestine is enlarged to increase the rate of gastric emptying.

    ■ Nursing Actions

      □ Provide the client with preoperative teaching and postoperative care.

      □ Place the client in a semi-Fowler's position to facilitate respiratory movements.

      □ Monitor the client's nasogastric output as appropriate and intervene to avoid abdominal distention (a scant amount of blood is expected in the first 12 to 24 hr). Notify the provider before repositioning or irrigating the nasogastric tube (disruption of sutures).

      □ Assess bowel sounds – diminished or absent with surgery and anesthesia. Monitor for return (3 to 5 per quadrant/min).

      □ Follow guidelines for reintroduction of fluids and foods. Healing of sutures is supported by NPO status. Generally, resumption of enteral intake begins with clear liquids and the client's diet is advanced as tolerated. Abdominal distention is avoided.

    ■ Client Education

      □ Educate the client regarding the need for vitamin and mineral supplementation after a gastrectomy, including vitamin B_{12}, vitamin D, calcium, iron, and folate.

- Client Outcomes

  - The client will experience no further bleeding.

  - The client will be able to verbalize medication regimen and foods that should be avoided.

Complications

- Perforation/Hemorrhage

  - When peptic ulcers perforate or bleed, it is an emergency situation.

    - Perforation presents as severe epigastric pain spreading across the abdomen. The abdomen is rigid, board-like, hyperactive to diminished bowel sounds, and has rebound tenderness. Perforation is a surgical emergency.

    - Gastrointestinal bleeding in the form of hematemesis or melena may cause symptoms of shock (hypotension, tachycardia, dizziness, confusion), and decreased hemoglobin.

  - Nursing Actions

    - Nurses should perform periodic assessments of the client's pain and vital signs to detect subtle changes that may indicate perforation or bleeding.

    - Nurses should report findings, prepare the client for endoscopic or surgical intervention, replace fluid and blood losses, insert nasogastric tube, provide saline lavages, and maintain the client's blood pressure.

- Pernicious Anemia

  - Pernicious anemia is due to a deficiency of the intrinsic factor normally secreted by the gastric mucosa.

    - Symptoms include pallor, glossitis, fatigue, and paresthesias.

  - Client Education

    - Routine lifelong vitamin B_{12} injections will be necessary.

- Dumping Syndrome

  - Dumping syndrome is a complication of gastric surgery that consists of vasomotor symptoms occurring in response to food ingestion. Symptoms result from the rapid emptying of gastric contents into the small intestine. In response to the sudden influx of a hypertonic fluid, the small intestine pulls fluid from the extracellular space to convert the hypertonic fluid to an isotonic fluid. This fluid shift causes a decrease in circulating volume, resulting in vasomotor symptoms (syncope, pallor, palpitations, dizziness, headache).

  - Gastric surgery, especially gastrojejunostomy (Billroth II), poses the greatest risk for dumping syndrome. Following gastric surgery, the reduced stomach has less ability to control the amount and rate of chyme that enters the small intestine after a meal.

○ Nursing Actions

  ■ Monitor for vasomotor symptoms:

	EARLY SYMPTOMS	LATE SYMPTOMS
Onset	Within 30 min after eating	90 min to 3 hr after eating
Cause	Rapid emptying	Excessive insulin release
Symptoms	• Nausea, vomiting, and dizziness • Tachycardia • Palpitations	• Hunger, dizziness, and sweating • Tachycardia and palpitations • Shakiness and feelings of anxiety • Confusion

  ■ Assist/instruct the client to lie down when vasomotor symptoms occur.

  ■ Administer medications as prescribed:

    □ Administration of powdered pectin or octreotide (Sandostatin) subcutaneously may be prescribed if symptoms are severe and not effectively controlled with dietary measures. Pectin slows the absorption of carbohydrates. Octreotide blocks gastric and pancreatic hormones, which can lead to symptoms of dumping syndrome.

    □ Antispasmodic medications (dicyclomine [Bentyl]).

    □ Acarbose (Prandase) will slow the absorption of carbohydrates.

    □ Malnutrition and fluid electrolyte imbalances may occur due to altered absorption. Monitor intake and output, laboratory values, and the client's weight.

○ Client Education

  ■ Instruct the client that lying down after a meal will slow the movement of food within the intestines.

  ■ Limit the amount of fluid ingested at one time.

  ■ Eliminate liquids with meals for 1 hr prior to and following a meal.

  ■ Consume a high-protein, high-fat, low-fiber, and a low to moderate carbohydrate diet.

  ■ Avoid milk, sweets, or sugars (fruit juice, sweetened fruit, milk shakes, honey, syrup, jelly).

  ■ Small, frequent meals rather than large meals.

CHAPTER 54: PEPTIC ULCER DISEASE

Ⓐ Application Exercises

Scenario: A nurse has admitted a client with a possible diagnosis of peptic ulcer disease. The client reports symptoms consistent with a gastric ulcer and has lost 15 lb in the past 3 months. Currently, the client is nauseated, has had two episodes of hematemesis, and his vital signs indicate hypovolemia.

1. For which of the following pathogens should the client be tested?

   A. Methicillin resistant *Staphylococcus aureus*

   B. *H. pylori*

   C. *Giardia lamblia*

   D. Ascariasis

2. The client is to be observed for signs of perforation. For which of the following should the nurse observe? (Select all that apply.)

   _____ Rigid abdomen

   _____ Tachycardia

   _____ Pain in the right shoulder

   _____ Elevated blood pressure

   _____ Circumoral cyanosis

   _____ Rebound tenderness

3. The client does experience a perforation and a Billroth II surgical procedure is performed. Which of the following instructions should the nurse give the client to prevent the occurrence of dumping syndrome?

   A. Eat three moderate-sized meals a day.

   B. Drink at least one glass of water with each meal.

   C. Eat a bedtime snack that contains a milk product.

   D. Increase pectin in the diet.

CHAPTER 54: PEPTIC ULCER DISEASE

(A) Application Exercises Answer Key

Scenario: A nurse has admitted a client with a possible diagnosis of peptic ulcer disease. The client reports symptoms consistent with a gastric ulcer and has lost 15 lb in the past 3 months. Currently, the client is nauseated, has had two episodes of hematemesis, and his vital signs indicate hypovolemia.

1. For which of the following pathogens should the client be tested?

    A. Methicillin resistant *Staphylococcus aureus*

    B. H. pylori

    C. *Giardia lamblia*

    D. Ascariasis

H. pylori is a bacteria that has been found to cause the majority of the cases of peptic ulcer disease. Methicillin resistant *Staphylococcus aureus* is a bacteria that infects skin and soft tissues. Giardia lamblia is a protozoa that typically invades the upper small intestine. Ascariasis is an infestation, typically of the small intestine, with roundworms.

(N) **NCLEX® Connection: Physiological Adaptation, Infectious Disease**

2. The client is to be observed for signs of perforation. For which of the following should the nurse observe? (Select all that apply.)

__X__	**Rigid abdomen**
__X__	**Tachycardia**
__X__	**Pain in the right shoulder**
_____	Elevated blood pressure
_____	Circumoral cyanosis
__X__	**Rebound tenderness**

Signs of perforation include findings related to the perforation itself (rigid abdomen, rebound tenderness, abdominal pain that radiates into the right shoulder, hematemesis) as well as the loss of blood (tachycardia, hypotension, syncope). Signs of perforation do not include circumoral cyanosis or elevated blood pressure.

(N) **NCLEX® Connection: Physiological Adaptation, Medical Emergencies**

3. The client does experience a perforation and a Billroth II surgical procedure is performed. Which of the following instructions should the nurse give the client to prevent the occurrence of dumping syndrome?

    A. Eat three moderate-sized meals a day.

    B. Drink at least one glass of water with each meal.

    C. Eat a bedtime snack that contains a milk product.

    D. Increase pectin in the diet.

The addition of pectin in the diet will delay the absorption of carbohydrates in the small intestine, decreasing the incidence of dumping syndrome. Encourage small, frequent meals rather than large meals, eliminate liquids with meals and for 1 hr prior to and following meals, and avoid milk products.

Ⓝ **NCLEX® Connection: Reduction of Risk Potential, Potential for Complications from Surgical Procedures and Health Alterations**

UNIT 7	NURSING CARE OF CLIENTS WITH GASTROINTESTINAL DISORDERS
Section	Upper Gastrointestinal Disorders
Chapter 55	Acute and Chronic Gastritis

 Overview

- The stomach is coated with a protective layer. Cox 1 enzymes produce mucosal prostaglandins that protect the lining of the stomach.

- Gastritis is an inflammation in the lining of the stomach.

- Inflammation is the result of an irritation to the stomach mucosa.

> **View Media Supplement:** *H. pylori* Gastritis (Image)

- Gastritis may be chronic or acute.

- Acute gastritis:

  o Sudden onset

  o Short duration

  o Severe acute gastritis may result in gastric bleeding

- Chronic gastritis:

  o Slow onset

  o Chronic profuse damage to stomach mucosa may cause parietal cell damage

  o Pernicious anemia

  o Extensive gastric mucosal wall damage may cause erosive gastritis (ulcers) and increase the risk of stomach cancer

Health Promotion and Disease Prevention

- Follow a prescribed diet.

- Watch for signs and symptoms of GI bleeding.

- Follow the prescribed medication regimen.

- Eat small, frequent meals.

- Report constipation, nausea, vomiting, or bloody stools.

Assessment

- Risk Factors

    o Bacterial infection: *Helicobacter pylori (H. pylori)*, salmonella, streptococci, staphylococci or Escherichia coli

    o Family member with *H. pylori* infection

    o Family history of gastritis

    o Prolonged use of NSAIDS, corticosteroids (stops prostaglandin synthesis)

    o Excessive alcohol use

    o Bile reflux disease

    o Autoimmune diseases (systemic lupus, rheumatoid arthritis)

    o Advanced age

    o Radiation therapy

    o Smoking

    o Caffeine

    o Excessive stress

    o Exposure to contaminated food or water

- Subjective Data

    o Dyspepsia, general abdominal discomfort, indigestion

    o Upper abdominal pain or burning may increase or decrease after eating

    o Nausea

    o Reduced appetite

    o Abdominal bloating or distention

    o Hematemesis (bloody emesis)

    o Erosive gastritis:

        ▪ Black, tarry stools, coffee ground emesis

        ▪ Acute abdominal pain

- Objective Data
  - Physical Assessment Findings
    - Vomiting
    - Weight loss
    - Stools or emesis test positive for occult blood
  - Laboratory Tests
    - Noninvasive tests
      - CBC to check for anemia (In women, Hgb less than 12 g/dL and RBC less than 4.2 cells/mcL; in men, Hgb less than 14 g/dL and RBC less than 4.7 cells/mcL)
      - Serum and stool antibody/antigen test for presence of *H. pylori*
      - C 13 Urea breath test: used to measure *H. pylori*
  - Diagnostic Procedures
    - Upper endoscopy
      - A small flexible scope is inserted through the mouth into the esophagus, stomach, and duodenum to visualize the upper digestive tract. This procedure allows for a biopsy, cauterization, removal of polyps, dilation, or diagnosis.
    - Nursing Actions
      - Verify or obtain a signed written consent for the procedure prior to sedation.
      - Establish intravenous access.
      - Monitor vital signs pre, intra, and post procedure.
      - Position the client on left side.
      - Monitor post-procedure for signs of perforation (severe abdominal pain, tachycardia, fever, nausea, vomiting).
      - Assess for gag reflex post-procedure.
    - Client Education
      - Instruct the client to maintain NPO status 6 to 8 hr prior to procedure.
      - Advise the client to have a ride home available after the procedure.
      - Inform the client that a local anesthetic will be sprayed onto the back of the throat.
      - Inform the client a mouth piece will be inserted.
      - Inform the client that he will be positioned on the left side during the procedure.

□   Instruct the client to not eat or drink post-procedure until gag reflex has returned.

□   Inform the client of a possible sore throat post-procedure.

□   Instruct the client to monitor for signs of perforation and have emergency contact numbers available.

Collaborative Care

- Nursing Care

  o Monitor fluid intake and urine output.

  o Provide intravenous fluids as prescribed.

  o Monitor electrolytes (diarrhea and vomiting may deplete electrolytes and cause dehydration).

  o Assist the client in identifying foods that may trigger symptoms.

  o Provide small, frequent meals and encourage the client to eat slowly.

  o Advise the client to avoid alcohol, caffeine, and foods that may cause gastric irritation.

  o Assist the client in identifying ways to reduce stress.

  o Monitor for signs of gastric bleeding (coffee ground emesis, black, tarry stools).

  o Monitor for signs of anemia (tachycardia, hypotension, fatigue, shortness of breath, pallor, feeling light headed or dizzy, chest pain).

- Medications

CLASSIFICATION/ACTION	MEDICATIONS	NURSING INTERVENTIONS	CLIENT EDUCATION
- Histamine$_2$ antagonists o Decreases gastric acid output by blocking gastric histamine$_2$ receptors	- nizatidine (Axid) - famotidine (Pepcid) - ranitidine (Zantac)	- Allow 1 hr before or after to give antacid. - Monitor for neutropenia and hypotension. - Administer IV slowly, too quickly may cause bradycardia and hypotension.	- Advise the client not to smoke or drink alcohol. - Advise the client to take oral dose with meals. - Advise the client to wait 1 hr prior to or following H$_2$ receptor antagonist to take an antacid. - Advise the client to monitor for signs of GI bleed (black stools, coffee ground emesis).

CLASSIFICATION/ACTION	MEDICATIONS	NURSING INTERVENTIONS	CLIENT EDUCATION

• Antacids
   ○ Increases gastric pH and neutralizes pepsin
   ○ Improves mucosal protection
	• Aluminum hydroxide (Amphojel)
	• Magnesium hydroxide with aluminum hydroxide (Maalox, Mylanta)
		• Do not give to clients with renal failure or renal dysfunction.
		• Monitor: Aluminum antacids for aluminum toxicity and constipation, magnesium antacids for diarrhea or hypermagnesemia.
			• Advise the client to take on an empty stomach.
			• Advise the client to wait 1 to 2 hr to take other medications.

• Proton pump inhibitor ○ Reduces gastric acid by stopping acid-producing proton pump	• Omeprazole (Prilosec) • Lansoprazole (Prevacid) • Rabeprazole sodium (Aciphex) • Pantoprazole (Protonix) • Esomeprazole (Nexium)	• These can cause nausea, vomiting, and abdominal pain. • Use filter for IV administration.	• Advise the client to allow 30 min before eating and not to crush or chew pills. • It can take up to 4 days for the client to see the effects. • Advise the client to take on an empty stomach.
• Prostaglandins ○ Reduces gastric acid secretion	• Misoprostol (Cytotec)	• This may be given with NSAIDs to prevent gastric mucosal damage. • This may cause abdominal pain and diarrhea.	• Advise the client to use contraceptives. • Advise the client not to take if there is a chance of becoming pregnant. • Advise the client to take with food to reduce gastric effects.

CLASSIFICATION/ACTION	MEDICATIONS	NURSING INTERVENTIONS	CLIENT EDUCATION
• Anti-ulcer/mucosal barrier ○ Inhibits acid and forms a protective coating over mucosa	• Sucralfate (Carafate)	• Allow 30 min before or after to give antacid.	• Advise the client to take on an empty stomach. • Advise the client not to smoke or drink alcohol. • Advise the client to continue to take medication even if symptoms subside. • Advise the client to notify the provider of tinnitus.
• Antibiotics ○ Eliminates *H. pylori* infection	• Clarithromycin (Biaxin) • Amoxicillin (Amoxil) • Tetracycline (Achromycin V) • Metronidazole (Flagyl)	• Monitor for increased abdominal pain and diarrhea. • Monitor electrolytes and hydration if fluid is depleted.	• Advise the client to complete prescribed dosage. • Advise the client to notify the provider of persistent diarrhea.

- Interdisciplinary Care

    ○ A nutritionist may be necessary to assist in the alterations to diet.

    ○ Supportive care may be needed to reduce stress, increase exercise, and stop smoking.

- Therapeutic Procedures

    ○ Upper endoscopy

- Surgical Interventions

    ○ May be needed to treat erosive gastritis unrelieved by nonsurgical interventions.

    ○ Vagotomy or highly selective vagotomy

        ▪ The vagus nerve is cut where it enters the stomach in order to decrease gastric acid. A highly selective vagotomy severs only the nerve fibers that control gastric acid secretion. Often done laparoscopically to reduce post-operative complications.

    ○ Pyloroplasty

        ▪ The outlet from the stomach to the duodenum is widened to increase gastric emptying. This is usually done at the same time as the vagotomy.

- Nursing Actions
  - Postoperative
    - Monitor for infection.
    - Monitor bowel sounds.
    - Provide pain medicine as needed.
    - Client may require stool softeners.
    - Monitor for alteration in fluids and electrolytes.
    - Monitor for diarrhea.
    - Slowly introduce foods.
    - Assess abdomen for distention and tenderness.
    - Monitor incision site for redness, discharge, and swelling.
  - Preoperative teaching
    - Include postoperative pain management, deep breathing, and anti-embolism care.
- Care after discharge
  - Eat small, frequent meals.
  - Follow the recommended diet.
  - Report constipation, nausea, vomiting, or bloody stools.
  - Take prescribed medications as instructed and monitor for adverse reactions.
- Client Outcomes
  - The client will maintain adequate nutritional intake.
  - The client will eat a healthy diet without abdominal distress.
  - The client will be pain free.
  - The client will identify methods to reduce stress.

Complications

- Gastric bleeding
  - Causes
    - Severe acute gastritis with deep tissue inflammation extending into the stomach muscle
    - In chronic erosive gastritis, bleeding may be slow or profuse as in a perforation of the stomach wall

- o Nursing Actions
  - Monitor vital signs and airway.
  - Provide fluid replacement and blood products.
  - Monitor CBC and clotting factors.
  - May need to insert a nasogastric (NG) tube for gastric lavage (irrigate with normal saline or water to stop active gastric bleed).
  - Confirm placement of NG tube prior to fluid instillation to prevent aspiration.
  - Monitor NG tube output.
  - Give IV medications (proton-pump inhibitors, H_2-receptor antagonists) as prescribed.
- o Client Education
  - Instruct the client to monitor for signs of slow gastric bleeding (coffee-ground emesis, black, tarry stools). Seek immediate medical attention with severe abdominal pain or vomiting blood. Take medications as directed.

- Gastric outlet obstruction
  - o Causes
    - Severe acute gastritis with deep tissue inflammation extending into the stomach muscle
  - o Nursing Actions
    - Monitor fluids and electrolytes.
    - Continuous vomiting may result in metabolic alkalosis (due to loss of hydrochloric acid) and severe fluid and electrolyte depletion.
    - Provide fluid and electrolyte replacement.
    - May need to insert a NG tube to empty stomach contents.
    - Prepare for a diagnostic endoscopy.
  - o Client Education
    - Instruct the client to seek medical attention for continuous vomiting, bloating, and nausea.

- Dehydration
  - o Causes
    - Loss of fluid due to vomiting or diarrhea
  - o Nursing Actions
    - Monitor fluid intake and urine output.
    - Provide intravenous fluids if needed.
    - Monitor electrolytes.

- ○ Client Education
    - Instruct the client to contact a health care provider for vomiting and diarrhea.
- Pernicious anemia
    - ○ Causes
        - Chronic gastritis may damage the parietal cells. This may lead to reduced production of intrinsic factor, which is necessary for the absorption of vitamin B_{12}.
        - Insufficient vitamin B_{12} may lead to pernicious anemia.
    - ○ Nursing Actions
        - Monitor for anemia.
        - Administer vitamin B_{12} injections monthly.
    - ○ Client Education
        - Instruct the client of the need for monthly vitamin B_{12} injections.

CHAPTER 55: ACUTE AND CHRONIC GASTRITIS

 Application Exercises

1. A nurse is assessing a client in the emergency department with a 36 hr history of severe vomiting and diarrhea. Which of the following findings should the nurse expect to find? (Select all that apply.)

_____ Hct of 55%

_____ Arterial blood gas: pH 7.30 and HCO_3^- 20

_____ Arterial blood gas: pH 7.50 and HCO_3^- 30

_____ Hgb of 10 g/dL

_____ Serum potassium of 3.0 mEq/L

2. A nurse is caring for a client diagnosed with chronic gastritis. Pernicious anemia may develop as a result of chronic gastritis due to

A. blood loss from erosion.

B. loss of intrinsic factor due to parietal cell damage.

C. reduced iron absorption due to breakdown of the gastric mucosal barrier.

D. autoimmune destruction of RBCs.

3. A nurse is providing discharge teaching to a client who has been prescribed aluminum hydroxide (Amphojel). The nurse should advise the client to

A. take the aluminum hydroxide with food.

B. monitor for diarrhea.

C. wait 1 to 2 hr before taking other oral medications.

D. avoid foods high in bulk (bran, fresh fruits).

4. A nurse is assessing a client diagnosed with acute gastritis. Which of the following should the nurse include in the plan of care for the client? (Select all that apply.)

_____ Monitor fluid intake and urine output.

_____ Monitor electrolytes.

_____ Provide large, infrequent meals.

_____ Administer ibuprofen for pain.

_____ Weigh the client daily.

5. A nurse is caring for a client with chronic gastritis and is scheduled to have a pyloroplasty. The nurse should know that the pyloroplasty will do which of the following?

A. Increase duodenal gastric emptying

B. Reduce gastric acid secretions

C. Increase gastric mucous protection

D. Reduce histamine secretion

CHAPTER 55: ACUTE AND CHRONIC GASTRITIS

 Application Exercises Answer Key

1. A nurse is assessing a client in the emergency department with a 36 hr history of severe vomiting and diarrhea. Which of the following findings should the nurse expect to find? (Select all that apply.)

__X__	**Hct of 55%**
_____	Arterial blood gas: pH 7.30 and HCO_3^- 20
__X__	**Arterial blood gas: pH 7.50 and HCO_3^- 30**
_____	Hgb of 10 g/dL
__X__	**Serum potassium of 3.0 mEq/L**

Severe vomiting may result in dangerous fluid and electrolyte depletion (as indicated by the elevated Hct and low potassium) and metabolic alkalosis (due to loss of hydrochloric acid, as indicated by pH 7.50 and HCO3 30).

 NCLEX® Connection: Reduction of Risk Potential, System Specific Assessment

2. A nurse is caring for a client diagnosed with chronic gastritis. Pernicious anemia may develop as a result of chronic gastritis due to

   A. blood loss from erosion.

   B. loss of intrinsic factor due to parietal cell damage.

   C. reduced iron absorption due to breakdown of the gastric mucosal barrier.

   D. autoimmune destruction of RBCs.

Parietal cell damage may lead to insufficient production of intrinsic factor, which is necessary for the absorption of vitamin B_{12}. Insufficient vitamin B_{12} may lead to pernicious anemia. Pernicious anemia does not result from blood loss due to erosion, reduced iron absorption, or autoimmune destruction of RBCs.

 NCLEX® Connection: Physiological Adaptation, Pathophysiology

3. A nurse is providing discharge teaching to a client who has been prescribed aluminum hydroxide (Amphojel). The nurse should advise the client to

   A. take the aluminum hydroxide with food.

   B. monitor for diarrhea.

   C. wait 1 to 2 hr before taking other oral medications.

   D. avoid foods high in bulk (bran, fresh fruits).

The client should be advised not to take oral medications within 1 to 2 hr of an antacid. Antacids may breakdown enteric-coated medications. Aluminum hydroxide may cause constipation. The client should be advised to increase dietary bulk, and to take the medication on an empty stomach.

 NCLEX® Connection: Pharmacological and Parenteral Therapies, Adverse Effects/ Contraindications/Side Effects/Interactions

4. A nurse is assessing a client diagnosed with acute gastritis. Which of the following should the nurse include in the plan of care for the client? (Select all that apply.)

   X   **Monitor fluid intake and urine output.**

   X   **Monitor electrolytes.**

         Provide large, infrequent meals.

         Administer ibuprofen for pain.

   X   **Weigh the client daily.**

Nursing care of a client with acute gastritis should include monitoring electrolytes, intake and output, daily weight, and provide small, frequent meals. Ibuprofen and other NSAIDs should be avoided to prevent further gastric irritation.

 NCLEX® Connection: Reduction of Risk Potential, Potential for Complications from Surgical Procedures and Health Alterations

5. A nurse is caring for a client with chronic gastritis and is scheduled to have a pyloroplasty. The nurse should know that the pyloroplasty will do which of the following?

A. Increase duodenal gastric emptying

B. Reduce gastric acid secretions

C. Increase gastric mucous protection

D. Reduce histamine secretion

A pyloroplasty is performed to widen the opening from the stomach to the duodenum, which increases gastric emptying. It does not increase gastric mucous protection or reduce histamine secretion. A vagotomy reduces gastric acid secretions.

 NCLEX® Connection: Reduction of Risk Potential, Potential for Complications from Surgical Procedures and Health Alterations

UNIT 7	NURSING CARE OF CLIENTS WITH GASTROINTESTINAL DISORDERS
Section	Lower Gastrointestinal Disorders
Chapter 56	Appendicitis

 Overview

- Appendicitis occurs when the vermiform appendix (a small projection of the cecum) becomes trapped with hard material (usually feces) that leads to a bacterial infection. The lumen of the appendix is blocked and edematous, which leads to abdominal pain.

- Appendicitis is the most common indication for emergency abdominal surgery.

- Appendicitis is not preventable, therefore early detection is important.

> **(M)** **View Media Supplement:** Appendicitis (Image)

Assessment

- Risk Factors

  ○ Appendicitis is seen most often in people between the ages of 10 to 30. Peak incidence is among adolescent males and individuals between 20 and 30 years of age.

  ○ Appendicitis is rare in older adult clients.

  ○ In the older adult, the symptoms of appendicitis are less pronounced. The client may delay seeking treatment, which increases the risk of perforation.

- Subjective Data and Objective Data

  ○ The order in which symptoms occur is important to aid in the diagnosis. With appendicitis, classical abdominal pain occurs first and nausea and vomiting later. The client reports cramping and pain around the umbilicus and in the epigastric area. As the condition progresses, the pain moves to the right lower quadrant (McBurney's point).

  ○ Anorexia, nausea, and vomiting may be reported by the client.

  ○ Rebound tenderness (pain after deep pressure is applied and released) over McBurney's point (located halfway between the umbilicus and anterior iliac spine).

  ○ Pain that is relieved by right hip flexion and increases with coughing and movement may indicate perforation with peritonitis.

o Muscle rigidity, tense positioning, and guarding may indicate perforation with peritonitis.

o Normal to low-grade temperature (higher suggests peritonitis)

o Laboratory Tests

- White blood cell (WBC) count and differential: Mild to moderate elevation of 10,000 to 18,000/mm³ with left shift is consistent with appendicitis; greater than 20,000/mm³ may indicate peritonitis.

o Diagnostic Procedures

- An ultrasound of the abdomen may show an enlarged appendix.

- Abdominal computed tomography (CT) may be diagnostic if symptoms are recurrent or prolonged. The CT may show the presence of fecal material in the appendix.

Collaborative Care

- Nursing Care

  o Surgical management includes an appendectomy, which can be done using a laparoscope (using several small incisions and an endoscope) or an open approach (requiring a larger abdominal incision).

  - Nursing Actions

    □ Preoperative

    ▸ Maintain nothing by mouth (NPO) status in the anticipation of surgery and to prevent GI stimulation.

    ▸ Administer IV fluids as prescribed.

    ▸ Encourage semi-Fowler's position to contain abdominal drainage in the lower abdomen.

    ▸ Avoid laxatives/enemas or application of heat to the abdomen, which can predispose the client to perforation.

    □ Postoperative

    ▸ Administer opioid analgesia (usually morphine sulfate) as ordered.

    ▸ Administer IV antibiotics as prescribed (surgical prophylaxis, perforation).

    ▸ Offer food as tolerated with return of bowel sounds.

    ▸ For peritonitis, monitor nasogastric (NG) tube drainage.

    ▸ For perforation or abscess, monitor surgical drains.

- Discharge Instructions
  - □ If the client does not have complications, he may be discharged 12 to 24 hr after the surgery.
  - □ Discharge instructions are similar to those for clients with other types of abdominal surgery.
  - □ The nurse should teach the client to:
    - ▸ Provide care to the surgical site.
    - ▸ How to recognize the signs and symptoms of wound infection.
    - ▸ Use of postoperative medications (purpose, guidelines, adverse effects).
    - ▸ Activity restrictions (lifting, driving, returning to work).
  - □ The nurse should assess the client's ability to care for himself and the client's support system.

- Client Outcomes
  - ○ The client will remain free of signs and symptoms of infection.
  - ○ The client will report that pain is controlled.
  - ○ The client's fluid and electrolyte status will be restored.
  - ○ The client will return to his regular ADLs

Complications

- Peritonitis, which is an inflammation of the peritoneum and viscera, can occur due to perforation of the appendix. The peritoneal area, which is normally sterile, becomes contaminated with bacteria and gastric juices from the gastrointestinal tract.
  - ○ When a client has appendicitis, the risk of perforation is greatest 24 hr following the onset of pain.

- Nursing Actions
  - ○ Assess and monitor for:
    - ▪ Fever
    - ▪ Tachycardia
    - ▪ Signs of dehydration
    - ▪ Distended or board-like abdomen
    - ▪ Nausea and vomiting
    - ▪ Rebound tenderness
    - ▪ Hiccups
  - ○ Report elevated WBC (20,000/mm³) and elevated neutrophil count.
  - ○ Monitor the client's hemodynamic status.

- o   Administer prescribed IV fluids and antibiotics.

- o   Maintain intermittent nasogastric suction.

- o   Provide oxygen by nasal cannula or mask to maintain adequate oxygenation.

- o   Measure intake and output.

- o   Administer medications to control pain, nausea, and vomiting.

- o   Place the client in a side-lying position with knees bent to decrease abdominal tension.

- o   Provide preoperative teaching if surgery is indicated.

- o   Provide postoperative care for laparoscopic procedure.

- Surgical Procedures

  - o   An exploratory laparotomy is performed to remove infected tissue and repair or removed the infected organ

  - o   Monitor output from drains.

  - o   Place the client in Fowler or semi-Fowler's position (this promotes comfort and allows the client to breathe easier).

  - o   Maintain and monitor nasogastric suction.

  - o   Keep the client NPO.

  - o   Monitor fluid and electrolyte status (be alert for signs of hypovolemia).

  - o   Intake and output may be monitored every hour immediately after surgery.

  - o   Use sterile technique to irrigate the peritoneal area via a catheter or drain (if prescribed by the provider).

  - o   The length of hospitalization for clients who have a laparotomy for peritonitis varies with the severity of the disease, and the client's response during the postoperative phase.

- Client Education

  - o   Instruct the client to provide care to the surgical site, which may include drains still in place.

  - o   Teach the client how to recognize the signs and symptoms of additional infection.

  - o   Teach the client use of postoperative medications (purpose, guidelines, adverse effects).

CHAPTER 56: APPENDICITIS

 Application Exercises

Scenario: A client is admitted to the emergency department with reports of abdominal pain. A diagnosis of acute appendicitis is suspected.

1. What additional nursing assessments are indicated? (Select all that apply.)

_____ Ask the client which occurred first: pain or nausea.

_____ Ask the client about the onset, duration, and intensity of the pain.

_____ Obtain the client's vital signs.

_____ Observe the client for periumbilical discoloration.

_____ Observe the client for a fruity breath odor.

2. Which of the following sites should the nurse use to assess McBurney's point?

A. In the right-lower quadrant, half-way between the anterior iliac crest and the umbilicus.

B. In the right-upper quadrant, half-way between the lower sternum and the umbilicus.

C. In the left-lower quadrant, half-way between the anterior iliac crest and the umbilicus.

D. In the left-upper quadrant, half-way between the lower sternum and the umbilicus.

3. In preparing the client for surgery, the nurse should anticipate which of the following interventions? (Select all that apply.)

_____ Administer an enema.

_____ Maintain NPO status.

_____ Administer IV fluids.

_____ Apply heat to the abdomen.

_____ Ensure the client signs surgical consent form.

4. The client returns to the nursing unit following surgery for a ruptured appendix. The client has an NG tube connected to low suction. An IV of 0.9% sodium chloride is infusing at 100 mL/hr. In providing postoperative care, the nurse should anticipate assisting with which of the following interventions? (Select all that apply.)

_____ Monitoring the abdominal incision

_____ Administering a full-liquid diet

_____ Administering opioid analgesics

_____ Measuring hourly intake and output

_____ Maintaining bed rest with frequent repositioning

CHAPTER 56: APPENDICITIS

 Application Exercises Answer Key

Scenario: A client is admitted to the emergency department with reports of abdominal pain. A diagnosis of acute appendicitis is suspected.

1. What additional nursing assessments are indicated? (Select all that apply.)

   __X__   **Ask the client which occurred first: pain or nausea.**

   __X__   **Ask the client about the onset, duration, and intensity of the pain.**

   __X__   **Obtain the client's vital signs.**

   _____   Observe the client for periumbilical discoloration.

   _____   Observe the client for a fruity breath odor.

The order of symptoms associated with appendicitis is important. Usually, pain precedes nausea and vomiting. The nurse may obtain a history, which includes obtaining additional information regarding pain. Vital signs are important to obtain as a baseline and tachycardia may be present. In the case of peritonitis, fever may be present. Periumbilical discoloration, and a fruity odor to the breath is not associated with appendicitis.

 NCLEX® Connection: Physiological Adaptation, Pathophysiology

2. Which of the following sites should the nurse use to assess McBurney's point?

   A. In the right-lower quadrant, half-way between the anterior iliac crest and the umbilicus.

   B. In the right-upper quadrant, half-way between the lower sternum and the umbilicus.

   C. In the left-lower quadrant, half-way between the anterior iliac crest and the umbilicus.

   D. In the left-upper quadrant, half-way between the lower sternum and the umbilicus.

The location is half-way between the anterior iliac crest and the umbilicus in the right-lower quadrant. This is the classic location for localized pain during the later stages of appendicitis.

 NCLEX® Connection: Reduction of Risk Potential, System Specific Assessment

3. In preparing the client for surgery, the nurse should anticipate which of the following interventions? (Select all that apply.)

   _____   Administer an enema.

   __**X**__   **Maintain NPO status.**

   __**X**__   **Administer IV fluids.**

   _____   Apply heat to the abdomen.

   __**X**__   **Ensure the client signs surgical consent form.**

The nurse should ensure that the client is maintained on NPO status, IV fluids are administered, and the surgical consent form has been signed. Enemas and heat to the abdomen are contraindicated as they can increase the risk of perforation.

 NCLEX® Connection: Reduction of Risk Potential, Potential for Complications from Surgical Procedures and Health Alterations

4. The client returns to the nursing unit following surgery for a ruptured appendix. The client has an NG tube connected to low suction. An IV of 0.9% sodium chloride is infusing at 100 mL/hr. In providing postoperative care, the nurse should anticipate assisting with which of the following interventions? (Select all that apply.)

   __**X**__   **Monitoring the abdominal incision**

   _____   Administering a full-liquid diet

   __**X**__   **Administering opioid analgesics**

   __**X**__   **Measuring hourly intake and output**

   _____   Maintaining bed rest with frequent repositioning

Routine postoperative care includes: monitoring the abdominal incision for drainage and signs of infection, administering opioid analgesics as prescribed for pain, and measuring intake and output for clients with an NG tube and IV infusion. A full-liquid diet is contraindicated for the client with an NG tube connected to suction. Progressive activity with ambulation is encouraged to facilitate peristalsis, promote postoperative recovery, and minimize the effects of immobility.

 NCLEX® Connection: Reduction of Risk Potential, Potential for Complications from Surgical Procedures and Health Alterations

UNIT 7	NURSING CARE OF CLIENTS WITH GASTROINTESTINAL DISORDERS
Section	Lower Gastrointestinal Disorders
Chapter 57	Intestinal Obstruction

Overview

- Intestinal obstruction can result from mechanical or nonmechanical causes. Mechanical obstruction usually requires surgery.

- Symptoms vary according to location.

  ○ Higher-level obstructions have colicky, intermittent pain, and profuse vomiting.

  ○ Lower-level obstructions tend to have vague, diffused, constant pain and significant abdominal distention.

- Bowel sounds will be hyperactive above obstruction and hypoactive below.

- Obstructions of the small intestine are the most common.

- Treatment focuses on fluid and electrolyte balance, decompressing the bowel, and relief/removal of the obstruction.

Assessment

- Risk Factors

  ○ Mechanical obstructions (90% of all obstructions) are the result of:

    ■ Encirclement or compression of intestine by adhesions, tumors, fibrosis (endometriosis), or strictures (Crohn's disease, radiation).

    ■ Twisting (volvulus) or telescoping (intussusception) of bowel segments.

    ■ Hernia (bowel becomes trapped in weakened area of abdominal wall).

    ■ Fecal impactions.

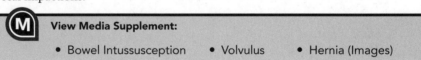

View Media Supplement:

- Bowel Intussusception   • Volvulus   • Hernia (Images)

  ○ Postsurgical adhesions are the most common cause of small bowel obstructions.

- o Carcinomas are the most common cause of large intestine obstructions.

- o Nonmechanical obstructions (paralytic ileus) are the result of decreased peristalsis secondary to:

  - ▪ Neurogenic disorders (manipulation of the bowel during major surgery and spinal fracture).

  - ▪ Vascular disorders (vascular insufficiency and mesenteric emboli).

  - ▪ Electrolyte imbalances (hypokalemia).

  - ▪ Inflammatory responses (peritonitis or sepsis).

- o Diverticulitis and tumors are common causes of obstruction in older adult clients.

- o Older adult clients are at a greater risk for fecal impactions. Bowel regimens can be effective in preventing impactions.

- Subjective and Objective Data

  - o Symptoms vary depending on the location of the obstruction.

SMALL BOWEL AND LARGE INTESTINE OBSTRUCTIONS	SMALL BOWEL OBSTRUCTIONS	LARGE INTESTINE OBSTRUCTIONS
Obstipation – the inability to pass a stool and/or flatus for more than 8 hr despite feeling the need to defecate	Pain is spasmodic and colicky	Pain is diffuse and constant
Abdominal distension	Visible peristaltic waves	Significant abdominal distension
High-pitched bowel sounds before site of obstruction (borborygmi) with hypoactive bowel sounds after, or overall hypoactive; absent bowel sounds later in process	Profuse, (projectile) sudden vomiting with fecal odor; vomiting relieves pain	Infrequent vomiting; the client can have diarrhea around an impaction

  - o Laboratory Tests

    - ▪ May reveal signs of dehydration (elevated hemoglobin and hematocrit) and an elevated white blood cell count with bowel strangulation.

    - ▪ Metabolic alkalosis with high obstruction of the small bowel, and metabolic acidosis with low obstruction of the large intestine.

    - ▪ Electrolytes

      - ▫ Small bowel obstruction: May have severe fluid and electrolyte imbalances

      - ▫ Large intestine obstruction: Usually have minimal fluid and electrolyte imbalances

o   Diagnostic Procedures

- X-ray: Flat plate and upright abdominal x-rays evaluate the presence of free air and gas patterns.

- Endoscopy helps determine the cause of obstruction.

- Computed tomography scan helps determine the cause and exact location of the obstruction.

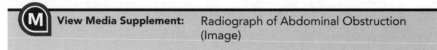

View Media Supplement: Radiograph of Abdominal Obstruction (Image)

Collaborative Care

- Nursing Care

  o   Nonmechanical cause of obstruction

  - Nothing by mouth with bowel rest

  - Assess bowel sounds

  - Provide oral care

  - Intravenous fluid and electrolyte replacement (particularly potassium)

  - Pain management once a diagnosis is made

  - Ambulation

  o   Mechanical cause of obstruction

  - Prepare the client for surgery and provide preoperative nursing care.

  - Withhold intake until peristalsis resumes.

- Therapeutic Procedures

  o   Nasogastric tube to decompress the bowel

  - Nursing Actions

    □   Maintain intermittent suction as prescribed.

    □   Assess NG tube patency and irrigate every 4 hr, or as prescribed.

    □   Measure gastric output.

    □   Monitor nasal area for skin breakdown.

    □   Monitor vital signs, skin integrity, weight, and I&O.

    □   Clamp the NG tube while ambulating.

- Surgical Interventions
  - Exploratory laparotomy – Determine the cause of obstruction and rectify if possible.
    - Nursing Actions
      - Provide pre and postoperative teaching and care.
      - Ensure the client understands the type of procedure (open or laparoscopic).
      - Monitor for hemodynamic instability.
      - Provide IV fluid replacement and maintenance.
      - Monitor bowel sounds and document.
      - Maintain NG tube patency and measure output.
      - Clamp NG tube as prescribed to assess the client's tolerance prior to removing.
      - Advance diet as tolerated when prescribed beginning with clear liquids – clamp tube after eating for 1 to 2 hr.
- Client Outcomes
  - The client's bowel sounds will return.
  - The client will be able to eat and drink without nausea and vomiting.

Complications

- Dehydration (potential hypotension; small bowel obstruction)
  - Causes
    - Persistent vomiting
  - Nursing Actions
    - Assess the client's hydration through hematocrit, BUN, orthostatic vital signs, skin turgor/mucous membranes, urine output, and specific gravity. Notify the provider of a fluid imbalance.
    - Administer IV fluids as prescribed.
- Electrolyte Imbalance (small bowel obstruction)
  - Causes
    - Persistent vomiting
  - Nursing Actions
    - Monitor the client's electrolytes, especially potassium levels.
    - Notify the provider of an electrolyte imbalance.
    - Administer IV fluids as prescribed to replace electrolytes.

- Metabolic Alkalosis
  - Causes
    - A higher level obstruction due to a loss of gastric hydrochloride and vomiting.
  - Nursing Actions
    - Monitor the client for hypoventilation from compensatory action by the lungs (confusion, hypercarbia)
    - Obtain arterial blood gas.
    - Notify the provider of abnormal values.
- Metabolic Acidosis
  - Causes
    - A lower level obstruction due to alkaline fluids not reabsorbed.
  - Nursing Actions
    - Monitor the client for deep, rapid respirations (compensatory action by the lungs), confusion, hypotension, and flushed skin.
    - Obtain arterial blood gas.
    - Notify the provider of abnormal values.

CHAPTER 57: INTESTINAL OBSTRUCTION

(A) Application Exercises

1. A nurse is caring for a client who is admitted to the hospital with a small bowel obstruction. Which of the following assessment data should the nurse report to the provider? (Select all that apply.)

_____ Reports of abdominal pain spasms rated at a "7"

_____ Profuse emesis prior to insertion of the nasogastric tube

_____ Urine specific gravity 1.040

_____ Hematocrit 60%

_____ Serum potassium 3.0 mEq/L

_____ Oral temperature 38.5° C (99.5° F)

_____ White blood cell count 10,000 mm³

2. A client is admitted with a small bowel obstruction, and a nasogastric tube (NG) is inserted. Which of the following actions is appropriate for the nurse to take? (Select all that apply.)

_____ Subtract the NG drainage from the client's output.

_____ Irrigate the NG with 20 mL normal saline every 8 hr.

_____ Assess the client's bowel sounds.

_____ Provide the client with oral care.

_____ Clamp the NG while the client ambulates to the bathroom.

3. A nurse is caring for a client who is admitted with a small bowel obstruction from adhesions. Which of the following findings are consistent with this diagnosis? (Select all that apply.)

_____ Vomitus greater than 500 mL and has a fecal odor

_____ Spasmodic and colicky abdominal pain

_____ Improved pain after vomiting

_____ Firm abdomen with rebound tenderness

_____ Laboratory values indicate metabolic acidosis

4. A nurse is caring for an older adult client in a nursing home. Which of the following findings indicates to the nurse that the client has a stool impaction causing a large intestine obstruction?

A. The client states he had a bowel movement yesterday.

B. The client is having small amounts of liquid stool.

C. The client has a slightly distended abdomen and is flatulent.

D. The client indicates he vomited once this morning.

CHAPTER 57: INTESTINAL OBSTRUCTION

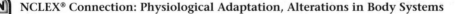 Application Exercises Answer Key

1. A nurse is caring for a client who is admitted to the hospital with a small bowel obstruction. Which of the following assessment data should the nurse report to the provider? (Select all that apply.)

_____ Reports of abdominal pain spasms rated at a "7"

_____ Profuse emesis prior to insertion of the nasogastric tube

__X__ **Urine specific gravity 1.040**

__X__ **Hematocrit 60%**

__X__ **Serum potassium 3.0 mEq/L**

_____ Oral temperature 38.5° C (99.5° F)

_____ White blood cell count 10,000 mm³

The urine specific gravity and hematocrit findings indicate significant dehydration and the potassium level is extremely low. The findings should be reported to the provider. Reports of abdominal pain spasms and profuse emesis are expected findings. The temperature and WBC count are within the expected reference range.

NCLEX® Connection: Physiological Adaptation, Alterations in Body Systems

2. A client is admitted with a small bowel obstruction, and a nasogastric tube (NG) is inserted. Which of the following actions is appropriate for the nurse to take? (Select all that apply.)

_____ Subtract the NG drainage from the client's output.

_____ Irrigate the NG with 20 mL normal saline every 8 hr.

__X__ **Assess the client's bowel sounds.**

__X__ **Provide the client with oral care.**

__X__ **Clamp the NG while the client ambulates to the bathroom.**

Nasogastric drainage, particularly in a small intestine obstruction, can be significant and is considered part of the output when planning fluid replacement. The NG is typically irrigated every 4 hr to maintain patency. Auscultating bowel sounds is part of the ongoing client assessment with an obstruction. An NG tube promotes breathing by the mouth and frequent oral care is needed. Clients can tolerate short-term clamping of the tube after the initial decompression. The client may be placed on a scheduled clamping before the tube is removed.

NCLEX® Connection: Physiological Adaptation, Alterations in Body Systems

3. A nurse is caring for a client who is admitted with a small bowel obstruction from adhesions. Which of the following findings are consistent with this diagnosis? (Select all that apply.)

  __X__   **Vomitus greater than 500 mL and has a fecal odor**

  __X__   **Spasmodic and colicky abdominal pain**

  __X__   **Improved pain after vomiting**

  _____   Firm abdomen with rebound tenderness

  _____   Laboratory values indicate metabolic acidosis

Profuse, projective, and fecal-smelling vomitus is consistent with a small bowel obstruction. Pain is usually colicky and is relieved temporarily after vomiting. A firm abdomen with rebound tenderness is a sign of peritonitis. The client's laboratory values most likely indicate metabolic alkalosis from the loss of gastric acid.

Ⓝ NCLEX® Connection: Physiological Adaptation, Alterations in Body Systems

4. A nurse is caring for an older adult client in a nursing home. Which of the following findings indicates to the nurse that the client has a stool impaction causing a large intestine obstruction?

A. The client states he had a bowel movement yesterday.

B. The client is having small amounts of liquid stool.

C. The client has a slightly distended abdomen and is flatulent.

D. The client indicates he vomited once this morning.

Liquid stool can, and frequently does, travel around an impaction. Since the client had a bowel movement yesterday, an impaction is unlikely. Having flatus resulting in mild distention is not a sign of a large intestine obstruction. Vomiting only once can result from various causes and does not necessarily indicate an impaction.

Ⓝ NCLEX® Connection: Physiological Adaptation, Pathophysiology

UNIT 7 NURSING CARE OF CLIENTS WITH GASTROINTESTINAL DISORDERS

Section Lower Gastrointestinal Disorders

Chapter 58 Inflammatory Bowel Disease

Overview

- Inflammatory bowel disease (IBD) is an umbrella term that includes chronic inflammatory GI diseases: ulcerative colitis, Crohn's disease, and diverticulitis. IBD is characterized by diarrhea (up to 20 stools during acute exacerbation), crampy abdominal pain, and exacerbations ("flare-ups")/remissions.

- Diverticulitis occurs when fecal matter becomes trapped in one or more diverticula resulting in inflammation and infection of the bowel mucosa. Diverticulitis is not to be confused with diverticulosis. Diverticulosis is a condition that develops in the colon where small pouches form. Many clients with diverticulosis never develop diverticulitis.

DISORDER	DESCRIPTION OF DISEASE PROCESS	RELEVANT INFORMATION
Ulcerative colitis	• Edema and inflammation of the rectum may progress to the sigmoid colon and may expand the length of the colon. This usually begins in the rectum and the distal colon involving the mucosa and submucosa.	• Bowel obstruction may occur and intestinal mucosal cell changes may cause colon cancer or insufficient production of intrinsic factor, which is necessary for the absorption of vitamin B_{12}. Insufficient amounts of vitamin B_{12} may lead to pernicious anemia.
Crohn's disease	• Crohn's disease is an inflammation and ulceration of the gastrointestinal tract, often at the distal ileum. • All bowel layers may become involved, and lesions are not continuous, but sporadic. • Fistulas are common with Crohn's disease.	• Crohn's disease can involve the entire GI tract from the mouth to the anus. • Malabsorption and malnutrition may develop when the jejunum and ileum become involved. Supplemental vitamins and minerals including vitamin B_{12} injections may be necessary.
Diverticulitis	• Diverticulitis is an inflammation of the diverticula (hernia in intestinal wall) that frequently occurs in the colon.	• Only about 10% of clients who have diverticula develop diverticulitis. Frequent episodes of inflammation from trapped feces or bacteria may lead to bleeding and infection. • Diverticula may bleed and the loss of blood may be minimal or severe. • Diverticula may perforate and cause peritonitis.

Assessment

- Risk Factors

    - Genetics – Both ulcerative colitis and Crohn's disease are familial diseases.

    - Culture – Ulcerative colitis is higher in Caucasians and persons with a Jewish heritage.

    - Gender and age – The incidence of ulcerative colitis peaks at two points in life: adolescent to young adult (more often in females) and with older adults (more often in males).

        - Crohn's disease may be diagnosed at any age.

        - Diverticulitis occurs more often in older adults and affects men more frequently than women.

    - Diet – A diet low in fiber may predispose a client to ulcerative colitis and the development of diverticula.

    - Smoking – The incidence of ulcerative colitis is higher in nonsmokers.

    - Other factors – Stress, autoimmunity, and infection may be causative agents for both ulcerative colitis and Crohn's disease.

DISORDER	SUBJECTIVE DATA	OBJECTIVE DATA
Ulcerative colitis	• Abdominal pain/cramping: Often left-lower quadrant pain • Anorexia and weight loss	• Fever • Diarrhea: May have up to 15 to 20 liquid stools/day ○ Mucus, blood, or pus may be present • Abdominal distension, tenderness and/or firmness upon palpitation • High-pitched bowel sounds • Rectal bleeding
Crohn's disease	• Abdominal pain/cramping: Often right-lower quadrant pain • Anorexia and weight loss	• Fever • Diarrhea: Five loose stools/day with mucous or pus • Abdominal distension, tenderness and/or firmness upon palpitation • High-pitched bowel sounds • Steatorrhea
Diverticulitis	• Abdominal pain in left-lower quadrant • Nausea and vomiting	• Fever • Chills • Tachycardia

| | LABORATORY FINDINGS | | |
LABORATORY TEST	ULCERATIVE COLITIS	CROHN'S DISEASE	DIVERTICULITIS
hematocrit and hemoglobin	Decreased	Decreased	Decreased
Erythrocyte sedimentation rate (ESR)	Elevated	Elevated	—
WBC	Elevated	Elevated	Elevated
C-reactive protein	Elevated	Elevated	—
Platelet counts	Elevated	Elevated	—
Serum albumin	Decreased	Decreased	—
Folic acid and B$_{12}$	—	Decreased	—
pANCA (perinuclear anti-neutrophil cytoplasmic antibody	Elevated	—	—
Antiglycan antibody	—	Elevated	—
Stool for occult blood	May be positive	May be positive	Positive
Urinalysis	—	WBC	Positive for RBCs
K+, Mg, and Ca	Decreased	Decreased	—

- o Diagnostic Procedures
  - Abdominal x-ray and CT scan
  - Barium enema: Barium is inserted into the rectum as a contrast medium for x-rays. This allows for the rectum and large intestine to be visualized, and is used to diagnose ulcerative colitis. A barium enema may show the presence of diverticulosis and is contraindicated in the presence of diverticulitis due to the risk of perforation.
  - Colonoscopy and sigmoidoscopy: A lighted, flexible scope is inserted into the rectum to visualize the rectum and large intestine.
- o Findings
  - Small intestine ulcerations and narrowing may be consistent with Crohn's disease.
  - Ulcerations and inflammation of the sigmoid colon and rectum may be significant for ulcerative colitis.
- o Nursing Actions
  - Monitor the client postprocedure for signs of bowel perforations (rectal bleeding, firm abdomen, tachycardia, hypotension).

- o Client Education
    - Instruct the client to remain NPO after midnight and provide bowel preparation instructions.
    - Inform the client of possible abdominal discomfort and cramping during the barium enema.
- o Nursing Actions
    - Monitor the client postprocedure for signs of bowel perforation (fever, rectal bleeding, severe abdominal pain).

Collaborative Care

- Nursing Care
    - o Ulcerative colitis and Crohn's disease
        - Educate the client in eating foods that are high in protein and calories, and low in fiber.
        - Instruct the client to avoid caffeine and alcohol, and take a multivitamin that contains iron.
        - Advise the client that small frequent meals may reduce the occurrence of symptoms.
        - Inform the client that dietary supplements that are high in protein and low in fiber may be used.
        - Monitor for an electrolyte imbalance, especially potassium. Diarrhea can cause a loss of fluids and electrolytes.
        - Monitor fluids and assess for dehydration.
        - Educate the client regarding the use of vitamin supplements and B_{12} injections, if needed.
        - Assist the client in identifying foods that trigger symptoms.
        - Instruct the client to seek emergency care for signs of bowel obstruction or perforation (fever, severe abdominal pain, vomiting).
    - o Diverticulitis
        - A client with a mild case of diverticulitis may be treated at home. A health care provider may prescribe antibiotics, analgesics, antispasmodics, and rest.
        - The client's oral intake is limited to clear liquids initially, but may progress to a high-fiber, low-fat diet.
        - The client is hospitalized when symptoms are more severe (severe pain, high fever). The client is NPO, has nasogastric suctioning, is receiving IV fluids, IV antibiotics, total parenteral nutrition, and opioid analgesics for pain.

CLASSIFICATION/THERAPEUTIC INTENT	NURSING CONSIDERATIONS/CLIENT EDUCATION

5-aminosalicyllic acid (5-ASA)
• Sulfonamide
• Anti-inflammatory
  ○ Reduces inflammation of the intestinal mucosa
Medications:
• Sulfasalazine (Azulfidine)
• Olsalazine (Dipentum) for clients intolerant to sulfasalazine
Disorders:
• Ulcerative colitis
• Crohn's disease
	• Sulfasalazine is given orally.
	• These medications may be contraindicated if the client has a sulfa allergy.
	• Monitor CBC, renal, and hepatic function.
	• Advise the client of the following:
	  ○ Take with food.
	  ○ Avoid sun exposure.
	  ○ Increase fluid intake.
	  ○ Urine and skin may appear yellow or brown.
	  ○ Color may damage soft contact lenses. Notify the provider if sore throat, rash, bruising, and/or fever occur.

5-ASA • Anti-inflammatory Medication: • Mesalamine (Asacol, Pentasa, Rowasa) Disorder: • Ulcerative colitis	• Asacol and Pentasa may be given orally. • Rowasa is given by retention enema or rectal suppository. • These medications may be contraindicated if the client has a sulfa allergy. • Monitor CBC, renal, and hepatic function. • The suppository should be firm at the time of insertion. • The client should retain the suppository for at least 1 hr to promote effectiveness. • The client should retain rectal suspension for at least 4 hr. • Educate the client on when and how to take the medication. • The adverse effects are not as serious as sulfasalazine. • Inform the client to report headache or gastrointestinal problems (abdominal discomfort, diarrhea).

Corticosteroids
• Used to reduce inflammation and pain
Medications:
• Prednisone (Delta-son)
• Budesonide (Entocort)
• Hydrocortisone Enema-Cortenema
• Rectal foam (Cortifoam)
• IV corticosteroids for fulminant disease (occurring suddenly)
Disorders:
• Ulcerative colitis
• Crohn's disease
	• Use corticosteroids in low doses to minimize adverse effects.
	• Monitor blood pressure.
	• Reduce systemic dose slowly.
	• Monitor electrolytes and glucose.
	• This medication may slow healing.
	• Advise the client to:
	  ○ Take oral dose with food.
	  ○ Avoid discontinuing dose suddenly.
	  ○ Report unexpected increase in weight or other signs of fluid retention.
	  ○ Avoid crowds and other exposures to infectious diseases.

CLASSIFICATION/THERAPEUTIC INTENT	NURSING CONSIDERATIONS/CLIENT EDUCATION
Immunosuppressants • The mechanism of action in treatment of IBD is unknown. Medication: • Cyclosporine (Sandimmune) and methotrexate (Rheumatrex) for severe refractory disease (resistant to treatment) Disorders: • Ulcerative colitis • Crohn's disease	• Teach clients to avoid crowds and other chances of exposures to infectious diseases and to report signs of infection. • Advise the client to monitor for signs of bleeding, bruising, or infection. • Monitor kidney and hepatitic function.
Immunomodulators • Acts by suppressing the immune response • An antibody used to reduce tumor necrosis factor Medications: • Infliximab (Remicade) • Certolizumab (Cimzia) Disorders: • Crohn's disease • Ulcerative colitis	• Follow directions for IV use with care and in accordance with agency policy. • Many adverse effects are possible, including chills, fever, hypertension, dysrhythmias, and low levels of blood cells. • Monitor liver enzymes and hemoglobin and hematocrit. • Teach clients to avoid crowds and other chances of exposures to infectious diseases and to report signs of infection. The client is at risk for development or reactivation of tuberculosis. • Advise the client to monitor for signs of bleeding, bruising, or infection.
Antidiarrheals • Used to suppress the number of stools Medications: • Diphenoxylate hydrochloride and atropine (Lomotil) • Loperamide (Imodium) Disorders: • Crohn's disease • Ulcerative colitis	• These medications are used to decrease risk of fluid volume deficit and electrolyte imbalance. They also reduce discomfort. • Observe the client for signs of respiratory depression, especially in the older adult client. • Observe the client for signs of toxic megacolon (hypotension, abdominal distension, decrease or absence of bowel sounds). • Due to the central nervous system effects, the client should be taught to avoid hazardous activities until the response to the medication is established.
Antibiotics used to treat infections • Metronidazole (Flagyl) • Ciprofloxacin (Cipro)	

- Interdisciplinary Care

  o Refer the client for nutritional counseling.

  o The client may benefit from complementary therapy (biofeedback, massage, yoga).

  o The client may need a mental health referral for assistance with coping.

- Surgical Interventions

  o Clients who do not have success with medical treatment or who have complications (bowel perforation, colon cancer) are candidates for surgery.

  o Surgical Procedure for Ulcerative Colitis

    ▪ Colectomy with or without ileostomy

  o Surgical Procedures for Crohn's Disease

    ▪ Stricturoplasty may be performed laparoscopically in some cases

    ▪ Surgical repair of fistulas or in response to other complications related to the disease (perforation)

  o Surgical Procedures for Diverticulitis

    ▪ Double-barrel colostomy, but may be temporary

  o Preoperative Care

    ▪ Preoperative care is similar to care for clients with other abdominal surgeries.

    ▪ Reinforce teaching on the type of surgery to be performed.

    ▪ If the creation of stoma is planned, collaborate with an enterostomal therapy nurse regarding care related to the stoma.

    ▪ Administer antibiotic bowel prep (neomycin sulfate), if prescribed.

    ▪ Administer cleansing enema or laxative, if prescribed.

  o Postoperative Care

    ▪ Postoperative care is similar to care for clients with other types of abdominal surgery.

    ▪ The client will be NPO and have a nasogastric tube to suction, unless the surgery was performed laparoscopically.

    ▪ An ileostomy may drain as much as 1,000 mL/day. Prevent fluid volume deficit (Administer IV fluids if the client is NPO. Oral hydration may be administered later in the course of recovery).

- Care After Discharge

  o Refer the client with ostomy to an enterostomal therapist and to an ostomate support group.

- Client Outcomes

  o The client's bowel elimination patterns will improve.

  o The client will be able to carry out ADLs.

  o The client's nutritional status will improve.

  o The client will identify family and community resources to aid in coping with a chronic illness.

Complications

- Complications of ulcerative colitis, Crohn's disease, and diverticulitis include bleeding and fluid and electrolyte imbalance. Peritonitis may occur due to perforation of the bowel. Abscess formation may occur as a complication of diverticular disease and Crohn's disease.

- Nursing Actions

  - Place the client in Fowler or semi-Fowler's position (this promotes comfort and allows for the client to breathe easier).

  - Administer oxygen as prescribed. Turn, cough, deep breathe.

  - Maintain and monitor nasogastric suction.

  - Keep the client NPO.

  - Monitor fluid and electrolyte status (be alert for signs of hypovolemia).

  - Administer IV antibiotics as prescribed.

  - If surgery is performed:

    - Intake and output may be monitored every hour immediately after surgery.

    - Use sterile technique to irrigate the peritoneal area via a catheter or drain (if ordered by the provider).

- Bleeding

  - Bleeding occurs due to deterioration of the bowel.

- Nursing Actions

  - Observe the client for indications of rectal bleeding.

  - Monitor vital signs.

  - Check laboratory values, especially hematocrit, hemoglobin, and coagulation factors.

- Client Education

  - Instruct the client to report rectal bleeding.

  - Explain to the client the importance of bed rest.

- Fluid and electrolyte imbalance

  - Fluid and electrolyte imbalance occurs due to loss of fluid through diarrhea and vomiting, and may occur with nasogastric suctioning.

- Nursing Actions

  - Monitor laboratory values and provide replacement therapy.

  - Monitor weight.

  - Assess for signs of fluid volume deficit (poor skin turgor).

- Client Education

  o Instruct the client to record and report the number of loose stools.

  o Encourage the client to obtain adequate fluid intake.

  o Advise the client to follow the prescribed diet.

  o Inform the client of abscess and fistula formation:

    ▪ Abscess and fistula formation occurs due to the destruction of the bowel wall, leading to an infection.

- Nursing Actions

  o Monitor fluid and electrolytes.

  o Observe for signs of dehydration.

  o Provide a diet high in protein and calories, and low in fiber.

  o Administer a vitamin supplement.

  o Consult with an enterostomal therapist to develop a plan to prevent skin breakdown and promote wound healing.

  o Ensure the function of drainage devices if used.

  o Toxic megacolon:

    ▪ Toxic megacolon occurs due to inactivity of the colon. Massive dilation of the colon occurs and the client is at risk for perforation.

- Nursing Actions

  o Maintain nasogastric suction.

  o Administer IV fluids and electrolytes.

  o Administer prescribed medications (antibiotics, corticosteroids).

  o Prepare the client for surgery (usually an ileostomy) if the client does not begin to show signs of improvement within 72 hr or less.

IRRITABLE BOWEL SYNDROME

Overview

- Irritable bowel syndrome (IBS) is a disorder of the gastrointestinal system.

- IBS differs from ulcerative colitis and Crohn's disease in that it does not cause structural damage to the GI tract and does not involve an inflammatory process.

- Additionally, it does not predispose the client to cancer.

Health Promotion and Disease Prevention

- Encourage the client to avoid food that contains dairy, eggs, and wheat products.

- Encourage the client to avoid alcoholic and caffeinated beverages. Beverages containing fructose and sorbitol should be avoided.

- Encourage the client to drink 2 to 3 L/fluid per day from food and fluid sources.

- Encourage the client to increase the amount of daily fiber intake (approximately 30 to 40 mg/day).

Assessment

- Risk Factors

  - Female

  - Stress

  - Eating large meals containing a large amount of fat

  - Caffeine

  - Alcohol

Subjective and Objective Data

- Cramping pain in abdomen

- Abdominal pain due to changes in bowel pattern and consistency

- Nausea with meals or passing stool

- Anorexia

- Abdominal bloating

- Belching

- Diarrhea

- Constipation

Laboratory Tests

- CBC, serum albumin, erythrocyte sedimentation rate (ESR), and occult stools are all laboratory findings that are obtained with clients with IBS.

Diagnostic Tests

- Difficult to diagnose with specific tests. A Diagnosis is made by the presence of specific characteristics including: abdominal pain accompanied by changes in bowel patterns, abdominal distention, feeling that defecation is not complete, and the presence of mucus with stools.

Collaborative Care

- Nursing Care

  ○ Teach strategies to reduce stress.

  ○ Instruct the client to limit the intake of irritating agents (gas-forming foods, caffeine, alcohol).

  ○ Encourage a diet high in fiber.

Medications

- Classification and Therapeutic Intent

  ○ Alosetron (Lotronex) is an IBS specific medication that selectively blocks 5-HT4 receptors that innervate the viscera and result in increased firmness in stools, and decrease the urgency and frequency of defecation.

  ○ Indicated for irritable bowel syndrome with diarrhea (IBS-D) in women that has lasted more than 6 months and is resistant to conventional management.

- Nursing Considerations

  ○ This medication is contraindicated for clients with chronic constipation, history of bowel obstruction, Crohn's disease, ulcerative colitis, impaired intestinal circulation, or thrombophlebitis.

  ○ The dosage will start as once a day and may be increased to BID.

- Client Education

  ○ Instruct the client that symptoms should resolve within 1 to 4 weeks, but will return 1 week after medication is discontinued.

- Classification and Therapeutic Intent

  ○ Lubiprostone (Amitiza) is an IBS specific medication that increases fluid secretion in the intestine to promote intestinal motility. This is indicated for irritable bowel syndrome with constipation (IBS-C).

- Nursing Considerations

  ○ These medications are contraindicated for clients with a history of bowel obstruction, Crohn's disease, ulcerative colitis, or diverticulitis.

- Client Education

  ○ Instruct the client to take with food to decrease nausea.

CHAPTER 58: INFLAMMATORY BOWEL DISEASE

(A) Application Exercises

1. A nurse is reviewing the laboratory findings for a client who has an acute exacerbation of Crohn's disease. Which of the following laboratory findings is indicative of Crohn's disease? (Select all that apply.)

_____ Elevated hematocrit

_____ Elevated erythrocyte sedimentation rate (ESR)

_____ Elevated WBC

_____ Elevated folic acid

_____ Elevated serum albumin

2. A client is prescribed prednisone following an exacerbation of IBD. Which of the following client findings is the highest priority?

A. The client is having difficulty sleeping.

B. The client's morning blood glucose is 140 mg/dL.

C. The client reports having a sore throat.

D. The client indicates a gain in weight.

3. A nurse is reinforcing teaching for a client who has a prescription for sulfasalazine (Azulfidine). Which of the following should the nurse include in the teaching?

A. "Take the medication 1 or 2 hr after eating."

B. "Avoid taking the medication if you are allergic to penicillin."

C. 'Notify the provider if you experience a sore throat."

D. "This medication may cause your stools to turn black."

CHAPTER 58: INFLAMMATORY BOWEL DISEASE

 Application Exercises Answer Key

1. A nurse is reviewing the laboratory findings for a client who has an acute exacerbation of Crohn's disease. Which of the following laboratory findings is indicative of Crohn's disease? (Select all that apply.)

	Elevated hematocrit
X	**Elevated erythrocyte sedimentation rate (ESR)**
X	**Elevated WBC**
	Elevated folic acid
	Elevated serum albumin

In Crohn's disease, the ESR and WBC are elevated due to the inflammatory aspects of the disease. The hematocrit is low due to chronic blood loss. Malabsorption leads to a decrease in folic acid and serum albumin.

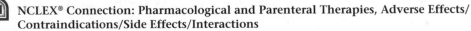 NCLEX® Connection: Physiological Adaptation, Pathophysiology

2. A client is prescribed prednisone following an exacerbation of IBD. Which of the following client findings is the highest priority?

A. The client is having difficulty sleeping.

B. The client's morning blood glucose is 140 mg/dL.

C. The client reports having a sore throat.

D. The client indicates a gain in weight.

The greatest risk to the client taking prednisone is the risk of infection due to immunosuppression. Report of a sore throat may indicate an infection, therefore this is the highest priority finding. Difficulty sleeping, a slightly elevated blood glucose level, and weight gain are important but not the highest priority.

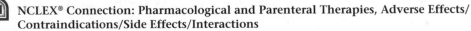 NCLEX® Connection: Pharmacological and Parenteral Therapies, Adverse Effects/Contraindications/Side Effects/Interactions

3. A nurse is reinforcing teaching for a client who has a prescription for sulfasalazine (Azulfidine). Which of the following should the nurse include in the teaching?

   A. "Take the medication 1 or 2 hr after eating."

   B. "Avoid taking the medication if you are allergic to penicillin."

   C. "Notify the provider if you experience a sore throat."

   D. "This medication may cause your stools to turn black."

A client taking sulfasalazine may have a depressed immune system and is more vulnerable to infection. The client should notify the provider of a sore throat. Sulfasalazine should be taken with food and may be contraindicated for clients allergic to sulfa. Sulfasalazine is not contraindicated for clients who have an allergy to penicillin and does not change the color of stools.

Ⓝ NCLEX® Connection: Pharmacological and Parenteral Therapies, Adverse Effects/ Contraindications/Side Effects/Interactions

UNIT 7	NURSING CARE OF CLIENTS WITH GASTROINTESTINAL DISORDERS
Section	Lower Gastrointestinal Disorders
Chapter 59	Colorectal Cancer

Overview

- Colorectal cancer (CRC) is cancer of the rectum or colon. Most CRCs are adenocarcinoma, a tumor that arises from a gland in the epithelial layer of the colon.

- Adenocarcinoma grows slowly and begins as a polyp. If caught early when it is still benign, it can be removed during a colonoscopy. If left untreated, the polyp will grow and the risk of malignancy increases. Many times, the client is asymptomatic but occult blood is discovered in the stool during a rectal exam.

- CRC can metastasize (through blood or lymph) to the liver (most common), lungs, brain, or bones. Spreading can occur as a result of peritoneal seeding (during surgical resection of tumor).

- The most common location of CRC is the rectosigmoidal region.

Health Promotion/Disease Prevention

- CRC can be cured with early detection. Regular colorectal screenings and fecal occult blood tests should be done annually for individuals 50 years of age or older, or earlier and more frequently if there is a family history of CRC.

- Undergo a colonoscopy every 10 years after a baseline colonoscopy. If polyps are found, colonoscopies need to be done more frequently.

- Eat a diet high in fruits, vegetables, and whole grains.

- Decrease the intake of fats and meat proteins.

- Drink alcohol in moderation and stop smoking.

Assessment

- Risk Factors

  - CRC is more common in women, rectal cancer is more common in men
  - Adenomatous colon polyps
  - Family history of CRC
  - Inflammatory Bowel Disease (ulcerative colitis, Crohn's disease)
  - High-fat, low-fiber diet
  - Older than 50 years of age

- Subjective and Objective Data

  - Blood in stool
  - Change in bowel habits (constipation, diarrhea)
  - Cramps and/or gas
    - Palpable mass
    - Weight loss and fatigue
    - Vomiting
    - Abdominal distention
    - Abnormal bowel sounds indicative of obstruction (high-pitched tingling bowel sounds)

  - Laboratory Tests
    - Fecal Occult Blood Test (FOBT) – two stool samples within three consecutive days. False-positive results can occur with the ingestion of some foods or drugs. In general, meat, NSAIDs, and vitamin C are avoided for the 48 hr prior to testing.
    - Carcinoembryonic Antigen (CEA) serum test – CEA levels are elevated in most individuals with CRC.
    - Hct and Hgb decreased due to intermittent bleeding

  - Diagnostic Procedures
    - Sigmoidoscopy/Colonoscopy provides a definitive diagnosis of CRC.
      - This scope procedure permits visualization of tumors, removal of polyps, and tissue biopsy.
    - Barium enemas; CT scans of the abdomen, pelvis, lungs, and liver; chest x-rays; and liver scans may be done to further identify the specific location of cancer and to identify sites of metastases.

Collaborative Care

- Surgical Interventions

    o Colon resection, colectomy, colostomy, and abdominoperineal (AP) resection surgeries may be performed to remove all or portions of CRC.

    o CRC occurs in stages from 0 to IV according to the tissue depth of the lesion, and whether it has spread to local or distant sites.

    o Colectomy (surgical removal of part of the colon) with an end-to-end anastomosis or placement of external stoma is performed

    o An external stoma or colostomy may be temporary or permanent.

- Nursing Actions

    o Provide postoperative care to prevent complications

    o Postoperatively, if the client has a stoma, assess the color and integrity of the stoma (an immediate postoperative stoma should be reddish pink, moist, and may have a small amount of visible blood; report any evidence of stoma ischemia or necrosis).

View Media Supplement: Healthy Stoma (Image)

    o Maintain nasogastric suction (decompression).

    o Slowly progress the diet after suctioning is discontinued and monitor the client's response and bowel sounds.

    o Provide client education regarding activity limits (no lifting or use of stool softeners to avoid straining).

    o Provide ostomy teaching (signs of ischemia to report, expected output, appliance management) if applicable.

    o Support the client who is experiencing disturbed body image.

    o Management of a colostomy may be more difficult with older adult clients because of impaired vision and the need for fine motor skills.

- Client Education

    o Preoperatively

        ▪ Educate the client regarding preoperative diet (clear liquids several days prior to surgery).

        ▪ Instruct the client to complete bowel prep with cathartics as prescribed.

        ▪ Inform the client of the administration of antibiotics (neomycin, metronidazole [Flagyl]) to eradicate intestinal flora.

    o Postoperatively

        ▪ Educate the client regarding the care of the incision, activity limits, and ostomy care, if applicable.

- Interdisciplinary Care

  o Stoma nurse referral for instruction on care of colostomy

  o Referral to ostomy support group

- Therapeutic Procedures

  o Chemotherapy

    ▪ Classification and Therapeutic Intent

      ☐ Adjuvant therapy may be given to decrease the chance of metastases for stage II, and distant metastases for type III cancers.

      ☐ If stage IV cancer is found, chemotherapy is routinely given.

      ☐ Targeted medication therapy – Monoclonal antibodies (MABs)

      ☐ Angiogenesis inhibitors (inhibits growth of new blood vessels to tumors): bevacizumab (Avastin)

      ☐ Tyrosine kinase inhibitors (decreases cell proliferation and increases cell death of certain cancers): cetuximab (Erbitux) and panitumumab (Vectibix)

    ▪ Radiation therapy

      ☐ Radiation therapy is given in conjunction with chemotherapy to improve prognosis (usually used for rectal cancer to prevent lymph node involvement and recurrence).

- Client Outcomes

  o The client will be cancer free without recurrence for 5 years.

  o The client will adapt to bowel redirective surgery (colostomy).

Complications

- Recurrence

  o Causes

    ▪ Recurrence of tumor at surgical or distant site (metastasis)

  o Nursing Actions

    ▪ Support the client with prognosis.

    ▪ Ensure that the client understands treatment options.

CHAPTER 59: COLORECTAL CANCER

 Application Exercises

1. A nurse is caring for an older adult client with colon cancer. The client had the cancer resected and a transverse colostomy established. Which of the following assessment data indicate that the client was at risk for colon cancer? (Select all that apply.)

_____ Family history of CRC

_____ Personal history of Crohn's disease

_____ Consumption of a diet that was low in fat and high in fiber

_____ Age

_____ Gluten intolerance

_____ Caucasian

2. Postoperative care for a client following a colon resection for colorectal cancer includes which of the following? (Select all that apply.)

_____ Report to the provider that the stoma is red in color and has serosanguineous discharge.

_____ Monitor and treat pain, and evaluate pain-relief measures.

_____ Start a full liquid diet upon return to medical unit.

_____ Provide wound care using surgical aseptic technique.

_____ Advise the client to use stool softeners to prevent straining.

3. A nurse is providing education regarding colon cancer to a group of women ranging from 45 to 65 years of age. Which of the following statements by the nurse is appropriate to include?

A. "Colonoscopies for individuals with no family history of cancer should begin at age 45."

B. "Colonoscopies should be routinely done every 5 years on clients who do not have polyps."

C. "Fecal occult blood tests should be done annually at age 50."

D. "Fecal occult blood tests are diagnostic of colon cancer."

CHAPTER 59: COLORECTAL CANCER

 Application Exercises Answer Key

1. A nurse is caring for an older adult client with colon cancer. The client had the cancer resected and a transverse colostomy established. Which of the following assessment data indicate that the client was at risk for colon cancer? (Select all that apply.)

   X   **Family history of CRC**

   X   **Personal history of Crohn's disease**

   _____   Consumption of a diet that was low in fat and high in fiber

   X   **Age**

   _____   Gluten intolerance

   _____   Caucasian

A family history of colorectal cancer, a history of an inflammatory bowel disease (Crohn's), and age over 50 are risk factors for CRC. The consumption of a diet low in fat and high in fiber is protective against CRC, and there is no relationship between gluten intolerance and CRC. African Americans are at an increased risk for CRC, not Caucasians.

 NCLEX® Connection: Reduction of Risk Potential, System-Specific Assessment

2. Postoperative care for a client following a colon resection for colorectal cancer includes which of the following? (Select all that apply.)

   _____   Report to the provider that the stoma is red in color and has serosanguineous discharge.

   X   **Monitor and treat pain, and evaluate pain-relief measures.**

   _____   Start a full liquid diet upon return to medical unit.

   X   **Provide wound care using surgical aseptic technique.**

   X   **Advise the client to use stool softeners to prevent straining.**

Pain should be routinely monitored, treated, and evaluated for treatment efficacy. Surgical aseptic technique should be used for wound care to prevent infection. Straining the stool can put undue stress on the surgical incision and lead to wound dehiscence. The client's stoma should be reddish pink in color, moist, and may have a small amount of serosanguineous drainage during the first few days after surgery. Oral intake should start with ice chips, then clear liquids, and advance as tolerated.

 NCLEX® Connection: Physiological Adaptation, Alterations in Body Systems

3. A nurse is providing education regarding colon cancer to a group of women ranging from 45 to 65 years of age. Which of the following statements by the nurse is appropriate to include?

    A. "Colonoscopies for individuals with no family history of cancer should begin at age 45."

    B. "Colonoscopies should be routinely done every 5 years on clients who do not have polyps."

    C. "Fecal occult blood tests should be done annually at age 50."

    D. "Fecal occult blood tests are diagnostic of colon cancer."

Colonoscopies should begin by at least age 45 for individuals who have a family history of cancer, and at age 50 for those who do not. Colonoscopies should be done every 10 years if polyps are not found. Fecal occult blood tests should be done annually starting at age 50. However, fecal occult blood test are not diagnostic of colon cancer, and a colonoscopy will need to be done to confirm the diagnosis.

Ⓝ **NCLEX® Connection: Reduction of Risk Potential, Diagnostic Tests**

UNIT 7	NURSING CARE OF CLIENTS WITH GASTROINTESTINAL DISORDERS
Section	Gallbladder and Pancreas Disorders
Chapter 60	Cholecystitis and Cholelithiasis

(@) Overview

- Cholecystitis is an inflammation of the gallbladder wall.

- Cholecystitis is most often caused by gallstones (cholelithiasis) obstructing the cystic and/or common bile ducts (bile flow from the gallbladder to the duodenum) causing bile to back up and the gall bladder to become inflamed.

- Cholelithiasis is the presence of stones in the gall bladder related to either the precipitation of bile or cholesterol into stones.

- Bile is used for the digestion of fats. It is produced in the liver and stored in the gall bladder.

- Cholecystitis can be acute or chronic, and can obstruct the pancreatic duct causing pancreatitis. It can also cause the gall bladder to rupture with secondary peritonitis.

Health Promotion and Disease Prevention

- Low-fat diet

- BMI below 30

- Cholesterol below 200 mg/dL

- Lipid profile within expected reference range

Assessment

- Risk Factors

  o More common in females

  o High-fat diet

  o Obesity (impaired fat metabolism, high cholesterol levels)

  o Genetic predisposition

(G) o Older than 60 years of age (more likely to develop gallstones)

- o Individuals who have type 1 diabetes mellitus (high triglycerides)

- o Low-calorie, liquid protein diets

- o Rapid weight loss (increases cholesterol)

- Subjective Data

  - o An episode of cholecystitis is characterized by:

    - Sharp pain in the right upper quadrant of the abdomen, often radiating to the right shoulder.

    - Pain with deep inspiration during right subcostal palpation (Murphy's sign).

    - Intense pain (increased heart rate, pallor, diaphoresis) caused by biliary colic with nausea and vomiting after ingestion of a large quantity of high-fat food.

    - Rebound tenderness.

    - Dyspepsia, eructation (belching), and flatulence.

    - Fever.

- Objective Data

  - o Physical Assessment Findings

    - Jaundice, clay-colored stools, steatorrhea (fatty stools), dark urine, and pruritus (accumulation of bile salts in the skin) may be seen in clients with chronic cholecystitis (due to biliary obstruction).

    - Older adult clients may have diabetes mellitus and have atypical presentations of cholecystitis (absence of pain or fever).

  - o Laboratory Tests

    - White blood cell count (elevations with left shift indicate inflammation)

    - Direct, indirect, and total serum bilirubin (elevated if bile duct obstruction)

    - Amylase and lipase (elevated if pancreatic involvement)

    - Aspartate aminotransferase (AST), lactate dehydrogenase (LDH), and alkaline phosphatase (elevated if liver dysfunction) may indicate the common bile duct is obstructed.

    - Serum cholesterol (elevated above 200 mg/dL)

  - o Diagnostic Procedures

    - A right-upper quadrant (RUQ) ultrasound visualizes gall stones and a dilated common bile duct.

    - An abdominal x-ray or CT scan can visualize calcified gallstones and an enlarged gall bladder.

    - A hepatobiliary scan (HIDA) assesses the patency of the biliary duct system after an IV injection of contrast.

- An endoscopic retrograde cholangiopancreatography (ERCP) allows for direct visualization through the use of an endoscope that is inserted through the esophagus and into the common bile duct via the duodenum. A sphincterotomy with gall stones removal may be done during this procedure.

- A percutaneous transhepatic cholangiography involves the direct injection of contrast into the biliary tract through the use of a flexible needle. The gallbladder and ducts can be visualized.

Collaborative Care

- Nursing Care

    o Administer analgesics as needed and prescribed.

- Medications

    o Meperidine (Demerol) or hydromorphone (Dilaudid) are analgesics that are preferred over morphine, as morphine sulfate may increase biliary spasms.

        - Analgesic and biliary antispasmodic

        - Nursing Considerations

            □ Monitor for seizures in older adults receiving meperidine.

    o Anticholinergics – dicyclomine (Bentyl)

        - Decrease ductal tone and biliary spasms

        - Nursing Considerations

            □ Monitor for constipation, urinary hesitancy/retention.

            □ Monitor for confusion in older adults.

    o Bile Acid – chenodiol (Chenix), ursodiol (Ursodeoxycholic Acid)

        - Bile acid used to gradually dissolve cholesterol-based gall stones

        - Nursing Considerations

            □ Chenodiol – Monitor for excessive diarrhea and hepatotoxicity.

            □ Ursodiol has few side effects.

        - Client Education

            □ Chenodiol – Inform the client that routine liver function tests must be done.

- Therapeutic Procedures

    - Extracorporeal shock wave lithotripsy (ESWL) – Shock waves are used to break up stones. This may be used more on nonsurgical candidates who have small, cholesterol-based stones and are of normal weight.

    - Nursing Actions

        □ Prepare the client for immersion in water (fluid filled bag may be used in place of immersion).

    - Client Education

        □ Inform the client that several procedures may be required to break up all stones.

- Surgical Interventions

    o Cholecystectomy – removal of the gallbladder with a laparoscopic or an open approach.

    o The client is usually discharged within 24 hr if a laparoscopic approach is used. An open approach requires the client to be hospitalized for 2 to 3 days.

        - Nursing Actions

            □ Laparoscopic approach

                ▸ Provide immediate postoperative care.

            □ Open approach

                ▸ A T-tube may be placed in the common bile duct. This is only required when there is exploration of the common bile duct intraoperatively.

                ▸ The use of T-tubes has significantly decreased due to the laparoscopic approach.

            □ Care of the T-tube

                ▸ Monitor and record drainage (initially bloody, then green-brown bile).

                ▸ Initially, the T-tube may drain more than 400 mL/day and then gradually decrease in amount.

                ▸ The client should report an absence of drainage with symptoms of nausea and pain (may indicate obstruction in the T-tube).

                ▸ The client should report sudden increases in drainage or amounts exceeding 1,000 mL/day.

                ▸ Inspect the surrounding skin for signs of infection or bile leakage.

                ▸ Maintain flow by gravity and do not raise above level of gallbladder.

                ▸ Empty the drainage bag every 8 hr.

- ▸ Clamp the tube 1 to 2 hr before and after meals to assess the tolerance to food post cholecystectomy, and prior to removal.

- ▸ Assess stools for color (stools will be clay-colored until biliary flow is reestablished).

- ▸ Monitor for bile peritonitis (pain, fever, jaundice).

- ▸ Monitor and document the client's response to food.

- ■ Client Education

  - □ Laparoscopic approach

    - ▸ Educate the client regarding free air pain following laparoscopic surgery (under the right clavicle, shoulder, scapula), and that ambulation is helpful for this type of pain.

    - ▸ Educate the client regarding pain control and incision care.

    - ▸ Educate the client regarding complications (infection, bile leak [pain, vomiting, abdominal distension]).

    - ▸ Activities are often resumed in 1 week.

  - □ Open approach

    - ▸ Activity precautions for 4 to 6 weeks.

    - ▸ The T-tube is usually left in 1 to 2 weeks postoperatively.

    - ▸ Report sudden increase in drainage, foul odor, pain, fever, or jaundice.

    - ▸ Take showers instead of baths until T-tube is removed.

    - ▸ Clamp 1 to 2 hr before and after meals to prepare for removal.

    - ▸ The color of stools should return to brown in about a week, and diarrhea is common.

- ■ Dietary Counseling

  - □ Encourage a low-fat diet (reduce dairy and avoid fried foods, chocolate, nuts, gravies).

  - □ Promote weight reduction.

  - □ If an obstruction is present, fat-soluble vitamins and bile salts may be prescribed to enhance absorption and aid with digestion.

  - □ Avoid gas-forming foods (beans, cabbage, cauliflower, broccoli).

  - □ Small, frequent meals may be tolerated.

  - □ Prepare for the care of T-tube at home if indicated.

- • Client Outcomes

  - ○ The client will resume a regular diet without experiencing abdominal pain.

Complications

- Obstruction of the bile duct

    o This can cause ischemia, gangrene, and a rupture of the gallbladder wall. A rupture of the gallbladder wall can cause a local abscess or peritonitis (rigid, board-like abdomen, guarding), which requires a surgical intervention and administration of broad spectrum antibiotics.

- Bile peritonitis

    o This can occur if adequate amounts of bile are not drained from the surgical site. This is a rare complication, but it may be fatal.

    o Nursing Actions

        ▪ Monitor the client for pain, fever, and jaundice.

        ▪ Report to the provider immediately.

CHAPTER 60: CHOLECYSTITIS AND CHOLELITHIASIS

Ⓐ Application Exercises

Scenario: A client is admitted with severe upper abdominal pain following a family dinner celebration. She reports frequent belching and is febrile.

1. Which of the following food choices might have triggered a cholecystitis attack? (Select all that apply.)

_____ Ice cream

_____ Brownie with nuts

_____ Fruit salad

_____ Turkey

_____ Broccoli with cheese sauce

_____ Potatoes and gravy

_____ Deviled eggs and mayonnaise

2. Which of the following client laboratory findings indicates a biliary obstruction? (Select all that apply.)

_____ Conjugated (direct) serum bilirubin 0.6 mg/dL

_____ Serum cholesterol 278 mg/dL

_____ Unconjugated (indirect) serum bilirubin 0.4 mg/dL

_____ Total serum bilirubin 1 mg/dL

_____ Yellow sclera

_____ Light-colored bowel movements

_____ Steatorrhea (fatty stools)

_____ Dilute yellow urine

3. A nurse is caring for a client who is post open cholecystectomy with T-tube placement. Which of the following instructions should the nurse include when providing discharge teaching? (Select all that apply.)

_____ Take baths rather than showers.

_____ Clamp T-tube for 1 to 2 hr before and after meals.

_____ Keep the drainage system above the level of the gallbladder.

_____ Avoid heavy lifting and strenuous activity.

_____ Empty drainage bag every 8 hr.

CHAPTER 60: CHOLECYSTITIS AND CHOLELITHIASIS

(A) Application Exercises Answer Key

Scenario: A client is admitted with severe upper abdominal pain following a family dinner celebration. She reports frequent belching and is febrile.

1. Which of the following food choices might have triggered a cholecystitis attack? (Select all that apply.)

X	**Ice cream**
X	**Brownie with nuts**
_____	Fruit salad
_____	Turkey
X	**Broccoli with cheese sauce**
X	**Potatoes and gravy**
X	**Deviled eggs and mayonnaise**

Foods (ice cream, brownies, cheese sauce, gravy, mayonnaise) that are high in fat should be avoided. Fruits and turkey are not high in fat and are usually better tolerated.

(N) **NCLEX® Connection: Basic Care and Comfort, Nutrition and Oral Hydration**

2. Which of the following client laboratory findings indicates a biliary obstruction? (Select all that apply.)

X	**Conjugated (direct) serum bilirubin 0.6 mg/dL**
X	**Serum cholesterol 278 mg/dL**
_____	Unconjugated (indirect) serum bilirubin 0.4 mg/dL
_____	Total serum bilirubin 1 mg/dL
X	**Yellow sclera**
X	**Light-colored bowel movements**
X	**Steatorrhea (fatty stools)**
_____	Dilute yellow urine

An elevated serum bilirubin and cholesterol indicate biliary obstruction. Yellow sclera indicates jaundice secondary to an elevated bilirubin, and light-colored stools indicate bile is not being secreted into the small intestine. Steatorrhea occurs as fat is no longer broken down by bile salts. Serum bilirubin 0.4 mg/dL and total serum bilirubin 1 mg/dL are within the expected reference range. The urine would most likely be dark in color.

(N) **NCLEX® Connection: Physiological Adaptation, Pathophysiology**

3. A nurse is caring for a client who is post open cholecystectomy with T-tube placement. Which of the following instructions should the nurse include when providing discharge teaching? (Select all that apply.)

_____	Take baths rather than showers.
__X__	**Clamp T-tube for 1 to 2 hr before and after meals.**
_____	Keep the drainage system above the level of the gallbladder.
__X__	**Avoid heavy lifting and strenuous activity.**
__X__	**Empty drainage bag every 8 hr.**

The T-tube should be clamped 1 to 2 hr before and after meals to assess tolerance to food post cholecystectomy, and prior to removal. Due to the abdominal incision, the client should avoid heavy lifting to prevent evisceration. The drainage bag attached to the T-tube should be emptied every 8 hr. Soaking in bath water is contraindicated due to the increased risk for introduction of organisms and infection. The drainage system should not be placed above the level of the gallbladder due to the risk of infection from the reflux of drainage from the tube into the wound bed.

Ⓝ NCLEX® Connection: Reduction of Risk Potential, Therapeutic Procedures

UNIT 7	NURSING CARE OF CLIENTS WITH GASTROINTESTINAL DISORDERS
Section	Gallbladder and Pancreas Disorders
Chapter 61	Pancreatitis and Pancreatic Cancer

◎ Overview

- The pancreas's islets of Langerhans secrete insulin and glucagon. The pancreatic tissues secrete digestive enzymes that break down carbohydrates, proteins, and fats.

PANCREATITIS

◎ Overview

- Pancreatitis is an autodigestion of the pancreas from premature activation (before reaching the intestines) of pancreatic digestive enzymes (exact mechanism unknown). It can result in inflammation, necrosis, and hemorrhage.

- Classic signs and symptoms of an acute attack include severe, constant, and knife-like pain (left upper quadrant, mid-epigastric, and/or radiating to the back) that is unrelieved by nausea and vomiting.

- Acute pancreatitis is an inflammation of the pancreas from activated pancreatic enzymes autodigesting the pancreas. Severity varies, but overall mortality is 10% to 20%.

- Chronic pancreatitis is a progressive, destructive disease of the pancreas with the development of calcification and necrosis, possibly resulting in hemorrhagic pancreatitis. Mortality can be as high as 50%.

Health Promotion and Disease Prevention

- Avoid excessive alcohol consumption

- Eat a diet low-fat diet

Assessment

- Risk Factors

  o Two primary causes of pancreatitis are alcoholism and biliary tract disease (gallstones can cause a blockage where the common bile duct and pancreatic duct meet).

  o Pancreatitis is a possible complication of endoscopic retrograde cholangiopancreatography (ERCP).

- o Triggering factors include an intake of large amounts of fat and/or alcohol.

- o The primary cause of chronic pancreatitis is alcoholism. This may occur more often in older adults as age-related changes reduce the ability to physiologically handle alcohol. Gallbladder disease can also cause pancreatitis.

- Subjective Data

  - o Sudden onset of severe, boring pain

    - ■ Epigastric, radiating to back, left flank, or left shoulder

    - ■ Worse when lying down or while eating

    - ■ Not relieved with vomiting

  - o Pain relieved somewhat by fetal position

  - o Nausea and vomiting

  - o Weight loss

- Objective Data

  - o Physical Assessment Findings

    - ■ Seepage of blood-stained exudates into tissue

      - □ Ecchymoses on the flanks (Turner's sign)

      - □ Bluish periumbilical discoloration (Cullen's sign)

View Media Supplement:
- Turner's Sign (Image)
- Cullen's Sign (Image)

    - ■ Generalized jaundice

    - ■ Paralytic ileus

    - ■ Hyperglycemia

    - ■ Ascites

    - ■ Tetany

      - □ Trousseau's sign (hand spasm when blood pressure cuff is inflated)

      - □ Chvostek's sign (facial twitching when facial nerve is tapped)

  - o Laboratory Tests

    - ■ Serum amylase (rises within 12 hr, lasts 4 days) and serum lipase (rises slower but lasts up to 2 weeks).

      - □ Urine amylase remains elevated for up to 2 weeks.

      - □ Rises in enzymes indicate pancreatic cell injury.

□ Memory aid: In pancreatitis, the "ases" (aces) are high.

□ For amylase and lipase to be considered positive, the enzyme rise must be significant (2 to 3 times the normal value for amylase, and 3 to 5 times the normal value for lipase). The degree of enzyme elevation does not directly correlate with the severity of the disease.

- White blood cell count (WBC): Elevated due to infection and inflammation

- Serum calcium and magnesium levels: Decreased due to fat necrosis with pancreatitis

- Serum liver enzymes and bilirubin levels: Elevated with associated biliary dysfunction

- Serum glucose level: Elevated due to a decrease in insulin production from the pancreas.

○ Diagnostic Procedures

- Computed tomography (CT) scan with contrast: Reliably diagnostic of acute pancreatitis

Collaborative Care

- Nursing Care

  ○ Rest the pancreas.

  - NPO – no food until pain free

  - Administer antiemetic as needed

  - Nasogastric tube – gastric decompression

  - Total parenteral nutrition (TPN) or jejunal feedings (less risk of hyperglycemia)

  - When diet is resumed: bland, low-fat diet with no stimulants (caffeine); small, frequent meals

  - No alcohol consumption

  - No smoking

  - Limit stress

  - Pain management

  ○ Position the client for comfort (fetal, side-lying, the head of the bed elevated, sitting up or leaning forward).

  ○ Administer analgesics and other medications as prescribed.

  ○ Monitor blood glucose levels and provide insulin as needed (potential for hyperglycemia).

  ○ Monitor hydration levels (orthostatic blood pressure, intake and output, laboratory values).

  ○ Provide IV fluids and electrolyte replacement as prescribed.

- Medications
    - Opioid analgesics: morphine sulfate (Morphine)
        - Given for acute pain.
        - Nursing Considerations
            - Large doses of intravenous opioids are often needed for pain management.
            - Meperidine (Demerol) is discouraged in older adult clients due to the risk of seizures.
    - Antibiotics: imipenem (Primaxin)
        - Antibiotics may be used, but are generally indicated for clients with acute necrotizing pancreatitis.
        - Nursing Considerations
            - Monitor for signs of infection.
    - Anticholinergics – dicyclomine (Bentyl)
        - This is given to decrease intestinal motility and the flow of pancreatic enzymes.
        - Spasmolytics – papaverine (Pavabid)
            - This medication relaxes smooth muscle.
    - Histamine receptor antagonists – ranitidine (Zantac) and proton pump inhibitors – omeprazole (Prilosec)
        - This is given to decrease gastric acid secretion.
    - Pancreatic enzymes (pancreatin [Donnazyme], pancrelipase [Viokase])
        - This aids with the digestion of fats and proteins when taken with meals and snacks.
- Interdisciplinary Care
    - Dietary referral for post pancreatitis diet and nutritional supplements when oral intake resumed
- Therapeutic Procedures
    - ERCP to create an opening in the sphincter of Oddi if pancreatitis is caused by gallstones
- Surgical Interventions
    - Cholecystectomy if pancreatitis is a result of cholecystitis and gallstones
    - Pancreaticojejunostomy (Roux-en-Y) reroutes drainage of pancreatic secretions into jejunum

- Care After Discharge

  o Home health services may be indicated for clients regarding nutritional needs, possible wound care, and assistance with ADLs.

  o Alcoholics Anonymous (AA) may be indicated for the client or family member who is an alcoholic.

- Client Outcomes

  o The client will be able to tolerate an oral diet without the precipitation of pain or nausea.

  o The client's WBC count and pancreatic enzymes will return to values within the expected reference range.

Complications

- Hypovolemia

  o Causes

    ▪ Up to 6 L can be third-spaced; retroperitoneal loss of protein-rich fluid from proteolytic digestion

  o Nursing Actions

    ▪ Monitor vital signs, electrolytes, and provide IV fluid and electrolyte replacement.

- Chronic pancreatitis

  o Causes

    ▪ Alcohol abuse

  o Client Education

    ▪ Encourage the client to avoid alcohol intake and caffeinated beverages, and to participate in alcoholic support groups.

- Pancreatic Infection: Pseudocyst (outside pancreas); abscess (inside pancreas)

  o Causes

    ▪ Leakage of fluid out of damaged pancreatic duct

  o Nursing Actions

    ▪ Monitor for rupture and hemorrhage.

    ▪ Maintain sump tube if placed for drainage of cyst.

    ▪ Monitor skin around tube for breakdown secondary to corrosive enzymes.

- Type 1 diabetes mellitus

  o Causes

    ▪ Total destruction of the pancreas that regulates insulin produced by the beta cells

- o Nursing Actions
  - Monitor blood glucose closely.
  - Administer insulin as needed.
- o Client Education
  - Inform the client about long-term diabetic management.
- Left lung effusion and atelectasis
  - o Causes
    - Splinting of chest due to pain upon coughing and deep breathing
    - Pancreatic ascites
  - o Nursing Actions
    - Monitor for hypoxia and provide ventilatory support.

- This is a more common complication in older adults and may precipitate pneumonia
- Coagulation defects (disseminated intravascular coagulopathy)
  - o Causes
    - Release of thromboplastic endotoxins secondary to necrotizing hemorrhagic pancreatitis
  - o Nursing Actions
    - Monitor bleeding times.

PANCREATIC CANCER

Overview

- Pancreatic carcinoma has vague symptoms and is usually diagnosed in late stages after liver or gallbladder involvement.
- It has a high mortality rate (less than 20% live longer than 1 year after diagnosis).

Assessment

- Risk Factors
  - o The cause is unknown, but there is a possible inherited risk.
  - o The highest incidence occurs:
    - For people between 60 and 80 years of age.
    - Tobacco use.
  - o Chronic pancreatitis

- o Diabetes mellitus
- Subjective Data
  - o Pain that radiates to the back and is unrelieved by change in position, and is more severe at night
  - o Fatigue
  - o Anorexia
  - o Pruritus
- Objective Data
  - o Physical Assessment Findings
    - ■ Weight loss
    - ■ Palpable abdominal mass
    - ■ Hepatomegaly
    - ■ Jaundice (late sign)
    - ■ Clay colored stools
    - ■ Dark urine
    - ■ Ascites
  - o Laboratory Tests
    - ■ Carcinoembryonic antigen (CEA): Elevated
    - ■ Serum amylase and lipase: Elevated
    - ■ Serum alkaline phosphatase and bilirubin levels: Elevated
  - o Diagnostic Procedures
    - ■ Ultrasound visualization of tumor
    - ■ Computed tomography (CT): visualization of the tumor to determine size, location, and metastases
    - ■ ERCP is the most definitive and allows for the placement of a drain or stent for biliary drainage
    - ■ Abdominal paracentesis can allow testing of abdominal fluid for malignant cells

Collaborative Care

- Nursing Care
  - o Care of a client who has pancreatic cancer usually focuses on palliation and not curative measures
    - ■ Treat pain with opioid analgesics
    - ■ Employ other comfort measures as appropriate

- o Monitor glucose levels and administer insulin as prescribed.
- o Provide nutritional support (enteral supplements, TPN).
- Medications
  - o Opioid analgesics
    - Pain management is the priority intervention. Generally, large doses of opioids (morphine) are given.
    - Nursing Considerations
      - □ Assess the client's level of pain and administer analgesic as prescribed.
      - □ Monitor the client's needs for analgesics frequently.
    - Client Education
      - □ Advise the client to ask for analgesics before the pain becomes severe.
- Interdisciplinary Care
  - o Palliative care
  - o Cancer support group
- Therapeutic Procedures
  - o Chemotherapy may be used to shrink tumor size. Several medications are given to improve the results.
    - Nursing Actions
      - □ Monitor for myelosuppression and pancytopenia.
  - o Radiation may be used to shrink tumor size.
    - Nursing Actions
      - □ Monitor the client for fatigue and diarrhea.
      - □ A biliary stent is needed for the client with a biliary obstruction.
- Surgical Interventions
  - o Partial pancreatectomy – small tumors. This procedure may be done laparoscopically.
  - o Whipple procedure – removal of the head of the pancreas, duodenum, parts of the jejunum and stomach, gallbladder, and possibly the spleen. The pancreatic duct is connected to the common bile duct, and the stomach is connected to the jejunum. This procedure may be done laparoscopically.
    - Nursing Actions (pre, post)
      - □ Provide postoperative care (Refer to Chapter 110: Postoperative).
      - □ Monitor NG tube output and ensure unimpeded drainage from NG and surgical drains. Observe for bloody or bile-tinged drainage which could indicate anastomotic disruption.

- □ Place the client in semi-Fowler's position to facilitate lung expansion and to prevent stress on the suture line.

- □ Provide IV replacement of fluid and blood losses as appropriate.

- □ Assess breath sounds and respirations and facilitate deep breathing. Encourage the use of incentive spirometer and administer oxygen as needed.

- □ Monitor blood glucose and administer insulin as needed.

- ■ Client Education (pre, post)

  - □ Instruct the client to support measures for pain, anorexia, weight loss, and community resources.

- Client Outcomes

  - ○ The client's pain will be managed with analgesics.

  - ○ The client will be able to maintain adequate oral or enteral nutrition.

  - ○ The client and client's family will be able to verbalize a realistic prognosis and related care needs.

Complications

- Fistulas

  - ○ Cause

    - ■ Breakdown of a site of anastomosis

  - ○ Nursing Actions

    - ■ Report drainage that is not serosanguineous from the drain, or drainage from the wound to the provider immediately.

- Peritonitis

  - ○ Cause

    - ■ Internal leakage of corrosive pancreatic fluid

  - ○ Nursing Actions

    - ■ Monitor for signs and symptoms of peritonitis (elevated fever, WBC, abdominal pain, abdominal tenderness/rebound tenderness, alteration in bowel sounds, shoulder tip pain).

    - ■ Provide antibiotics as prescribed.

CHAPTER 61: PANCREATITIS AND PANCREATIC CANCER

(A) Application Exercises

1. Which of the following nursing interventions is appropriate for a client diagnosed with acute pancreatitis? (Select all that apply.)

_____ Drink plenty of fluids.

_____ Avoid alcohol.

_____ Avoid smoking.

_____ Encourage relaxation.

_____ Place the client in a supine position for maximum comfort.

_____ Practice pursed-lip breathing.

2. A client is admitted to the hospital with a diagnosis of acute pancreatitis. Which of the following client assessments should the nurse follow up on first?

A. History of cholelithiasis

B. Serum amylase levels are three times the normal value

C. Reports severe pain radiating to the back that is rated at an "8"

D. Hand spasm present when the nurse is taking the blood pressure

3. A client had a Whipple procedure 3 days ago for pancreatic cancer. Which of the following client assessments should the nurse report to the provider?

A. Bowel sounds are auscultated 10/min and the client is nauseated

B. Wound edges are slightly edematous, reddish, and soft

C. The client reports abdominal pain radiating to the shoulder and the abdomen is rigid

D. WBC 9,000/mm³ and hemoglobin is 10.2 g/dL

CHAPTER 61: PANCREATITIS AND PANCREATIC CANCER

(A) Application Exercises Answer Key

1. Which of the following nursing interventions is appropriate for a client diagnosed with acute pancreatitis? (Select all that apply.)

    _____   Drink plenty of fluids.

    __X__   **Avoid alcohol.**

    __X__   **Avoid smoking.**

    __X__   **Encourage relaxation.**

    _____   Place the client in a supine position for maximum comfort.

    _____   Practice pursed-lip breathing.

The client is initially NPO and fluids are needed by an IV route. Avoiding alcohol and smoking, and encouraging the client to relax are appropriate interventions. Clients are more comfortable with the head of the bed elevated, sitting leaning forward, or laying in a fetal position. Pursed-lip breathing is used to extend the exhalation for air trapping with COPD clients. Clients with pancreatitis are encouraged to deep breathe.

(N) **NCLEX® Connection: Physiological Adaptation, Alterations in Body Systems**

2. A client is admitted to the hospital with a diagnosis of acute pancreatitis. Which of the following client assessments should the nurse follow up on first?

A. History of cholelithiasis

B. Serum amylase levels are three times the normal value

C. Reports severe pain radiating to the back that is rated at an "8"

D. Hand spasm present when the nurse is taking the blood pressure

The greatest risk to the client is hypocalcemia due the risk of cardiac dysrhythmias. Hand spasms that are present when the nurse is taking the blood pressure and Trousseau's sign indicate hypocalcemia and should be followed up on first. History of cholelithiasis, elevated serum amylase, and reports of pain are all important but not the priority.

(N) **NCLEX® Connection: Reduction of Risk Potential, System-Specific Assessment**

3. A client had a Whipple procedure 3 days ago for pancreatic cancer. Which of the following client assessments should the nurse report to the provider?

A. Bowel sounds are auscultated 10/min and the client is nauseated

B. Wound edges are slightly edematous, reddish, and soft

C. The client reports abdominal pain radiating to the shoulder and the abdomen is rigid

D. WBC 9,000/mm³ and hemoglobin is 10.2 g/dL

Abdominal pain and a rigid abdomen are classic signs and symptoms of peritonitis and require further investigation. The bowel sounds are within normal range (5 to 35/min) and would be anticipated to be hypoactive 3 days postoperative along with nausea. Wound edges may show minor inflammation. Slight elevation of WBC is expected after surgery due to inflammation, and hemoglobin may be low due to the malnourished state of the client.

Ⓝ NCLEX® Connection: Reduction of Risk Potential, System-Specific Assessment

UNIT 7	NURSING CARE OF CLIENTS WITH GASTROINTESTINAL DISORDERS
Section	Liver Disorders

Chapter 62   Hepatitis and Cirrhosis

(O) Overview

- Hepatitis is an inflammation of the liver.

- Hepatitis is caused by an infectious organism that enters the body through a chemical (alcohol, medications) or by a toxin (poisonous mushrooms).

- Cirrhosis occurs secondary to the inflammation of the liver, which replace functional liver tissue with fibrotic, scar tissue.

- Cirrhosis is caused by infections (hepatitis, alcohol abuse, inflammatory disorders).

HEPATITIS

(O) Overview

- Hepatitis is an inflammation of the liver.

- Viral hepatitis can be acute or chronic.

- Non-infectious hepatitis may occur secondary to exposure to a chemical or medication.

- There are five major categories of viral hepatitis (hepatitis F and G have been identified but are uncommon).

  o   Hepatitis A virus (HAV)

  o   Hepatitis B virus (HBV)

  o   Hepatitis C virus (HCV)

  o   Hepatitis D virus (HDV)

  o   Hepatitis E virus (HEV)

- All of the hepatitis viruses can cause an acute or short-term illness, and may become a chronic debilitating disease with increasing severity in symptoms over a long period of time. However, hepatitis A rarely results in long-term problems.

- Individuals with hepatitis are carriers and can spread the disease without showing any symptoms.

- People with hepatitis should never donate blood, body organs, or other body tissue.

- It is required to report all cases of hepatitis to the health department.

Health Promotion and Disease Prevention

- Encourage hepatitis prevention activities:

    o Community health educational interventions on transmission and exposure

    o Hepatitis B vaccination prophylaxis for all health care workers

    o Proper use of standard precautions

    o Use of needleless system when delivering medications and parenteral solutions

    o Use of personal protective equipment appropriate to type of exposure (gown, gloves, goggles)

    o Report hepatitis outbreaks to health authorities

- Frequent hand hygiene (before eating, after using the toilet)

- If traveling in underdeveloped countries, drink bottled water and limit sharing of bed linens and eating utensils

Assessment

- Risk Factors

TYPE	ROUTE OF TRANSMISSION	RISK FACTORS
Hepatitis A (HAV)	Oral-fecal route	• Ingestion of contaminated food/water • Daycares and communal living facilities
Hepatitis B (HBV)	Blood	• Drug abuse • Sexual contact • Health care work
Hepatitis C (HCV)	Blood	• Drug abuse • Sexual contact
Hepatitis D (HDV)	Co-infection with HBV	• Drug abuse
Hepatitis E (HEV)	Oral-fecal route	• Ingestion of contaminated water

    o High risk behaviors

        ▪ Percutaneous exposure (dirty needles, sharp instruments, body piercing, tattooing, use of another person's drug paraphernalia or personal hygiene tools)

        ▪ Unprotected sexual intercourse with a hepatitis-infected person, sex with multiple partners, and/or anal sex

- ■ Unscreened blood transfusions (prior to 1992)

- ■ Hemodialysis

- ■ Ingestion of food prepared by a hepatitis-infected person who does not practice proper sanitation precautions

- ■ Travel/residence in underdeveloped country (using tap water to clean food products, drinking contaminated water)

- ■ Eating and/or living in crowded environments (correctional facilities, dormitories, universities, long-term care facilities, military base housing)

- Subjective Data

  - o Influenza-like symptoms

    - ■ Headache

    - ■ Fatigue

    - ■ Arthralgia and myalgia (joint and muscle pain, respectively)

    - ■ Pruritus

- Objective Data

  - o Physical Assessment Findings

    - ■ Low grade fever

    - ■ Right upper quadrant abdominal pain

    - ■ Nausea and vomiting

    - ■ Jaundice

    - ■ Dark urine

  - o Laboratory Tests

    - ■ Enzyme-linked immunosorbent assay (ELISA), or recombinant immunoblot assay (RIBA) may be done if hepatitis C is suspected. Assays confirm the presence of antibodies to hepatitis C.

    - ■ Serum liver enzymes: Elevated

      - □ Alanine aminotransferase (ALT): Elevated (expected reference range – 8 to 20 units/L; 3 to 35 IU/L); most definitive for assessment of liver tissue damage.

      - □ Aspartate aminotransferase (AST): Elevated (expected reference range – 5 to 40 units/L)

      - □ Alkaline phosphatase (ALP): Elevated (expected reference range – 42 to 128 units/L; 30 to 85 IU/L)

- Serum bilirubin: elevated

  □ Bilirubin – direct (conjugated): elevated (expected reference range – 0.1 to 0.3 mg/dL)

  □ Bilirubin – indirect (unconjugated): elevated (expected reference range – 0.2 to 0.8 mg/dL)

  □ Bilirubin – total: elevated (expected reference range – 0.1 to 1.0 mg/dL)

  □ Albumin: decreased (expected reference range – 3.5 to 5 g/dL)

- Serologic markers: Identifies the presence of the virus (HAV, HBsAg and Anti HBc IgM, HCV, HDV, HEV). Serum presence of HBsAg for longer than 6 months indicates chronic hepatitis and/or hepatitis carrier status.

- Hepatitis antibody serum testing related to strain of hepatitis: anti-HAV, HBsAb, anti-HCV, anti-HDV, anti-HEV. Serum presence of HBsAb indicates immunity to HBV following the recovery from hepatitis B, or a successful vaccination.

  o Diagnostic Procedures

    - Abdominal films are used to visualize possible hepatomegaly, ascites, and spleen enlargement.

    - Liver biopsy: This is the most definitive, and is used to identify the intensity of the infection, and the degree of tissue damage.

      □ Nursing Actions

        ▸ Witness informed consent for liver biopsy.

        ▸ Review and explain to the client the biopsy procedure and what is expected following the procedure.

        ▸ Require the client to lie on the affected surgical side for a short period of time after the biopsy has been taken.

        ▸ Monitor the client's blood pressure and heart rate post procedure to detect bleeding.

Collaborative Care

- Nursing Care

  o Most clients will be cared for in the home unless they are acutely ill.

  o Enforce standard and contact precautions to include:

    - A private room or a room with other clients with the same infection.

    - Gloves and gowns worn by the nurses and visitors while in the client's room.

    - The use of disposable equipment or dedicated equipment and disposal of infectious dressing material into a single, nonporous bag without touching the outside of the bag.

  o Distinguish between blood born and GI. Use universal precautions with all, but private room is seldom available and would not be advocated for hepatitis B or C.

- ○ Limit the client's activity (bed rest, rest periods) in order to promote hepatic healing.

- ○ Provide dietary education regarding a high-carbohydrate, high-calorie, low to moderate fat, and low to moderate protein diet, and small, frequent meals to promote nutrition and healing. Food aversion may make this difficult.

- ○ To promote hepatic rest and the regeneration of tissue, only necessary medications are administered. Cautious, if any, use of acetaminophen due to the potential for liver damage.

- ○ Administer interferon as prescribed for HBV and HCV. Monitor clients receiving interferon for side effects of flu-like symptoms, alopecia, and bone marrow suppression. Monitor CBC and administer an antiemetic as needed during interferon therapy.

- ○ Educate the client and family regarding measures to prevent the transmission of the disease with others at home (avoid sexual intercourse until hepatitis antibody testing is negative).

- ○ Provide comfort measures.

- • Medications

  - ○ Immunoglobulin – may be prescribed for household members and sexual partners of clients with hepatitis A. Prophylactic injections may be given to individuals traveling to high-risk countries.

  - ○ Biologic response modifiers (BMRs)

    - ■ Peginterferon alfa-2a (Pegasys) Interferon alfa-2b (Intron-A) – administered to clients with chronic hepatitis B (Intron-A) or C (Pegasys, Intron-A) for several months to induce remission

    - ■ Nursing Considerations

      - □ Note dose – given in millions of units (10 MU [10 million units])

      - □ Monitor for bone marrow suppression and depression.

    - ■ Client Education

      - □ Inform the client of possible flu-like symptoms after each injection

  - ○ Antivirals: lamivudine (Epivir), adefovir (Hepsera) or ribavirin (Rebetol) – may be given for clients with chronic hepatitis B to decrease the incidence of cirrhosis, or clients waiting for a liver transplant. A combination of Peginterferon alfa-2a and ribavirin is used in clients with hepatitis C to attain sustained virologic response (decreased viral load).

    - ■ Nursing Considerations

      - □ Monitor clients taking adefovir for nephrotoxicity.

- Client Education
  - Inform the client that acute exacerbation of hepatitis B may occur if medication is abruptly discontinued.
  - Advise clients taking ribavirin and their sexual partners to not get pregnant while taking this medication.

- Interdisciplinary Care

  - Infection control services may be consulted.

  - Client Education

    - Instruct the client to avoid alcohol and all drugs not prescribed by the provider.

    - Instruct the client to avoid sexual intercourse until tests are negative for hepatitis.

- Client Outcomes

  - The client will recover from hepatitis A without liver damage.

  - The client's viral load of hepatitis B and C will be suppressed.

  - Clients with hepatitis B and C will not experience liver failure.

Complications

- Chronic hepatitis

  - Results from hepatitis B, C, or D.

  - Increases the client's risk for liver cancer

- Fulminating hepatitis

  - This is a fatal form of hepatitis due to the inability of the liver cells to regenerate with the progression of the necrotic process.

  - This disease results in hepatic encephalopathy and death.

  - Nursing Actions

    - Monitor the client for neurological changes, manage fluid and electrolytes, and provide comfort measures.

- Cirrhosis of the liver (See next section in this chapter)

  - Continued episodes of chronic hepatitis result in scarring and permanent injury to the liver, and are a risk factor for liver cancer.

- Liver cancer

- Liver failure

  - Chronic hepatitis, liver abscesses, and fatty liver infiltration all result in changes within the healthy liver and cause irreversible damage.

CIRRHOSIS

 Overview

- Cirrhosis refers to extensive scarring of the liver caused by necrotic injury or a chronic reaction to inflammation over a prolonged period of time. Normal liver tissue is replaced with fibrotic tissue that lacks function.

- Portal and periportal areas of the liver are primarily involved affecting the liver's ability to handle the flow of bile. The development of new bile channels causes an overgrowth of tissue and liver scarring/enlargement. Jaundice is often the result.

Health Promotion and Disease Prevention

- Encourage the client not to drink alcohol and to engage in an alcohol recovery program.

Assessment

- Risk Factors

  - Alcohol abuse

  - Chronic viral hepatitis (hepatitis B, C, or D)

  - Autoimmune hepatitis (destruction of the liver cells by the immune system)

  - Steatohepatitis (fatty liver disease causing chronic inflammation)

  - Damage to the liver caused by drugs, toxins, and other infections

  - Chronic biliary cirrhosis (bile duct obstruction, bile stasis, hepatic fibrosis)

  - Cardiac cirrhosis resulting from severe right heart failure inducing necrosis and fibrosis due to lack of blood flow

  - Obesity

- Subjective Data

  - Fatigue

  - Weight loss, abdominal pain, and distention

  - Pruritus (severe itching of skin)

  - Confusion or difficulty thinking (due to the build-up of waste products in the blood and brain that the liver is unable to get rid of)

  - Personality and mentation changes, emotional lability, euphoria, sometimes depression

- Objective Data

    o Physical Assessment Findings

        ▪ Gastrointestinal bleeding (enlarged veins [varices] develop and burst, causing vomiting and passing of blood in bowel movements)

        ▪ Ascites (bloating or swelling due to fluid build-up in abdomen and legs)

        ▪ Jaundice (yellowing of skin) and icterus (yellowing of the eyes)

        ▪ Petechiae (round, pinpoint, red-purple lesions), ecchymosis (large yellow and purple blue bruises), nose bleeds, hematemesis, melena (decreased synthesis of prothrombin, deteriorating hepatic function)

        ▪ Palmar erythema (redness, warmth of the palms of the hands)

        ▪ Spider angiomas (red lesions vascular in nature with branches radiating on the nose, cheeks, upper thorax, shoulders)

        ▪ Dependent peripheral edema of extremities and sacrum

        ▪ Asterixis (liver flapping tremor) – coarse tremor characterized by rapid, nonrhythmic extension, and flexion of the wrists and fingers

        ▪ Fetor hepaticus (liver breath) – fruity or musty odor

    o Laboratory Tests

        ▪ Serum liver enzymes: elevated initially

            □ Alanine aminotransferase (ALT): expected reference range – 8 to 20 units/L; 3 to 35 IU/L

            □ Aspartate aminotransferase (AST): expected reference range – 5 to 40 units/L

            □ Alkaline phosphatase (ALP): expected reference range – 42 to 128 units/L; 30 to 85 IU/L

            □ ALT and AST are elevated initially due to hepatic inflammation, and return to normal when liver cells are no longer able to create an inflammatory response. ALP increases in cirrhosis due to intrahepatic biliary obstruction.

        ▪ Serum bilirubin: elevated

            □ Bilirubin – direct (conjugated): elevated (expected reference range – 0.1 to 0.3 mg/dL)

            □ Bilirubin – indirect (unconjugated): elevated (expected reference range – 0.2 to 0.8 mg/dL)

            □ Bilirubin – total: elevated (expected reference range – 0.1 to 1.0 mg/dL)

            □ Bilirubin levels are elevated in cirrhosis due to the inability of the liver to excrete bilirubin.

        ▪ Serum proteins and serum albumin (expected reference range 3.5 to 5 g/dL) are lowered due to the lack of hepatic synthesis.

        ▪ Hematological tests: CBC, WBC, and platelets are decreased secondary to anemia.

- PT/INR is prolonged due to decreased synthesis of prothrombin.

- Ammonia levels (expected reference range 15 to 110 mg/dL) rise when hepatocellular injury (cirrhosis) prevents the conversion of ammonia to urea for excretion.

- Serum creatinine levels (expected reference range 0.6 to 1.2 mg/dL) may increase due to deteriorating kidney function which may occur as a result of advanced liver disease.

- Diagnostic Procedures

  - Abdominal films and ultrasonography

    - This is used to visualize possible hepatomegaly, ascites, and spleen enlargement.

  - Liver biopsy (most definitive)

    - A liver biopsy identifies the progression and extent of the cirrhosis.

    - To minimize the risk of hemorrhage, a radiologist may perform the biopsy through the jugular vein, which is threaded to the hepatic vein to obtain tissue for a microscopic evaluation.

    - This is done under fluoroscopy for safety as this procedure can be problematic for cirrhosis clients due to an increased risk for bleeding complications.

    - Nursing Actions

      ‣ Obtain the client's consent for a liver biopsy.

      ‣ Review and explain to the client the biopsy procedure and what is expected following the procedure.

      ‣ Require the client to lie on the affected surgical side for a short period of time following the biopsy.

  - Esophagogastroduodenoscopy (EGD)

    - This is performed under moderate (conscious) sedation to detect the presence of esophageal varices.

Collaborative Care

- Nursing Care

  - Assess/Monitor

    - Respiratory status – Monitor oxygen level. Provide comfort measures by positioning the client to ease respiratory effort (may be compromised by plasma volume excess and ascites). Have the client sit in a chair or elevate the head of the bed to 30°.

    - Skin integrity – Monitor the client closely for skin breakdown. Implement measures to prevent pressure ulcers. Pruritus will cause the client to scratch. Encourage washing with cold water and applying lotion to decrease the itching.

- Vital signs – Monitor the client for signs of fluid volume excess and keep strict intake and output. Restrict fluids and sodium if prescribed and weigh daily.

- Neurological status – Monitor the client for deteriorating mental status and dementia consistent with hepatic encephalopathy. Lactulose may need to be given to aid in excretion of ammonia.

- Nutritional status – Encourage a high caloric, high protein (unless has hepatic encephalopathy) diet and supplemental vitamins (B complex), folic acid, and iron.

- Gastrointestinal status – In the presence of ascites, measure abdominal girth daily. Mark the location of tape for consistency.

- Pain status – Assess the client's pain and administer analgesics and gastrointestinal antispasmodics as needed.

    ○ Observe the client for potential bleeding complications. Give blood transfusions (packed red blood cells, fresh frozen plasma) to replace blood volume and clotting factors as ordered by the provider. Monitor the trends in hemoglobin and hematocrit levels and note coagulation studies (aPTT, PT/INR).

    ○ Provide medications as prescribed.

- Medications

    ○ As the metabolism of most medications is dependent upon a functioning liver, general medications are administered sparingly, especially opioids, sedatives, and barbiturates.

    ○ Diuretics are administered to decrease ascites.

    ○ Proton pump inhibitors and H_2 receptor antagonist are administered to decrease gastric acid secretion and the risk of gastrointestinal bleeding.

    ○ Lactulose is administered to promote ammonia excretion via the stool.

    ○ Neomycin and metronidazole (Flagyl) are administered to remove intestinal bacteria, which produces ammonia.

- Interdisciplinary Care

    ○ A dietary consult may be needed if hepatic encephalopathy requires a low-protein diet.

    ○ Initiate appropriate referrals (social services, Alcoholics Anonymous, Al-Anon).

- Therapeutic Procedures

    ○ Paracentesis

        - Used to relieve ascites.

    ○ Injection sclerotherapy/variceal band ligation

        - The varices are either sclerosed or banded endoscopically.

        - There is a decreased risk of hemorrhage with banding.

- Surgical Interventions

  - Transjugular intrahepatic portosystemic shunt (TIPS)

    - This is done to control ascites and variceal bleeding.

  - Surgical bypass shunting procedures

    - This is a last resort for clients with portal hypertension and esophageal varices. The ascites are shunted from the abdominal cavity to the superior vena cava.

  - Liver transplantation

    - Portions of healthy livers from trauma victims or living donors may be used for transplant.

    - The transplanted liver portion will regenerate and grow in size based on the needs of the body.

    - The client must meet the transplant criteria to be eligible.

    - Nursing Actions (pre, post)

      □ Administer immunosuppressant therapy as ordered to prevent organ rejection.

      □ Protect the client from infection.

      □ Monitor the client for symptoms of organ rejection (jaundice, fever, right upper abdominal pain)

    - Client Education

      □ Clients with severe cardiac and respiratory disease, metastatic malignant liver cancer, and a continued history of alcohol/substance abuse are not candidates for liver transplantation.

  - Client Education

    - Encourage the client abstain from alcohol and engage in alcohol recovery program.

      □ Helps prevent further scarring and fibrosis of liver

      □ Allows healing and regeneration of liver tissue

      □ Prevents irritation of the stomach and esophagus lining

      □ Helps decrease the risk of bleeding

      □ Helps to prevent other life-threatening complications

    - Follow diet guidelines:

      □ High-calorie, moderate-fat diet

      □ Low-sodium diet (if the client has excessive fluid in the peritoneal cavity)

      □ Low-protein (if encephalopathy, elevated ammonia)

      □ Small, frequent, well-balanced nutritional meals

      □ Supplemental vitamin enriched liquids (Ensure, Boost)

         □   Replacement and administration of vitamins due to the inability of the liver to store them

         □   Fluid intake restrictions if serum sodium is low

- Client Outcomes

  o The client's hematocrit and electrolytes will return to their expected reference range.

  o The client will demonstrate orientation to person, place, and time.

  o The client's abdominal girth will demonstrate a decrease in circumference.

Complications

- Portal systemic encephalopathy (PSE)

  o Clients who have a poorly functioning liver are unable to convert ammonia and other waste products to a less toxic form. These products are carried to the brain and cause neurological symptoms. Clients are treated with medications such as lactulose to reduce the ammonia levels in the body via intestinal excretion. Reductions in dietary protein are indicated as ammonia is formed when protein is broken down by intestinal flora.

  o Nursing Actions

    ▪ Administer lactulose as prescribed, and monitor serum ammonia and potassium levels during treatment.

    ▪ Assess for changes in the level of consciousness and orientation.

    ▪ Report asterixis (flapping of the hands) and fetor hepaticus (liver breath) immediately to the provider.

  o Client Education

    ▪ Instruct the client to follow a protein-restricted or vegetable protein diet.

- Esophageal varices

  o Causes

    ▪ Portal hypertension (elevated blood pressure in veins that carry blood from the intestines to the liver) is caused by impaired circulation of blood through the liver. Collateral circulation is subsequently developed creating varices in the upper stomach and esophagus. Varices are fragile and can bleed easily.

  o Nursing Actions

    ▪ Assist with saline lavage (vasoconstriction), esophagogastric balloon tamponade, blood transfusions, ligation and sclerotherapy, and shunts to stop bleeding and reduce the risk for hypovolemic shock.

    ▪ Monitor the client's hemoglobin level and vital signs.

- Acute graft rejection post liver transplantation

  ○ This typically occurs between 4 and 10 days after surgery.

  ○ Symptoms of rejection include:

    ▪ Tachycardia

    ▪ Upper right flank pain

    ▪ Jaundice

    ▪ Laboratory results indicative of liver failure

  ○ Causes

    ▪ Graft versus host disease (GVHD) – recipient's bone marrow creates T-cells to attack the new organ

  ○ Nursing Actions

    ▪ Prevention interventions include the administration of immunosuppressants (cyclosporine [Sandimmune]).

    ▪ The administration of increased doses of immunosuppressants is an appropriate response to rejection symptoms.

    ▪ Monitor for infection (due to immunosuppression) and bleeding (due to the lack of clotting factors being produced by liver).

  ○ Client Education

    ▪ Inform the client of the importance of taking immunosuppressants and monitoring white blood cell count.

    ▪ Instruct the client to report signs of rejection to the provider immediately.

CHAPTER 62: HEPATITIS AND CIRRHOSIS

(A) Application Exercises

Scenario: A client with a history of chronic biliary disease is admitted to the acute care facility with reports of anorexia, vomiting, chronic indigestion, and abdominal pain. The client's liver is enlarged and her abdomen is protruding. The client's liver enzymes are elevated. Based on her history, physical examination, and laboratory values, the client is diagnosed with cirrhosis of the liver.

1. What is the significance and cause of the client's enlarged and protruding abdomen?

2. Why is the client at an increased risk for developing difficulty breathing?

3. Which of the following client findings should alert the nurse that the client has impending hepatic coma?

_____ Inability to state she is in the hospital

_____ Asterixis

_____ Anorexia

_____ Ascites

_____ Fetor hepaticus

4. A client presents to the clinic with an elevated temperature and reports poor appetite and diarrhea for the past 2 weeks that is unrelieved by antidiarrheal medicine. She works at a daycare center with children. Which of the following types of hepatitis should the nurse anticipate is most likely the cause of these symptoms?

   A. Hepatitis A
   B. Hepatitis B
   C. Hepatitis C
   D. Hepatitis E

5. Which of the following laboratory findings is supportive of a diagnosis of hepatitis?

   A. ALT 45 units/L
   B. WBC 7,800/mm³
   C. Total bilirubin 1.0 mg/dL
   D. Albumin 4.9 g/dL

6. The nurse is providing care instruction for a client with hepatitis B and her family. Which of the following information would be appropriate for this client? (Select all that apply.)

_____ Limit physical activity.

_____ Avoid alcohol.

_____ Take acetaminophen for comfort.

_____ Have family members wear masks.

_____ Take supplemental vitamins.

CHAPTER 62: HEPATITIS AND CIRRHOSIS

 Application Exercises Answer Key

Scenario: A client with a history of chronic biliary disease is admitted to the acute care facility with reports of anorexia, vomiting, chronic indigestion, and abdominal pain. The client's liver is enlarged and her abdomen is protruding. The client's liver enzymes are elevated. Based on her history, physical examination, and laboratory values, the client is diagnosed with cirrhosis of the liver.

1. What is the significance and cause of the client's enlarged and protruding abdomen?

The client's large, protruding abdomen is consistent with the ascites that is commonly associated with cirrhosis. Ascites is due to portal hypertension, decreased synthesis of albumin, and an obstruction of hepatic lymph flow.

 NCLEX® Connection: Physiological Adaptation, Pathophysiology

2. Why is the client at an increased risk for developing difficulty breathing?

The client's ascites, if not relieved by paracentesis, will place pressure on her lungs and internal organs, placing her at risk for difficulty breathing.

 NCLEX® Connection: Physiological Adaptation, Pathophysiology

3. Which of the following client findings should alert the nurse that the client has impending hepatic coma?

  __X__   **Inability to state she is in the hospital**
  __X__   **Asterixis**
  _____   Anorexia
  _____   Ascites
  __X__   **Fetor hepaticus**

Impending signs of a hepatic coma are deterioration in neurological status, abnormal flapping of the hands (asterixis), and foul breath (fetor hepaticus). Anorexia and ascites are findings of cirrhosis and may accompany hepatic coma, but may also exist in the absence of hepatic coma.

 NCLEX® Connection: Physiological Adaptation, Medical Emergencies

4. A client presents to the clinic with an elevated temperature and reports poor appetite and diarrhea for the past 2 weeks that is unrelieved by antidiarrheal medicine. She works at a daycare center with children. Which of the following types of hepatitis should the nurse anticipate is most likely the cause of these symptoms?

    A. Hepatitis A

    B. Hepatitis B

    C. Hepatitis C

    D. Hepatitis E

    Because the client works in a daycare center with children, it's most likely she has hepatitis A. HAV usually resolves on its own.

    Ⓝ NCLEX® Connection: Physiological Adaptation, Infectious Disease

5. Which of the following laboratory findings is supportive of a diagnosis of hepatitis?

    A. ALT 45 units/L

    B. WBC 7,800/mm^3

    C. Total bilirubin 1.0 mg/dL

    D. Albumin 4.9 g/dL

    A normal ALT range is 8 to 20 units/L. An ALT (Alanine aminotransferase) level is a definitive serum test for detecting liver damage. Infection usually results in elevations in WBC above 10,000/mm^3. A total bilirubin level of 1.0 mg/dL and an albumin level of 4.9 g/dL are within normal ranges.

    Ⓝ NCLEX® Connection: Reduction of Risk Potential, Laboratory Values

6. The nurse is providing care instruction for a client with hepatitis B and her family. Which of the following information would be appropriate for this client? (Select all that apply.)

      X   **Limit physical activity.**

      X   **Avoid alcohol.**

      _____   Take acetaminophen for comfort.

      _____   Have family members wear masks.

      X   **Take supplemental vitamins.**

    Clients who have hepatitis B should limit physical activity to promote healing. Alcohol should be avoided to prevent further damage to the liver. Clients who have hepatitis B should be encouraged to consume a high-caloric, high-protein diet with supplemental vitamins (B complex), folic acid, and iron. Acetaminophen should be avoided due to the potential for liver damage. Masks are not necessary as hepatitis B is a blood borne pathogen.

    Ⓝ NCLEX® Connection: Physiological Adaptation, Illness Management

UNIT 7	NURSING CARE OF CLIENTS WITH GASTROINTESTINAL DISORDERS
Section	Liver Disorders
Chapter 63	Liver Cancer

 Overview

- Liver cancer or hepatocellular carcinoma (HCC) is the most frequently occurring type of liver cancer. HCC is a primary liver cancer, not metastatic liver cancer.

Health Promotion and Disease Prevention

- Avoid excessive alcohol intake.

- Eat a low-fat diet and maintain a BMI less than 30.

- Receive a hepatitis B vaccination.

- Take precautions against hepatitis B and C (recognize that multiple sexual partners, IV drug use, and the sharing of needles all increase risk).

Assessment

- Risk Factors

  - Cirrhosis

    - Chronic hepatitis B infection

    - Chronic hepatitis C infection

    - Alcoholic liver disease

    - Hemochromatosis (inability to breakdown iron)

  - Male

  - Tobacco use

  - Metastasis from another site

- Subjective Data

  - Abdominal pain

  - Loss of appetite

  - Weakness and fatigue

- Objective Data
  - Physical Assessment Findings
    - Weight loss
    - Enlarged liver on palpation
    - Jaundice
    - Ascites
    - Pruritus
    - Encephalopathy
  - Laboratory Tests
    - Alpha-fetoprotein (AFP), a tumor marker, is elevated in primary liver cancer.
    - The alkaline phosphatase (ALP), serum aspartate aminotransferase (AST), and albumin and bilirubin are elevated in both primary and metastatic cancer.
    - An elevated CEA along with an elevated AFP can be used to discriminate metastatic from primary liver cancer.
    - Prothrombin time predicts the severity of cirrhosis
  - Diagnostic Procedures
    - An ultrasound and computerized tomography can be used to visualize a tumor.
    - A liver biopsy is the most definitive diagnostic procedure and is done through the skin (percutaneously) with a biopsy needle.
      - If there is a risk for hemorrhage, an interventional radiologist can perform the biopsy through the jugular vein to the hepatic vein to obtain tissue for microscopic evaluation.
      - This is done under fluoroscopy.
      - Nursing Actions
        - Obtain coagulation studies as prescribed.
        - Obtain client consent for the liver biopsy.
        - Review and explain to the client the biopsy procedure and what is expected following the procedure.
      - Client Education
        - Instruct the client to lie on the affected side after the biopsy in order for hemostasis to occur.

Collaborative Care

- Nursing Care
  - Observe the client for potential bleeding complications.
    - Give blood transfusions (packed red blood cells and fresh frozen plasma) to replace blood volume and clotting factors as ordered by the provider.
    - Monitor trends in hemoglobin and hematocrit levels.
    - Monitor coagulation studies (aPTT, PT/INR).
  - Encourage the client to follow diet guidelines.
    - High-calorie, moderate fat diet
    - Low-sodium diet (if ascites is present)
    - Low-protein diet (if there is encephalopathy, elevated ammonia)
    - Small, frequent, well-balanced nutritional meals
    - Vitamin-enriched supplements (Ensure, Boost)
    - Replacement and administration of vitamins due to the inability of the liver to store them
    - Restriction of fluid intake (if serum sodium is low)
  - Encourage the client to avoid drinking alcohol as this will:
    - Help prevent further scarring and fibrosis of the liver.
    - Allow healing and regeneration of the liver tissue.
    - Prevent irritation of the stomach and esophagus lining.
    - Help decrease the risk of bleeding.
    - Help to prevent other life-threatening complications.
  - Monitor for:
    - Abdominal discomfort and increase in ascites (measure abdominal girth daily)
    - Anorexia and weight loss
    - Signs of biliary obstruction (jaundice)
    - Pain
    - Fluid and electrolyte status
    - Hepatic function
    - Nutritional status
  - Provide medications as prescribed.
    - As the metabolism of most drugs is dependent upon a functioning liver, medications generally are administered sparingly (especially opioids, sedatives, and barbiturates).

- Medications

  o Systemically delivered chemotherapy has been found to be largely ineffective in treating tumors of the liver or prolonging life. Therefore, more direct delivery methods are used.

  o Hepatic arterial infusion (HAI) is the direct infusion of chemotherapy via a catheter into the tumor. The client may go home with a catheter in place if continuous infusion is desired.

  o Client Education

    ▪ Instruct the client and family to watch for signs of infection of the pump, hepatic toxicity (jaundice, liver functions tests), and immunosuppression (fatigue, decreased WBC).

    ▪ Inform the client of the side effects of chemotherapy.

- Interdisciplinary Care

  o Initiate referrals (social services, hospice, home health, Alcoholics Anonymous).

- Therapeutic Procedures

  o Hepatic artery embolization/chemoembolization: Using a catheter threaded through the femoral artery and up to the liver, particles are injected into the arteries that supply blood to the tumor. If a chemotherapeutic drug is included, this procedure is called chemoembolization.

    ▪ Nursing Actions

      ▫ Monitor the client for bleeding.

  o Radiofrequency ablation involves the use of an electric current that is directly delivered to the tumor via thin needles.

  o Percutaneous alcohol injections involves the direct injection of alcohol into the tumor mass, resulting in cell death.

  o Cryotherapy uses liquid nitrogen injected directly into the tumor to destroy the tumor.

    ▪ Nursing Actions

      ▫ Monitor the client for hypothermia, bile leak, and hemorrhage.

      ▫ Monitor urine for myoglobinuria.

  o External radiation is not generally used as healthy liver tissue does not tolerate high doses of radiation.

- Surgical Interventions

  - Surgical resection: If liver cancer involves only one lobe of the liver, surgical removal may be indicated. A liver-lobe resection can result in a survival rate of up to 5 years.

    - Nursing Actions

      - Support nutritional status.

      - Inform the client about diagnostic tests that will be done to determine if the liver cancer has metastasized (chest x-ray, PET scan, MRI, laparoscopy).

      - Provide preoperative teaching and postoperative care.

      - Monitor the client for hypoglycemia after surgery. This may require dextrose 10% in water.

      - Monitor the client for bleeding and replace fluids and blood as necessary.

  - Liver transplantation: May be an option for clients who have small primary tumors

    - Immunosuppressants that are given after the transplant may increase the risk for recurrence of cancer.

- Client Outcomes

  - The client's tumor will be surgically, chemically, or mechanically removed or demonstrate a decrease in size.

  - The client's appetite and nutritional status will improve.

Complications

- Acute graft rejection post liver transplantation

CHAPTER 63: LIVER CANCER

(A) Application Exercises

Scenario: A client is being evaluated for possible primary hepatocellular carcinoma. The client is slightly jaundiced and has been experiencing nausea, anorexia, and abdominal pain. The client's provider has discovered a small abdominal mass in the right upper quadrant. The client's serum sodium level is 140 mEq/L and ammonia level is 40 mg/dL. There is no evidence of hepatic encephalopathy or ascites at this time.

1. When the nurse reviews the client's chart, which of the following laboratory findings support the diagnosis of primary liver cancer? (Select all that apply.)

_____ Elevated alpha-fetoprotein (AFP)

_____ Alkaline phosphatase (ALP) 189 units/L

_____ Hemoglobin 14 g/dL

_____ Serum total bilirubin 1.0 mg/dL

_____ Decreased albumin 3.5g/dL

2. Which of the following dietary modifications should the nurse include in the client's plan of care? (Select all that apply.)

_____ High-calorie, moderate fat diet

_____ Low-sodium diet

_____ Low-protein diet

_____ Small, frequent, well-balanced nutritional meals

_____ Supplemental vitamin-enriched liquids

_____ Replacement and administration of vitamins

_____ Fluid restriction

3. A nurse is caring for a client who had a lobe of the liver removed due to liver cancer. Which of the following should the nurse monitor postoperatively?

A. Urine specific gravity

B. Amylase

C. Blood glucose

D. D-dimer

CHAPTER 63: LIVER CANCER

 Application Exercises Answer Key

Scenario: A client is being evaluated for possible primary hepatocellular carcinoma. The client is slightly jaundiced and has been experiencing nausea, anorexia, and abdominal pain. The client's provider has discovered a small abdominal mass in the right upper quadrant. The client's serum sodium level is 140 mEq/L and ammonia level is 40 mg/dL. There is no evidence of hepatic encephalopathy or ascites at this time.

1. When the nurse reviews the client's chart, which of the following laboratory findings support the diagnosis of primary liver cancer? (Select all that apply.)

    X   **Elevated alpha-fetoprotein (AFP)**

    X   **Alkaline phosphatase (ALP) 189 units/L**

    _____   Hemoglobin 14 g/dL

    _____   Serum total bilirubin 1.0 mg/dL

    _____   Decreased albumin 3.5g/dL

AFP and ALP are elevated in a client who has liver cancer. The hemoglobin, and serum total bilirubin levels are within the expected reference range. The albumin level is low, but within the expected reference range. This level would be increased in a client with liver cancer.

 NCLEX® Connection: Reduction of Risk Potential, Laboratory Values

2. Which of the following dietary modifications should the nurse include in the client's plan of care? (Select all that apply.)

    X   **High-calorie, moderate fat diet**

    _____   Low-sodium diet

    _____   Low-protein diet

    X   **Small, frequent, well-balanced nutritional meals**

    X   **Supplemental vitamin-enriched liquids**

    X   **Replacement and administration of vitamins**

    _____   Fluid restriction

The client's sodium level is within the expected reference range and there is no evidence of ascites at this time, therefore a low-sodium diet and fluid restriction is not necessary. The client's ammonia level is normal and there is no evidence of hepatic encephalopathy, therefore a low-protein diet is not indicated.

 NCLEX® Connection: Basic Care and Comfort, Nutrition and Oral Hydration

3. A nurse is caring for a client who had a lobe of the liver removed due to liver cancer. Which of the following should the nurse monitor postoperatively?

    A. Urine specific gravity

    B. Amylase

    C. Blood glucose

    D. D-dimer

The client's blood glucose should be closely monitored due decreased gluconeogenesis during the first 48 hr. Changes in the client's urine specific gravity, amylase, and D-dimer are not expected.

NCLEX® Connection: Reduction of Risk Potential, Potential for Complications of Diagnostic Tests/Treatments/Procedures

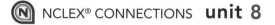

UNIT 8: NURSING CARE OF CLIENTS WITH RENAL DISORDERS

- Diagnostic and Therapeutic Procedures
- Renal System Disorders

NCLEX® CONNECTIONS

When reviewing the chapters in this unit, keep in mind the relevant sections of the NCLEX® outline, in particular:

CLIENT NEEDS: BASIC CARE AND COMFORT

Relevant topics/tasks include:
- Elimination
  - Use alternative methods to promote voiding.
- Nonpharmacological Comfort Interventions
  - Assess the client's need for pain management and intervene as needed using non-pharmacological comfort measures.
- Nutrition and Oral Hydration
  - Provide/maintain special diets based on the client's diagnosis/nutritional needs and cultural considerations.

CLIENT NEEDS: REDUCTION OF RISK POTENTIAL

Relevant topics/tasks include:
- Diagnostic Tests
  - Apply knowledge of related nursing procedures and psychomotor skills when caring for clients undergoing diagnostic testing.
- Laboratory Values
  - Educate the client about the purpose and procedure of prescribed laboratory tests.
- Potential for Complications of Diagnostic Tests/Treatments/Procedures
  - Intervene to manage potential circulatory complications.

CLIENT NEEDS: PHYSIOLOGICAL ADAPTATION

Relevant topics/tasks include:
- Alterations in Body Systems
  - Perform and manage care of the client receiving peritoneal dialysis.
- Hemodynamics
  - Manage the care of a client receiving hemodialysis.
- Unexpected Response to Therapies
  - Promote the recovery of the client from unexpected responses to therapy.

UNIT 8	NURSING CARE OF CLIENTS WITH RENAL DISORDERS
Section	Diagnostic and Therapeutic Procedures
Chapter 64	**Renal Diagnostic Procedures**

Overview

- Renal assessment and diagnostic procedures are used to evaluate kidney function by testing indicators such as an intravenous (IV) bolus, CT scan or magnetic resonance imaging (MRI). By testing the kidney function, diagnosis of disease and efficacy of treatment can be determined.

- Renal diagnostic procedures that nurses should be knowledgeable about include:

  o   Radiography (x-ray)

  o   CT scan

  o   MRI

  o   IV bolus

  o   Voiding cystourethrography (VCUG)

  o   Excretory urography

  o   Renal biopsy

  o   Cystoscopy

  o   Renal scan

  o   Ultrasound

Procedures

TEST	PURPOSE	NURSING INTERVENTIONS
Radiography	• An x-ray of the kidneys, ureters, and bladder (KUB) (may also be prescribed as a "flat plate") • Allows for visualization of these structures	• Ask a female client if she is pregnant. Inform client that clothes over the area will need to be removed as well as all jewelry and medallions • IV contrast dye (iodine-based) may be used to enhance images. Determine the client's allergy to iodine. Dye can cause renal failure. Always check the client's creatinine levels. Parenteral fluid can be given for prevention
CT scan	Provides cross-sectional images of the kidney to assess the size of the kidney and to assess for obstruction, cysts, or masses on the kidney	• Same as KUB
MRI	Useful in staging cancer, similar to CT	• The client will lie down and have to remain still for test
IV bolus	Used to detect renal stones and location, as well as assess renal function	• Not to be done during pregnancy • Relieving bowels produces better images • IV bolus contrast dye (iodine based) may be used to enhance images. Determine the client's allergy to iodine. Dye can cause renal failure
VCUG	Used to outline the bladder's shape and to detect urinary reflux	• This process can increase the risk of an infection. Monitor the client for infection for the first 72 hr after the procedure
Excretory urography	Used to detect obstruction, assess for a parenchymal mass, and assess size of the kidney	• Same as KUB
Renal biopsy	Removal of a sample of tissue by excision or needle aspiration for cytological (histological) examination	• The client receives sedation and is monitored for this procedure. • The client must lie on back postoperatively for 6 hr to prevent bleeding. Check for signs of bleeding and infection

TEST	PURPOSE	NURSING INTERVENTIONS
Cystoscopy	Used to discover abnormalities of the bladder wall and/or occlusions of the ureter or urethra	• The client is given anesthesia for the procedure. • Check for signs of bleeding and infection. Monitor the client for infection for the first 72 hr after the procedure
Renal scan	Used to assess renal blood flow and function	• 48 hr prior to the procedure, ACE inhibitors should not be given. • Medications can be given during the test. Watch for hypotension and make sure the client is well hydrated
Ultrasound	Used to assess the size of kidney or for an obstruction in the lower urinary tract	• Minimal risk for the client. Good option if not able to do the excretory urography

- Complications

  - Bleeding

    - Bleeding can result from some of the above tests noted and should be monitored closely.

    - Nursing Actions

      - If bleeding does occur, notify the provider immediately.

  - Hematuria

    - Blood in the urine is one of the most common complications with a renal biopsy.

    - Nursing Actions

      - Monitor the client's urinary output closely. Note the color and amount. If bright red blood or clots are observed, notify the provider immediately.

  - Renal failure

    - Using contrast dye can place the client at risk for renal failure.

    - Nursing Actions

      - Always check the client's creatinine level prior to the procedure.

      - Parenteral fluid can be given for prevention of renal failure if needed.

  - Infection

    - Infection can be a result of some of the above tests noted and needs to be monitored for the first 48 to 72 hr after the procedure.

    - Nursing Actions

      - Notify the provider if the client has a temperature, is unable to void, or reports pain.

CHAPTER 64: RENAL DIAGNOSTIC PROCEDURES

(A) Application Exercises

1. A nurse is caring for a client undergoing a KUB, an x-ray of the kidneys, ureters, and bladder. Which of the following should the nurse include in the teaching?

    A. "This test will take most of the day."

    B. "You may experience some discomfort during the test."

    C. "You will be in the prone position for the test."

    D. "This test will determine if you have a kidney stone."

2. A nurse is caring for a client who has just had a renal biopsy. Which of the following complications is the most immediate risk to the client?

    A. Infection

    B. Bleeding

    C. Hematuria

    D. Renal failure

CHAPTER 64: RENAL DIAGNOSTIC PROCEDURES

 Application Exercises Answer Key

1. A nurse is caring for a client undergoing a KUB, an x-ray of the kidneys, ureters, and bladder. Which of the following should the nurse include in the teaching?

>   A. "This is a specific test and will take most of the day."
>
>   B. "You may experience some discomfort during the test."
>
>   C. "You will be in the prone position for the test."
>
>   **D. "This test will determine if you have a kidney stone."**

>   **A KUB can identify kidney stones and other abnormalities, such as shape, strictures, or obstructions. This test is very brief unless a contrast dye is used, in which case the client will be monitored for side effects. There is no discomfort experienced during this test and the client should be positioned supine.**

 NCLEX® Connection: Reduction of Risk Potential, Therapeutic Procedures

2. A nurse is caring for a client who has just had a renal biopsy. Which of the following complications is the most immediate risk to the client?

>   A. Infection
>
>   **B. Bleeding**
>
>   C. Hematuria
>
>   D. Renal failure

>   **The most immediate risk to the client is bleeding into the muscle or the kidney due to the invasiveness of the procedure. Infection, hematuria and renal failure may be complications, but may not develop immediately.**

 NCLEX® Connection: Reduction of Risk Potential, Potential for Complications of Diagnostic Tests/Treatments/Procedures

UNIT 8	NURSING CARE OF CLIENTS WITH RENAL DISORDERS
Section	Diagnostic and Therapeutic Procedures
Chapter 65	Hemodialysis and Peritoneal Dialysis

@ Overview

- Functions of dialysis

  o Rids the body of excess fluid and electrolytes.

  o Achieves acid-base balance.

  o Eliminates waste products.

  o Restores internal homeostasis by osmosis, diffusion, and ultrafiltration.

- Dialysis can sustain life for clients who have both acute and chronic renal failure.

- Dialysis does not replace the hormonal functions of the kidneys.

- The two types of dialysis are hemodialysis and peritoneal dialysis.

Hemodialysis

- Hemodialysis shunts the client's blood from the body through a dialyzer and back into circulation. Vascular access is needed for hemodialysis.

- Indications

  o Diagnoses

    ▪ Renal insufficiency

    ▪ Acute renal failure

    ▪ Chronic renal failure

    ▪ Drug overdose

    ▪ Persistent hyperkalemia

    ▪ Hypervolemia unresponsive to diuretics

  o Client Presentation

    ▪ Subjective data

      □ Fatigue, numbness and tingling of extremities, shortness of breath, anorexia, and dry itchy skin

- ■ Objective data

    - □ Lethargy, decreased attention span, seizures, tremors, hypertension, heart failure (edema of hands and feet, dyspnea, distended jugular veins), anemia, vomiting, pulmonary edema, cardiac dysrhythmias, pallor, bruising, halitosis, diminished or dark-colored urine

- Client Outcomes

    - o The client will achieve and maintain a desired fluid and electrolyte balance, be free of infection, and maintain an active lifestyle with minimum restrictions.

- Preprocedure

    - o Nursing Actions

        - ■ Assess patency of the access site (presence of bruit, palpable thrill, distal pulses, and circulation).

        - ■ Avoid taking blood pressure, administering injections, performing venipunctures or inserting IV lines on an arm with an access site. Elevate the extremity following surgical development of AV fistula to reduce swelling.

        - ■ Assess vital signs, laboratory values (BUN, serum creatinine, electrolytes, Hct), and weight.

        - ■ Discuss with the primary care provider any medications that need to be withheld until after dialysis. Dialyzable medications and medications that lower blood pressure are usually withheld.

    - o Client Education

        - ■ The client should be instructed about the procedure. Advise the client that hemodialysis is usually done three times per week, for 3 to 5 hr sessions. Two needles are inserted, one into an artery and the other into a vein.

        - ■ Instruct the client to notify the nurse of muscle cramps, headache, nausea, or dizziness that occurs during the procedure.

- Intraprocedure

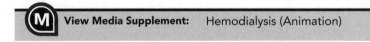

View Media Supplement: Hemodialysis (Animation)

    - o Nursing Actions

        - ■ Monitor vital signs and laboratory values during dialysis. Monitor for bleeding, such as oozing from insertion site. Monitor coagulation studies.

        - ■ Administer anticoagulants as prescribed.

        - ■ Have protamine sulfate ready to reverse heparin, if needed.

        - ■ Provide emotional support. Offer activities, such as books, magazines, music, cards, or television, to occupy the client.

- Postprocedure

  - Nursing Actions

    - Monitor vital signs, laboratory values (BUN, serum creatinine, electrolytes, Hct), and weight. Decreases in blood pressure, weight, and laboratory values are expected following dialysis.

    - Assess for:

      □ Complications (hypotension, clotting of vascular access, headache, muscle cramps, bleeding, disequilibrium syndrome)

      □ Indications of bleeding, and/or infection at the access site

      □ Nausea, vomiting, and change in level of consciousness

      □ Signs of hypovolemia

    - Avoid invasive procedures for 4 to 6 hr after dialysis due to the risk of bleeding related to an anticoagulant.

  - Client Education

    - Teach the client to:

      □ Avoid lifting heavy objects with access-site arm.

      □ Avoid carrying objects that compress the extremity.

      □ Avoid sleeping on top of the extremity with the access device.

      □ Perform hand exercises that promote fistula maturation.

      □ Check the access site at intervals following dialysis. Apply light pressure if bleeding. Notify the provider if the site continues to bleed after 30 min following dialysis.

- Complications

  - Clotting/infection of access site

    - Anticoagulants are often given to prevent blood clots from forming. Infections of the access site are likely introduced during cannulation.

      □ Advanced age is a risk factor for access site complications related to chronic illnesses and/or fragile veins.

    - Nursing Actions

      □ Use surgical aseptic technique during cannulation.

      □ Avoid compression of access site and venipuncture or blood pressure on extremity with access site.

      □ Administer anticoagulants as prescribed.

      □ Assess graft site for palpable thrill or audible bruit indicating vascular flow.

      □ Assess the access site for redness, swelling, or drainage. Monitor for fever.

- Client Education

  - Instruct the client to monitor the access site for signs of an infection such as fever, redness, drainage or swelling.

  - Teach the client to check the graft for patency by checking for thrill or bruit. Advise client to contact the primary care provider for absence of thrill/bruit and for signs of infection.

  - Advise the client to prevent any constriction of extremity with the vascular access.

- Disequilibrium syndrome

  - Disequilibrium syndrome is caused by too rapid a decrease of BUN and circulating fluid volume. It may result in cerebral edema and increased ICP.

    - Early recognition of disequilibrium syndrome is essential. Signs include nausea, vomiting, change in level of consciousness, seizures, and agitation.

    - Advanced age is a risk factor for dialysis disequilibrium and hypotension due to rapid changes in fluid and electrolyte status.

  - Nursing Actions

    - Use a slow dialysis exchange rate, especially for older adult clients and those being treated with hemodialysis for the first time.

    - Administer anticonvulsants/barbiturates if needed.

  - Client Education

    - Advise the client to alert the nurse of early signs of disequilibrium syndrome, such as nausea and headache.

- Hypotension

  - Rapid fluid depletion during dialysis may cause hypotension. Other causes include antihypertensives and splanchnic vasodilation due to food ingestion during dialysis.

  - Nursing Actions

    - Carefully replace fluid volume with transfusion of intravenous fluids or colloid as prescribed. Slow the dialysis exchange rate.

    - Lower the head of the client's bed.

    - For severe hypotension that is unresponsive to fluid replacement, discontinue the dialysis.

  - Client Education

    - Advise the client to notify the nurse of headache, nausea, or dizziness during dialysis. Advise the client not to eat during dialysis.

- Anemia

  - Blood loss and removal of folate during dialysis may contribute to an existing anemia that often occurs with chronic renal failure (caused by decreased RBC production due to decreased erythropoietin secretion).

- Nursing Actions

  - Administer prescribed medication therapy (erythropoietin) to stimulate the production of red blood cells.

  - Monitor Hgb and RBC level.

  - Monitor for hypotension and tachycardia.

  - Transfuse blood products if prescribed.

- Client Education

  - Advise the client to take medications and supplements as prescribed.

  - Educate the client about diet and nutrition, including foods high in folate (beans, green vegetables).

- Infectious Diseases

  - Blood transfusions and frequent blood access due to hemodialysis pose a risk for transmission of bloodborne diseases such as HIV and hepatitis B and C.

  - Nursing Actions

    - Maintain sterility of equipment.

    - Use standard precautions.

    - Administer medications, especially erythropoietin, as prescribed.

  - Client Education

    - Advise the client to take medications and supplements as prescribed.

    - Educate the client about diet and nutrition, including foods high in folate (beans, green vegetables).

Peritoneal Dialysis

- Peritoneal dialysis involves instillation of fluid into the peritoneal cavity. The peritoneum serves as the filtration membrane.

  - The client should have an intact peritoneal membrane, without adhesions from infection or multiple surgeries.

- Indications

  - Peritoneal dialysis is indicated for clients requiring dialysis who:

    - Are unable to tolerate anticoagulation.

    - Have difficulty with vascular access.

- Client Outcomes

  - The client will achieve and maintain a desired fluid and electrolyte balance, be free of infection, and maintain an active lifestyle with minimum restrictions.

- Preprocedure

  - Nursing Actions

    - Assess dry weight (obtained when dialysate is drained), serum electrolytes, creatinine, BUN, and blood glucose.

    - Determine the client's ability to perform self-peritoneal dialysis.

  - Client Education

    - The client should be instructed about the procedure. The client may feel fullness when the dialysate is dwelling. There may be discomfort initially with dialysate infusion.

    - Continuous ambulatory peritoneal dialysis (CAPD) is usually is done 7 days a week for 4 to 8 hr. Clients may continue normal activities during CAPD.

- Intraprocedure

  (M) View Media Supplement: Peritoneal Dialysis (Animation)

  - Nursing Actions

    - Monitor the client's vital signs frequently during initial dialysis of clients in a hospital setting.

    - Monitor the client's serum glucose level.

    - Record the amount of inflow compared to outflow of dialysate.

    - Monitor the color (clear, light yellow is expected) and amount (expected to equal or exceed amount of dialysate inflow) of outflow.

    - Monitor for signs of infection (fever; bloody, cloudy, or frothy dialysate return; drainage at access site) and for complications (respiratory distress, abdominal pain, insufficient outflow, discolored outflow).

    - Check the access site dressing for wetness (risk of dialysate leakage).

    - Warm the dialysate prior to instilling. Avoid the use of microwaves, which cause uneven heating.

    - Follow prescribed times for infusion, dwell, and outflow.

    - Maintain surgical asepsis of the catheter insertion site and when accessing the catheter.

    - Keep the outflow bag lower than the client's abdomen (drain by gravity, prevent reflux).

    - Reposition the client if inflow or outflow is inadequate.

    - Carefully milk peritoneal dialysis catheter if fibrin clot has formed.

    - Provide emotional support to the client and family.

- Postprocedure

  - Nursing Actions

    - Monitor weight, serum electrolytes, creatinine, BUN, and blood glucose.

  - Client Education

    - Teach the client home care of the access site.

      □ Instruct the client and family how to perform peritoneal dialysis exchanges at home. Provide support for home peritoneal dialysis with home visits and support groups, such as the National Kidney Foundation. Instruct the client to follow instructions carefully and to take all medications as directed.

      □ Older adult clients may be unable to care for a peritoneal access site due to cognitive or physical deficits.

- Complications

  - Peritonitis

    - Peritoneal dialysis can allow micro-organisms into the peritoneum and cause peritonitis.

    - Nursing Actions

      □ Maintain surgical asepsis during the procedure.

      □ Monitor for infection, such as fever, purulent drainage, redness or swelling and cloudy or discolored drained dialysate.

    - Client Education

      □ Educate the client to use strict sterile technique during exchanges.

      □ Instruct the client to notify the provider with any sign of infection.

  - Infection at the access site

    - Infection at the access site may be related to leakage of dialysate. Access site infections may cause peritonitis.

      □ Advanced age is a risk factor for access site complications related to chronic illnesses and/or fragile veins.

    - Nursing Actions

      □ Maintain surgical asepsis of access site.

      □ Assess site for wetness from a leaking catheter.

      □ Monitor for infection, such as fever, purulent drainage, redness or swelling.

    - Client Education

      □ Educate the client to use strict sterile technique during exchanges.

      □ Instruct the client to notify the provider with any sign of infection.

      □ Advise the client to assess the site for leaks and prevent tugging or twisting of tubing.

- ○ Protein Loss

  - Peritoneal dialysis may remove needed protein from the blood as well as excess fluid, wastes, and electrolytes.

  - Nursing Actions

    - □ Increase dietary intake of protein.

    - □ Monitor serum albumin level.

  - Client Education

    - □ Instruct the client to follow recommended renal diet with an increase in dietary protein.

- ○ Hyperglycemia

  - Hyperglycemia can result due to the hyperosmolarity of the dialysate.

    - □ Glucose may be absorbed from the dialysate into the blood.

    - □ Hyperlipidemia may also occur.

  - Nursing Actions

    - □ Monitor serum glucose.

    - □ Administer insulin for glycemic control.

    - □ Provide lipid therapy for triglyceride control.

  - Client Education

    - □ Instruct the client to check serum glucose.

    - □ Instruct the client to follow a recommended diet.

- ○ Poor dialysate inflow or outflow

  - The tubing may become obstructed or twisted, causing a decrease in flow.

  - Nursing Actions

    - □ Reposition the client if inflow or outflow is inadequate.

    - □ Milk tubing to break up fibrin clot.

    - □ Check tubing for kinks or closed clamps.

    - □ Tell the client to avoid constipation by using stool softeners and consuming a diet high in fiber.

  - Client Education

    - □ Advise the client to check the tubing for kinks, and instruct him how to remove a fibrin clot.

    - □ Remind the client to monitor the in and out flow and to change position or lower or raise the dialysate bag as needed to improve flow.

    - □ Prevent constipation with diet and stool softeners, if needed.

CHAPTER 65: HEMODIALYSIS AND PERITONEAL DIALYSIS

(A) Application Exercises

1. One goal of renal dialysis for a client who has chronic renal failure is to

    A. restore kidney function.

    B. replace hormonal function of the kidneys.

    C. allow the client to have an unrestricted diet.

    D. balance serum electrolytes.

2. Which of the following actions should the nurse take immediately prior to initiating hemodialysis? (Select all that apply.)

    _____ Determine current medications being taken by the client.

    _____ Assess AV fistula for bruit.

    _____ Calculate total urine output for the previous shift.

    _____ Assess dietary intake.

    _____ Obtain weight.

    _____ Check serum electrolytes.

    _____ Obtain vital signs.

3. Which of the following actions should a nurse implement following a client's hemodialysis procedure? (Select all that apply.)

    _____ Check BUN and serum creatinine.

    _____ Assess for headache and/or confusion.

    _____ Obtain weight.

    _____ Administer IV antibiotic.

    _____ Obtain serum electrolytes.

    _____ Assess access site for indications of bleeding.

    _____ Evaluate blood pressure on side of AV fistula.

4. A client who has polycystic kidney disease is admitted to the acute care facility with reports of fever and flu-like symptoms. The client is scheduled to receive hemodialysis in 1 hr. His vital signs are: temperature 38.3° C (101° F) orally, pulse 90/min, respirations 26/min, and blood pressure 160/90 mm Hg. Does the client's current health status contraindicate the scheduled hemodialysis?

CHAPTER 65: HEMODIALYSIS AND PERITONEAL DIALYSIS

 Application Exercises Answer Key

1. One goal of renal dialysis for a client who has chronic renal failure is to

A. restore kidney function.

B. replace hormonal function of the kidneys.

C. allow the client to have an unrestricted diet.

D. balance serum electrolytes.

Renal dialysis removes excess fluids, electrolytes, waste products, and restores acid-base balance. Dialysis does sustain the life of clients with renal failure, but it does not or restore kidney function, nor replace hormonal functions, which are permanently lost. Medications such as erythropoietin can be given to stimulate the production of red blood cells, a hormonal function that is lost with renal failure. Clients who have chronic renal failure and are receiving dialysis need to restrict fluid intake, and maintain a diet that is often high protein and low in sodium, potassium, and phosphorus.

NCLEX® Connection: Physiological Adaptation, Alterations in Body Systems

2. Which of the following actions should the nurse take immediately prior to initiating hemodialysis? (Select all that apply.)

X	**Determine current medications being taken by the client.**
X	**Assess AV fistula for bruit.**
_____	Calculate total urine output for the previous shift.
_____	Assess dietary intake.
X	**Obtain weight.**
X	**Check serum electrolytes.**
X	**Obtain vital signs.**

Prior to hemodialysis, the nurse should evaluate the client's current medications and determine which medications should be held until after dialysis. It is also important to check the AV fistula and obtain pre-dialysis vital signs, weight, and serum electrolytes. The client's total urine output and dietary intake is not needed immediately prior to hemodialysis.

NCLEX® Connection: Physiological Adaptation, Illness Management

3. Which of the following actions should a nurse implement following a client's hemodialysis procedure? (Select all that apply.)

   __X__   **Check BUN and serum creatinine.**

   __X__   **Assess for headache and/or confusion.**

   __X__   **Obtain weight.**

   _____   Administer IV antibiotic.

   __X__   **Obtain serum electrolytes.**

   __X__   **Assess access site for indications of bleeding.**

   _____   Evaluate blood pressure on side of AV fistula.

Following hemodialysis, the nurse should check laboratory results including BUN, creatinine, and electrolytes. The client should be weighed and assessed for nausea, headache, or confusion. Often, the client is hypotensive following dialysis. Use caution when standing the client, in case of orthostatic hypotension. Monitor the AV access site for bleeding for 1 hr following dialysis. There is no indication to administer an antibiotic. Do not take blood pressure, administer injections, perform venipuncture or insert an IV on an arm that has an AV fistula.

(N) NCLEX® Connection: Physiological Adaptation, Illness Management

4. A client who has polycystic kidney disease is admitted to the acute care facility with reports of fever and flu-like symptoms. The client is scheduled to receive hemodialysis in 1 hr. His vital signs are: temperature 38.3° C (101° F) orally, pulse 90/min, respirations 26/min, and blood pressure 160/90 mm Hg. Does the client's current health status contraindicate the scheduled hemodialysis?

The client's current fever and flu-like symptoms are not a contraindication to hemodialysis. His illness does place him at an increased risk for complications such as infection, fluid volume deficit, and nausea and vomiting.

(N) NCLEX® Connection: Physiological Adaptation, Illness Management

UNIT 8	NURSING CARE OF CLIENTS WITH RENAL DISORDERS
Section	Diagnostic and Therapeutic Procedures
Chapter 66	Renal Transplant

Overview

- End-stage renal disease, when the kidneys can no longer function, may be treated with a renal transplant. Transplantation may greatly improve the quality of life for a person who is otherwise dependent on dialysis.

- The recipient's tissue must be matched with a donor's.

    o Donors for renal transplantation may be living, non heart-beating, or cadaver donors.

    o In-depth tissue typing includes assessment of blood type (ABO) compatibility and histocompatibility, including human leukocytic antigen (HLA) and other minor antigens.

    o Clients receiving a donor kidney from a living, related donor – with matching tissue type – have the greatest chance of graft survival.

- The donated kidney is surgically implanted in the client.

Transplantation Procedure

- Indications

    o Diagnoses

        ▪ Client indications of end-stage renal disease necessitating renal transplantation:

            □ Anuria

            □ Proteinuria

            □ Marked azotemia (elevated BUN and serum creatinine)

            □ Severe electrolyte imbalance (hyperkalemia, hypernatremia)

            □ Fluid volume excess conditions (heart failure, pulmonary edema)

            □ Uremic lung

- o Risks
  - Conditions that increase the risks involved in renal transplantation surgery, lifelong immunosuppression, and organ rejection:
    - □ Age younger than 2 years
    - □ Age older than 70 years
      - ▸ Older adult clients are more likely to have advanced heart disease and malignancies, which make them less than ideal candidates for renal transplantation surgery.
    - □ Advanced, untreatable cardiac disease
    - □ Active cancer
    - □ Chemical dependency
    - □ Chronic infections or systemic diseases (HIV, hepatitis C)
    - □ Coagulopathies and certain immune disorders
- o Client Presentation
  - Signs and symptoms of end-stage renal disease may include: anorexia, decreased attention span, fatigue, seizures, tremor, heart failure, edema of hands and feet, dyspnea, distended jugular veins, anemia, vomiting, pulmonary edema, hypertension, cardiac dysrhythmias, numbness and tingling, pallor, dry itchy skin, bruising, halitosis, and diminished or dark-colored urine.

- Client Outcomes
  - o The client will achieve and maintain a desired fluid and electrolyte balance, be free of infection, and maintain an active lifestyle with minimum restrictions.

- Preprocedure
  - o Nursing Actions
    - Schedule preoperative laboratory assessments, including blood chemistry studies, CBC and differential, bleeding times, urine culture, blood type, and crossmatch.
    - Administer preoperative medications as prescribed, including prophylactic antibiotics and induction of immunosuppressant therapy, such as methylprednisolone sodium succinate (Solu-Medrol) and cyclosporine (Neoral).
    - The client is usually dialyzed within 24 hr of surgery.
  - o Client Education
    - Prepare the client mentally and emotionally for the procedure.
    - Advise the client that compliance with the posttransplant interventions (lifelong immunosuppression) and risk factor reduction (smoking cessation, blood pressure and blood glucose control) are crucial to the success of the transplantation.

- Intraprocedure
  - ○ Nursing Actions
    - ■ Provide padding to the client's bony prominences to provide comfort and prevent skin breakdown.
    - ■ Communicate surgical progress to the client's family members, if appropriate.
    - ■ Assist in monitoring urine output and blood loss.
    - ■ Document appropriate surgical events.
    - ■ Assist in arranging postoperative unit placement and communicate postoperative needs of the client.
- Postprocedure
  - ○ Nursing Actions
    - ■ Assess/monitor
      - ◻ Vital signs every 15 min initially and advance to every hour (follow institutional protocol)
        - ▸ Maintain the client's blood pressure within prescribed parameters.
      - ◻ Intake and output at least hourly
        - ▸ Urine output should be greater than 30 mL/hr. Notify the provider of oliguria as evidenced by urine output of 100 to 400 mL in 24 hr.
      - ◻ Urine appearance and odor hourly (initially pink and bloody, gradually returning to normal in a few days to several weeks)
      - ◻ Daily urinalysis to check for protein, WBCs, RBCs, ketones, glucose, specific gravity, and pH
      - ◻ Daily weight
      - ◻ For fluid and electrolyte imbalances, such as hypervolemia, hypovolemia, hypokalemia, and hyponatremia
      - ◻ For signs of infection, such as dyspnea, fever, incisional drainage, and redness
      - ◻ For signs of organ rejection
      - ◻ Surgical dressing for bloody drainage
    - ■ Administer intravenous fluids as prescribed, usually calculated to replace hourly urine output.
    - ■ Administer oral fluids and discontinue IV fluid once bowel function returns and fluids are tolerated.
    - ■ Encourage the client to turn, cough, and deep breathe to prevent atelectasis and pneumonia.

- Provide urinary catheter care
    - Attach the large indwelling urinary catheter to bedside drainage.
    - Maintain continuous bladder irrigation as prescribed.
    - Remove the urinary catheter as soon as possible to decrease the risk of infection.
- Intervene for oliguria as prescribed. Diuretics and/or dialysis may be necessary until kidney function is satisfactory.
- Administer immunosuppressive medications to prevent rejection.
    - Monitor for side effects, such as infection and fluid retention.
- Immediately notify the surgeon if any signs of organ rejection appear.
- Administer stool softeners to prevent straining and constipation (risk associated with bowel manipulation during abdominal surgery and the effects of general anesthetics and analgesics).
- Arrange for counseling for the client and family if necessary.
- Arrange for posttransplant follow-up appointments and interventions.
  - Client Education
    - Instruct the client to monitor and report signs of infection, such as fever, incisional drainage, and redness.
    - Instruct the client to adhere to the pharmacological regimen.
    - Instruct the client and family about prescribed diet and activity level.
- Complications
  - Organ rejection
    - Clients undergoing renal transplant face the possibility of organ rejection.
    - Nursing Actions
        - Monitor for and report signs of rejection immediately.
            - Hyperacute – occurs within 48 hr after surgery. Findings include fever, hypertension, and pain at the transplant site. Treatment is immediate removal of the donor kidney.
            - Acute – occurs 1 week to 2 years after surgery. Findings include oliguria, anuria, low-grade fever, hypertension, tenderness over the transplanted kidney, lethargy, azotemia, and fluid retention. Treatment involves increased doses of immunosuppressive medications.
            - Chronic – occurs gradually over months to years. Findings include gradual return of azotemia, fluid retention, electrolyte imbalance, and fatigue. Treatment is conservative (monitor kidney status, continue immunosuppressive therapy) until dialysis is required.

- Client Education
  - Teach the client to monitor for signs of rejection and to contact the primary care provider immediately.
  - Instruct the client to adhere to the pharmacological regimen.
- Acute tubular necrosis (ATN)
  - A delay in transplanting the donor kidney after harvesting may result in hypoxic injury of the donor kidney.
  - Nursing Actions
    - Monitor the client's urine output, serum creatinine, and BUN levels to detect failure of the transplanted kidney.
    - Report hourly output volumes of less than 30 mL/hr.
    - Assist the client with dialysis as indicated.
    - Prepare the client for a renal biopsy to distinguish ATN from organ rejection.
  - Client Education
    - Advise the client that dialysis may be needed until the donor kidney heals.
- Renal Artery Stenosis
  - Renal artery stenosis is due to scarring of surgical anastomosis.
  - Nursing Actions
    - Monitor for and report hypertension, bruit over artery anastomosis site, and decreased renal function, such as oliguria and elevated BUN and creatinine.
    - Prepare the client for a renal scan to verify the status of renal blood flow.
    - Angioplasty and/or surgical intervention may be necessary.
  - Client Education
    - Advise the client to monitor for peripheral edema and have blood pressure checked often.
- Thrombosis
  - A blood clot may form in a major vessel of the transplanted kidney.
  - Nursing Actions
    - Monitor the client for and report a sudden decease in urine output.
    - Prepare the client for emergency surgery.
  - Client Education
    - Keep the client informed about the risk of a blood clot.
    - Advise the client to inform the provider of a sudden decrease in urine output.

- ○ Infection
    - Infection is the most common cause of first-transplant-year morbidity and mortality.
    - Nursing Actions
        - □ Give high priority to infection control measures, such as frequent hand hygiene.
        - □ Monitor for and report signs of a localized (wound) or systemic infection (pneumonia, sepsis).
    - Client Education
        - □ Instruct the client to monitor and report signs of infection, such as fever, incisional drainage, and redness. Later signs of infection may include fatigue and discomfort. Report any signs of infection to the primary care provider.
        - □ Educate the client and family about the increased risk for infection during immunosuppressant therapy and infection control measures, such as frequent hand hygiene and avoiding crowds and people who have a communicable disease. The client may need to wear a facemask when out in public.
        - □ Instruct the client to adhere to the pharmacological regimen.

CHAPTER 66: RENAL TRANSPLANT

Ⓐ Application Exercises

Scenario: A 40-year-old male client with end-stage renal disease underwent a renal transplant 4 days ago. His urinary catheter has been removed and the client is able to void. He is being started on oral fluids today. If he tolerates fluids, his intravenous electrolyte infusion will be discontinued.

1. Which of the following should be included in the postoperative nursing care for this client? (Select all that apply.)

_____ Obtaining daily weights

_____ Restricting oral fluids

_____ Replacing hourly urine output with IV fluids

_____ Elevating the head of the bed

_____ Monitoring serum electrolytes

2. The client is given the stool softener docusate sodium (Colace). Why is this intervention necessary following kidney transplantation?

3. What findings should cause the nurse to suspect organ rejection? What kind of rejection can occur at this time? What is a priority intervention?

CHAPTER 66: RENAL TRANSPLANT

 Application Exercises Answer Key

Scenario: A 40-year-old male client with end-stage renal disease underwent a renal transplant 4 days ago. His urinary catheter has been removed and the client is able to void. He is being started on oral fluids today. If he tolerates fluids, his intravenous electrolyte infusion will be discontinued.

1. Which of the following should be included in the postoperative nursing care for this client? (Select all that apply.)

   X   **Obtaining daily weights**

   _____   Restricting oral fluids

   X   **Replacing hourly urine output with IV fluids**

   _____   Elevating the head of the bed

   X   **Monitoring serum electrolytes**

Daily weights are important to assess fluid status. Fluid intake and output should be closely monitored in a client after a renal transplant. A client who has a high volume of urine output may have IV fluids recalculated hourly to replace hourly urine output. Fluid replacement is necessary to prevent dehydration and hypotension, which may reduce kidney perfusion. Electrolyte loss may occur with diuresis and should be monitored. There is no indication to elevate the head of the client's bed.

 NCLEX® Connection: Reduction of Risk Potential: Potential for Complications from Surgical Procedures and Health Alterations

2. The client is given the stool softener docusate sodium (Colace). Why is this intervention necessary following kidney transplantation?

Stool softeners such as docusate sodium are necessary to prevent constipation, because manipulation of the bowel during surgery and decreased activity after surgery can exacerbate constipation. They also prevent straining, which should be avoided.

 NCLEX® Connection: Physiological Adaptation: Illness Management

3. What findings should cause the nurse to suspect organ rejection? What kind of rejection can occur at this time? What is a priority intervention?

Signs of organ rejection include malaise, oliguria, anuria, fever, tachycardia, an enlarged tender kidney, boggy kidney on palpation, weight gain, hypertension, decreased urine output, abnormal chemistry studies, abnormal renal biopsy, and abnormal radionuclide scan. Rejection after the first 48 hr and up to 2 years following transplant is acute rejection. Administration of increased doses of immunosuppressants is a priority intervention.

 NCLEX® Connection: Physiological Adaptation: Medical Emergencies

UNIT 8	NURSING CARE OF CLIENTS WITH RENAL DISORDERS
Section	Renal System Disorders
Chapter 67	Acute and Chronic Glomerulonephritis

Overview

- Glomerulonephritis is an inflammation of the glomerular capillaries, usually following a streptococcal infection. It is an immune complex disease, not an infection of the kidney.

- Glomerulonephritis exists as an acute, latent, and chronic disease.

- Acute glomerulonephritis (AGN)

  o Insoluble immune complexes develop and become trapped in the glomerular tissue producing swelling and capillary cell death.

  o Prognosis varies depending upon the specific cause, but spontaneous recovery generally occurs after the acute illness.

- Chronic glomerulonephritis (CGN)

  o CGN can occur without a previous history or known onset.

  o This involves the progressive destruction of glomeruli and eventual hardening (sclerosis).

  o CGN is the third leading cause of end-stage renal disease (ESRD), with the prognosis varying depending on the specific cause.

View Media Supplement: Glomerulonephritis (Image)

Health Promotion and Disease Prevention

- Consume a diet low in sodium and restrict fluid intake. Consult a health care provider regarding diet restrictions.

Assessment

- Risk Factors

  o Immunological reactions

    ▪ Primary infection with group A beta-hemolytic streptococcal infection (most common)

    ▪ Systemic lupus erythematosus

- - ○ Vascular injury (hypertension)

    ○ Metabolic disease (diabetes mellitus)

    ○ Excessively high protein and high sodium diets

    ○ Older adult clients may report vague symptoms (nausea, fatigue, joint aches) which may mask glomerular disease.

    ○ Older adult clients tend to have decreased working nephrons and are at increased risk for chronic renal failure.

  - Subjective and Objective Data

    ○ Renal symptoms

      - Decreased urine output

      - Smoky or coffee-colored urine (hematuria)

      - Proteinuria

    ○ Fluid volume excess symptoms

      - Shortness of breath

      - Orthopnea

      - Bibasilar rales

      - Periorbital edema

      - Mild to severe hypertension

    ○ Changes in the level of consciousness

    ○ Anorexia/nausea

    ○ Headache

    ○ Back pain

    ○ Fever (AGN)

    ○ Pruritus (CGN)

    ○ Laboratory Tests

      - Throat culture to identify possible streptococcus infection

      - Serum BUN (elevated: 100 to 200 mg/dL; expected reference range: 10 to 20 mg/dL) and Creatinine (elevated: greater than 6 mg/dL; expected reference range: males: 0.6 to 1.2 mg/dL, and females: 0.5 to 1.1mg/L)

      - Creatinine clearance (decreased: 50 mL/min/m^2; expected reference range: males: 90 to 139 mL/min/m^2, females: 80 to 125 mL/min/m^2)

      - Urinalysis: proteinuria, hematuria, cell debris (red cells and casts), increased urine specific gravity

      - Electrolytes: hyperkalemia, hypoalbuminemia, and hyperphosphatemia

- Antistreptolysin-O (ASO) titer (positive indicating the presence of strep antibodies)

- Erythrocyte sedimentation rate (ESR) (elevated indicating active inflammatory response)

- White blood cell count (elevated indicating inflammation and presence of active strep infection)

- Glomerular filtration rate (GFR): filtration rate of kidneys, best indicator of kidney function.

  o Diagnostic Procedures

- X-ray of kidney, ureter, bladder (KUB), and renal ultrasound (to detect structural abnormalities [atrophy])

- Renal biopsy (to confirm or rule out diagnosis)

- In acute glomerulonephritis, dialysis can be an intervention to treat severe uremia (large amounts of urea and other nitrogenous waste found in the blood)

Collaborative Care

- Nursing Care

  o Monitor the client's daily weight and note any recent weight gain.

  o Monitor intake and output.

  o Observe the client for changes in urinary pattern.

  o Monitor serum electrolytes, BUN, and creatinine.

  o Observe the client's skin for pruritus.

  o Maintain bed rest to decrease metabolic demands.

  o Maintain prescribed dietary restrictions.

- Fluid restriction (24 hr output + 500 mL).

- Sodium restriction.

- Protein restriction (if azotemia is present = increased BUN).

- Medications

  o Administer antibiotics on time to maintain blood levels for an effective elimination of the strep infection.

  o Administer diuretics to reduce edema.

  o Use vasodilators to decrease blood pressure.

  o Administer corticosteroids to decrease the inflammatory response.

- Interdisciplinary Care

  o Nephrology services may be consulted to manage renal function.

  o Nutritional services may be consulted for diet modifications and fluid restriction.

- Therapeutic Procedures

  o Plasmapheresis (filters antibodies out of circulating blood volume)

    ■ Nursing Actions

      □ Monitor the client carefully during and following the procedure.

      □ Take appropriate interventions to reduce the risk of coagulation.

    ■ Client Education

      □ Encourage the client to rest in order to conserve energy.

- Care after Discharge

  o Home care services may be indicated if the client is homebound or living in a nursing facility.

  o Outpatient services are routinely set-up to follow the client's medications and status.

  o Laboratory services are routinely set-up to follow the client's renal function.

  o Client Education

    ■ Instruct the client to take medications as prescribed.

    ■ Instruct the client to weigh daily, at the same time, and to notify the provider for a weight gain of 2 lb in 24 hr or 5 lb in 1 week.

    ■ Advise the client to maintain fluid and sodium restriction – a dietary consult may be necessary.

    ■ Educate the client and family regarding the illness and encourage the expression feelings.

- Client Outcomes

  o The client will be free from pain.

  o The client will maintain fluid balance.

  o The client will improve tolerance to activity.

  o The client will follow a medication regimen.

Complications

- Uremia
  - Symptoms include muscle cramps, fatigue, pruritus, anorexia, and a metallic taste in mouth.
  - Nursing Actions
    - Intervene to maintain skin integrity.
    - Assist with dialysis.
- Pulmonary edema, congestive heart failure, pericarditis
  - Nursing Actions
    - Monitor for dyspnea, crackles, edema, and decreased cardiac output.
    - Intervene accordingly (oxygen, diuretics, inotropic medications).
- Anemia
  - Nursing Actions
    - Monitor hemoglobin.
    - Administer iron and erythropoietin as indicated.

CHAPTER 67: ACUTE AND CHRONIC GLOMERULONEPHRITIS

Ⓐ Application Exercises

1. Interpret the following laboratory test results:

TEST	RESULT	NORMAL RANGE	INTERPRETATION
Serum Creatinine	2.2 mg/dL	0.6 to 1.2 mg/dL	
Serum BUN	30 mg/dL	10 to 20 mg/dL	
24 hr Urine Creatinine Clearance	52 mL/min	80 to 140 mL/min	

2. Order from 1 to 5 the sequence of pathological events that occurs in glomerulonephritis.

_____ Edema

_____ Salt and water retention

_____ Glomerular-capillary membrane damage

_____ Hematuria and proteinuria

_____ Immune response with antibody production

3. Which of the following clinical findings are expected in clients with glomerulonephritis? (Select all that apply.)

_____ Fever

_____ Peripheral edema

_____ Polyuria

_____ Irregular pulse

_____ Hypotension

_____ Weight gain

_____ Headache

_____ Proteinuria

_____ Dyspnea

_____ Bradycardia

CHAPTER 67: ACUTE AND CHRONIC GLOMERULONEPHRITIS

 Application Exercises Answer Key

1. Interpret the following laboratory test results:

TEST	RESULT	NORMAL RANGE	INTERPRETATION
Serum Creatinine	2.2 mg/dL	0.6 to 1.2 mg/dL	Indicates decreased renal function.
Serum BUN	30 mg/dL	10 to 20 mg/dL	Indicates decreased renal function.
24 hr Urine Creatinine Clearance	52 mL/min	80 to 140 mL/min	Indicates reduced renal blood flow.

The findings are all out of the expected reference range for these tests. This indicates a decrease in the productivity of the renal system.

NCLEX® Connection: Reduction of Risk Potential, Laboratory Values

2. Order from 1 to 5 the sequence of pathological events that occurs in glomerulonephritis.

<u> 5 </u>   Edema

<u> 4 </u>   Salt and water retention

<u> 2 </u>   Glomerular-capillary membrane damage

<u> 3 </u>   Hematuria and proteinuria

<u> 1 </u>   Immune response with antibody production

The sequence of pathological events should occur in this order: immune response with antibody production, glomerular-capillary membrane damage, hematuria and proteinuria, salt and water retention, and edema.

NCLEX® Connection: Physiological Adaptation, Pathophysiology

3. Which of the following clinical findings are expected in clients with glomerulonephritis? (Select all that apply.)

   X   **Fever**

   X   **Peripheral edema**

_____   Polyuria

_____   Irregular pulse

_____   Hypotension

   X   **Weight gain**

   X   **Headache**

   X   **Proteinuria**

   X   **Dyspnea**

_____   Bradycardia

A fever, peripheral edema, weight gain, headache, proteinuria, and dyspnea are all expected clinical findings. Irregular pulse, bradycardia, polyuria, and hypotension are not expected clinical findings.

Ⓝ NCLEX® Connection: Reduction of Risk Potential, System Specific Assessment

UNIT 8	NURSING CARE OF CLIENTS WITH RENAL DISORDERS
Section	Renal System Disorders
Chapter 68	Nephrotic Syndrome and Acute and Chronic Renal Failure

Overview

- There are several disorders that affect the renal system and its ability to function.

- Some of these disorders include acute and chronic renal failure, and nephrotic syndrome.

NEPHROTIC SYNDROME

Overview

- Nephrotic syndrome is a group of symptoms.

- Glomerular capillaries are damaged from immune complex deposits, nephrotoxic antibodies, or non-immunological insults.

- Damaged glomerular capillaries are permeable to serum proteins, resulting in decreased serum osmotic pressure.

- Nephrotic syndrome is characterized by proteinuria, hypoalbuminemia, and edema.

Health Promotion and Disease Prevention

- Clients should consume a diet low in sodium and restrict fluid intake, and consult with a health care provider regarding diet restrictions.

Assessment

- Risk Factors

  o Immunologic disorders

  o Toxic injury to the kidney

  o Neoplasms

  o Multisystem diseases (diabetes mellitus)

  o Infections

  o Hyperlipidemia

- ○ Diseases of the vascular system

    Ⓖ

- ○ Chronic illnesses can increase the potential of nephrotic syndrome in the older adult client.

- ○ Renal function decreases with aging, which increases the risk for nephrotic syndrome.

- Subjective Data

    - ○ Edema (periorbital, dependent)

    - ○ Irritability

    - ○ Malaise, fatigue

    - ○ Anorexia, nausea

- Objective Data

    - Proteinuria

    - Hematuria

    - Hypertension

    - Anasarca (generalized edema)

    - Foamy urine

    - Oliguria

    - Anemia (hemoglobin 12 g/dL or less)

    - Azotemia (increased BUN)

    - Uremia (symptoms of renal failure)

    - Loss of skin integrity related to edema

    - ○ Laboratory Tests

        - Urinalysis/24 hr urine collection

            - □ Protein as high as +3 or +4 (> 3.5 g in 24 hr)

            - □ Casts

        - Serum lipid levels

            - □ Elevated serum cholesterol (> 200 mg/dL)

            - □ Elevated triglycerides

            - □ Elevated low-density and very low-density lipoproteins

        - Serum albumin

            - □ Less than 3 g/dL

        - Serum blood urea nitrogen (BUN), creatinine, and glomerular filtration rate (GFR) levels may indicate minimal to extensive loss of kidney function.

            - □ BUN and creatinine levels rise, while GFR levels decrease with the loss of kidney function.

- o Diagnostic Procedures
  - ■ Kidney biopsy
    - □ Minimal to extensive damage
    - □ Fatty deposits in tubules
    - □ Epithelium changes
    - □ Hypercellularity
    - □ Glomerular sclerosis
    - □ Immunoglobulins in capillary walls
    - □ Nursing Action
      - ‣ Explain the reason for the test.
      - ‣ Prepare the client for the test.
      - ‣ Collect specimens accurately.

Collaborative Care

- • Nursing Care
  - o Report abnormal findings to the provider.
  - o Provide periods of rest with activities.
  - o Provide emotional support.
  - o Encourage adequate nutritional intake within restriction guidelines.
    - ■ Encourage lowering sodium intake.
    - ■ Adjust protein intake according to protein loss in urine over 24 hr.
    - ■ Provide high biologic value protein (lean meat, fish, poultry, dairy).
    - ■ Provide small, frequent feedings due to the client's loss of appetite.
  - o Administer medications as prescribed.
  - o Assess skin and provide skin care.
- • Medications
  - o Loop diuretics: furosemide (Lasix), bumetanide (Bumex)
    - ■ Nursing Considerations
      - □ Administer IV furosemide (Lasix) no faster than 20 mg/min.
      - □ Loop diuretics are indicated for renal impairment.
    - ■ Client Education
      - □ Instruct the client to take the medication with food.
      - □ Inform the client that the medication may cause hypotension.

- o Angiotensin-converting enzyme (ACE) inhibitors: captopril (Capoten)
    - This is used to block the production of angiotensin II, resulting in the excretion of sodium and water.
    - Nursing Considerations
        - □ Monitor the client for increased potassium level.
        - □ Monitor the client for hypotension.
        - □ Use carefully on clients with renal impairment related to leukocyte depletion, and watch for infection.
    - Client Education
        - □ Inform the client that the medication may cause a dry cough.
- o Anticoagulants: Heparin, warfarin (Coumadin)
    - This can be used to decrease proteinuria and renal insufficiency.
    - Nursing Considerations
        - □ Monitor the client's PT levels for an appropriate Coumadin dose.
    - Client Education
        - □ Instruct the client to monitor for signs of bleeding (dark stools, bruising easily).
- o Erythropoietin alfa (Epogen, Procrit)
    - This is used to stimulate the production of red blood cells and is given for anemia.
    - Nursing Considerations
        - □ Monitor hemoglobin and hematocrit.
        - □ Monitor the client's blood pressure.
        - □ This is contraindicated for clients with uncontrolled hypertension.
    - Client Education
        - □ Instruct the client to have blood drawn twice a week to monitor hemoglobin and hematocrit.
- Interdisciplinary Care
    - o Nephrology services may be consulted for renal impairment.
    - o Nutritional services may be consulted for dietary modifications.

- Care after Discharge

    o Nutritional services may be consulted for dietary modifications.

    o Client Education

        ▪ Instruct the client to consume a diet low in sodium and restrict fluid intake.

        ▪ Inform the client to consult with the provider regarding diet restrictions.

        ▪ Encourage the client to provide periods of rest with activities.

        ▪ Encourage the client to take medications as prescribed.

        ▪ Instruct the client to notify the provider for a possible increased risk for bleeding.

    o Client Outcomes

        ▪ The client will adhere to a prescribed medication regimen.

        ▪ The client will have a decrease in anxiety.

        ▪ The client will have an increase in activity level.

        ▪ The client will maintain an oral fluid restriction regimen.

Complications

- Respiratory Compromise

    o Nursing Actions

        ▪ Assess and monitor breath sounds, respiratory rate.

- Peritonitis

    o Nursing Actions

        ▪ Assess and monitor bowel sounds.

        ▪ Monitor for infection (rigid, tender abdomen, fever, elevated white blood cell count).

- Renal Failure

    o Nursing Actions

        ▪ Assess and monitor renal status (BUN, serum creatinine, urinalysis).

        ▪ Prepare the client for dialysis, if indicated.

- Shock/Death

    o Nursing Actions

        ▪ Assess and monitor for early indications of shock.

        ▪ Implement life-saving measures.

ACUTE AND CHRONIC RENAL FAILURE

@ Overview

- The kidneys regulate fluid, acid-base, and electrolyte balance, while also, eliminating wastes from the body.

- Renal failure may be diagnosed as acute or chronic. Acute renal failure can result in chronic renal failure without aggressive treatment, or when complicating pre-existing conditions exist.

- Acute Renal Failure (ARF) is the sudden cessation of renal function that occurs when blood flow to the kidneys is significantly compromised.

  o ARF is a leading cause of death among hospitalized clients and 50% is due to an iatrogenic cause.

  o ARF is comprised of four phases:

    ▪ Onset – begins with the onset of the event and lasts for hours to days.

    ▪ Oliguria – begins with the renal insult and lasts for 1 to 3 weeks.

    ▪ Diuresis – begins when the kidneys start to recover and can last for 2 to 6 weeks.

    ▪ Recovery – continues until renal function is fully restored and can take up to 12 months.

  o Prerenal failure from volume depletion or prolonged reduction of blood pressure is the most common cause of acute renal deterioration and is usually reversible with prompt intervention.

- Clinical manifestations occur abruptly with ARF.

- Chronic Renal Failure (CRF) is a progressive, irreversible kidney disease.

  o End-stage renal failure exists when 90% of the functioning nephrons have been destroyed and are no longer able to maintain fluid, electrolyte, or acid-base homeostasis.

  o CRF is comprised of five stages:

    ▪ Stage 1: Minimal kidney damage with normal GFR

    ▪ Stage 2: Mild kidney damage with mildly decreased GFR

    ▪ Stage 3: Moderate kidney damage with moderate decrease in GFR

    ▪ Stage 4: Severe kidney damage with severe decrease in GFR

    ▪ Stage 5: Kidney failure and end-stage renal disease with little or no glomerular filtration

  o Dialysis or kidney transplantation can maintain life, but neither are cures for CRF.

- A client diagnosed with CRF may be asymptomatic except during periods of stress (infection, surgery, trauma). As renal failure progresses, clinical manifestations become apparent.

Health Promotion and Disease Prevention

- Encourage clients to drink at least 3L daily. Consult with the provider regarding prescribed fluid restriction, if needed.

- Promote smoking cessation.

Assessment

- Risk Factors of ARF:

  ○ African Americans, Native Americans, and Asians have the highest incidence of end-stage renal disease.

  ○ Risk factors for acute renal failure include prerenal, intrarenal, and postrenal causes.

  ○ Prerenal – occurs before damage to the kidney occurs

    ▪ Hypovolemia resulting from:

      □ Hemorrhage

      □ Dehydration

      □ Prolonged vomiting or diarrhea

  ○ Decreased cardiac output resulting in reduced renal perfusion can be caused by:

    ▪ Myocardial infarction

    ▪ Cardiogenic shock

    ▪ Cardiac arrhythmias

    ▪ Heart failure

    ▪ Pericardial tamponade

    ▪ Open-heart surgery

  ○ Decreased peripheral vascular resistance is associated with:

    ▪ Renal artery stenosis

    ▪ Septic shock

    ▪ Anaphylaxis

    ▪ Neurological injury

  ○ Renal vascular obstruction can be caused by:

    ▪ Thrombosis of renal arteries or veins

    ▪ Embolism

  ○ Intrarenal – occurs within the kidney and the damage is usually irreversible (acute tubular necrosis)

- Nephrotoxic injury can be caused by:
    - Specific antibiotics
    - NSAIDs
    - Burns (myoglobin)
    - Organic solvents
    - Contrast dye
    - Heavy metals
    - Hemolytic transfusion reactions
- Acute glomerulonephritis
    - Acute pyelonephritis
    - Toxemia of pregnancy
    - Malignant hypertension
    - Systemic lupus erythematosus
    - Interstitial nephritis

- Postrenal – obstruction of structures leaving the kidney
    - Renal calculi
    - Urinary tract obstruction
    - Prostate cancer
    - Bladder cancer
    - Trauma
    - Strictures
    - Spinal cord disease
- Risk factors and causes of CRF:
    - Acute renal failure
    - Diabetes mellitus
    - Chronic glomerulonephritis
    - Nephrotoxic medications (gentamicin, NSAIDS) or chemicals
    - Hypertension, especially if African-American
    - Autoimmune disorders (systemic lupus erythematosus)
    - Polycystic kidney
    - Pyelonephrosis
    - Renal artery stenosis
    - Recurrent severe infections

Ⓖ

- o Older adult clients are at an increased risk for renal failure related to the decreased number of functioning nephrons, decreased GFR, and water and sodium-conserving and compensating mechanisms.

- o An increased incidence of chronic renal failure may be related to the prevalence of diabetes mellitus, hypertension, and the use of NSAIDs in older adult clients.

- Subjective Data

  - o Fatigue

  - o Lethargy

  - o Restless leg syndrome

  - o Depression

  - o Intractable hiccups

- Objective Data

  - o In most cases, findings of renal failure are related to fluid volume overload and include:

    - Renal – polyuria, nocturia (early), oliguria, anuria (late), proteinuria, hematuria, and dilute urine color when present

    - Cardiovascular – hypertension, peripheral edema, pericardial effusion, congestive heart failure, cardiomyopathy, and orthostatic hypotension

    - Respiratory – dyspnea, tachypnea, uremic pneumonitis, lung crackles, Kussmaul respirations, and pulmonary edema

    - Hematologic – anemia, bruising, and bleeding

    - Neurologic – lethargy, insomnia, confusion, encephalopathy, seizures, tremors, ataxia, paresthesias, and coma

    - Gastrointestinal – nausea, anorexia, vomiting, metallic taste, stomatitis, diarrhea, uremic halitosis, and gastritis

    - Skin – decreased skin turgor, yellow cast to skin, dry, pruritus, bruising, and uremic frost (late)

    - Musculoskeletal – osteomalacia (softening of bone), muscle weakness, pathologic fractures, and muscle cramps

    - Reproductive – erectile dysfunction

  - o Laboratory Tests

    - Urinalysis

      - □ Hematuria, proteinuria, and alterations in specific gravity

      - □ Serum creatinine

        - ▸ Gradual increase of 1 to 2 mg/dL per every 24 to 48 hr for acute renal failure (ARF)

        - ▸ Gradual increase over months to years for chronic renal failure (CRF) exceeding 4 mg/dL

- Blood urea nitrogen (BUN)
  - 80 to 100 mg/dL within 1 week with ARF
  - Gradual increase with elevated serum creatinine over months to years for CRF
  - 180-200 mg/dL with (CRF)
- Serum electrolytes
  - Decreased sodium (dilutional) and calcium, increased potassium, phosphorus, and magnesium
- Complete blood count (CBC)
  - Decreased hemoglobin and hematocrit from anemia secondary to the loss of erythropoietin in CRF
- Diagnostic Procedures
  - Radiology
    - Demonstrates disease processes, obstruction, and arterial defects
    - Renal ultrasound
    - Kidneys, ureter, and bladder (KUB)
    - Computerized tomography (CT)
    - Aortorenal angiography
    - Cystoscopy
    - Retrograde pyelography
    - Renal biopsy

Collaborative Care

- Nursing Care
  - Abnormal findings to be reported and monitored include:
    - Urinary elimination patterns (amount, color, odor, and consistency)
    - Vital signs (blood pressure may be increased or decreased)
    - Weight – 1 kg (2.2 lb) daily weight increase is approximately 1 L of fluid retained
    - Assess and monitor vascular access or peritoneal dialysis insertion site
  - Provide the client a diet that is high in carbohydrates and moderate in fat.
  - Restrict the client's intake of fluids (based on urinary output).
  - Balance the client's activity and rest.
  - Prepare the client for hemodialysis, peritoneal dialysis, and hemofiltration if indicated.
  - Provide skin care to the client in order to increase comfort and prevent breakdown.

- Protect the client from injury.

- Provide emotional support to the client and family.

- Encourage the client to ask questions and discuss fears.

- Encourage the client to diet, exercise, and take medication to control hyperlipidemia.

- Administer medications as prescribed.

- For clients with ARF, nurses should:

  - Identify and assist with correcting the underlying cause.

  - Prevent prolonged episodes of hypotension and hypovolemia.

  - Prepare for fluid challenge and diuretics during prerenal period of azotemia if the client is showing signs of fluid volume deficit.

  - Restrict fluid intake during oliguric phase.

  - Restrict dietary intake of protein, sodium, and potassium during oliguric phase (this restriction is for the client not requiring dialysis).

- For clients with CRF, nurses should:

  - Obtain a detailed medication and herb history to determine the client's risk for continued renal insult.

  - Control protein intake based on the client's stage of renal failure and type of dialysis.

  - Restrict the client's dietary sodium, potassium, phosphorous, and magnesium.

  - Encourage the client with diabetes mellitus to adhere to strict blood glucose control as uncontrolled diabetes is a major risk factor for renal failure.

- Medications

  - Cardiac Glycoside (Digoxin) increases contractility of the myocardium and promotes cardiac output.

    - Nursing Considerations

      - Take apical pulse for 1 min prior to giving the medication. Notify the provider if the client's heart rate is less than 60/min.

    - Client Education

      - Instruct the client to take apical pulse for 1 full minute daily, prior to self-administration of the medication.

      - Instruct the client to notify the provider if apical pulse is less than 60/min.

      - Instruct the client to notify the provider immediately if vision changes (blurred vision, seeing more yellow color), or if there is a sensitivity to light or behavior changes. These are signs of digoxin toxicity and need immediate attention.

- ○ Sodium Polystyrene (Kayexalate) to increase elimination of potassium
  - ▪ Nursing Considerations
    - □ Monitor levels of potassium.
    - □ Monitor vital signs.
    - □ Use cautiously with clients who have heart failure, hypertension, or edema.
    - □ Monitor clients who are taking digoxin cautiously.
- ○ Erythropoietin alfa (Epogen, Procrit) to stimulate production of red blood cells, given for anemia
  - ▪ Nursing Considerations
    - □ Monitor hemoglobin and hematocrit.
    - □ Monitor the client's blood pressure.
    - □ This is contraindicated for clients with uncontrolled hypertension.
    - □ Use medication cautiously in clients who have bone marrow cancer.
  - ▪ Client Education
    - □ Instruct the client to have blood drawn twice weekly to monitor hemoglobin and hematocrit.
- ○ Iron supplement (Ferrous Sulfate)
  - ▪ Increases the level of iron in blood.
  - ▪ Nursing Considerations
    - □ Administer medication after dialysis (if applicable).
    - □ Stool softener should be used as this medication causes constipation.
  - ▪ Client Education
    - □ Instruct the client to take the medication with food.
- ○ Aluminum hydroxide gel (Amphojel)
  - ▪ A phosphate binder is used to increase the elimination of phosphate.
  - ▪ Nursing Considerations
    - □ Stool softener should be used as this medication causes constipation.
    - □ This is contraindicated in clients with gastrointestinal disorders.
  - ▪ Client Education
    - □ Encourage the client to report signs of constipation.

- o Diuretics (except in ESRD) (Lasix)
  - ■ This is uses to excrete excess fluid.
  - ■ Nursing Considerations
    - □ Monitor intake/output.
    - □ Monitor blood pressure.
  - ■ Client Education
    - □ Encourage the client to weigh daily.
    - □ Instruct the client to notify the provider if experiencing thirst, coughing, or light-headedness.

- • Interdisciplinary Care
  - o Nephrology services may be consulted to manage dialysis or renal failure.
  - o Nutritional services may be consulted to manage the nutritional needs of the client.

- • Therapeutic Procedures
  - o Hemodialysis

- • Care after Discharge
  - o Nephrology services may be indicated if the client is to receive outpatient dialysis.
  - o Refer the client to a community support group relating to the disease.
  - o Nutritional services may be consulted for the client's dietary needs.
  - o Refer the client to a smoking cessation support group and counseling, if needed.

- • Client Education
  - o Instruct the client to monitor the daily intake of carbohydrates, proteins, sodium, and potassium, according to the provider.
  - o Instruct the client to monitor fluid intake according to fluid restriction prescribed by the provider.
  - o Instruct the client to avoid antacids containing magnesium.
  - o Encourage the client to take rest periods from activity.
  - o Educate the client receiving hemodialysis or peritoneal dialysis on an outpatient basis.
  - o Educate the client on how to measure blood pressure and weight at home.
  - o Encourage the client to ask questions and discuss fears.
  - o Encourage the client to diet, exercise, and take medication as prescribed.
  - o Advise the client to notify the provider if observe signs of skin breakdown.

- Client Outcomes

  o The client will maintain a fluid balance.

  o The client will improve tolerance to activity.

  o The client will report a decrease in anxiety.

  o The client will follow a medication regimen.

  o The client will have no signs of skin breakdown.

Complications

- Potential complications of renal failure include: electrolyte imbalance, dysrhythmias, fluid overload, metabolic acidosis, and secondary infection.

COMPLICATION	NURSING ACTIONS
Hyperkalemia	• Administer Kayexalate or insulin as prescribed.
Hypertension	• Administer antihypertensives and diuretics as prescribed.
Seizures	• Implement seizure precautions and administer antiepileptics as prescribed.
Cardiac dysrhythmias	• Provide life-support interventions for life-threatening dysrhythmias. • Monitor the client for and report non-lethal dysrhythmias.
Pulmonary edema	• Prepare the client for hemodialysis.
Infection	• Maintain the client's surgical asepsis of invasive lines, monitor breath sounds, and turn the client every 2 hr. • Monitor the client for signs of localized and systemic infections and report.
Metabolic acidosis	• Prepare the client for hemodialysis.
Uremia	• Prepare the client for hemodialysis.

CHAPTER 68: NEPHROTIC SYNDROME AND ACUTE AND CHRONIC RENAL FAILURE

 Application Exercises

1. Beginning with the first event, identify the sequence of pathological events that occurs in a client with nephrotic syndrome.

    _____   Proteinuria

    _____   Generalized edema

    _____   Renal insult

    _____   Increased glomerular permeability

    _____   Decreased serum protein

2. A nurse is caring for a client with nephrotic syndrome. The client asks the nurse why her legs and feet are swollen. How can the nurse best address the client's concerns?

3. Which of the following signs and symptoms should the nurse monitor for in a client with nephrotic syndrome? (Select all that apply.)

    _____   Malnutrition

    _____   Hematuria

    _____   Infection

    _____   Peritonitis

    _____   Hyperkalemia

    _____   Hypotension

    _____   Fever

4. Which of the following assessments should be made while the client is in acute renal failure? (Select all that apply.)

    _____   Cardiac enzymes

    _____   Blood glucose

    _____   Blood pressure

    _____   Serum electrolytes

    _____   Serum creatinine

    _____   Arterial blood gases

    _____   Urine output

5. Prioritize the following nursing interventions according to how they occur in a client diagnosed with renal failure.

    _____   Monitor serum potassium level.

    _____   Turn the client every 2 hr.

    _____   Offer emotional support to the family.

    _____   Assess breath sounds.

CHAPTER 68: NEPHROTIC SYNDROME AND ACUTE AND CHRONIC RENAL FAILURE

 Application Exercises Answer Key

1. Beginning with the first event, identify the sequence of pathological events that occurs in a client with nephrotic syndrome.

__3__	**Proteinuria**
__5__	**Generalized edema**
__1__	**Renal insult**
__2__	**Increased glomerular permeability**
__4__	**Decreased serum protein**

According to the sequence of pathological events, a client with nephrotic syndrome will first experience renal insult, leading to an increase in glomerular permeability along with proteinuria. The client will next exhibit a decrease in serum protein in the blood followed by generalized edema throughout the body.

 NCLEX® Connection: Physiological Adaptation, Pathophysiology

2. A nurse is caring for a client with nephrotic syndrome. The client asks the nurse why her legs and feet are swollen. How can the nurse best address the client's concerns?

The nurse should explain that the client's kidneys are not able to rid her body of excess fluids that collect in the tissues. The nurse should reassure the client that interventions will be implemented to help rid her body of fluids while her kidneys heal.

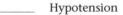 NCLEX® Connection: Physiological Adaptation, Pathophysiology

3. Which of the following signs and symptoms should the nurse monitor for in a client with nephrotic syndrome? (Select all that apply.)

__X__	**Malnutrition**
__X__	**Hematuria**
__X__	**Infection**
__X__	**Peritonitis**
__X__	**Hyperkalemia**
_____	Hypotension
__X__	**Fever**

Malnutrition, hematuria, infection, peritonitis, hyperkalemia, and fever should all be signs and symptoms related to a client with nephrotic syndrome. Hypotension would not be indicated in the client.

 NCLEX® Connection: Reduction of Risk Potential, System Specific Assessment

4. Which of the following assessments should be made while the client is in acute renal failure? (Select all that apply.)

_____	Cardiac enzymes
__X__	**Blood glucose**
__X__	**Blood pressure**
__X__	**Serum electrolytes**
__X__	**Serum creatinine**
__X__	**Arterial blood gases**
__X__	**Urine output**

Blood glucose, blood pressure, serum electrolytes, serum creatinine, arterial blood gases, and urine output should all be indicated for a client with acute renal failure. Cardiac enzymes is not indicated for the client.

(N) NCLEX® Connection: Reduction of Risk Potential, System Specific Assessment

5. Prioritize the following nursing interventions according to how they occur in a client diagnosed with renal failure.

__1__	**Monitor serum potassium level.**
__3__	**Turn the client every 2 hr.**
__4__	**Offer emotional support to the family.**
__2__	**Assess breath sounds.**

According to the sequence of events, the first intervention the nurse should take for a client in renal failure is to monitor the client's potassium level. The nurse should then listen to the client's breath sounds to assess for a possible respiratory infection. Next, the nurse should turn the client every 2 hr since the client may be weak and unable to turn himself. This also promotes circulation to the body. The family will require emotional support due to the client's disease, which can be acute or chronic and may require dialysis or surgery with the medication regimen.

(N) NCLEX® Connection: Physiological Adaptation, Pathophysiology

UNIT 8	NURSING CARE OF CLIENTS WITH RENAL DISORDERS
Section	Renal System Disorders
Chapter 69	Infections of the Renal System

Overview

- There are three components to the urinary system: the ureter, bladder, and urethra. The goal of the urinary system is to promote optimal kidney function. Two infections that affect the renal system are urinary tract infections, and pyelonephritis.

URINARY TRACT INFECTION

Overview

- A urinary tract infection (UTI) refers to any portion of the lower urinary tract. This includes:

  o Cystitis.

  o Urethritis.

  o Prostatitis.

- An upper UTI refers to conditions including pyelonephritis.

- UTIs are caused by Enterobacteriaceae micro-organisms (Klebsiella, Proteus), Pseudomonas, Serratia, and most commonly, Escherichia coli.

- Untreated UTIs may lead to urosepsis, which can cause septic shock and death.

Assessment

- Risk Factors

  o Female gender

    ▪ Short urethra predisposes women to UTIs

    ▪ Close proximity of the urethra to the rectum

    ▪ Decreased estrogen in aging women promotes atrophy of the urethral opening toward the rectum (increases the risk of urosepsis in women)

    ▪ Sexual intercourse

- ■ Frequent use of feminine hygiene sprays, tampons, sanitary napkins, and spermicidal jellies

- ■ Pregnancy

- ■ Women who have poorly fitted diaphragms

- ■ Hormonal influences within the vaginal flora

- ■ Synthetic underwear and pantyhose

- ■ Wet bathing suits

- ■ Frequent submersion into baths or hot tubs

- o Indwelling urinary catheters (significant source of infection in clients who are hospitalized)

- o Stool incontinence

- o Bladder distention

- o Urinary conditions (anomalies, stasis, calculi, residual urine)

- o Possible genetic links

- o Disease (diabetes mellitus)

- Ⓖ o Older adult clients have an increased risk of bacteremia, sepsis, and shock.

- o Renal complications increase for older adult clients due to a decreased number of functioning nephrons and fluid intake.

- • Subjective Data

  - o Lower back or lower abdominal discomfort and tenderness over the bladder area

  - o Nausea

  - o Urinary frequency and urgency

  - o Dysuria, bladder cramping, or spasms

  - o Perineal itching

  - o Hematuria (red-tinged, smoky, coffee colored urine)

  - o Pyuria

- • Objective Data

  - o Fever

  - o Vomiting

  - o Voiding in small amounts

  - o Nocturia

  - o Urethral discharge

  - o Cloudy or foul smelling urine

- ○ Laboratory Tests
  - ■ Urinalysis and urine culture and sensitivity
    - □ Nursing Actions
      - ▸ Instruct the client regarding proper technique for the collection of a clean catch urine specimen.
      - ▸ Collect catheterized urine specimens using sterile technique.
    - □ Expected findings include:
      - ▸ Bacteria, sediment, white blood cells (WBC), and red blood cells (RBC).
      - ▸ Positive leukocyte esterase (85% to 90% specific).
      - ▸ Positive nitrate (95% specific).
  - ■ WBC count and differential if urosepsis is suspected
    - □ White blood cell count at or above 10,000/mm³ with a shift to the left (indicating an increased number of immature cells in response to infection).
  - ■ Rule out sexually transmitted diseases.
- ○ Diagnostic Procedures
  - ■ Cystoscopy is used for complicated UTIs.

Collaborative Care

- • Nursing Care
  - ○ Promote fluid intake up to 3L daily.
  - ○ Consult with the provider regarding prescribed fluid restrictions if needed.
  - ○ Administer medications as prescribed.
  - ○ Encourage clients to urinate every 3 to 4 hr instead of waiting until the bladder is completely full.
  - ○ Encourage clients to bathe daily to promote good body hygiene.
  - ○ Avoid the use of indwelling catheters if possible. This reduces the risk for infection.
- • Medications
  - ○ Fluoroquinolones (Ciprofloxacin), nitrofurantoin (Macrobid), or sulfonamides (Bactrim or Septra) are antibiotics used to treat urinary infections.
    - ■ Nursing Considerations
      - □ If sulfonamide is prescribed, ask the client if there he/she is allergic to sulfa.
    - ■ Client Education
      - □ Educate the client regarding the need to take all of the prescribed antibiotics even if symptoms subside.
      - □ Encourage the client to take the medication with food.

- ○ Phenazopyridine is bladder analgesic used to treat UTIs.
  - ▪ Nursing Considerations
    - ▫ The medication will not treat the infection, but will help relieve bladder discomfort.
    - ▫ Inform the client that the medication will turn urine orange.
  - ▪ Client Education
    - ▫ Encourage the client to take the medication with food.
- **Interdisciplinary Care**
  - ○ Urology services may be consulted for managing UTIs.
- **Care after Discharge**
  - ○ Urology services may be consulted for management of long-term antibiotic therapy for chronic UTIs.
- **Client Education**
  - ○ Instruct the client to drink at least 3L of fluid daily.
  - ○ Instruct the client to bathe daily to promote good body hygiene.
  - ○ Advise the client to empty bladder every 3 to 4 hr instead of waiting until the bladder is completely full.
  - ○ Advise the client to urinate before and after intercourse.
  - ○ Advise the client to drink cranberry juice as an alternative to water to decrease the risk of infection.
  - ○ Advise the client to empty the bladder as soon as there is an urgency to void.
  - ○ Instruct female clients to:
    - ▫ Wipe the perineal area from front to back.
    - ▫ Avoid using bubble baths, or feminine products or toilet paper containing perfumes.
    - ▫ Avoid sitting in wet bathing suits.
    - ▫ Avoid wearing pantyhose with slacks or tight clothing.
- **Client Outcomes**
  - ○ The client will be free from pain.
  - ○ The client will be free of infection.
  - ○ The client will take the medication as prescribed.
  - ○ The client will drink at least 3 L daily to decrease the risk of infection.

Complications

- Urethral obstruction, pyelonephritis, chronic renal failure, urosepsis, septic shock, and death

  - Nursing Actions

    - Monitor/assess the client.

    - Report abnormal data promptly.

    - Maintain medication schedules to assure adequate medication blood levels to eradicate infection.

PYELONEPHRITIS

Overview

- Pyelonephritis is an infection and inflammation of the renal pelvis, calyces, and medulla. The infection usually begins in the lower urinary tract with organisms ascending into the renal pelvis.

- Escherichia coli organisms are the cause of most acute cases of pyelonephritis.

- Repeated infections create scarring that changes the blood flow to the kidney, glomerulus, and tubular structure.

- Filtration, reabsorption, and secretion are impaired, which results in a decrease in renal function.

- Acute pyelonephritis is an active bacterial infection that can cause:

  - Interstitial inflammation.

  - Tubular cell necrosis.

  - Abscess formation in the capsule, cortex, or medulla.

  - Temporarily altered renal function (this rarely progresses to renal failure).

- Chronic pyelonephritis is the result of repeated infections that cause progressive inflammation and scarring.

  - This can result in the thickening of the calyces and postinflammatory fibrosis with permanent renal tissue scarring.

  - It is more common with obstructions, urinary anomaly, and vesicoureteral urine reflux.

  - Reflux of urine occurs at the junction where the ureter connects to the bladder.

Assessment

- Risk Factors

    (G)

    - Women over 65 years of age
    - Older men with prostate problems
    - Chronic urinary stone disorders
    - Spinal cord injury
    - Pregnancy
    - Congenital malformations
    - Bladder tumors
    - Chronic illness (diabetes mellitus, hypertension, chronic cystitis)

    (G)

    - A decrease in vascular flow in older adult clients may decrease blood flow to the kidneys.
    - Urine pH increases in older adult clients and promotes bacterial growth.
    - Incomplete bladder emptying is more common among older adult clients.
    - Older adult clients may exhibit gastrointestinal or pulmonary symptoms instead of febrile responses.

- Subjective Data

    - Chills
    - Colicky-type abdominal pain
    - Nausea
    - Malaise, fatigue
    - Burning, urgency, and frequency with urination
    - Costovertebral tenderness

- Objective Data

    - Fever, tachycardia, tachypnea, hypertension
    - Flank and back pain
    - Vomiting
    - Nocturia
    - Inability to concentrate urine or conserve sodium (chronic pyelonephritis)
    - Asymptomatic Bacteremia

- Laboratory Tests

  - Urinalysis and urine culture and sensitivity

    - Monitor for:

      - Dark color, cloudy appearance, and foul odor

      - Bacteria, sediment, white blood cells, and red blood cells

      - Positive leukocyte esterase (85% to 90% specific)

      - Positive nitrate (95% specific)

  - WBC count and differential: A white blood cell count at or above 10,000/mm^3 with a shift to the left indicates an increased number of immature cells in response to an infection.

  - Blood cultures will be positive for the presence of bacteria if a systemic infection is present.

  - Serum creatinine and blood urea nitrogen (BUN) are elevated during acute episodes and consistently elevated with chronic infection.

  - C-reactive protein is elevated during exacerbating inflammatory processes.

    - Erythrocyte sedimentation rate (ESR) is elevated during acute or chronic inflammation.

- Diagnostic Procedures

  - An X-ray of the kidneys, ureters, and bladder (KUB) may demonstrate calculi or structural abnormalities.

  - Gallium scan should be used to identify active pyelonephritis or an abscess related to specific enzymes present.

  - Intravenous pyelogram (IVP) may demonstrate calculi, structural, or vascular abnormalities.

    - Nursing Actions

      - Assess renal function and allergy to contrast dye prior to the procedure.

    - Client Education

      - Inform the client that bowel preparation may be prescribed prior to the procedure for image clarity.

      - Inform the client of hydration prior to the procedure and that diuretic administration following the procedure may be prescribed to reduce the risk of nephrotoxicity.

Collaborative Care

- Nursing Care

  o Assess/Monitor:

    ■ Nutritional status.

    ■ Intake and output.

    ■ Fluid and electrolyte balance.

    ■ Pain status.

    ■ Temperature

    ■ The onset, quality, duration, and severity of the pain.

  o Increase fluid intake to 2 to 3 L/day unless contraindicated.

  o Administer antipyretic as needed.

  o Provide emotional support.

  o Assist with personal hygiene.

- Medications

  o Opioid analgesics (opioid agonists), morphine sulfate, and morphine

    ■ Opioid agents are used to treat moderate to severe pain. These drugs act on the mu and kappa receptors that help alleviate pain. Activation of these receptors produces analgesia (pain relief), respiratory depression, euphoria, sedation, and a decrease in GI motility.

    ■ Use cautiously with clients who have asthma or emphysema due to the risk of respiratory depression.

    ■ Nursing Considerations

      □ Assess the client's pain every 4 hr.

      □ Watch the client for signs of respiratory depression, especially in older adults. If respirations are 12 or less, stop the medication and notify the provider immediately.

      □ Monitor the client's vital signs closely for sign of hypotension and decreased respirations.

      □ Assess the client's level of sedation (drowsiness, LOC [level of consciousness]).

    ■ Client Education

      □ Encourage the client to suck on hard candies to help with dry mouth.

      □ Encourage the client to drink plenty of fluids to help prevent constipation.

- Non-steroidal anti-inflammatory agents (NSAIDs), Ibuprofen
  - These are used to treat mild to moderate pain, fever, and inflammation.
  - Nursing Considerations
    - Encourage clients to take with food to decrease GI distress.
    - Observe for signs of bleeding.
  - Client Education
    - Instruct the client to watch for signs of bleeding.
    - Instruct the client to notify the provider if signs of gastric discomfort of ulceration occur.
- Antibiotics: nitrofurantoin (Macrodantin)
  - Antibiotic used to treat UTIs.
  - Nursing Considerations
    - Encourage clients to notify the provider immediately if persistent cough begins after starting the medication.
    - Inform clients that the medication may turn urine color brown.
  - Client Education
    - Encourage the client to take with food.

- Interdisciplinary Care
  - Urology services may be consulted to manage pyelonephritis.
  - Nutritional services may be consulted to promote adequate calories for the client.
- Surgical Interventions
  - Pyelolithotomy
    - This is the removal of a stone from the kidney.
    - Nursing Actions
      - Inform the client of the purpose of the surgery and expected outcomes.
      - Intravenous antibiotics and analgesics are usually administered for this procedure.
  - Nephrectomy
    - This is the removal of the kidney.
    - Nursing Actions
      - Inform the client of the purpose of the surgery and expected outcomes.
      - Intravenous antibiotics and analgesics are usually administered for this procedure.

- ○ Ureteroplasty
  - ▪ This is done to repair or revise the ureter.
  - ▪ Nursing Actions
    - ☐ Inform the client of the purpose of the surgery and expected outcomes.
    - ☐ Intravenous antibiotics and analgesics are usually administered for this procedure.
- • Care after Discharge
  - ○ Home care services may be indicated if the client needs assistance with medications or nutritional therapy.
  - ○ Follow up with the provider as directed
- • Client Education
  - ○ Educate the client regarding adequate nutritional status.
  - ○ Encourage the client to drink at least 3 L of fluids daily unless otherwise indicated by the provider.
  - ○ Instruct the client to take medications as prescribed.
  - ○ Instruct the client to notify the provider if acute onset of pain occurs or a fever is present.
  - ○ Encourage the client and family to express their fears and anxiety related to the disease.
  - ○ Encourage the client to take rest periods as needed from activity.
- • Client Outcomes
  - ○ The client will be free from pain.
  - ○ The client will have a decrease in anxiety.
  - ○ The client will be compliant with a medication regimen.
  - ○ The client will have an increase in activity level.

Complications

- • Septic Shock
  - ○ Nursing Actions
    - ▪ Identify signs (hypotension, tachycardia, fever).
    - ▪ Initiate life-support interventions as needed.

- Renal Failure
  - Nursing Actions
    - Monitor intake and output.
    - Monitor renal function studies for elevations in BUN and creatinine.
    - Encourage increased fluid intake.
- Hypertension
  - Nursing Actions
    - Monitor blood pressure for trends.
    - Report changes from baseline.

INFECTIONS OF THE RENAL SYSTEM

CHAPTER 69: INFECTIONS OF THE RENAL SYSTEM

Ⓐ Application Exercises

1. Which of the following findings should the nurse expect to see when reviewing the laboratory report of a client with pyelonephritis? (Select all that apply.)

_____ Elevated BUN

_____ Decreased C-reactive protein

_____ Positive leukocyte esterase

_____ Decreased ESR

_____ Bacteriuria

_____ Decreased serum protein

2. Which of the following clients is at risk for developing pyelonephritis? (Select all that apply.)

_____ A client who is pregnant

_____ A client who just had a catheterized urine specimen obtained

_____ A client who has not voided for 8 hr postoperatively

_____ A client who has a neurogenic bladder

_____ A client who has diabetes mellitus

3. A nurse is caring for a client who is diagnosed with a urinary tract infection. The client reports pain and a burning sensation upon urination, and cloudy urine with an odor. Which of the following actions should the nurse take?

A. Offer a warm sitz bath.

B. Encourage increased fluids.

C. Obtain a set of vital signs.

D. Administer an antibiotic.

CHAPTER 69: INFECTIONS OF THE RENAL SYSTEM

 Application Exercises Answer Key

1. Which of the following findings should the nurse expect to see when reviewing the laboratory report of a client with pyelonephritis? (Select all that apply.)

X	**Elevated BUN**
_____	Decreased C-reactive protein
X	**Positive leukocyte esterase**
_____	Decreased ESR
X	**Bacteriuria**
_____	Decreased serum protein

An elevated BUN, positive leukocyte esterase, and bacteriuria are all expected findings in a client with pyelonephritis. A decreased C-reactive protein, ESR, and serum protein are not expected findings.

 NCLEX® Connection: Reduction of Risk Potential, Laboratory Values

2. Which of the following clients is at risk for developing pyelonephritis? (Select all that apply.)

X	**A client who is pregnant**
_____	A client who had a catheterized urine specimen obtained
_____	A client who has not voided for 8 hr postoperatively
X	**A client who has a neurogenic bladder**
X	**A client who has diabetes mellitus**

Pregnancy, a neurogenic bladder, and diabetes mellitus are all risk factors for developing pyelonephritis. A client who had a catheterized urine specimen obtained or has not voided for 8 hr postoperatively, is not at risk for developing pyelonephritis.

 NCLEX® Connection: Reduction of Risk Potential, Potential for Alterations in Body Systems

3. A nurse is caring for a client who is diagnosed with a urinary tract infection. The client reports pain and a burning sensation upon urination, and cloudy urine with an odor. Which of the following actions should the nurse take?

A. Offer a warm sitz bath.

B. Encourage increased fluids.

C. Obtain a set of vital signs.

D. Administer an antibiotic.

The greatest risk to the client is injury from the UTI. The first action the nurse should take is to administer the prescribed antibiotic. Offering a warm sitz bath, encouraging increased fluid intake, and obtaining the client's vital signs are important, but not the first action the nurse should take.

 NCLEX® Connection: Physiological Adaptation, Infectious Disease

UNIT 8	NURSING CARE OF CLIENTS WITH RENAL DISORDERS
Section	Renal System Disorders
Chapter 70	Renal Calculi

 Overview

- Urolithiasis is the presence of calculi (stones) in the urinary tract.

- The majority of stones (75%) are composed of calcium phosphate or calcium oxalate, but may contain other substances (uric acid, struvite, cystine).

- A diet high in calcium is not believed to increase the risk of stone formation unless there is a preexisting metabolic disorder or renal tubular defect.

- Reoccurrence is increased (35% to 50%) in individuals with calcium stones who have a family history, or whose first occurrence of urinary calculi is prior to the age of 25.

- Most clients can expel stones without invasive procedures. Factors that influence whether a stone will pass spontaneously or not include the composition, size, and location of the stone.

> **(M) View Media Supplement:** Renal Calculus (Image)

Assessment

- Risk Factors

  o The cause of urolithiasis is unknown.

  o There is an increased incidence of urolithiasis in males.

  o Urolithiasis formation is associated with:

    ▪ Urinary tract lining that is usually damaged.

    ▪ Urine flow that is decreased and concentrated containing particles (calcium).

    ▪ Decreased inhibitor substances in the urine.

    ▪ Metabolic defects including:

      □ Increased intestinal absorption or decreased renal excretion of calcium.

      □ Increased oxalate production (genetic) or ingestion from foods.

      □ Increased production or decreased clearance of purines (contributing to increased uric-acid levels).

- Stone formation can be attributed to high alkalinity or acidity in the urine.

- Urinary stasis, urinary retention, immobilization, and dehydration contribute to an environment favorable for stone formation.

Ⓖ
- Decreased fluid intake or increased incidence of dehydration among older adult clients may increase the risk of stone formation.

- Subjective Data

  - Severe pain (renal colic)

    - Pain intensifies as stone moves through the ureter.

    - Flank pain suggests stones are located in the kidney or ureter.

    - Flank pain that radiates to the abdomen, scrotum, testes, or vulva is suggestive of stones in the ureter or bladder.

  - Urinary frequency or dysuria (occurs with stones in the bladder)

  - Fever

- Objective Data

  - Diaphoresis

  - Pallor

  - Nausea/vomiting

  - Vital signs: Tachycardia, tachypnea, increased or decreased blood pressure with pain

  - Oliguria/anuria (occurs with stones that obstruct urinary flow)

  - Hematuria (smoky-looking urine)

  - Laboratory Tests

    - Urinalysis is used to detect:

      - The odor of the urine and increased urine turbidity if infection is present.

      - Increased RBCs, WBCs, and bacteria.

      - Crystals noted on microscopic exam.

      - Elevated WBC if infection is present.

      - Abnormal serum calcium, phosphate, and uric-acid levels in the presence of metabolic disorders/defects.

- o Diagnostic Procedures
  - Radiology examination
    - □ KUB (x-ray of kidney, ureters, bladder), noncontrast helical CT scan, or IVP (intravenous pyelogram) is used to confirm the presence and location of stones. IVP is contraindicated if there is a urinary obstruction.
  - CT or MRI
    - □ A CT or MRI is used to identify cystine or uric-acid stones, which cannot be seen on standard x-rays.
  - A renal ultrasound or cystoscopy may confirm the diagnosis.

Collaborative Care

- Nursing Care
  - o Report abnormal findings to the provider.
  - o Provide preoperative and postoperative care as indicated.
  - o Assess/Monitor for:
    - Pain status.
    - Intake and output.
    - Urinary pH.
  - o Administer prescribed medications.
  - o Strain all urine to check for passage of the stone and save the stone for laboratory analysis.
  - o Encourage increased oral intake to 3 L/day unless contraindicated.
  - o Administer intravenous fluids as prescribed.
  - o Encourage ambulation to promote passage of the stone.
- Medications
  - o Analgesics
    - Opioids (morphine sulfate)
      - □ Used for the acute onset of stones within the first 24 hr
      - □ Opioid agents are used to treat moderate to severe pain. These drugs act on the mu and kappa receptors that help alleviate pain. Activation of these receptors produce analgesia (pain relief), respiratory depression, euphoria, sedation, and decrease in GI motility.
      - □ Use cautiously with clients who have asthma or emphysema due to the risk of respiratory depression.

- □ Nursing Considerations
  - ▸ Assess the client's pain every 4 hr.
  - ▸ Watch the client for signs of respiratory depression, especially in older adult clients. If respirations are 12 or less, stop the medication and notify the provider immediately.
  - ▸ Monitor the client's vital signs closely for signs of hypotension and decreased respirations.
  - ▸ Assess the client's level of sedation (drowsiness, LOC [level of consciousness]).
- □ Client Education
  - ▸ Encourage the client to suck on hard candies to help with dry mouth.
  - ▸ Encourage the client to drink plenty of fluids to help prevent constipation.
- ■ NSAIDS ([ketorolac], Toradol)
  - □ Used to treat mild to moderate pain, fever, and inflammation.
  - □ Nursing Considerations
    - ▸ Observe for signs of bleeding.
  - □ Client Education
    - ▸ Instruct the client to watch for signs of bleeding.
    - ▸ Instruct the client to notify the provider if signs of gastric discomfort of ulceration occur.
- ○ Spasmolytic drugs
  - ■ Oxybutynin chloride (Ditropan)
    - □ Used to help alleviate pain with a neurogenic or overactive bladder.
  - ■ Nursing Considerations
    - □ Ask the client if there is a history of glaucoma, as this medication increases intraocular pressure.
    - □ Monitor for dizziness and tachycardia.
    - □ Monitor for urinary retention.
  - ■ Client Education
    - □ Instruct the client report problems voiding or constipation.
    - □ Inform the client to report palpitations.
    - □ Inform client that dizziness and dry mouth are common with the medication.

- ○ Antibiotics, gentamicin (Garamycin) and cephalexin (Keflex)
    - ▪ This is given if an infection is present in order to treat bacteria.
    - ▪ Nursing Considerations
        - □ Administer medication with food to decrease GI distress.
    - ▪ Client Education
        - □ Inform the client that urine may have foul odor related to the antibiotic.
        - □ Instruct the client to report loose stools related to the medication.

- • Interdisciplinary Care
    - ○ Urology services may be consulted for management of urolithiasis.
    - ○ Nutritional services may be consulted for dietary modifications concerning foods related to stone formation.

- • Therapeutic Procedures
    - ○ Extracorporeal shock wave lithotripsy (ESWL)
        - ▪ Uses sound, laser, or shock-wave energies to break the stone into fragments.
        - ▪ Requires moderate (conscious) sedation and ECG monitoring during the procedure.
        - ▪ Nursing Actions
            - □ Educate the client regarding ESWL.
            - □ Assess gross hematuria following the procedure.
            - □ Strain urine following the procedure.
            - □ Provide pain relief following procedure.
        - ▪ Client Education
            - □ Inform the client that bruising is normal at the site where waves are applied.
            - □ Explain to the client that there will be hematuria postprocedure.

- • Surgical Interventions
    - ○ Stenting
        - ▪ Stenting is the placement of a small tube in the ureter during a ureteroscopy to dilate the ureter, enlarging the passageway for the stone to be passed.
    - ○ Retrograde ureteroscopy
        - ▪ Retrograde ureteroscopy uses a basket, forceps, or loop on the end of the ureteroscope to grasp and remove the stone.
    - ○ Percutaneous ureterolithotomy/nephrolithotomy
        - ▪ Percutaneous ureterolithotomy/nephrolithotomy is the insertion of an ultrasonic or laser lithotripter into the ureter or kidney to grasp and extract the stone.

- o Open surgery
  - ■ Open surgery uses a surgical incision to remove the stone. This surgery is used for large or impacted stones (staghorn calculi), or for stones not removed by other approaches.
  - ■ Ureterolithotomy (into the ureter).
  - ■ Pyelolithotomy (into the kidney pelvis)
  - ■ Nephrolithotomy (into the kidney)
- Care after Discharge
  - o Nutritional services may be consulted for dietary modifications concerning foods related to stone formation.
- Client Education
  - o Educate the client regarding the role of diet and medications in the treatment and prevention of urinary stones.
    - ■ Calcium phosphate
      - □ Limit intake of food high in animal protein (reduction of protein intake decreases calcium precipitation).
      - □ Limit sodium intake.
      - □ Reduced calcium intake (dairy products) is individualized.
      - □ Medications
        - ‣ Thiazide diuretics (hydrochlorothiazide) are used to increase calcium reabsorption.
        - ‣ Orthophosphates are used to decrease urine saturation of calcium oxalate.
        - ‣ Sodium cellulose phosphate is used to reduce the intestinal absorption of calcium.
    - ■ Calcium oxalate
      - □ Avoid oxalate sources: Spinach, black tea, rhubarb, cocoa, beets, pecans, peanuts, okra, chocolate, wheat germ, lime peel, and Swiss chard.
      - □ Limit sodium intake.
    - ■ Struvite (magnesium ammonium phosphate)
      - □ Avoid high-phosphate foods (dairy products, red and organ meats, whole grains).

- Uric acid (urate)
    - □ Decrease intake of purine sources (organ meats, poultry, fish, gravies, red wine, sardines).
    - □ Medications
        - ‣ Allopurinol (Zyloprim) is used to prevent the formation of uric acid.
        - ‣ Potassium or sodium citrate or sodium bicarbonate is used to alkalinize the urine.
- Cystine
    - □ Limit animal protein intake.
    - □ Medications
        - ‣ Alpha mercapto propionylglycine (AMPG) is used to lower urine cystine.
        - ‣ Captopril (Capoten) is used to lower urine cystine.

- Client Outcomes
    - ○ The client will have a decrease in anxiety.
    - ○ The client will be free from pain.
    - ○ The client will be free from infection.
    - ○ The client will take the medication as prescribed and follow dietary restrictions.

Complications

- Obstruction
    - ○ A stone may block the passage of urine into the kidney, ureter, or bladder. The client's urinary output may be greatly diminished or absent.
    - ○ Nursing Action
        - Notify the provider immediately.
        - Prepare the client for removal of the stone.
- Hydronephrosis
    - ○ This occurs when a stone has blocked a portion of the urinary tract. The urine becomes backed up and causes distension of the kidney.
    - ○ Nursing action
        - Notify the provider immediately.
        - Prepare the client for removal of the stone.

CHAPTER 70: RENAL CALCULI

 Application Exercises

1. A male client is admitted to the nursing unit with a diagnosis of right renal calculus. Upon assessment, the client reports nausea with moderate right flank pain that radiates to his right testicle. His admission vitals are: blood pressure 142/86 mm Hg, heart rate 96/min, respirations 24/min, and temperature 37.2° C (99° F). What additional nursing assessment is indicated specific to this client's diagnosis of renal calculus?

2. A nurse is caring for a client who is admitted to the nursing unit with a diagnosis of left renal calculus. She has an indwelling urinary catheter and is receiving 0.9% sodium chloride IV infusing at 150 mL/hr. Which of the following assessment findings indicates intervention by the nurse?

   A. Flank pain that radiates to the lower abdomen

   B. Nausea that is controlled with prescribed medication

   C. No urine output for 2 hr

   D. The client reports feeling "sweaty"

3. A client is scheduled for extracorporeal shock wave lithotripsy (ESWL). Which of the following statements by the client demonstrates a correct understanding of the procedure?

   A. "I will be fully awake during the procedure."

   B. "Lithotripsy will reduce my chances of stone reoccurrence."

   C. "I will report any bruising that occurs to my doctor."

   D. "Straining my urine following the procedure is important."

4. A nurse is completing discharge instructions for a client who spontaneously passed a urinary calcium phosphate stone. Which of the following foods should the nurse instruct the client to avoid? (Select all that apply.)

   _____ Organ meats

   _____ Tea

   _____ Cheese

   _____ Soy sauce

   _____ Fish

   _____ Red meat

   _____ Rhubarb

   _____ Red wines

   _____ Dairy products

   _____ Whole grains

   _____ Spinach

5. A client is to be discharged home after a spontaneous passage of a calcium phosphate stone. The nurse informs the client of ways to prevent reoccurrence. Which of the following should be included in the discharge plan? (Select all that apply.)

_____ Limit the intake of foods high in animal protein.

_____ Reduce sodium intake in diet.

_____ Avoid drinking fluids at bedtime.

_____ Limit physical activity throughout the day.

_____ Report burning or dysuria to the provider.

_____ Increase fluid intake to 3 L/day.

_____ Strain all urine.

6. Match the appropriate medications to the types of calculi listed below.

_____ Calcium phosphate   A. Allopurinol (Zyloprim)

_____ Calcium oxalate   B. Captopril (Capoten)

_____ Uric acid (urate)   C. Thiazide diuretic

_____ Cystine   D. Vitamin B_6 (pyridoxine)

CHAPTER 70: RENAL CALCULI

 Application Exercises Answer Key

1. A male client is admitted to the nursing unit with a diagnosis of right renal calculus. Upon assessment, the client reports nausea with moderate right flank pain that radiates to his right testicle. His admission vitals are: blood pressure 142/86 mm Hg, heart rate 96/min, respirations 24/min, and temperature 37.2° C (99° F).What additional nursing assessment is indicated specific to this client's diagnosis of renal calculus?

Diet history and assessment of fluid intake patterns

A personal or family history of calculi

Altered patterns of elimination, including dysuria, frequency, or oliguria

Detailed pain assessment, including intensity, location, and character

Observation of urinary output, including amount and presence of stones, hematuria

 NCLEX® Connection: Reduction of Risk Potential, System Specific Assessment

2. A nurse is caring for a client who is admitted to the nursing unit with a diagnosis of left renal calculus. She has an indwelling urinary catheter and is receiving 0.9% sodium chloride IV infusing at 150 mL/hr. Which of the following assessment findings indicates intervention by the nurse?

A. Flank pain that radiates to the lower abdomen

B. Nausea that is controlled with prescribed medication

C. No urine output for 2 hr

D. The client reports feeling "sweaty"

The lack of urine output may indicate an obstruction and requires an immediate intervention by the nurse. Nausea, flank pain that radiates to the abdomen, and sweating are all common occurrences associated with a renal calculus.

NCLEX® Connection: Reduction of Risk Potential, System Specific Assessment

3. A client is scheduled for extracorporeal shock wave lithotripsy (ESWL). Which of the following statements by the client demonstrates a correct understanding of the procedure?

A. "I will be fully awake during the procedure."

B. "Lithotripsy will reduce my chances of stone reoccurrence."

C. "I will report any bruising that occurs to my doctor."

D. "Straining my urine following the procedure is important."

Straining the urine will allow for analysis of the stone. The other statements indicate a need for additional teaching.

NCLEX® Connection: Reduction of Risk Potential, Therapeutic Procedures

4. A nurse is completing discharge instructions for a client who spontaneously passed a urinary calcium phosphate stone. Which of the following foods should the nurse instruct the client to avoid? (Select all that apply.)

_____ Organ meats

_____ Tea

__X__ **Cheese**

__X__ **Soy sauce**

_____ Fish

__X__ **Red meat**

_____ Rhubarb

_____ Red wines

_____ Dairy products

_____ Whole grains

_____ Spinach

Cheese, soy sauce, and red meat all contain calcium phosphate and should be avoided by the client. The other food options do not need to be avoided by the client as they do not contain calcium phosphate.

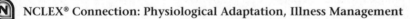 NCLEX® Connection: Physiological Adaptation, Illness Management

5. A client is to be discharged home after a spontaneous passage of a calcium phosphate stone. The nurse informs the client of ways to prevent reoccurrence. Which of the following should be included in the discharge plan? (Select all that apply.)

__X__ **Limit the intake of foods high in animal protein.**

__X__ **Reduce sodium intake in diet.**

_____ Avoid drinking fluids at bedtime.

_____ Limit physical activity throughout the day.

__X__ **Report burning or dysuria to the provider.**

__X__ **Increase fluid intake to 3 L/day.**

_____ Strain all urine.

Limiting the intake of foods high in animal protein, reducing sodium intake, reporting burning or dysuria to the provider, and increasing fluid intake to 3 L/day should be included in the nurse's discharge teaching. The other options are not indicated for the client.

NCLEX® Connection: Physiological Adaptation, Illness Management

6. Match the appropriate medications to the types of calculi listed below.

C	Calcium phosphate	A. Allopurinol (Zyloprim)
A,D	Calcium oxalate	B. Captopril (Capoten)
A	Uric acid (urate)	C. Thiazide diuretic
B	Cystine	D. Vitamin B_6 (pyridoxine)

Ⓝ NCLEX® Connection: Pharmacological and Parenteral Therapies, Expected Actions/Outcomes

UNIT 8	NURSING CARE OF CLIENTS WITH RENAL DISORDERS
Section	Renal System Disorders

Chapter 71   Voiding Disorders

Overview

- There are six major types of urinary incontinence:

    o   Stress – The loss of small amounts of urine when laughing, sneezing, or lifting. Stress incontinence is related primarily to weak pelvic muscles, urethra, or surrounding tissues.

    o   Urge – The inability to stop urine flow long enough to reach the bathroom. Urge incontinence is related to an overactive detrusor muscle with increased bladder pressure.

    o   Overflow –Urinary retention associated with bladder overdistention and frequent loss of small amounts of urine. Overflow incontinence is related to obstruction of the urinary outlet or an impaired detrusor muscle.

    o   Reflex – The involuntary loss of a moderate amount of urine usually without warning. Reflex incontinence is related to hyperreflexia of the detrusor muscle, usually from altered spinal cord activity.

    o   Functional – The inability to make it to the bathroom to urinate. Functional incontinence is related to physical, cognitive, or social impairment.

    o   Total incontinence – The unpredictable, involuntary loss of urine that does not generally respond to treatment.

- Urinary incontinence is a significant contributing factor to altered skin integrity and falls, especially in older adults.

Assessment

- Risk Factors

    o   Female

    o   History of multiple pregnancies and vaginal births, aging, chronic urinary retention, urinary bladder spasm, renal disease, and chronic bladder infection (cystitis)

    o   Neurological disorders: Parkinson's disease, cerebrovascular accident, spinal cord injury, multiple sclerosis

    o   Medication therapy: Diuretics, narcotics, anticholinergics, calcium channel blockers, sedative/hypnotics, and adrenergic antagonists

- o Obesity

- o Confusion, dementia, immobility, and depression

- o Older adult client (due to physiological changes secondary to aging)

- o Decreased estrogen levels and decreased pelvic-muscle tone

- o Risks may be attributed to immobility, chronic degenerative diseases, dementia, diabetes mellitus, stroke, and medications

- o Urinary incontinence is associated with a risk for falls, fractures, pressure ulcers, and depression.

- Subjective Data

  - o Loss of urine when laughing, coughing, or sneezing

  - o Enuresis (bed-wetting)

  - o Bladder spasms

  - o Urinary retention

  - o Frequency, urgency, nocturia

- Objective Data

  - o Laboratory Tests

    - Urinalysis and urine culture/sensitivity – to rule out urinary tract infection (presence of RBCs, WBCs, microorganisms).

    - Serum creatinine and BUN – to assess renal function (elevated with renal dysfunction).

  - o Diagnostic Procedures

    - Postvoid residual urine using a pelvis ultrasonographic scanner or postvoid catheterization– to rule out urinary retention (greater than 100 mL retained urine post voiding)

    - Voiding cystourethrography (VCUG)

      - □ Used to assess the size, shape, support, and function of the urinary bladder, identify obstruction (prostate), and postvoid residual urine

    - Urodynamic Testing

      - □ Cystourethroscopy

        - ▸ Visualization of the inside of the bladder

      - □ Cystometrogram (CMG)

        - ▸ Measures pressure inside the bladder while urine is filling

      - □ Uroflowmetry

        - ▸ Measures rate and degree of bladder emptying

          □   Urethral pressure profilometry (UPP)

                ▸   Compares urethral pressure to bladder pressure during certain activities (coughing, lifting)

- Electromyography (EMG)

          □   Measures strength of pelvic muscle contractions

- Ultrasound

          □   Used to detect bladder abnormalities and/or residual urine

Collaborative Care

- Nursing Care

    o Establish a toileting schedule.

    o Monitor fluid intake during the daytime, and decrease fluid intake prior to bedtime.

    o Remove or control barriers to toileting.

    o Apply and monitor electrical stimulation of the pelvic floor muscles if ordered.

    o Provide incontinence garments.

    o Apply an external or condom catheter to males.

    o Avoid the use of indwelling urinary catheters.

    o Provide incontinence care.

    o Teach the client:

        - To keep an incontinence diary.

        - How to perform Kegel exercises. Tighten pelvic muscles for a count of 10, relax slowly for a count of 10, and repeat in sequences of 15 in the lying-down, sitting, and standing positions.

        - Bladder compression techniques (Credé, Valsalva, double-voiding, splinting).

        - To avoid caffeine and alcohol consumption as these produce diuresis and the urge to urinate.

        - The side effects of prescribed medications that may stimulate voiding.

        - Vaginal cone therapy to strengthen pelvic muscles (stress incontinence).

- Medications

    o Antibiotics

        - Gentamicin (Garamycin) and cephalexin (Keflex) are given if an infection is present to treat bacteria.

        - Nursing Considerations

            □ Administer medication with food to decrease GI distress.

- Client Education
  - Inform client that urine may have foul odor related to the antibiotic.
  - Instruct the client to report loose stools related to the medication.
  - Encourage the client to complete the full course of therapy even if symptoms resolve.
- Tricyclic antidepressants
  - Nortriptyline (Pamelor) contains anticholinergic effects which can relieve urinary incontinence.
  - Nursing Considerations
    - Medication can cause dizziness.
    - Monitor blood pressure and signs of orthostatic hypotension.
    - This medication should not be given if the client is on MAO inhibitors.
  - Client Education
    - Encourage the client to get up slowly.
- Urinary antispasmodics or anticholinergic agents
  - Oxybutynin (Ditropan) and dicyclomine (Bentyl) are used to decrease urgency and help alleviate pain with a neurogenic or overactive bladder.
  - Nursing Considerations
    - Ask the client if there is a history of glaucoma.
    - The medication increases intraocular pressure.
    - Monitor for dizziness and tachycardia.
    - Inform client that dry mouth and constipation are common with this medication.
    - Monitor for urinary retention.
  - Client Education
    - Instruct the client to report problems voiding or constipation.
    - Instruct the client to report palpitations.
    - Inform the client that dizziness and dry mouth are common with this medication.
- Phenazopyridine (Pyridium)
  - This is a bladder analgesic used to treat urinary tract infections.
  - Nursing Considerations
    - The medication will not treat infection but will help with bladder discomfort.
    - Remind the client that the medication will turn urine orange.

▫ Monitor for a decrease in hemoglobin and hematocrit.

▫ This is contraindicated in clients with hepatic disorders or renal insufficiency.

■ Client Education

▫ Encourage the client to take with food.

▫ Inform the client that the medication turns urine orange in color.

▫ Instruct the client to notify the provider immediately if skin becomes yellow-tinged.

○ Hormone replacement therapy

■ This is controversial, but it increases blood supply to the pelvis.

● Interdisciplinary Care

○ Urology services may be consulted for urinary incontinence.

● Therapeutic Procedures

○ Bladder training program

■ Urinary bladder training increases the bladder's ability to hold urine and the client's ability to suppress urination.

■ Nursing Actions

▫ The client should void at scheduled intervals.

▫ Gradually increase voiding intervals if the client has no incontinence episodes for 3 days until the optimal 4 hr interval is achieved.

■ Client Education

▫ Remind the client to consciously hold urine until the scheduled toileting time.

▫ Encourage the client to keep track of voiding times.

○ Urinary habit training

■ Urinary habit training helps clients with limited cognitive ability to establish a predictable pattern of bladder emptying.

■ Nursing Actions

▫ The client should void at scheduled intervals.

■ Client Education

▫ Inform the client that the toileting schedules are based on voiding patterns.

▫ Encourage the client to maintain a voiding schedule according to the pattern in which no incontinence occurs (every 2 hr).

- o Intermittent urinary catheterization
  - Intermittent urinary catheterization is periodic catheterization to empty the bladder. Intermittent catheterization is recommended over an indwelling urinary catheter due to the risk of infection. Indwelling urinary catheters should be used only when the client is at risk for skin breakdown, or when other options have failed. The use should be temporary.
  - Nursing Actions
    - □ The frequency of catheterization is adjusted to maintain an output of 300 mL or less.
    - □ Explain the procedure to the client.
  - Client Education
    - □ Encourage the client to maintain a voiding schedule according to the pattern in which no incontinence occurs (every 2 hr).
- Surgical Interventions
  - o Anterior vaginal repair, retropubic suspension, pubovaginal sling, and/or insertion of an artificial sphincter
    - Catheters (suprapubic and/or urinary) are typically inserted and maintained until the client has a postvoid residual of less than 50 mL. Traction (with tape) is applied to the catheter to prevent movement of the bladder.
    - Suprapubic catheters are surgically inserted into the abdomen above the pubic bone and in the bladder. This can be performed under a local anesthetic and the catheter is sutured in place. The care for the catheter tubing and drainage bag is the same as for an indwelling catheter.
    - Nursing Actions
      - □ Monitor the client's output closely and for any signs of infection (color of urine, sediment, level of output).
      - □ Keep the catheter patent at all times.
      - □ Determine the client's ability to detect the urge to void.
    - Client Education
      - □ Educate the client regarding proper skin care around the insertion site.
      - □ Educate the client regarding proper care and emptying of the catheter bag.
  - o Periurethral collagen injections to bladder neck
- Care after Discharge
  - o In order to alleviate stress incontinence, nutritional services may be consulted for dietary modifications if the client is obese.
  - o Home care services may be consulted to provide intermittent catheter, portable commode, or stool riser. Handrails can be installed to assist the client in bathroom needs.

     ○ Client Education

- Instruct the client to drink at least 2 to 3 L of fluid daily.

- Instruct the client to try and hold urine, and stay in schedule with bladder training.

- Advise the client to try cranberry juice to decrease the risk of infection.

- Encourage the obese client to participate in a weight reduction program to improve stress incontinence.

- Instruct the client to take medications as prescribed to help with incontinence.

- Educate the client regarding the proper use of an intermittent catheterization, if required.

- Encourage the client to express feelings regarding incontinence.

- **Client Outcomes**

  ○ The client will have decrease in anxiety.

  ○ The client will demonstrate the proper use of incontinence products.

  ○ The client will follow a bladder training program.

  ○ The client will be free from infection.

  ○ The client will take medications as prescribed, and follow dietary restrictions.

Complications

- **Skin Breakdown** (related to chronic exposure to urine)

  ○ Nursing Actions

    - Keep the skin clean and dry.

    - Assess for signs of breakdown.

    - Apply protective barrier creams.

    - Implement bladder retraining program.

- **Social Isolation**

  ○ Nursing Actions

    - Assist the client with measures to conceal urinary leaking (peri-pad, external catheter, adult incontinence garments).

    - Offer emotional support.

CHAPTER 71: VOIDING DISORDERS

(A) Application Exercises

Scenario: A female client visits her provider and reports losing control of urine whenever she coughs, laughs, or sneezes. The client relates a history of three vaginal births, but no serious accidents or illnesses.

1. What type of urinary incontinence is the client experiencing? Explain your answer.

2. Which of the following collaborative interventions are appropriate to control or eliminate the client's incontinence? (Select all that apply.)

    _____ Limit total daily fluid intake.

    _____ Decrease or avoid caffeine.

    _____ Increase the intake of calcium supplements.

    _____ Avoid the intake of alcohol.

    _____ Use Credé maneuver.

    _____ Maintain prescribed hormone therapy.

3. Why is the use of an indwelling catheter contraindicated for long-term control of urinary incontinence?

CHAPTER 71: VOIDING DISORDERS

 Application Exercises Answer Key

Scenario: A female client visits her provider and reports losing control of urine whenever she coughs, laughs, or sneezes. The client relates a history of three vaginal births, but no serious accidents or illnesses.

1. What type of urinary incontinence is the client experiencing? Explain your answer.

Stress incontinence is the loss of small amounts of urine with sneezing, laughing, lifting, or an increase in intra-abdominal pressure. It is primarily related to weak pelvic muscles, urethra, or surrounding tissues.

 NCLEX® Connection: Physiological Adaptation, Pathophysiology

2. Which of the following collaborative interventions are appropriate to control or eliminate the client's incontinence? (Select all that apply.)

_____ Limit total daily fluid intake.

__X__ **Decrease or avoid caffeine.**

_____ Increase the intake of calcium supplements.

__X__ **Avoid the intake of alcohol.**

_____ Use Credé maneuver.

__X__ **Maintain prescribed hormone therapy.**

Decreasing or avoiding the intake of caffeine and alcohol, and maintaining a prescribed hormone therapy, are all appropriate interventions for the client. The other options should not be indicated for the client.

 NCLEX® Connection: Physiological Adaptation, Illness Management

3. Why is the use of an indwelling catheter contraindicated for long-term control of urinary incontinence?

Indwelling urinary catheters increase the risk for infection and subsequent urosepsis in older adults, and should be avoided whenever possible.

 NCLEX® Connection: Physiological Adaptation, Illness Management

UNIT 9: NURSING CARE OF CLIENTS WITH REPRODUCTIVE DISORDERS

- Female Reproductive Disorders
- Male Reproductive Disorders

NCLEX® CONNECTIONS

When reviewing the chapters in this unit, keep in mind the relevant sections of the NCLEX® outline, in particular:

CLIENT NEEDS: BASIC CARE AND COMFORT

Relevant topics/tasks include:
- Elimination
  - Perform irrigations.
  - Evaluate whether the client's elimination is restored/maintained.

CLIENT NEEDS: REDUCTION OF RISK POTENTIAL

Relevant topics/tasks include:
- Diagnostic Tests
  - Compare the client's diagnostic findings with pretest results.
- Laboratory Values
  - Educate the client about the purpose and procedure of prescribed laboratory tests.
- Potential for Alterations in Body Systems
  - Monitor the client's output for changes from baseline.

CLIENT NEEDS: PHYSIOLOGICAL ADAPTATION

Relevant topics/tasks include:
- Alterations in Body Systems
  - Assess the client for signs and symptoms of adverse effects of radiation therapy.
- Illness Management
  - Identify client data that needs to be reported immediately.
- Pathophysiology
  - Understand general principles of pathophysiology.

UNIT 9	NURSING CARE OF CLIENTS WITH REPRODUCTIVE DISORDERS
Section	Female Reproductive Disorders
Chapter 72	Diagnostic and Therapeutic Procedures for Female Reproductive Disorders

Overview

- Diagnostic procedures used to evaluate the structure, condition, and function of a female client's reproductive tissues and organs:

  o Pelvic exam with Papanicolaou (Pap) test

  o Colposcopy and cervical biopsy

  o Cone biopsy

  o Endometrial biopsy

  o Serologic studies

  o Mammography

  o Hysterectomy

- Biopsies can also serve as therapeutic purposes in removing abnormal tissue. Another therapeutic procedure that nurses should be knowledgeable about is a hysterectomy.

Pelvic Exam with Papanicolaou (Pap) Test

- Bimanual examination of the cervix, uterus, fallopian tubes, and ovaries is performed by the provider. The provider inserts two gloved fingers into the vagina and traps the reproductive structures between the fingers of the one hand and the fingers of the opposite hand that is on the abdomen. Palpation of the structures is done during this time.

- For a Pap test, the cervix is scraped with a wooden spatula, cytology brush, cotton-tipped applicator, or a combination of these tools, and specimens are placed on glass slides with a fixative applied prior to delivery to the laboratory.

  o All women should undergo a Pap test for cervical cancer on a regular basis. The frequency of this test is related to several factors.

  o A Pap test can also detect the presence of fungal, viral, and parasitic disorders.

  o False positives may be obtained in the presence of infection

- Indications

  o Begin testing at age 21 or within 3 years of becoming sexually active.

- ○ A yearly Pap test should be performed until age 30. If all tests have been negative, a longer period of time such as every 2 to 3 years may be recommended by the provider.

- ○ Pap tests may be discontinued after cervical removal during a hysterectomy or at age 65 if they have been normal for the past several years.

- ○ Potential Diagnoses

  - ■ Analysis of the Pap smear will yield either a "negative" result or description of cell abnormalities as outlined by either the Bethesda or cervical intraepithelial neoplasia (CIN) systems.

    - □ ASC-US – normal atypical squamous cells of undetermined significance (considered mildly abnormal)

    - □ ASC-H – atypical squamous cells of which high-grade squamous intraepithelial lesions cannot be excluded (indicates high risk of being precancerous)

    - □ LSIL – low-grade squamous intraepithelial lesion (indicates mild abnormality that demonstrates early changes in shape and size of squamous cells)

    - □ HSIL – high-grade squamous intraepithelial lesion (indicates a more severe abnormality in size and shape of cells that can progress to invasive cancer)

    - □ AGC – atypical glandular cells (indicates a change in the glandular cells of the cervix rather than the squamous cells)

    - □ AIS – adenocarcinoma in situ (indicates the presence of precancerous cells in the glandular tissue)

- • Preprocedure

  - ○ Nursing Actions

    - ■ Ask the client if she has douched in the past 24 hr.

    - ■ Inform the client that use of vaginal medications or sexual intercourse within the last 24 hr may alter test results.

    - ■ Have the client empty her bladder.

    - ■ Place the client in the lithotomy position and drape appropriately.

    - ■ Explain to the client how the procedure will be carried out.

    - ■ Have all necessary equipment available (cervical scraping tools, glass slides, fixative, perineal pad).

- • Intraprocedure

  - ○ Nursing Actions

    - ■ Have ready the necessary equipment for the provider during procedure.

    - ■ Transfer specimens to slides and apply fixative to slides.

- Postprocedure
  - Nursing Actions
    - Provide the client with perineal pad and tissues.
  - Client Education
    - Inform the client that minimal bleeding may occur from the cervix.
    - Inform the client of the time frame for results to be available.

Colposcopy and Cervical Biopsy

- After application of acetic acid to the cervix, a colposcope is used to inspect the cervix and take a cervical biopsy. All suspicious areas are biopsied and sent to a laboratory for microscopic examination.

- Indications
  - Pap tests that demonstrate atypical or abnormal cells must be followed up with a colposcopy and cervical biopsy.

- Preprocedure
  - Nursing Actions
    - Preprocedure care is the same as that for a Pap test, except a sterile biopsy cup will be needed instead of the other equipment.

- Postprocedure
  - Nursing Actions
    - Postprocedure care is the same as that for a Pap test.
  - Client Education
    - Instruct the client to abstain from sexual intercourse and avoid using a douche, vaginal creams, or tampons until all discharge has stopped (usually about 2 weeks).

- Complications
  - Bleeding
    - Heavy bleeding can result from the excision of tissue.
    - Nursing Actions
      - Assess the client for heavy bleeding.
    - Client Education
      - Instruct the client to notify the provider for abnormal vaginal bleeding.
  - Infection
    - Infection can result from this invasive procedure.

- ■ Nursing Actions
  - □ Assess the client for fever, chills, severe pain, foul odor, or purulent vaginal discharge.
- ■ Client Education
  - □ Instruct the client to notify the provider regarding these symptoms.

Cone Biopsy

- A cone biopsy is an extensive cervical biopsy that excises a cone-shaped sample of tissue. This is done to remove potentially harmful cells, which can, in some cases, be examined.

  - Anesthesia may or may not be used for this procedure.

  - Margins of the excised tissue must be examined to ensure removal of all cancerous cells.

  - A cone biopsy can be performed using a scalpel, laser, or loop electrosurgical excision procedure (LEEP). A LEEP uses an electric current, and laser surgery uses a laser beam that vaporizes abnormal tissues.

  - Cryotherapy is another treatment that is used to eliminate abnormal cells. Extreme cold is used to freeze the cancer, ultimately causing necrosis of tissue. No tissue for biopsy is available for either the laser or cryotherapy.

- Indications

  - A cone biopsy is done if a cervical lesion is clearly visible.

- Postprocedure

  - Nursing Actions

    - ■ Postprocedure care is the same as that for a Pap test.

  - Client Education

    - ■ Instruct the client to abstain from sexual intercourse and avoid using a douche, vaginal creams, or tampons until all discharge has stopped (usually about 2 weeks).

Endometrial Biopsy

- A thin, hollow tube is inserted through the cervix, and a curette or suction equipment is used to obtain the endometrial tissue sample.

- Indications

  - Potential Diagnoses

    - ■ Endometrial biopsies are done to assess for uterine cancer as well as evaluate for menstrual irregularities and potential causes of infertility.

  - Client Presentation

    - ■ Abnormal or postmenopausal bleeding

- Preprocedure

  - Nursing Actions

    - Give the client pain reliever 30 min prior to the procedure.

    - Witness consent.

  - Client Education

    - Educate the client about the procedure.

      - Biopsies are done with the client awake.

      - Some discomfort and cramping will be felt by the client.

    - Have the client empty her bladder.

- Postprocedure

  - Nursing Actions

    - Postprocedure care is the same as that for a Pap test.

  - Client Education

    - Instruct the client to abstain from sexual intercourse and avoid using a douche, vaginal creams, or tampons until all discharge has stopped (usually about 2 weeks).

    - Have the client notify the provider of heavy vaginal bleeding, fever, severe pain, and/or foul discharge.

- Complications

  - Bleeding

    - Heavy vaginal bleeding is a potential complication of an endometrial biopsy.

    - Nursing Actions

      - Assess the client for heavy bleeding.

    - Client Education

      - Instruct the client to notify the provider of abnormal vaginal bleeding.

  - Infection

    - Infection can result from this invasive procedure.

    - Nursing Actions

      - Assess the client for fever, chills, severe pain, foul odor, and purulent vaginal discharge.

    - Client Education

      - Instruct the client to notify the provider regarding these symptoms.

Serologic Studies

- There are two serologic (blood) studies that can be used to screen for syphilis.

    o Venereal disease research laboratory (VDRL) – the oldest test for syphilis that is still performed

    o Rapid plasma regain (RPR) – a newer test for syphilis and has replaced the VDRL test in many institutions

- Indications

    o Client Presentation

        ■ Primary chancre – a firm, painless skin ulceration localized at point of initial exposure, and heals without treatment (clients still positive for syphilis)

        ■ Local lymph node swelling

        ■ Secondary symptoms – headache, anorexia, rash on trunk and extremities, fever, sore throat, malaise, and weight loss

- Interpretation of Findings

    o Both tests are done using a sample of blood and reported as nonreactive (negative for syphilis) or reactive (positive for syphilis).

    o False positives may occur secondary to infection, pregnancy, malignancies, and autoimmune disorders.

    o If either test comes back as reactive, diagnosis should be done by confirming the results using one of the following tests:

        ■ Fluorescent treponemal antibody absorbed (FTA-ABS)

        ■ Treponema pallidum particle agglutination assay (TPPA)

Mammography

- A mammogram is an x-ray of the breast that is used as a screening tool for breast cancer. Tumors that are too small to be palpated can be visualized on a mammogram.

    o During a mammogram, a woman's breast is mechanically compressed both vertically and horizontally by the x-ray machine while radiologic pictures are taken of each breast.

- Indications

    o Mammograms should be done every 1 to 2 years beginning at age 40 for wellness screening. If there is a family history of breast cancer, mammograms should begin at an earlier age.

    o They are also performed to evaluate a lesion or lump.

- Interpretation of Findings

    o If a suspicious lesion is identified, this finding is usually followed up by a fine needle aspiration or open biopsy.

- Preprocedure

  - Nursing Actions

    - Instruct the client to avoid the use of deodorant or powders in the axillary region or on the breasts prior to the exam.

    - Tell the client she should not have a mammogram if she is pregnant.

  - Client Education

- Intraprocedure

  - Nursing Actions

    - Radiologic technicians are often the members of the health care team that perform mammograms.

- Postprocedure

  - Client Education

    - Instruct the client to return every 1 to 2 years for a follow-up mammogram.

    - If follow-up is needed, the client will be contacted.

Hysterectomy

- A hysterectomy is the removal of the uterus and, in some cases, removal of the ovaries and fallopian tubes.

  - There are three methods of performing a hysterectomy

    - Abdominal approach, also known as a total abdominal hysterectomy

    - Vaginal approach

    - Laparoscopy-assisted vaginal hysterectomy

- Indications

  - Diagnoses

    - Uterine cancer

    - Noncancerous conditions – fibroids, endometriosis (inflammation of the endometrium), and genital prolapse – that cause pain, bleeding, or emotional stress

  - Client Presentation

    - Painful intercourse

    - Hypermenorrhea

    - Pelvic pressure

    - Urinary urgency or frequency

    - Constipation

- Preprocedure

  - Nursing Actions

    - Maintain NPO status.

    - Ensure that informed consent has been obtained.

  - Client Education

    - Teach the client how to turn, cough, and deep breathe.

    - Instruct the client how to use an incentive spirometer.

- Postprocedure

  - Nursing Actions

    - Postoperatively, the nurse must monitor the client for vaginal bleeding. Excess bleeding is more than one saturated pad in 4 hr.

    - An indwelling urinary catheter is generally inserted intraoperatively and in place for the first 24 hr postoperatively.

    - Priority assessments and interventions following a total abdominal hysterectomy:

      - Monitor the client's vital signs (fever, hypotension).

      - Monitor the client's breath sounds (risk of atelectasis; turn, cough, and deep breathe; use of incentive spirometry; ambulation).

      - Monitor the client's bowel sounds (risk of paralytic ileus).

      - Monitor the client's urine output (call the provider if less than 30 mL/hr).

      - Provide IV fluid and electrolyte replacement (until bowel sounds return).

      - Monitor the client's incision (infection, integrity, risk of dehiscence).

      - Monitor the client for signs of thrombophlebitis (warmth, tenderness, edema).

      - Take thromboembolism precautions (sequential compression devices, ambulation).

      - Monitor the client's blood loss (Hgb and Hct).

  - Client Education

    - Instruct the client about a well-balanced diet that is high in protein and vitamin C for wound healing, and high in iron if the client is anemic.

    - Instruct the client to restrict activity (heavy lifting, strenuous activity, driving, stairs, sexual activity) for 4 to 6 weeks.

- Complications

  - Hypovolemic shock

    - Hypovolemic shock due to blood loss is a potential complication following a hysterectomy.

- Nursing Actions
  - Monitor the client's Hgb and Hct.
  - Provide fluid replacement therapy and/or blood transfusions as indicated.
- Psychological reactions
  - Psychological reactions can occur months to years after surgery.
  - Nursing Actions
    - Encourage the client to discuss the positive aspects of life.
    - Understand that occasional sadness in the client is normal, but persistent sadness or depression indicates a need for counseling assistance.
  - Client Education
    - Encourage the client to attend at a support group.

CHAPTER 72: DIAGNOSTIC AND THERAPEUTIC PROCEDURES FOR FEMALE REPRODUCTIVE DISORDERS

 Application Exercises

1. A nurse is preparing a client for her first Papanicolaou (Pap) test. Which of the following statements is appropriate for the nurse to make?

    A. "You should urinate immediately after the procedure is over."

    B. "You will not feel any discomfort."

    C. "You may experience some bleeding after the procedure."

    D. "You will need to hold your breath during the procedure."

2. A client's RPR has come back positive from the laboratory. Which of the following tests should the nurse anticipate will be necessary to confirm the diagnosis of syphilis?

    A. VDRL

    B. PSA

    C. TPPA

    D. AFB

3. A nurse is giving instructions to a client before a mammogram. Which of the following should the nurse instruct the client to avoid prior to the procedure?

    A. Facial makeup

    B. Deodorant

    C. Sexual intercourse

    D. Exercise

CHAPTER 72: DIAGNOSTIC AND THERAPEUTIC PROCEDURES FOR FEMALE REPRODUCTIVE DISORDERS

 Application Exercises Answer Key

1. A nurse is preparing a client for her first Papanicolaou (Pap) test. Which of the following statements is appropriate for the nurse to make?

   A. "You should urinate immediately after the procedure is over."

   B. "You will not feel any discomfort."

   C. "You may experience some bleeding after the procedure."

   D. "You will need to hold your breath during the procedure."

   It is normal and expected for a small amount of bleeding to occur after the procedure secondary to the scraping of the cervix. It is unnecessary for the client to urinate immediately after the procedure. Some discomfort may be felt when the speculum is introduced and the cervical scraping is done. The client should breath normally or take a few deep breaths during the procedure.

 NCLEX® Connection: Reduction of Risk Potential: Diagnostic Tests

2. A client's RPR has come back positive from the laboratory. Which of the following tests should the nurse anticipate will be necessary to confirm the diagnosis of syphilis?

   A. VDRL

   B. PSA

   C. TPPA

   D. AFB

   After a positive RPR, a client should have a TPPA blood test done to confirm the diagnosis of syphilis. VDRL is another screening test for syphilis, PSA is done to screen for prostate cancer, and AFB is the test done on sputum for acid-fast bacillus

 NCLEX® Connection: Reduction of Risk Potential: Diagnostic Tests

3. A nurse is giving instructions to a client before a mammogram. Which of the following should the nurse instruct the client to avoid prior to the procedure?

   A. Facial makeup

   B. Deodorant

   C. Sexual intercourse

   D. Exercise

   A client should not apply deodorant prior to a mammogram because it can show up on the film as a shadow that could be mistaken for a lesion. Using facial makeup, sexual intercourse, and exercising are not contraindicated prior to having a mammogram.

 NCLEX® Connection: Reduction of Risk Potential: Diagnostic Tests

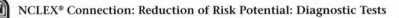

UNIT 9	NURSING CARE OF CLIENTS WITH REPRODUCTIVE DISORDERS
Section	Female Reproductive Disorders
Chapter 73	Menstrual Disorders and Menopause

Overview

- The average age of menarche (first menses) in the United States is 13 years of age. If an adolescent has not begun having periods by 15 years of age, possible causes should be investigated.

- Menstrual cycles are typically 28 days long, with a range from 21 to 35 days. The first day of menstruation is day 1 of a menstrual cycle. Ovulation typically occurs around day 14. Bleeding begins 14 days after ovulation and typically lasts 4 to 5 days, but it can continue for up to 7 days.

- Menstrual cycles continue until menopause or surgical removal of the uterus. Menopause is the time when ovulation ceases and menstrual cycles become irregular and eventually stop. The median age of onset of menopause is 51 years of age.

MENSTRUAL DISORDERS

Overview

- Painful menstruation, or dysmenorrhea, is common in adolescents and young women. In many women, this pain is significantly decreased after the birth of a child.

- Dysfunctional uterine bleeding (DUB) is believed to be due to a hormonal imbalance and may include menorrhagia and metrorrhagia. Menorrhagia is excessive bleeding (in amount and duration), possibly with clots and for longer than 7 days. Metrorrhagia is bleeding between menstrual periods more frequently than every 21 days. It is more common in women who are entering menopause and adolescent females who have begun menstruating in the past 1 to 2 years.

- Amenorrhea is the absence of menses. In a woman who has had menstrual cycles, this can be a sign of a medical disorder. A common cause is low percentage of body fat in women who are involved in sports or women who over exercise.

- Premenstrual syndrome (PMS) is the appearance of a number of symptoms immediately prior to menstruation. The monthly fluctuation of hormones as well as a change in the level of serotonin has been considered a possible cause for these symptoms. Symptoms can usually be treated with medication and dietary changes, and the ability to function is not significantly affected.

- Premenstrual dysphoric disorder (PMDD) is similar to premenstrual syndrome, but the symptoms occur for at least 2 consecutive cycles and are so severe they interfere with a women's ability to function. The symptoms include depression, irritability, changes in appetite, abdominal bloating, fatigue, emotional lability, and fluid retention. Treatment includes decreasing intake of sugar, salt, and alcohol, as well as increasing exercise. Antidepressants have been helpful for some women who experience severe PMDD.

- Endometriosis is characterized by an over growth of endometrial tissue that extends outside the uterus into the fallopian tubes, onto the ovaries, and into the pelvis. Blockage of the fallopian tubes by endometrial tissue is a common cause of infertility.

Assessment

- Subjective data

  - Menstrual history (age of first menses, monthly cycle)

  - Report of premenstrual depression, irritability, changes in appetite, abdominal bloating, fatigue, emotional lability, or fluid retention

  - Characteristics of flow

  - Characteristics and location of pain during menstrual cycle

  - Painful intercourse

  - Objective data

    - Pelvic tenderness during palpation of the lower abdomen and the pelvic examination

    - Metabolic disorders (hypothyroidism)

  - Laboratory tests

    - Hemoglobin and hematocrit

      - May be below reference range due to excessive blood loss

  - Diagnostic procedures

    - Endometrial biopsy

      - Determines the relationship between menstrual flow and the hormone cycle, as well as possible pathologic reasons for bleeding, such as uterine cancer

    - Transvaginal ultrasound

      - Can identify the presence of uterine fibroids or leiomyomas

Collaborative Care

- Medications

    o Hormonal contraceptives

        ▪ May be used to decrease symptoms of PMS and PMDD

        ▪ May be the initial treatment for endometriosis

    o Leuprolide (Lupron) – synthetic luteinizing hormone

        ▪ Suppresses estrogen and testosterone production in the body, making it an effective treatment for endometriosis (promotes atrophy of ectopic tissue)

        ▪ Can cause birth defects, so a reliable form of contraception should be used

        ▪ May cause decreased libido and increased risk of osteoporosis

    o NSAIDs – Ibuprofen (Motrin)

        ▪ May be given for endometriosis to inhibit production of prostaglandins

        ▪ Aids in treatment of pain and discomfort related to PMS and PMDD

    o SSRIs

        ▪ May be used if other treatments for PMDD are unsuccessful

- Surgical Interventions

    o DUB

        ▪ Endometrial ablation

            □ Used to remove endometrial tissue in the uterus

            □ The tissue may be removed by laser, heat, electricity, or cryotherapy

    o Endometriosis

        ▪ Laparoscopic removal of ectopic tissue and adhesions

            □ A laser may be used to remove tissue.

- Client Outcomes

    o DUB

        ▪ The client will re-established a menstrual cycle of approximately 28 days, with menstruation lasting no more than 7 days.

    o PMDD

        ▪ The client will be able to continue with regular activities of daily living.

    o Endometriosis

        ▪ The client will experience less pain and discomfort and be able to become pregnant if desired.

Complications

- Ectopic pregnancy

  o Due to the presence of endometrial tissue outside of the uterus, the ovum may implant in the fallopian tubes or abdominal cavity.

  o As the ovum increases in size, the fallopian tube may rupture and the client may bleed to death.

  o The fallopian tube may need to be surgically removed if bleeding is severe or the tube is irreparably damaged.

  o If ectopic pregnancy is identified prior to rupture of the fallopian tube, a salpingostomy may be performed to remove the fetus, or a medication (methotrexate [Rheumatrex]) may be given to terminate the pregnancy and promote reabsorption of the fetal products.

MENOPAUSE

Overview

- Menopause is the cessation of menses. Menses will appear on an infrequent cycle for a period of time that does not exceed 2 years. Menopause is considered complete when no menses have occurred for 12 months.

- Menopause may be natural or surgically induced.

Assessment

- Subjective and Objective Data

  o Vasomotor symptoms – Hot flashes and irregular menses

  o Genitourinary – Atrophic vaginitis, vaginal dryness, and incontinence

  o Psychologic – Mood swings, changes in sleep patterns, and decreased REM sleep

  o Skeletal – Decreased bone density

  o Cardiovascular – Decreased HDL and increased LDL

  o Dermatologic – Decreased skin elasticity and loss of hair on head and in the pubic area

  o Reproductive – Breast tissue changes

  o Laboratory Tests

    ▪ Follicle stimulating hormone (FSH) – Increased during menopause

    ▪ Blood, urine, and saliva hormone levels (estrogens, progesterone, dehydroepiandrosterone sulfate [DHEA-S], testosterone)

- ○ Diagnostic Procedures

    - Pelvic examination with Papanicolaou (PAP) smear to rule out cancer in cases of abnormal bleeding

    - Breast examination with mammogram to rule out cancer in cases of a palpable change from predominantly glandular tissue to fatty tissue

    - Biopsy of uterine lining in cases of undiagnosed abnormal uterine bleeding in a woman over 40 years of age or in a woman whose menses has stopped for a year and bleeding has begun again

    - Bone mass measurements to determine a baseline measurement of density and strength and subsequently confirm the development of osteopenia/osteoporosis

Collaborative Care

- Medications

    - ○ Hormone replacement therapy (HRT)

        - HRT may be prescribed to help control symptoms associated with the estrogen deficiency that occurs during and after menopause. Estrogen deficiency symptoms (hot flashes, atrophy of vaginal tissues, osteoporosis) occur naturally as part of the aging process during menopause. For a woman who has a uterus, HRT will include estrogen and progesterone. For a woman who no longer has a uterus (following a hysterectomy), HRT will only include estrogen.

        - Many different preparations of HRT are available (oral, transdermal, intravaginal, intramuscular). HRT may be prescribed as a continuous, combined estrogen-progesterone therapy or a variety of cyclic patterns.

        - Based on their individual risk factors and health care needs, women should discuss the risks and benefits of using HRT with their health care providers.

        - If a woman and her health care provider believe that the use of HRT is required for management of menopausal symptoms, the best recommendation is to use HRT on a short-term basis, generally less than 5 years.

        - HRT is not indicated for prophylaxis of heart disease and generally is not prescribed for women at high risk for heart disease.

        - Risk factors that increase the incidence of adverse effects from HRT

            - □ Pregnancy – HRT should not be taken during pregnancy, due to the risk of teratogenic effects.

            - □ Smoking

            - □ Cancer

                - ▸ Cancer of the breast or family history of breast cancer

                - ▸ Cancer of the uterus

                - ▸ Undiagnosed abnormal vaginal bleeding

- □ Embolism
  - ‣ Active thrombophlebitis
  - ‣ Thromboembolic disorder or history of thrombus
  - ‣ Stroke
  - ‣ Heart disease or high risk for heart disease (hypertension)
- ■ Nursing Actions
  - □ Assess/Monitor
    - ‣ Increased blood pressure
    - ‣ Breast tenderness, lumps, or abnormalities
    - ‣ Vaginal bleeding
    - ‣ Venous thrombosis
- ■ Client Education
  - □ Reinforce to the client the advantages and disadvantages of HRT.
  - □ Instruct the client in self-administration of HRT.
  - □ Advise the client to immediately quit smoking if applicable.
  - □ Teach the client how to prevent and assess the development of venous thrombosis.
    - ‣ Avoid wearing knee-high stockings and clothing or socks that are restrictive.
    - ‣ Note and report symptoms of unilateral leg pain, edema, warmth, and redness.
    - ‣ Avoid sitting for long periods of time.
    - ‣ Take short walks throughout the day to promote circulation.
    - ‣ Perform frequent ankle pumps, and move and stretch legs.
  - □ Schedule annual physicals, pelvic examinations, and mammograms.
  - □ Schedule bone density tests when ordered.
  - □ Instruct the client about atypical presentation of myocardial infarction signs and symptoms in women (abdominal pain, vague chest symptoms, arm pain, pain between the shoulders) and instruct the client to seek assistance immediately.
  - □ If oral therapy causes nausea, taking pills with food may help.
  - □ If the client is using vaginal creams or suppositories of estrogen compounds, be sure to refrain from inserting them prior to intercourse, or the client's partner may absorb some of the product.

- ■ Alternative therapies
    - □ Dong quai and black cohosh have been found effective in some women. Research regarding their usefulness has been inconsistent.
    - □ Phytoestrogens interact with estrogen receptors in the body. Vegetables such as dandelion greens, alfalfa sprouts, black beans, and soy beans contain phytoestrogens.
    - □ Vitamin E has been reported to decrease hot flashes in some women.
  - ○ Client Education
    - ■ HRT is beneficial in the prevention of age-related problems.
      - □ Osteoporosis
      - □ Atrophic vaginitis, which is characterized by vaginal burning and bleeding, pruritus, and painful intercourse may improve with HRT. Vaginal instillations of estrogen may be an option and may result in less systemic absorption.
      - □ Older adult clients may also decrease the risk of osteoporosis by performing regular weight bearing exercises; increasing intake of high-protein and high-calcium foods; avoiding alcohol, caffeine, and tobacco; and taking calcium with vitamin D supplements.
- • Client Outcomes
  - ○ The client will report a decrease in estrogen deficiency symptoms.
  - ○ The client's bone scans will not demonstrate demineralization.

Complications

- • Embolic complications (risk increased by concurrent smoking)
  - ○ Myocardial infarction, especially during the first year of therapy
  - ○ Stroke
  - ○ Venous thrombosis – Thrombophlebitis, especially during the first year of therapy
- • Cancer
  - ○ In some studies, long-term use of HRT has been found to increase the risk for breast cancer.
  - ○ Long-term use of estrogen-only HRT increases the risk for ovarian and endometrial cancer, but this risk is decreased with 12 or more days of progesterone per month.

CHAPTER 73: MENSTRUAL DISORDERS AND MENOPAUSE

(A) Application Exercises

Scenario: A 51-year-old nulliparous female presents to the women's health clinic with reports of hot flashes and irregular menses. She states that she cannot sleep at night because the hot flashes awaken her. She is requesting hormone replacement therapy (HRT) for relief of menopausal symptoms. She stopped using oral contraceptive pills several years ago when her husband passed away. She has not been sexually active since his death. This is her first visit to a health care provider in 3 years.

1. What assumptions may the nurse make about the client's irregular menses?

2. What diagnostic tests should the nurse anticipate this client will need prior to initiating HRT?

3. While the nurse is collecting data from the client, the history reveals the information provided below. Which of the following should be considered as a possible contraindication for HRT with this client? (Select all that apply.)

> _____ Type 2 diabetes mellitus
> _____ Family history of osteoporosis
> _____ Smokes one pack per day
> _____ History of blood clot
> _____ Family history of breast cancer

4. A nurse is discussing with a client the implications of her new diagnoses of endometriosis. Which of the following should the nurse include?

   A. Increased susceptibility for pelvic inflammatory disease (PID)

   B. Infertility

   C. Risk for multiple births

   D. Contraindication for use of contraceptives

5. A client who does not wish to begin HRT but would like to try something for her hot flashes may be counseled to try which of the following?

   A. Ginkgo biloba

   B. Black cohosh

   C. St. John's wort

   D. Kava kava

CHAPTER 73: MENSTRUAL DISORDERS AND MENOPAUSE

 Application Exercises Answer Key

Scenario: A 51-year-old nulliparous female presents to the women's health clinic with reports of hot flashes and irregular menses. She states that she cannot sleep at night because the hot flashes awaken her. She is requesting hormone replacement therapy (HRT) for relief of menopausal symptoms. She stopped using oral contraceptive pills several years ago when her husband passed away. She has not been sexually active since his death. This is her first visit to a health care provider in 3 years.

1. What assumptions may the nurse make about the client's irregular menses?

The client is probably menopausal. Her menses are irregular and she is experiencing the vasomotor symptoms and sleep disturbance commonly associated with menopause.

 NCLEX® Connection: Physiological Adaptation, Pathophysiology

2. What diagnostic tests should the nurse anticipate this client will need prior to initiating HRT?

Because the client has not received medical care for 3 years, she will most likely need a complete physical exam, including a clinical breast exam, pelvic exam, Papanicolaou smear, and mammogram. She will also need a CBC and cholesterol testing. Some providers obtain a follicle stimulating hormone level to determine if the client is menopausal.

 NCLEX® Connection: Reduction of Risk Potential, Diagnostic Tests

3. While the nurse is collecting data from the client, the history reveals the information provided below. Which of the following should be considered as a possible contraindication for HRT with this client? (Select all that apply.)

_____	Type 2 diabetes mellitus
_____	Family history of osteoporosis
X	**Smokes one pack per day**
X	**History of blood clot**
X	**Family history of breast cancer**

Smoking can increase the risk for thrombus and should be discouraged prior to beginning therapy. Since venous thrombi can develop as a side effect of HRT, clients who have experienced a blood clot before should not be placed on HRT therapy. Clients who have a family history of breast cancer should consider other options until research can determine if there is a relationship between HRT and increased risk for breast cancer. Type 2 diabetes and a family history of osteoporosis are not contraindications for HRT.

NCLEX® Connection: Pharmacological and Parenteral Therapies, Adverse Effects/ Contraindications/Side Effects/Interactions

4. A nurse is discussing with a client the implications of her new diagnoses of endometriosis. Which of the following should the nurse include?

    A. Increased susceptibility for pelvic inflammatory disease (PID)

    B. Infertility

    C. Risk for multiple births

    D. Contraindication for use of contraceptives

Endometriosis is an overgrowth of endometrial tissue that can block the fallopian tubes causing infertility. The risk for PID is not increased, nor is the risk for multiple births. Contraceptives are sometimes prescribed to treat endometriosis due to the suppression of endometrial growth.

 NCLEX® Connection: Reduction of Risk Potential, Potential for Alterations in Body Systems

5. A client who does not wish to begin HRT but would like to try something for her hot flashes may be counseled to try which of the following?

    A. Ginkgo biloba

    B. Black cohosh

    C. St. John's wort

    D. Kava kava

Black cohosh has been found to be effective in relieving hot flashes in some women. Ginkgo biloba, St. John's wort and kava kava have not been found to be effective in relieving hot flashes in women who are menopausal.

 NCLEX® Connection: Physiological Adaptation, Illness Management

UNIT 9	NURSING CARE OF CLIENTS WITH REPRODUCTIVE DISORDERS
Section	Female Reproductive Disorders
Chapter 74	**Disorders of Female Reproductive Tissue**

Overview

- A cystocele is a protrusion of the posterior bladder through the posterior vaginal wall. It is caused by weakened pelvic muscles and/or structures.

    o For a cystocele with mild signs and symptoms, medical treatment may be attempted. If this is not successful, surgery may be indicated.

- A rectocele is a protrusion of the anterior rectal wall through the posterior vaginal wall. It is caused by a defect of the pelvic structures a difficult delivery, or a forceps delivery.

    o For a rectocele with mild signs and symptoms, medical treatment may be attempted. If this is not successful, surgery may be indicated.

Health Promotion and Disease Prevention

- Instruct the client to avoid traumatic vaginal childbirth with an early and adequate episiotomy.

- Inform the client of measures to prevent atrophic vaginitis and the advantages of prevention.

- Advise clients who are at risk to lose weight if obese.

- Instruct clients to eat high-fiber diets and drink adequate fluids to prevent constipation.

- Administer estrogen therapy to prevent uterine atrophy and atrophic vaginitis if the client is not at risk for complications from hormone therapy (cardiovascular or embolic history)

Assessment

- Risk Factors
  - Cystocele
    - Obesity
    - Advanced age (loss of estrogen)
    - Chronic constipation
    - Family history
    - Childbearing
    - Hysterectomy
  - Rectocele
    - Pelvic structure defects
    - Obesity
    - Aging
    - Family history
    - Difficult childbirth necessitating repair of a tear
    - Forceps delivery
    - Previous hysterectomy
  - Cystocele and rectocele develop in older adult females, usually following menopause.
  - Older adult clients are more susceptible to constipation and chronic bearing down during elimination, which can displace weakened structures.
- Subjective Data
  - Cystocele
    - Urinary frequency and/or urgency
    - Stress incontinence
    - Urinary tract infection
    - Sense of vaginal fullness
  - Rectocele
    - Constipation and/or the need to place fingers in the vagina to elevate the rectocele to complete evacuation of feces
    - Sensation of a mass in the vagina
    - Pelvic pressure or pain
    - Pain with intercourse
    - Pain in back or pelvis

- Objective Data

  o Diagnostic Procedures

    ▪ Cystocele

      □ A pelvic examination reveals a bulging of the anterior wall when the client is instructed to bear down.

      □ A voiding cystourethrography is performed to identify the degree of bladder protrusion and the amount of urine residual.

    ▪ Rectocele

      □ A pelvic examination reveals a bulging of the posterior wall when the client is instructed to bear down.

      □ A rectal examination and/or barium enema reveals the presence of a rectocele.

Collaborative Care

- Therapeutic Procedures

  o Vaginal pessary

    ▪ A removable rubber, plastic, or silicone device inserted into the vagina to provide support and block protrusion of other organs into the vagina

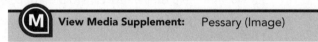

      View Media Supplement: Pessary (Image)

    ▪ Nursing Actions

      □ Teach the client how to insert, remove, and clean the device.

      □ Monitor for possible bleeding or fistula formation.

  o Kegel exercises

    ▪ Exercises done to strengthen the pelvic floor

    ▪ Client Education

      □ Teach the client how to perform the exercises.

        ‣ Tightening pelvic muscles for a count of 10.

        ‣ Relax slowly for a count of 10, pause for 10 to 15 seconds, repeat in sequences of 15.

        ‣ Perform while lying down, sitting, and standing.

        ‣ Perform 4 times daily.

        ‣ Keep abdominal muscles relaxed during contractions.

- Surgical Interventions
  - Cystocele
    - Anterior colporrhaphy
      - Using a vaginal approach, the pelvic muscles are shortened and tightened.
  - Rectocele
    - Posterior colporrhaphy
      - Using a vaginal/perineal approach, the pelvic muscles are shortened and tightened.
      - A biological mesh graft may be used to provide extra support to weakened tissue.
  - Anterior-Posterior repair
    - In some cases, surgery for both a cystocele and a rectocele is needed; this is called an anterior-posterior repair.
    - A hysterectomy may be performed at the same time as any of the procedures listed above.
    - Nursing Actions
      - Postoperative
        - Provide routine postoperative care to prevent complications.
        - Administer analgesics, antimicrobials, and stool softeners/laxatives as prescribed.
        - Provide perineal care at least twice daily following surgery and after every urination or bowel movement.
        - Apply an ice pack to the perineal area to relieve pain and swelling.
        - Suggest that the client take frequent sitz baths to soothe the perineal area.
        - Provide a liquid diet immediately following surgery followed by a low-residue diet until normal bowel function returns.
        - Recommend that the client drink at least 2,000 mL of fluid daily, unless contraindicated.
        - Following removal of the catheter, instruct the client to void every 2 to 3 hr to prevent a full bladder and stress on stitches.
        - The client may go home with an indwelling urinary catheter.

- Care After Discharge
  - Client Education
    - Instruct the client on how to care for an indwelling urinary catheter at home if applicable. Remind the client to thoroughly wash her hands before and after handling the catheter and to remove any crust or debris that has collected around the catheter.
    - Caution the client to avoid straining at defecation; sneezing; coughing; lifting; and sitting, walking, or standing for prolonged periods following surgery.
    - Instruct the client to tighten and support pelvic muscles when coughing or sneezing.
    - Advise the client of postoperative restrictions, including avoidance of strenuous activity, lifting anything weighing greater than 5 lb, and sexual intercourse.
    - Inform the client that if the provider did not schedule her for removal of stitches, they will be absorbed by the body, negating the need for removal.
- Client Outcomes
  - The client will not experience urine leakage when coughing, laughing, or bearing down.
  - The client will be able to have bowel movement without trapping of feces in the rectal pouch.

Complications

- Dyspareunia (painful sexual intercourse) is a possible surgical complication due to surgical alteration of the vaginal orifice.

CHAPTER 74: DISORDERS OF FEMALE REPRODUCTIVE TISSUE

 Application Exercises

1. What instructions should a nurse provide to a client concerning Kegel exercises for conservative management of a cystocele or rectocele? (Select all that apply.)

_____ Perform exercises four times a daily.

_____ Contract the circumvaginal and/or perirectal muscles.

_____ Hold the contraction for 6 to 10 seconds.

_____ Perform exercises every day.

_____ Follow each contraction with a 30-second relaxation period.

_____ Perform while sitting, lying, and standing.

_____ Tighten abdominal muscles during contractions.

2. A client is admitted to the gynecology unit for an anterior colporrhaphy. Which of the following client statements is consistent with the physiological alteration that necessitates this type of surgery?

A. "I have to push the feces out of a pouch in my vagina with my fingers."

B. "I have pain and bleeding when I have a bowel movement."

C. "I have had frequent urinary tract infections."

D. "I have pain during intercourse."

3. A nurse is preparing to discharge a client who has had an anterior and posterior colporrhaphy. Which of the following instructions should the nurse provide?

A. Do not bend over for at least 6 weeks.

B. Take showers, not tub baths, for at least 2 weeks.

C. Do not engage in intercourse for at least 6 weeks.

D. Expect to have a catheter in place for at least 2 weeks.

CHAPTER 74: DISORDERS OF FEMALE REPRODUCTIVE TISSUE

 Application Exercises Answer Key

1. What instructions should a nurse provide to a client concerning Kegel exercises for conservative management of a cystocele or rectocele? (Select all that apply.)

__X__	**Perform exercises four times a daily.**
__X__	**Contract the circumvaginal and/or perirectal muscles.**
__X__	**Hold the contraction for 6 to 10 seconds.**
__X__	**Perform exercises every day.**
_____	Follow each contraction with a 30-second relaxation period.
__X__	**Perform sitting, lying, and standing.**
_____	Tighten abdominal muscles during contractions.

Kegel exercises should be performed every day, at least 4 times a day. They are done using the circumvaginal and perirectal muscles. Contractions should be held for 6 to 10 seconds followed by a 10 to 15 second relaxation period. Exercises may be performed standing, sitting, or lying down. Abdominal muscles should be kept relaxed during the contractions.

Ⓝ NCLEX® Connection: Physiological Adaptation, Illness Management

2. A client is admitted to the gynecology unit for an anterior colporrhaphy. Which of the following client statements is consistent with the physiological alteration that necessitates this type of surgery?

A. "I have to push the feces out of a pouch in my vagina with my fingers."

B. "I have pain and bleeding when I have a bowel movement."

C. "I have had frequent urinary tract infections."

D. "I have pain during intercourse."

Clients with a cystocele experience frequent urinary tract infections due to the trapping of urine in the urovaginal pouch. Pushing feces out of a pouch in the vagina, pain and bleeding during urination, and pain during intercourse are consistent with a rectocele, not a cystocele.

Ⓝ NCLEX® Connection: Physiological Adaptation, Pathophysiology

3. A nurse is preparing to discharge a client who has had an anterior and posterior colporrhaphy. Which of the following instructions should the nurse provide?

    A. Do not bend over for at least 6 weeks.

    B. Take showers, not tub baths, for at least 2 weeks.

    C. Do not engage in intercourse for at least 6 weeks.

    D. Expect to have a catheter in place for at least 2 weeks.

The nurse should tell the client to not engage in intercourse for at least 6 weeks. There are no restrictions in regard to bending over. Tub baths are encouraged for comfort and hygiene, and the client's indwelling urinary catheter will be removed when swelling permits unimpeded urination, which is usually less than 2 weeks.

NCLEX® Connection: Reduction of Risk Potential, Potential for Complications from Surgical Procedures and Health Alterations

UNIT 9	NURSING CARE OF CLIENTS WITH REPRODUCTIVE DISORDERS
Section	Female Reproductive Disorders
Chapter 75	Cancers of the Female Reproductive System

Overview

- Cancer may affect the various parts of the female reproductive system

  o Breasts

  o Cervix

  o Uterus

  o Ovaries

- Breast cancer is the second leading cause of cancer deaths in women in the United States.

- Cervical cancer is a slow-growing cancer. With proper screening, it may be detected early and treated with good results.

- Uterine (endometrial) cancer is the fourth most common in women.

- The exact etiology of ovarian cancer is unknown; however, the more times a woman ovulates in her lifetime seems to be a risk factor since ovarian cancer is more prevalent in women with early menarche, late-onset menopause, nulliparity, and those who use infertility agents.

BREAST CANCER

Overview

- A combination of breast self-examination, a clinical breast exam, and mammography is effective in detecting early breast cancer and reducing mortality rates.

Health Promotion and Disease Prevention

- Screenings

  o All women over age 20 should conduct a monthly breast self-examination and schedule an annual clinical breast examination.

  o All women over age 40 should receive mammograms every 1 to 2 years.

- Instruct the client to eat five servings of fruits and vegetables daily.

- Instruct the client to maintain a healthy weight, and exercise regularly.

- Instruct the client to limit alcohol intake and avoid smoking.

Assessment

- Risk Factors

  o High genetic risk

    ▪ First-degree relative with breast cancer (parent, sibling, or child)

    ▪ Early age at diagnosis

  o Female sex (less than 1% of males develop breast cancer)

  o Age over 40

  o Early menarche

  o Late menopause

  o First pregnancy after age 30

  o Early or prolonged use of oral contraceptives

  o High-fat diet (possible risk)

  o Low-fiber diet (possible risk)

  o Excessive alcohol intake (possibly related to folic acid depletion)

  o Cigarette smoking

  o Exposure to low-level radiation

  o Hormone replacement therapy

  o Obesity

  o History of endometrial or ovarian cancer

  o Breast cancer rates are expected to increase over the next 50 years due to the increase in the older adult population.

  o Older adult clients are at greater risk of complications following surgery for cancer.

- Subjective Data

  o Breast pain or soreness

- Objective Data

  o Physical Assessment Findings

    ▪ Skin changes (peau d'orange)

View Media Supplement: Breast Changes: Peau d'orange (Image)

- ■ Dimpling
- ■ Breast tumors (usually small, irregularly shaped, firm, nontender, and nonmobile)
- ■ Increased vascularity
- ■ Nipple retraction or ulceration
- ■ Enlarged lymph nodes
- o Laboratory Tests
  - ■ BRCA1 and BRCA2 gene test
    - □ Recommended for women who have two first-degree relatives who were diagnosed with breast cancer before age 50 or women who have a family history of both breast and ovarian cancer.
    - □ A consent form is required before conducting the test.
    - □ Cannot be done within 3 months of a blood transfusion.
    - □ Test results are either positive or negative for presence of the gene.
  - ■ HER2 gene cell
    - □ A pathology report from a biopsy may determine if cancer cells contain the HER2 gene.
    - □ If the result is positive, this gene may be responsible for the rapidly cancerous growing cells.
    - □ Additional chemotherapy may be needed postoperatively.
- o Diagnostic Procedures
  - ■ Mammogram
  - ■ Biopsy-definitive diagnosis
    - □ An open biopsy is done by excising a small portion of the mass for histologic exam.
    - □ Fine needle aspiration is the removal of tissue or fluid from the breast mass through a large-bore needle.
    - □ The choice of treatment depends on the stage and size of the tumor, as well as nodal involvement.

Collaborative Care

- • Interdisciplinary Care
  - o Arrange for a visitor from Reach for Recovery to speak with the client.
  - o Refer the client to a community support group as appropriate.
  - o Refer the client to home health care services for care of drains and dressings and for help with ADLs.

- Therapeutic Procedures

  ○ Adjuvant therapy (radiation therapy, chemotherapy, or hormonal therapy) follows surgery to decrease the risk of reoccurrence.

    ■ Hormone therapy

      □ Gonadotropin-releasing hormone (GnRH)-leuprolide (Lupron)

        ▸ Inhibits estrogen synthesis.

        ▸ May be used in premenopausal women to stop or prevent the growth of breast tumors.

      □ Selective estrogen receptor modulators (SERMs)-tamoxifen (Nolvadex) and raloxifene (Evista)

        ▸ SERMs are used in women who are at high risk for breast cancer or who have advanced breast cancer.

        ▸ SERMs suppress the growth of remaining cancer cells postmastectomy or lumpectomy.

        ▸ Tamoxifen has been found to increase the risk of endometrial cancer, deep vein thrombosis, and pulmonary embolism; raloxifene does not share these side effects.

    ■ Chemotherapy/radiation therapy

      □ The decision to augment or replace a mastectomy procedure with chemotherapy and/or radiation therapy depends on several factors (client's age, hormone status related to menopause, genetic predisposition, and staging of disease).

      □ Clients who undergo chemotherapy are usually given a combination of several medications (Cytoxan, Adriamycin, and fluorouracil).

      □ Clients who have the HER2/neu gene may receive trastuzumab (Herceptin).

      □ Clients who have metastatic cancer may receive a vascular endothelial growth factor inhibitor, such as bevacizumab (Avastin).

      □ Stem-cell transplants are being researched in regard to treating clients who are at high risk of recurrence.

      □ Radiation therapy is usually reserved for clients who had a lumpectomy or breast-conserving procedure.

        ▸ Whole or partial breast radiation may be prescribed. Skin care will be a high priority due to radiation damage as well as generalized fatigue.

        ▸ Brachytherapy with radioactive seeds may also be an option.

        ▸ Intraoperative radiation therapy allows an intense dose of radiation to be delivered directly to the surgical site.

- Surgical Interventions
  - Surgical procedures include lumpectomy (breast-conserving), wide excision or partial mastectomy, total mastectomy, modified radical mastectomy, radical mastectomy, and reconstructive surgery .

     View Media Supplement: Total Mastectomy with Lymph Node Dissection (Image)

    - Nursing Actions
      - Provide routine postoperative care to prevent postoperative complications.
      - Have the client sit with the head of the bed elevated 30° when awake and support her arm on a pillow.
      - Have the client support her arm on the operative side with a sling while ambulating, and encourage good posture.
      - Encourage the client to lie on her unaffected side postoperatively to relieve pain.
      - Avoid administering injections, taking blood pressure, or drawing blood from the client's affected arm. Place a sign above the client's bed regarding these precautions.
      - Emphasize the importance of a well-fitting breast prosthesis for a client who has had a mastectomy.
      - Provide emotional support to the client and her family.
    - Client Education
      - Teach the client how to care for her incision and drainage tubes. (Drains are usually left in for 1 to 3 weeks.)
      - Advise the client to avoid placing her arm in a dependent arm position. This position will interfere with wound healing.
      - Encourage early arm and hand exercises (squeezing a rubber ball, elbow flexion and extension, and hand-wall climbing) to prevent lymphedema and to regain full range of motion.
      - Teach the client not to wear constrictive clothing and to avoid cuts and injuries to the affected arm.
      - Teach/reinforce teaching regarding breast self-examination.
      - Instruct the client to report numbness, pain, heaviness, or impaired motor function of the affected arm to the surgeon.
      - Encourage the client to discuss breast reconstruction alternatives with the surgeon.
        - ▸ Reconstruction may begin during the original breast removal procedure or after some healing has occurred.

- ▸ A tissue expander (a saline-filled implant that has a port through which additional saline can be injected, gradually expanding the tissue prior to permanent implant) is often placed during the original procedure.

- ▸ Saline or silicone implants are used for permanent placement.

- ▸ Autologous flaps may also be used for reconstruction.

- ▸ Nipple reconstruction may be done using tissue from the labia, abdomen, or inner thigh.

- Client Outcomes

  - ○ The client will regain full use of the arm on the side where the mastectomy occurred.

  - ○ The client will integrate the mastectomy scar or reconstructive appearance of the breast into her new body image.

Complications

- Tumor invasion

  - ○ A tumor invasion can occur in the lymphatic channels and seed cancer cells into the blood and lymphatic systems. The most common areas of metastases are the nearby bone, lungs, brain, and liver.

  - ○ Client Education

    - ▪ Reinforce the importance of continuing adjuvant therapy if prescribed.

    - ▪ Instruct the client about signs and symptoms of metastatic breast cancer and common locations.

CERVICAL CANCER

Overview

- The incidence of cervical cancer is increasing and affecting a younger population than in the past.

- Early cervical cancer is generally asymptomatic. Symptoms do not develop until the cancer has become invasive.

- Papanicolaou (Pap) tests are an effective screening tool for detecting the earliest changes associated with cervical cancer. Findings of a Pap smear are usually classified according to the Bethesda system.

Health Promotion and Disease Prevention

- All women should be tested for cervical cancer on a regular basis. The Papanicolaou (Pap) test is done to screen for cervical cancer. The frequency of this test is related to several factors, including age, results, and the presence of the cervix post hysterectomy.

- The client should limit the number of sexual partners.

- The client should use condoms during sex.

- The client should avoid smoking.

Assessment

- Risk Factors

    o   Early sexual activity (before 18 years of age)

    o   Client and/or male partner has had multiple sexual partners

    o   Male partner who had a female partner with cervical cancer

    o   Low economic status

    o   Family history of cervical cancer

    o   African American

    o   Chronic cervical inflammation/infections

    o   Infection with human papilloma virus (HPV), which is associated in 90% of cases

    o   History of sexually transmitted diseases

    o   Infection with HIV or other immunosuppressive disorder

    o   Cigarette smoking

    o   Intrauterine exposure to diethylstilbestrol during pregnancy

- Subjective Data

    o   Painless vaginal bleeding between periods

    o   Watery, blood-tinged vaginal discharge

    o   Unexplained weight loss

    o   Pelvic pain

    o   Pain during and after intercourse

- Objective Data

    o   Diagnostic Procedures

        ▪   Pap smear – microscopic examination of cervical cells

        ▪   Cervical biopsy (definitive) is performed for cytologic studies when a cervical lesion is identified. Biopsy is usually performed during colposcopy as a follow up to an abnormal Pap smear.

Collaborative Care

- Nursing Care

    o Treat anemia as indicated.

    o Administer antibiotics for pelvic, vaginal, or urinary tract infections.

    o Administer pain medications as prescribed.

    o Provide emotional support to the client and family.

- Interdisciplinary Care

    o Refer the client to a community support group as appropriate.

    o Refer the client to counseling if depressed or expressing concerns over sexuality.

- Therapeutic Procedures

    o Removal of the lesion by conization, cryotherapy, laser ablation, hysterectomy or a loop electrosurgical excision procedure.

        ■ Nursing Actions

            □ Prepare the client for the procedure indicated.

        ■ Client Education

            □ Teach the client signs and symptoms of infection.

            □ Inform the client that vaginal discharge, consistent with the type of procedure, is normal after the procedure.

            □ Teach the client about home care following special procedures (vaginal discharge, pain, avoiding douches, avoiding tampons, avoiding sexual intercourse, safety precautions, and postradiation treatments).

    o Radiation

        ■ Brachytherapy and external radiation therapy may be options for cancer that is no longer limited to local invasion.

        ■ Client Education

            □ Brachytherapy

            □ External radiation therapy

                ‣ Monitor the client for skin damage, especially in the perineal area.

- Surgical Interventions

    o Clients who have early stage cervical cancer may require a simple hysterectomy (one that removes the uterus and cervix) or a radical hysterectomy (one that removes the uterus, upper third of the vagina, uterosacral uterovesical ligaments, and pelvic nodes).

    o Clients with more extensive cancer may require a more extensive pelvic surgery called exenteration.

- Anterior exenteration involves removal of the uterus, cervix, fallopian tubes, vagina, ovaries, bladder, urethra, and pelvic lymph nodes. An ileal conduit will need to be established for urinary diversion.

- Posterior exenteration involves removal of the uterus, cervix, fallopian tubes, vagina, ovaries, anal canal, rectum, and descending colon. A colostomy will need to be established for bowel diversion.

- A total exenteration involves removal of all of the above organs and establishment of both urinary and bowel diversions.

- Nursing Actions

  □ Provide routine postoperative care to prevent complications.

  □ Manage drains as well as urinary and bowel diversions.

  □ Assess the client for body image disturbance and encourage speaking openly about it.

  □ Assess and discuss the client's understanding and expectations of treatment.

  □ Initiate social worker consultation to establish community referrals for home care needs (ostomy nurse, home health nurse, home health aide and emotional support).

- Client Education

  □ Teach the client signs and symptoms of wound infection and how to care for drains that may remain after discharge.

  □ Instruct the client about how to care for urinary and bowel diversion.

  □ Instruct the client about how to care for perineal wounds and expectations regarding discharge.

- Client Outcomes

  ○ The client will reestablish urinary and bowel function via a diversional method.

  ○ The client will reestablish positive self-image, integrating alterations caused by the surgical procedure.

Complications

  ○ Fistula development can occur after pelvic exenteration.

  ○ Kidney infections are also common secondary to the urinary diversion.

UTERINE (ENDOMETRIAL) CANCER

Overview

- Endometrial cancer is more common in older adult women and is related to prolonged exposure to estrogen.

- Estrogen therapy in postmenopausal women who have a uterus should include progesterone to decrease the risk of endometrial cancer.

Health Promotion and Disease Prevention

- Avoid the use of unopposed estrogen when considering postmenopausal hormone replacement therapy.

Assessment

- Risk Factors

    o Over 55 years of age

    o Obesity

    o Unopposed estrogen hormone replacement therapy

    o Nulliparity

    o Use of tamoxifen to prevent breast cancer

    o Late menopause

- Subjective Data

    o Irregular and/or postmenopausal bleeding

- Objective Data

    o Diagnostic Procedures

       ■ Endometrial biopsy

Collaborative Care

- Therapeutic Procedures

    o Radiation

       ■ Radiation therapy is given as adjuvant therapy, usually after a hysterectomy.

       ■ Brachytherapy and external radiation therapy may be options for cancer that is no longer limited to the uterus.

       ■ Client Education

          □ Brachytherapy and external radiation therapy

- Surgical Interventions

    o Treatment of endometrial cancer usually involves a total hysterectomy (uterus and cervix).

    o Removal of the fallopian tubes and ovaries (salpingectomy, oophorectomy) may also be done in the presence of a malignancy. The vagina is spared allowing sexual intercourse to continue.

       ■ Either an open, laparoscopic, or vaginal approach may be used for either of the above procedures.

- o   Nursing Actions

    - ▪   Provide routine postoperative care to prevent postoperative complications.

    - ▪   Observe for urinary retention and difficulty voiding due to proximity to the urethra (more common after vaginal hysterectomies).

    - ▪   A paralytic ileus may be more common due to manipulation of the bowel during surgery.

    - ▪   Discuss sexuality, surgically induced menopause, and other self-image issues with the client.

- o   Client Education

    - ▪   Instruct the client to avoid straining, driving, lifting more than 5 lb, douching, and participating in sexual intercourse until the provider gives release.

    - ▪   Instruct the client to immediately report signs and symptoms of infection, as well as vaginal discharge that is excessive or has a foul odor.

    - ▪   Discuss hormone replacement therapy options with the client if she is premenopausal.

- •   Client Outcomes

    - o   The client will reestablish positive self-image in regard to removal of the reproductive organs.

    - o   The client will not develop an infection of the incision or bladder.

OVARIAN CANCER

Overview

- •   Metastases frequently occur before the primary ovarian malignancy is diagnosed.

- •   The most reliable indicator of prognosis is related to the stage of the cancer at the time of diagnosis.

Health Promotion and Disease Prevention

- •   Birth control pills may offer protection against ovarian cancer.

Assessment

- •   Risk Factors

    - o   Over 40 years of age

    - o   Nulliparity or first pregnancy after 30 years of age

    - o   Family history of ovarian, breast, or colon cancer

    - o   History of dysmenorrhea or heavy bleeding

- o Endometriosis
- o High-fat diet (possible risk)
- o Hormone replacement therapy
- o Use of infertility medications
- o Older adult clients following surgery for cancer.

Ⓖ

- Subjective Data
  - o Abdominal pain or swelling
  - o Abdominal discomfort (dyspepsia, indigestion, gas, distention)
  - o Abdominal mass
  - o Urinary frequency

- Objective Data
  - o Laboratory Tests
    - Cancer antigen test (CA-125 antigen)
      - □ Elevates in the presence of damaged endometrial tissue
      - □ Also elevates in response to endometriosis, pregnancy, and fibroids
      - □ Elevated value is more than 35 units/mL
  - o Diagnostic Procedures
    - Bimanual examination may reveal an enlarged ovary. The finding may not be apparent until the ovarian tumor is 4 to 6 inches in size.
    - A vaginal ultrasound may also be helpful in determining the presurgical size and location of tumors as well as a 1 year follow up that evaluates success of treatment and recurrence or metastases of tumors.
    - Staging of ovarian cancer is determined at the time of the hysterectomy or exploratory laparotomy when the tumor is removed and examined by the pathologist.

Collaborative Care

- Interdisciplinary Care
  - o Arrange for the client to visit with a cancer survivor if possible.
  - o Provide the client with information about cancer support groups (Gilda's Club and National Ovarian Cancer Coalition).
  - o Provide information about hospice care when appropriate.

- Therapeutic Procedures

  - Chemotherapy (traditional or intraperitoneal)

    - Chemotherapy is always given for ovarian cancer, even if surgery was performed. Cisplatin and carboplatin are the most common chemotherapeutic mediations used for ovarian cancer.

    - Intracavitary chemotherapy involves the placement of an intraperitoneal catheter through which the chemotherapy is administered.

      - With client in a semi-Fowler's position, the chemotherapeutic agent is infused into the abdomen. Discomfort will be felt related to the pressure from the infusion, but may also indicate dislocation of the catheter.

      - "Dwell time" is the amount of time the agent remains in the abdominal cavity.

      - Agent is drained via the catheter after the prescribed amount of dwell time.

      - The client should be instructed to report signs and symptoms of infection, including peritonitis.

  - Pelvic or abdominal irradiation

    - Radiation is only used if the disease is localized to a small area or if palliative treatment of tumors is the goal.

- Surgical Interventions

  - A total abdominal hysterectomy with bilateral salpingectomy and oophorectomy (TAH with BSO) is the usual treatment for ovarian cancer.

    - A TAH with BSO also helps determine the extent of the disease as well as local and distant metastases. Staging of the cancer is done at this time.

    - Nursing Actions

      - Provide postoperative care and prevent postoperative complications.

      - Observe the client for urinary retention and difficulty voiding.

      - Paralytic ileus may be more common due to manipulation of the bowel during surgery.

      - Discuss sexuality, surgically induced menopause, and other self-image issues with the client.

      - Encourage the client to express feelings about the cancer and fears of death.

      - Help the client and family to develop coping strategies.

      - Monitor the client's progress through the stages of grief.

- Client Education

  □ Instruct the client to avoid straining, driving, lifting more than 5 pounds, douching, and participating in sexual intercourse until the provider gives release.

  □ Instruct the client to immediately report signs and symptoms of infection, as well as vaginal discharge that is excessive or has a foul odor.

- Client Outcomes

  o The client will experience a symptom-free period post surgery.

  o The client will experience minimal side effects from chemotherapy.

  o The client will set realistic personal goals in view of the stage of the disease and prognosis.

CHAPTER 75: CANCERS OF THE FEMALE REPRODUCTIVE SYSTEM

(A) Application Exercises

Scenario: A 47-year-old female client presents to the health screening clinic for the first time in 8 years. For the first time since the death of her husband 8 years ago, she is in a new relationship and is planning to resume sexual activity. Her medical history is significant for hypercholesteremia, which resolved with dietary changes and exercise. She lost 25 lb last year but has hypertension. Her body mass index is 25. She smokes three to four cigarettes daily. She engages in vigorous exercise four to five times a week. Family history is significant for the death of her mother at age 25 due to ovarian cancer. She has no siblings. She was married for 17 years prior to the death of her husband and was unable to conceive during that time. The couple did not seek infertility treatment. The client has had one sexual partner in her lifetime. Her menstrual history is: menarche at age 12, regular 31 day cycles, gravida 0.

1. Which of the following assessment findings place the client at risk for cancers of the reproductive system? (Select all that apply.)

   _____ Female gender

   _____ Over 40 years of age

   _____ Nullipara

   _____ Hypertensive

   _____ Previous history of obesity

   _____ Menarche at age 12

   _____ Cigarette smoking

   _____ Ovarian cancer in a first-degree relative

2. Which of the following diagnostic procedures should the nurse anticipate will need to be performed on the client to assess for ovarian cancer?

   A. Bimanual pelvic examination

   B. Pap smear

   C. Mammogram

   D. Stool for occult blood

3. A client is concerned that she may be at risk for breast cancer because she has had several relatives, including her mother, diagnosed with it. Her mother died of breast cancer at age 38. Which of the following tests should the nurse anticipate will be done to assess this client's risk?

   A. HER2 gene

   B. BRCA1 gene

   C. GnRH

   D. CA-125

4. A client who has advanced cervical cancer has undergone a posterior exenteration procedure. Which of the following should the nurse anticipate including in the client's plan of care?

    A. Make a referral to an ostomy nurse.

    B. Discuss contraceptive options.

    C. Administer vaginal irrigation daily.

    D. Change the bag on the ileal conduit daily.

CHAPTER 75: CANCERS OF THE FEMALE REPRODUCTIVE SYSTEM

 Application Exercises Answer Key

Scenario: A 47-year-old female client presents to the health screening clinic for the first time in 8 years. For the first time since the death of her husband 8 years ago, she is in a new relationship and is planning to resume sexual activity. Her medical history is significant for hypercholesteremia, which resolved with dietary changes and exercise. She lost 25 lb last year but has hypertension. Her body mass index is 25. She smokes three to four cigarettes daily. She engages in vigorous exercise four to five times a week. Family history is significant for the death of her mother at age 25 due to ovarian cancer. She has no siblings. She was married for 17 years prior to the death of her husband and was unable to conceive during that time. The couple did not seek infertility treatment. The client has had one sexual partner in her lifetime. Her menstrual history is: menarche at age 12, regular 31 day cycles, gravida 0.

1. Which of the following assessment findings place the client at risk for cancers of the reproductive system? (Select all that apply.)

   X   **Female gender**

   X   **Over 40 years of age**

   X   **Nullipara**

         Hypertensive

   X   **Previous history of obesity**

         Menarche at age 12

   X   **Cigarette smoking**

   X   **Ovarian cancer in a first-degree relative**

Female gender, age over 40, nulliparity, a previous history of obesity, cigarette smoking, and ovarian cancer in a first-degree relative are all risk factors for cancer of a reproductive organ. Hypertension is not a risk factor for reproductive cancer and menarche at age 13 is within the expected reference range (it is not considered early menarche).

Ⓝ **NCLEX® Connection: Physiological Adaptation: Alterations in Body Systems**

2. Which of the following diagnostic procedures should the nurse anticipate will need to be performed on the client to assess for ovarian cancer?

A. Bimanual pelvic examination

B. Pap smear

C. Mammogram

D. Stool for occult blood

Due to the location of ovarian cancer, a bimanual pelvic examination will need to be performed to assess for an ovarian mass or enlarged ovary. A pap smear is done to screen for cervical cancer, a mammogram is done to screen for breast cancer, and a stool for occult blood is done to screen for colon cancer.

Ⓝ **NCLEX® Connection: Reduction of Risk Potential: Diagnostic Tests**

3. A client is concerned that she may be at risk for breast cancer because she has had several relatives, including her mother, diagnosed with it. Her mother died of breast cancer at age 38. Which of the following tests should the nurse anticipate will be done to assess this client's risk?

    A. HER2 gene

    B. BRCA1 gene

    C. GnRH

    D. CA-125

The BRCA1 and BRCA2 genes are specific for breast cancer. They have been linked to breast cancer that occurs at a younger age in families. The HER2 gene is tested for on actual breast tissue after a biopsy or mastectomy has been done. The CA-125, or cancer antigen test, is diagnostic for ovarian cancer. GnRH is gonadotropin-releasing hormone and is given as a part of adjuvant therapy to decrease the risk of recurrent breast cancer.

 NCLEX® Connection: Reduction of Risk Potential: Diagnostic Tests

4. A client who has advanced cervical cancer has undergone a posterior exenteration procedure. Which of the following should the nurse anticipate including in the client's plan of care?

    A. Make a referral to an ostomy nurse.

    B. Discuss contraceptive options.

    C. Administer vaginal irrigation daily.

    D. Change the bag on the ileal conduit daily.

A client who has undergone a posterior exenteration will have a transverse colostomy. A referral to an ostomy nurse is appropriate to include in the plan of care. Since the client also had all reproductive organs removed, contraception does not need to be discussed and vaginal irrigations will not need to be done. Since the surgical procedure was a posterior exenteration, the bladder and urethra were spared.

 NCLEX® Connection: Reduction of Risk Potential: Potential for Complications of Diagnostic Tests/Treatments/Procedures

UNIT 9	NURSING CARE OF CLIENTS WITH REPRODUCTIVE DISORDERS
Section	Male Reproductive Disorders
Chapter 76	Diagnostic Procedures for Male Reproductive Disorders

Overview

- Changes to the prostate gland are common as men age, and routine diagnostic procedures should be performed to evaluate it.

  ○ Enlargement of the prostate gland is usually benign and is called benign prostatic hypertrophy.

  ○ Prostate cancer is the most common type of cancer in men.

- Diagnostic procedures for male reproductive disorders that nurses should be knowledgeable about

  ○ Prostatic specific antigen

  ○ Digital rectal exam

  ○ Transrectal ultrasound

Prostatic Specific Antigen (PSA) and Digital Rectal Exam (DRE)

- The PSA measures the amount of a protein produced by the prostate gland in the bloodstream.

  ○ The PSA is done on a sample of blood, and its value is reported.

  ○ A client who has an elevated PSA should undergo a DRE by a provider to validate the findings.

- The DRE is done by a provider in an office or clinic.

  ○ With the client leaning over the examination table, the provider places a gloved finger in the client's anus and palpates the posterior portion of the prostate gland through the rectal wall.

  ○ If the DRE reveals an abnormality, the location of the potentially cancerous prostate lesion is determined by ultrasonography and confirmed by a biopsy.

- Indications

  ○ Many providers recommend an annual PSA and DRE on men over 50 to better ensure early detection of prostate cancer. African-American men and men who have a family history of prostate cancer should begin screening at an earlier age.

- ○ Client Presentation

  - ■ As men age, their prostate glands enlarge. As the prostate gland enlarges, it encroaches on the urethra and causes diminished flow and retention of urine. Blood may also be found in the urine. These symptoms could be indicative of BPH or prostate cancer.

- Interpretation of Findings

  - ○ PSA

    - ■ An increase in PSA may indicate that a client has prostatic cancer.

      - □ The expected reference range for the PSA is from 2 to 4 ng/mL.

      - □ A PSA is considered elevated if its value is above 4 to 10 ng/mL.

  - ○ DRE

    - ■ Abnormal findings during the DRE include an abnormally large and hard prostate with an irregular shape or lumps.

Transrectal Ultrasound (TRUS)

- With the client in a left, side-lying position, a probe is inserted into the client's rectum, and sound waves are bounced off the surface of the prostate gland.

  - ○ The sound waves provide an image of the gland.

- Indications

  - ○ A TRUS is done if a client's PSA and/or DRE reveal a possible abnormality.

- Interpretation of Findings

  - ○ If an irregularity is found, the image from the TRUS will be used to guide a needle biopsy.

CHAPTER 76: DIAGNOSTIC PROCEDURES FOR MALE REPRODUCTIVE DISORDERS

 Application Exercises

1. An older adult client is having an annual physical exam at a provider's office. Which of the following client findings indicates additional follow up is needed in regard to the prostate gland? (Select all that apply.)

_____ PSA is 4.2 ng/mL.

_____ DRE reveals an enlarged prostate that is smooth and firm.

_____ The client reports a weak urine stream.

_____ The client reports urinating once during the night.

_____ Smegma is present below the glands of the penis.

2. A client's provider has decided to perform a transrectal ultrasound on him. Which of the following information is appropriate for the nurse to give the client regarding this procedure?

A. "This procedure will determine if you have prostate cancer."

B. "The provider will insert a finger into your anus during the procedure."

C. "Sound waves will be used to create a picture of your prostate."

D. "An anesthetic will be used prior to insertion of the biopsy needle."

CHAPTER 76: DIAGNOSTIC PROCEDURES FOR MALE REPRODUCTIVE DISORDERS

 Application Exercises Answer Key

1. An older adult client is having an annual physical exam at a provider's office. Which of the following client findings indicates additional follow up is needed in regard to the prostate gland? (Select all that apply.)

    X   **PSA is 4.2 ng/mL.**

    _____   DRE reveals an enlarged prostate that is smooth and firm.

    X   **The client reports a weak urine stream.**

    _____   The client reports urinating once during the night.

    _____   Smegma is present below the glans of the penis.

Follow up is indicated for this client because his PSA is above 4.0 ng/mL and he reports a weak urine stream. An enlarged prostate that is smooth and firm is normal for an older adult, because the prostate gland enlarges with age. Urinating once during the night is common in older adults due to redistribution of blood that may have been trapped in lower extremities during the day. Smegma is a normal secretion that can accumulate beneath the glans of the penis if not removed during hygiene.

 NCLEX® Connection: Reduction of Risk Potential: Diagnostic Tests

2. A client's provider has decided to perform a transrectal ultrasound on him. Which of the following information is appropriate for the nurse to give the client regarding this procedure?

A. "This procedure will determine if you have prostate cancer."

B. "The provider will insert a finger into your anus during the procedure."

C. "Sound waves will be used to create a picture of your prostate."

D. "An anesthetic will be used prior to insertion of the biopsy needle."

A TRUS is done using sound waves to create a picture of the prostate gland. It is done by introducing a transducer into the client's rectum and bouncing sound waves off the prostate to determine the presence of lumps or irregularities. This procedure cannot determine if a client has prostate cancer. Only a biopsy of the tissue can make this determination.

 NCLEX® Connection: Reduction of Risk Potential: Diagnostic Tests

UNIT 9	NURSING CARE OF CLIENTS WITH REPRODUCTIVE DISORDERS
Section	Male Reproductive Disorders
Chapter 77	Disorders and Cancers of the Male Reproductive System

Overview

- There are several disorders that are associated with the male reproductive system.

  o Testicular cancer

  o Benign prostatic hypertrophy

  o Prostate cancer

- Testicular cancer is the most common malignancy in men 15 to 35 years old.

- As an adult male ages, the prostate gland enlarges. When the enlargement of the gland begins to cause urinary dysfunction, it is called benign prostatic hypertrophy (BPH).

- Prostate cancer is a slow-growing cancer. Conservative treatment may be the treatment of choice for a client, based on how fast the cancer is growing, if the cancer has spread, and the client's age and life expectancy.

TESTICULAR CANCER

Overview

- The cause of testicular cancer is unknown.

Health Promotion and Disease Prevention

- Teach clients testicular self-examination (TSE).

- The client should perform the examination monthly after a shower and in front of a mirror.

- The client should look and feel for any lumps or change in the size, shape, or consistency of the testes by gently rolling them between the thumbs and fingers.

- Clients should begin TSE at age 15 or younger.

Assessment

- Risk Factors

    o Undescended testis (cryptorchidism)

    o Genetic disposition

    o Metastases

    o Age 15 to 34 (but can occur at any age)

- Subjective Data

    o Lumps and/or swelling of testes

    o Feeling of heaviness in the testicles

    o Evidence of metastasis (abdominal masses, gynecomastia, back pain)

- Objective Data

    o Enlarged testes without pain

    o Palpable lump

    o Swelling of lymph nodes in the groin

    o Laboratory Tests

        ▪ Bio-markers for testicular tumors – alpha-fetoprotein and human chorionic gonadotropin (hCG)

            ▫ Elevated values in testicular cancer

            ▫ May use for diagnostic purposes as well as for treatment efficacy

    o Diagnostic Procedures

        ▪ Ultrasonography

            ▫ Determines if palpable mass is solid or fluid-filled

        ▪ Computed tomography (CT) imaging scan, chest x-rays, and bone scans

            ▫ Evaluates the extent of the cancer

            ▫ Localized or metastasized to other organs in the body (brain, spinal cord and bones)

        ▪ Lymphangiography

            ▫ Evaluates spread to lymph nodes

Collaborative Care

- Surgical Interventions

  - Orchiectomy – removal of the testis (unilateral orchiectomy) is the treatment of choice for testicular cancer.

    - This procedure is performed using an inguinal incision.

    - Gel-filled prostheses are implanted in the scrotum after removal of diseased testes.

    - If the lymph nodes are involved or the risk of spread is high, retroperitoneal lymph node dissection may also be performed.

    - Depending on the type of tumor and stage of cancer, chemotherapy or radiation may be prescribed postoperatively.

    - Nursing Actions

      - Preoperative

        - Discuss with the client any concerns about sexual functioning.

          - Erectile and climactic functions are usually not affected.

          - Fertility may be affected. Arrange for sperm banking prior to surgery, if desired.

        - Discuss with the client what to expect in relation to incisions and pain.

        - Lymph node dissection will require larger and more extensive incision unless it is done laparoscopically.

      - Postoperative

        - Clients will require care typical for any type of abdominal surgery.

        - Monitor the client for postoperative complications and ileus, and manage pain with analgesics and ice packs.

        - Observe the client's incisions for signs and symptoms of infection.

    - Client Education

      - Instruct the client to report symptoms of infection.

      - Instruct the client to avoid heavy lifting and strenuous activity for the prescribed period of time.

      - Reinforce the importance of continuing to perform testicular self-examinations, and have the client promptly report any abnormal findings.

- Client Outcomes

  - The client will not have any recurrence of cancer.

  - The client will re-establish a positive body image.

BENIGN PROSTATIC HYPERTROPHY (BPH)

 Overview

- BPH can significantly impair the outflow of urine from the bladder making a client susceptible to infection and retention. Excessive amounts of urine retained can cause reflux of urine into the kidney, dilating the ureter and causing kidney infections.

Assessment

- Risk Factors

  o Age

  o Family history

- Subjective Data

  o Urinary hesitancy

  o Recurrent bladder infections

  o Urinary retention

  o Painless hematuria

- Objective Data

  o Small amounts of urine voided at one time with significant residue; weak stream, and posturination dribble

  o Nocturia

  o Hematuria and/or bacteruria

  o Elevated BUN and creatinine (indicates kidney damage)

  o Diagnostic Procedures

    ▪ A digital rectal exam (DRE) will reveal an enlarged, smooth prostate.

    ▪ A transrectal ultrasound (TRUS) and needle or aspiration biopsy will be taken of the prostate

      ☐ Both may be performed to definitively diagnose or rule out prostate cancer in the presence of an enlarged prostate.

Collaborative Care

- Nursing Care

  ▪ Client Teaching

    ☐ Frequent ejaculation has been found to release prostatic fluids, therefore, decreasing the size of the prostate.

□ Tell the client to avoid drinking large amounts of fluids at one time and urinate when the urge is initially felt.

□ Tell the client to avoid bladder stimulants, such as alcohol and caffeine.

□ Tell the client to avoid medications that cause decreased bladder tone, such as anticholinergics, decongestants, and antihistamines.

□ BPH may initially be treated conservatively with medication.

- Medications

    o The goal of medication for BPH is to re-establish an uninhibited urine flow out of the bladder.

        ■ Dihydrotestosterone (DHT) lowering medications – 5-alpha reductase inhibitor (5-ARI), such as finasteride (Proscar)

            □ DHT-lowering medications decrease the production of testosterone in the prostate gland.

            □ Decreasing a male client's DHT will often cause a decrease in the size of the prostate.

            □ Client Education

                ▸ Reinforce to the client that medication must be taken daily on a long-term basis.

                ▸ Inform the client that impotence and a decrease in libido are possible side effects.

        ■ Alpha-blocking agents – tamsulosin (Flomax)

            □ Alpha-adrenergic receptor antagonists cause relaxation of the bladder outlet and prostate gland.

            □ These agents cause less pressure to be placed on the urethra, therefore, re-establishing a stronger urine flow.

            □ Client Education

                ▸ Warn the client that postural hypotension may occur and that changes in position must be made slowly.

                ▸ Warn the client that concurrent use with cimetidine (Tagamet) can potentiate the hypotensive effect.

- Surgical Interventions

    o Clients who do not receive adequate relief from conservative measures may need to have a transurethral resection of the prostate (TURP) performed.

        ■ A TURP is performed using a resectoscope (similar to a cystoscope) that is inserted through the urethra and trims away excess prostatic tissue, enlarging the passageway of the urethra through the prostate gland.

- Nursing Actions
  - □ Preoperatively
    - ▸ Cardiovascular, respiratory, and renal systems should be carefully assessed prior to surgery.
    - ▸ Ensure that the client fully understands the procedure and what to expect postoperatively.
  - □ Postoperatively
    - ▸ Postoperative treatment usually includes placement of an indwelling three-way catheter.
      - ▷ The catheter drains urine and allows for instillation of a continuous bladder irrigation (CBI) of normal saline (isotonic) or another prescribed irrigating solution to keep the catheter free of obstruction.

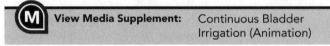

View Media Supplement: Continuous Bladder Irrigation (Animation)

      - ▷ The rate of the CBI is adjusted to keep the irrigation return pink or lighter. For example, if bright-red or ketchup-appearing (arterial) bleeding with clots is observed, the nurse should increase the CBI rate.
      - ▷ If the catheter becomes obstructed (bladder spasms, reduced irrigation outflow), turn off the CBI and irrigate with 50 mL of irrigation solution using a large piston syringe. Contact the primary care provider if unable to dislodge the clot.
      - ▷ Record the amount of irrigating solution instilled (generally very large volumes) and the amount of return. The difference equals urine output.
      - ▷ The catheter has a large balloon (30 to 45 mL) that is taped tightly to the leg, creating traction so that the balloon will apply firm pressure to the prostatic fossa to prevent bleeding. This makes the client feel a continuous need to urinate. Instruct the client to not void around the catheter as this causes bladder spasms. Avoid kinks in the tubing.
    - ▸ Monitor the client's vital signs and urinary output.
    - ▸ Administer/provide increased fluids to the client.
    - ▸ Monitor the client for bleeding (persistent bright-red bleeding unresponsive to increase in CBI and traction on the catheter or reduced Hgb levels) and report it to the primary care provider.
    - ▸ If blood is present, monitor the incision and change the dressing as appropriate.
    - ▸ Administer medications to the client as prescribed.
      - ▷ Analgesics (surgical manipulation or incisional discomfort)

▷ Antispasmodics (bladder spasms)

▷ Antibiotics (prophylaxis)

▷ Stool softeners (avoid straining)

▸ Discontinue CBI and catheter as prescribed. Monitor the client's urinary output. The initial voiding following removal may be uncomfortable, red in color and contain clots. The color of the urine should progress toward amber in 2 to 3 days. Instruct the client that expected output is 150 to 200 mL every 3 to 4 hr. The client should contact the provider if unable to void.

- Client Education

  □ Tell the client to avoid heavy lifting, strenuous exercise, straining, and sexual intercourse for the prescribed length of time (usually 2 to 6 weeks).

  □ Tell the client to drink 12 or more 8 oz glasses of water each day.

  □ Tell the client to avoid bladder stimulants, such as caffeine and alcohol.

  □ Tell the client that if urine becomes bloody, stop activity, rest, and increase fluid intake.

  □ Tell the client to contact the provider for persistent bleeding or obstruction (less than expected output or distention).

- Client Outcomes

  ○ The client's urine will be pink without clots postoperatively.

  ○ The client's flow of urine will allow the bladder to empty completely.

Complications

- TURP Complications

  ○ Urethral trauma, urinary retention, bleeding, and infection are complications associated with TURP.

  ○ Other complications include regrowth of prostate tissue and reoccurrence of bladder neck obstruction.

  ○ Nursing Actions

    - Monitor the client and intervene for bleeding.

    - Provide antibiotic prophylaxis to the client.

PROSTATE CANCER

Overview

- The incidence of prostate cancer increases with age.

- Symptoms are often similar to those of BPH.

Health Promotion and Disease Prevention

- Instruct the client to eat a diet low in animal fat and high in omega-3 fatty acids (fish), fruits, and vegetables.

- Instruct the client to have a PSA and DRE done yearly after age 50. African-American men and men who have a close relative who had prostate cancer may begin screenings earlier.

- Instruct the client to exercise regularly.

Assessment

- Risk Factors

  - Age greater than 65 years

  - Family history

  - African-American heritage

  - High-fat diet

  - BRCA2 mutation may be associated with an increase risk

- Subjective Data

  - Urinary hesitancy and weak stream

  - Recurrent bladder infections

  - Urinary retention

  - Blood in urine and semen

  - Painful ejaculation

- Objective Data

  - Small amounts of urine voided at one time with significant residue

  - Hematuria and/or bacteruria

  - Elevated BUN and creatinine (indicates kidney damage)

  - Laboratory Tests

    - Prostate-specific antigen (PSA) serum levels are elevated with prostate cancer (abnormal levels are greater than 4 ng/mL).

- o Diagnostic Procedures
  - ■ DRE – reveals a hard prostate with palpable irregularities
  - ■ TRUS – indicates the location of the lesion or lesions
  - ■ Needle or aspiration biopsy of the lesion – definitively diagnose or rule out prostate cancer
  - ■ Magnetic resonance imaging (MRI), computed tomography (CT) scans, and bone scans – assess for metastases

Collaborative Care

- Medications
  - o Hormone therapy
    - ■ Leuprolide acetate (Lupron) – gonadotropin-releasing hormone (GnRH)
      - □ Used in advanced prostate cancer to produce a chemical castration
      - □ Client Education
        - ‣ Warn the client that hot flashes are an adverse effect.
        - ‣ Tell the client that impotence and decreased libido may also be side effects.
        - ‣ The client should be monitored for osteoporosis, which can occur due to testosterone suppression.
    - ■ Flutamide (Eulexin) – androgen receptor blocker
      - □ Used in conjunction with a GnRH
      - □ Client Education
        - ‣ Warn the client that gynecomastia is a side effect.
        - ‣ The client's liver functions should be periodically monitored.
  - o Chemotherapy – may be used on clients whose cancer has spread or who have had little improvement with other therapies
    - ■ Docetaxel (Taxotere) – usually used to treat breast cancer
      - □ Client Education
        - ‣ Have the client's routine blood tests performed to monitor for neutropenia, leucopenia, thrombocytopenia, and anemia.
- Therapeutic Procedures
  - o Radiation therapy – external beam radiation therapy or implanted radioactive seeds (brachytherapy)
    - ■ Client Education
      - □ External radiation
      - □ Brachytherapy

- Surgical Interventions

  o Radical prostatectomy

    ▪ Involves the removal of the entire prostate gland, along with the seminal vesicles, the cuff at the bladder neck, and the regional lymph nodes

    ▪ Procedure of choice for treatment of prostate cancer

    ▪ May be done using a suprapubic, perineal, or retropubic approach

    ▪ A laparoscopic approach may be an option for treatment of localized prostate cancer

    ▪ Nursing Actions

      □ Preoperatively

        ‣ Ensure that the client fully understands the procedure and what to expect postoperatively.

      □ Postoperatively

        ‣ Clients will require care typical for any type of abdominal surgery.

        ‣ Monitor the client for postoperative complications and ileus, and manage his pain with analgesics and ice packs.

        ‣ Observe the client's incisions for signs and symptoms of infection.

        ‣ Provide catheter care and administer bladder antispasmodics to the client as prescribed.

        ‣ If the client has a suprapubic prostatectomy, a suprapubic catheter, in addition to the urethral catheter, will be placed. Usually, it will be removed when residual urine measurements are less than 75 mL.

    ▪ Client Education

      □ Instruct the client to report symptoms of infection.

      □ Teach the client catheter care if he will be going home with one in place.

      □ Tell the client to avoid heavy lifting and strenuous activity for the prescribed period of time.

      □ Instruct the client to avoid tub baths for at least 2 to 3 weeks.

- Client Outcomes

  o The client's incisions will heal without infection.

  o The client will redefine sexuality.

Complications

- A radical prostatectomy puts the client at risk for the following complications

  ○ Irreversible erectile dysfunction

  - This is due to pudendal nerve damage during the operation. In certain circumstances, the surgeon may be able to perform a nerve-sparing prostatectomy.

  - Nursing Actions

    □ Refer the client to other individuals who have had this same surgery and outcome.

  - Client Education

    □ Recommend to the client that he attend a community support group.

  ○ Refractory postoperative urinary incontinence

  - This requires implantation of an artificial urinary sphincter (AUS). An AUS is a device that prevents incontinence and allows the client some control over his bladder elimination pattern.

  - Teach the client to perform perineal exercises to reduce urinary incontinence.

CHAPTER 77: DISORDERS AND CANCERS OF THE MALE REPRODUCTIVE SYSTEM

 Application Exercises

1. When instructing a client about how to perform a testicular self-examination, the nurse should provide which of the following instructions? (Select all that apply.)

_____ Examine testicles while lying down.

_____ Examine testicles following a shower.

_____ Roll testes between thumb and fingers.

_____ Report changes in the size, shape, or consistency of the testes.

_____ Examine testes every 6 months.

2. Label each of the following findings as characteristic of prostate (P) or testicular cancer (T).

_____ Testicular lump

_____ Elevated alpha-fetoprotein (AFP)

_____ Elevated prostate-specific antigen (PSA)

_____ Urinary hesitancy

_____ Recurrent bladder infections

_____ Urinary retention

_____ Painless hematuria

3. A nurse is caring for a client who has undergone a transurethral resection of the prostate (TURP). Which of the following actions should the nurse take in relation to each of the client findings below?

CLIENT FINDINGS	NURSING RESPONSES
Urine output is bright red and contains more clots.	
Volume of urine output decreases and the client reports an extreme need to urinate.	
The client reports a constant need to urinate.	

4. A nurse is caring for a client who is preparing to undergo a radical prostatectomy. Which of the following complications should be discussed with the client prior to the surgery?

A. Bowel incontinence

B. Urethral strictures

C. Impotence

D. Constipation

CHAPTER 77: DISORDERS AND CANCERS OF THE MALE REPRODUCTIVE SYSTEM

 Application Exercises Answer Key

1. When instructing a client in testicular self-examination, the nurse should provide which of the following instructions? (Select all that apply.)

_____	Examine testicles while lying down.
X	**Examine testicles following a shower.**
X	**Roll testes between thumb and fingers.**
X	**Report changes in the size, shape, or consistency of the testes.**
_____	Examine testes every 6 months.

A testicular self-examination should be performed monthly following a shower by rolling the testes between the thumb and fingers while in front of a mirror. Any lumps or changes in the size, shape, or consistency of the testes should be reported to the primary care provider.

NCLEX® Connection: Reduction of Risk Potential, Diagnostic Tests

2. Label each of the following findings as characteristic of prostate (P) or testicular cancer (T).

T	Testicular lump
T	Elevated alpha-fetoprotein (AFP)
P	Elevated prostate-specific antigen (PSA)
P	Urinary hesitancy
P	Recurrent bladder infections
P	Urinary retention
P	Painless hematuria

All of the findings listed above, except testicular lump and elevated alpha-fetoprotein, are characteristics of prostate cancer. Testicular lumps and an elevated alpha-fetoprotein are characteristics of testicular cancer.

NCLEX® Connection: Reduction of Risk Potential, System-Specific Assessment

3. A nurse is caring for a client who has undergone a transurethral resection of the prostate (TURP). Which of the following actions should the nurse take in relation to each of the client findings below?

CLIENT FINDINGS	NURSING RESPONSES
Urine output is bright red and contains large clots.	**Increase CBI.** **Increase fluid intake.** **Contact the primary care provider if persistent.**
Volume of urine output decreases and client reports feeling an extreme need to urinate.	**Irrigate with 50 mL using a piston syringe (more pressure).** **Contact the provider if not able to resolve.**
Client reports a constant need to urinate.	**Explain the impact of the catheter balloon size and traction.** **Rule out obstruction.** **Administer antispasmodics as prescribed.**

 NCLEX® Connection: Reduction of Risk Potential, Potential for Complications from Surgical Procedures and Health Alterations

4. A nurse is caring for a client who is preparing to undergo a radical prostatectomy. Which of the following complications should be discussed with the client prior to the surgery?

    A. Bowel incontinence

    B. Urethral strictures

    C. Impotence

    D. Constipation

Due to the possibility of damaging the pudendal nerve during the operation, impotence is a potential complication. Bowel incontinence, urethral strictures, and constipation are not complications related to a radical prostatectomy.

 NCLEX® Connection: Reduction of Risk Potential, Potential for Complications from Surgical Procedures and Health Alterations

UNIT 10: NURSING CARE OF CLIENTS WITH MUSCULOSKELETAL DISORDERS

- Diagnostic and Therapeutic Procedures
- Musculoskeletal Disorders

NCLEX® CONNECTIONS

When reviewing the chapters in this unit, keep in mind the relevant sections of the NCLEX® outline, in particular:

CLIENT NEEDS: BASIC CARE AND COMFORT

Relevant topics/tasks include:
- Assistive Devices
  - Assess the client's use of assistive devices.
- Mobility/Immobility
  - Apply and maintain devices used to promote venous return.

CLIENT NEEDS: REDUCTION OF RISK POTENTIAL

Relevant topics/tasks include:
- Potential for Alterations in Body Systems
  - Identify the client with an increased risk for insufficient vascular perfusion.
- Potential for Complications of Diagnostic Tests/ Treatments/Procedures
  - Intervene to prevent potential neurological complications.
- System Specific Assessment
  - Assess the client for peripheral edema.

CLIENT NEEDS: PHYSIOLOGICAL ADAPTATION

Relevant topics/tasks include:
- Alterations in Body Systems
  - Provide wound care and/or assist with dressing change.
- Illness Management
  - Promote and provide continuity of care in illness management activities.
- Medical Emergencies
  - Notify the provider about the client's unexpected response/ emergency situation.

UNIT 10	NURSING CARE OF CLIENTS WITH MUSCULOSKELETAL DISORDERS
Section	Diagnostic and Therapeutic Procedures
Chapter 78	Musculoskeletal Diagnostic Procedures

Overview

- Imaging studies are the primary diagnostic procedures used for musculoskeletal disorders.

- Evaluation of the conduction of electrical impulses in muscles may also be assessed in the presence of muscle weakness.

- Endoscopic studies (arthroscopy) are done to assess the condition of a joint and may simultaneously repair tears and other joint defects that are identified.

- Musculoskeletal diagnostic procedures that nurses should be knowledgeable about:

  o Arthroscopy

  o Bone scans

  o Dual-energy x-ray absorptiometry scans

  o Electromyography and nerve conduction studies

Arthroscopy

- Arthroscopy is an endoscopic procedure done to visualize the internal structures of a joint.

- The knee and shoulder joints are the ones most commonly scoped.

- With the knee flexed, small incisions are made through which the scope is passed.

- Number and placement of incisions depend on the area of the joint needing to be visualized and the extent of the needed repair needed.

- Arthroscopy cannot be done if infection is present in the joint.

- Indications

  o Potential Diagnoses

    ■ A client who has sustained injuries to his joints may undergo arthroscopy to ascertain the extent of damage, during which time, repair may also be done using the endoscope (torn ligament or meniscus).

- o Client Presentation
  - Joint swelling, pain, and crepitus
  - Joint instability
- Preprocedure
  - o Nursing Actions
    - Teach the client postprocedure exercises or refer him to a physical therapist (straight leg raising, quadriceps setting isometrics).
    - Ensure that the client has signed the informed consent form.
  - o Client Education
    - Postoperative joint exercises
- Postprocedure
  - o Nursing Actions
    - Teach the client postprocedure care as arthroscopy is done on an outpatient basis.
    - Assess the neurovascular status of the client's limb prior to discharge.
  - o Client Education
    - Ice and elevate the client's extremity for 24 hr.
    - Instruct the client to take a prescribed analgesic for pain.
    - Apply a splint or sling if prescribed.
    - Have the client use crutches if limited weight bearing is prescribed.
    - Monitor the color and temperature of the client's extremity as well as pain and sensation.
    - Notify the provider of any changes.
- Complications
  - o Infection
    - Complications are uncommon after this procedure, but infection may occur as with any procedure that disrupts the integrity of the skin.
    - Client Education
      - □ Notify the provider immediately of any signs of infection, such as swelling, redness, or fever.

Bone Scan

- Bone scans are done when a client's entire skeletal system is to be evaluated.

- It is done using a radionuclide such as gallium or thallium.

- Radionuclide is injected 4 to 6 hr before scanning.

- The scan takes 30 to 60 min during which time the client must lay still.

- Indications

  - Potential Diagnoses

    - Osteoporosis

    - Primary or metastatic bone cancer

    - Bone pain of unknown origin

  - Client Presentation

    - Bone pain

- Preprocedure

  - Nursing Actions

    - Inform the client about how the procedure will be done.

  - Client Education

    - Tell the client to lie still during the length of the procedure.

- Postprocedure

  - Client Education

    - Following the procedure, the client does not need to take any radioactive precautions.

    - Encourage the client to drink fluids to increase excretion of radionuclide.

Dual-Energy X-ray Absorptiometry (DEXA) Scans

- DEXA scans are done to estimate the density of a client's bone mass and presence/extent of osteoporosis.

- These scans are usually done on the wrist, hip, or spine.

- Contrast material is not used.

- A DEXA scan uses two beams of radiation and findings are analyzed by a computer and interpreted by a radiologist. The client receives a score that relates their amount of bone density to other people in their age group and gender.

- The client will lie on an x-ray table while a scan of a selected area is done.

- Indications
  - Potential Diagnoses
    - Osteoporosis
    - Postmenopausal state (baseline may be done at age 40)
  - Client Presentation
    - Loss of height
    - Bone pain
    - Fractures
- Preprocedure
  - Nursing Actions
    - Inform the client about how the procedure will be done.
  - Client Education
    - Avoid taking a calcium supplement 24 hr prior to the procedure.
- Postprocedure
  - Client Education
    - Follow up with the provider regarding supplements and medications that may be needed if bone loss is present.

Electromyography and Nerve Conduction Studies

- Electromyography (EMG) and nerve conduction studies are done to determine the presence and cause of muscle weakness.
- EMG
  - Thin needles are placed in the muscle under study and attached to an electrode.
  - An electrode is attached to an oscilloscope and electrical activity is recorded during a muscle contraction.
- Nerve conduction study
  - Flat electrodes are taped on the skin.
  - Low, electrical currents are sent through the electrodes and muscle response to the stimulus is recorded.
- Indications
  - Potential Diagnoses
    - Lower motor neuron disease (amyotrophic lateral sclerosis, myasthenia gravis)
    - Peripheral nerve disorders (carpal tunnel, Guillain Barré)

- Preprocedure

  - Nursing Actions

    - Inform the client about what to expect.

    - Inform the client to avoid caffeine products before the exam.

    - Ask if the client is taking an anticoagulant or muscle relaxants (contraindicated for this procedure).

    - Have the client sign the consent form.

  - Client Education

    - Discomfort may be felt during needle insertion and when electrical current is sent through electrodes.

    - The client may be asked to flex his muscle while the needle is inserted.

- Postprocedure

  - Client Education

    - Inform the client that some bruising may occur at needle insertion sites.

    - Have the client report swelling or tenderness at any of the sites to provider.

    - Instruct the client to apply ice to the insertion sites to reduce swelling and pain.

CHAPTER 78: MUSCULOSKELETAL DIAGNOSTIC PROCEDURES

(A) Application Exercises

1. A client is scheduled for a dual-energy x-ray absorptiometry (DEXA) scan. The nurse recognizes that this has been prescribed in relation to which of the following client factors?

    A. Rheumatoid arthritis

    B. Age of 55

    C. Mother had osteoarthritis

    D. Body mass index is 30

2. A nurse should provide which of the following information to a client who is preparing to undergo a bone scan?

    A. "The entire procedure will only take about 1 hour."

    B. "You will be placed in a tube-like structure during the exam."

    C. "You will need to take precautions with your urine for 24 hr."

    D. "A radioactive substance will be injected into a vein."

3. A nurse is preparing a client for an arthroscopy during which time a repair of the meniscus is planned. Which of the following should the nurse include in the client's preoperative teaching? (Select all that apply.)

    _____ The affected extremity will be placed in a cast after the procedure.

    _____ Incisions must be monitored for infection at home.

    _____ Ice should be applied to the joint for 24 hr.

    _____ Joint should be placed in a dependent position.

    _____ Isometric exercises of the affected extremity should be performed.

CHAPTER 78: MUSCULOSKELETAL DIAGNOSTIC PROCEDURES

(A) Application Exercises Answer Key

1. A client is scheduled for a dual-energy x-ray absorptiometry (DEXA) scan. The nurse recognizes that this has been prescribed in relation to which of the following client factors?

    A. Rheumatoid arthritis

    B. Age of 55

    C. Mother had osteoarthritis

    D. Body mass index is 30

Postmenopausal women often have their bone mass monitored to identify osteoporosis prior to significant loss of bone mass. At age 55, this client is likely postmenopausal. There is no relationship between osteoporosis and osteoarthritis or rheumatoid arthritis. A body mass index (BMI) of 30 has no relationship to bone mass.

(N) NCLEX® Connection: Reduction of Risk Potential: Diagnostic Tests

2. A nurse should provide which of the following information to a client who is preparing to undergo a bone scan?

    A. "The entire procedure will only take about 1 hour."

    B. "You will be placed in a tube-like structure during the exam."

    C. "You will need to take precautions with your urine for 24 hour."

    D. "A radioactive substance will be injected into a vein."

A bone scan is done using a radionuclide such as gallium or thallium. Since the radionuclide must be absorbed by the bone prior to the procedure, the client must wait several hours after injection before the scan can be completed. An MRI is the procedure that uses a tube-like structure, and radioactive precautions do not need to be taken with the client's urine.

(N) NCLEX® Connection: Reduction of Risk Potential: Diagnostic Tests

3. A nurse is preparing a client for an arthroscopy during which time a repair of the meniscus is planned. Which of the following should the nurse include in the client's preoperative teaching? (Select all that apply.)

　　　　　　The affected extremity will be placed in a cast after the procedure.

　　X　　**Incisions must be monitored for infection at home.**

　　X　　**Ice should be applied to the joint for 24 hr.**

　　　　　　Joint should be placed in a dependent position.

　　X　　**Isometric exercises of the affected extremity should be performed.**

During the arthroscopy, small incisions will be made through which the arthroscope will be inserted. These must be monitored for infection postoperatively. Ice should be applied for 24 hr and isometric exercises of the muscles in the affected extremity should begin as soon as possible. The extremity should be elevated, not placed in a dependent position, to reduce swelling. Splints, not casts, are placed postprocedure.

(N) **NCLEX® Connection: Reduction of Risk Potential: Potential for Complications of Diagnostic Tests/Treatments/Procedures**

UNIT 10	NURSING CARE OF CLIENTS WITH MUSCULOSKELETAL DISORDERS

Section   Diagnostic and Therapeutic Procedures

Chapter 79   Musculoskeletal Surgical Procedures

Overview

- Most musculoskeletal surgical procedures are performed to repair damaged joints, in particular the knees and the hips.

- Arthroplasty refers to the surgical removal of a diseased joint and replacement with prosthetics or artificial components made of metal and/or plastic.

- Total joint arthroplasty, which can also be called total joint replacement, involves replacement of all components of an articulating joint.

- Musculoskeletal surgical procedures that nurses should be knowledgeable about:

  ○ Knee arthroplasty

  ○ Hip arthroplasty

Knee and Hip Arthroplasty

- Total knee arthroplasty involves the replacement of the distal femoral component, the tibia plate, and the patellar button. Total knee arthroplasty is a surgical option when conservative measures fail.

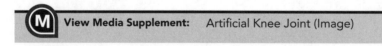
View Media Supplement: Artificial Knee Joint (Image)

- Unicondylar knee replacements are done when the client's joint may be diseased in one compartment of the joint.

- Total hip arthroplasty involves the replacement of the acetabular cup, the femoral head, and the femoral stem.

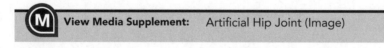
View Media Supplement: Artificial Hip Joint (Image)

- Hemiarthroplasty refers to half of a joint replacement. Fractures of the femoral neck can be treated with the replacement of the femoral component only.

- Indications

  - Diagnoses

    - Knee and hip arthroplasty is used to treat degenerative disease (osteoarthritis, rheumatoid arthritis).

      - Clients who generally require total-joint arthroplasty are older than 65 years.

  - Client Presentation

    - Pain when bearing weight on the joint (walking, running)

    - Joint crepitus and stiffness

    - Joint swelling (primarily occurs in the knees)

- Desired Therapeutic Outcome

  - The goal of both hip and knee arthroplasty is to eliminate pain, restore joint motions, and improve the client's functional status and quality of life.

- Preprocedure

  - Nursing Actions

    - Review diagnostic test results.

      - CBC, urinalysis, electrolytes, BUN, creatinine – Assess the client's surgical readiness, and rule out anemia, infection, or organ failure. Epoetin alfa may be prescribed preoperatively to increase Hgb.

      - Chest x-ray – Rule out pulmonary surgical contraindications (infection, tumor).

      - ECG – Gather a baseline rhythm to identify cardiovascular surgical contraindications (dysrhythmia).

    - Determine if there are contraindications to the procedure.

      - Recent or active infection

      - Arterial impairment to the affected extremity

      - The client's inability to follow the post-surgery regimen

      - A comorbid condition (unstable cardiac or respiratory conditions)

      - Risk for venous thromboembolism should also be considered prior to joint replacement surgery (previous history, obesity, advanced age, use of medications that increase risk such as hormone replacement therapy, NSAIDs)

      - Prophylactic broad-spectrum antibiotic if prescribed

- o Client Education

    - ▪ Postoperative care (incentive spirometry, transfusion, surgical drains, dressing, pain control, transfer, exercises, activity limits)

    - ▪ Autologous blood donation (client donates blood prior to procedure to be used postoperatively)

    - ▪ Postoperative exercises of surgical extremity

- ● Intraprocedure

    - o General or spinal anesthesia may be used.

    - o Joint components are removed and replaced with artificial components.

    - o Components may or may not be cemented in place. Components that do not use cement allow the bone to grow into the prosthesis to stabilize it. Weight bearing is delayed several weeks until femoral shaft has grown into prosthesis.

    - o Artificial joints have a limited life span ranging from 10 to 20 years.

- ● Postprocedure

    - o Nursing Actions

        - ▪ Knee arthroplasty

            - □ Provide postoperative care and prevent postoperative complications.

            - □ Older adult clients are at a higher risk for medical complications related to chronic conditions, including hypertension, diabetes mellitus, coronary artery disease, and obstructive pulmonary disease.

            - □ A continuous passive motion machine is used to promote motion in the knee and prevent scar tissue formation. It is usually placed and initiated immediately after surgery. It provides passive range of motion from full extension to the prescribed amount of flexion. The prescribed duration of its use should be followed, but it should be turned off during meals.

            - □ Positions of flexion of the knee are limited to avoid flexion contractures. Avoid knee gatch and pillows placed behind the knee.

            - □ Provide medications as prescribed.

                - ▸ Analgesics – opioids (epidural, PCA, IV, oral), NSAIDs

                - ▸ A continuous peripheral nerve block – Continuous infusion of local anesthetic directly into sciatic or femoral nerve

                    - ▹ A continuous peripheral nerve block provides localized pain relief.

                    - ▹ Monitor the client for systemic effects of local anesthetic, such as hypotension, bradycardia, restlessness or seizure.

                - ▸ Antibiotics – Prophylaxis and postoperatively

                - ▸ Anticoagulant – Aspirin; low-molecular weight heparin, such as enoxaparin (Lovenox); warfarin (Coumadin)

□ Ice or cold therapy may be applied to reduce postoperative swelling.

□ Monitor the client's neurovascular status of surgical extremity every 2 to 4 hr (movement, sensation, color, pulse).

□ Assess the client frequently for overt bleeding and signs of hypovolemia, such as hypotension and tachycardia.

- Hip arthroplasty

  □ Provide postoperative care and prevent postoperative complications.

  □ The older adult client is at a higher risk for medical complications related to chronic conditions including hypertension, diabetes mellitus, coronary artery disease, and obstructive pulmonary disease.

  □ Monitor the client for bleeding.

    ▸ Check the dressing site frequently, noting any evidence of bleeding. Monitor and record drainage from surgical drains.

    ▸ Monitor daily laboratory values, including Hgb and Hct levels. The client's Hgb and Hct may continue to drop 24 to 48 hr after surgery. Autologous blood from presurgery donation or blood salvaged intraoperatively or postoperatively using special collection devices may be used for postoperative blood replacement. Blood transfusions are relatively common for Hgb levels less than 9 g/dL.

  □ Monitor the neurovascular status of the surgical extremity every 2 to 4 hr (movement, sensation, color, pulse).

  □ Provide medications as prescribed.

    ▸ Analgesics – Opioids (epidural, PCA, IV, oral), NSAIDs

    ▸ Antibiotics – Prophylaxis and postoperatively

    ▸ Anticoagulant – Aspirin; low-molecular weight heparin, such as enoxaparin (Lovenox); warfarin (Coumadin)

  □ Early Ambulation

    ▸ Transfer the client out of bed from his unaffected side into a reclining wheelchair.

    ▸ The client's weight-bearing status is determined by the orthopedic surgeon and by choice of cemented (usually partial/full weight-bearing as tolerated) versus noncemented prostheses (usually only partial weight-bearing until after a few weeks of bone growth).

    ▸ Use assistive devices (walker) and adaptive devices (raised toilet seat) when caring for client.

▢ Client position – Place the client supine with his head slightly elevated and his affected leg in neutral position. A pillow or abduction device may be place between legs when turning him to the unaffected side or if he is noncompliant with restrictions. The client should not be turned to his operative side, which could cause hip dislocation.

▢ Use total hip precautions to prevent dislocation of new joint.

DO	DON'T
Use elevated seating/raised toilet set.	Avoid flexion of hip greater than 90°.
Use straight chairs with arms.	Avoid low chairs.
Use an abduction pillow between the client's legs while in bed (and with turning).	Do not cross the client's legs.
Externally rotate the client's toes.	Do not internally rotate the client's toes.

○ Client Education

■ Knee and hip arthroplasty

▢ The client will require extensive physical therapy to regain mobility. The client may be discharged to home or an extended care facility for rehabilitation. If discharged to home, outpatient or in-home therapy must be provided. Home care should be available for 4 to 6 weeks.

▢ Monitor signs and symptoms of incisional infection (fever, increased redness, swelling, purulent drainage) and care for the incision (clean daily with soap and water).

▢ Monitor for signs and symptoms of deep vein thrombosis (swelling, redness, pain in calf), pulmonary embolism (shortness of breath, chest pain), and bleeding if the client is taking an anticoagulant.

▢ Hip arthroplasty – Follow position restrictions to avoid dislocation (See table above.). Arrange for and instruct the client about the use of raised toilet seats, and care items (long-handled shoehorn, dressing sticks).

▢ Knee arthroplasty – Dislocation is not common following total knee arthroplasty. Kneeling and deep-knee bends are however, limited indefinitely.

- Complications
  - Deep vein thrombosis
    - Deep vein thrombosis is a complication and can result in a pulmonary embolism.
    - Nursing Actions
      - Monitor the client for symptoms of pulmonary embolism, including acute onset of dyspnea, tachycardia, and pleuritic chest pain.
      - Deep vein thrombosis prophylaxis includes pharmacological management, the use of anti-embolic stockings and sequential compression devices, ankle exercises while in bed, and early mobilization with physical and occupational therapy.
    - Hip dislocation and subluxation
      - Since the muscle surrounding the hip joint has been cut to expose and replace the diseased joint, the client is at risk for hip dislocation.
    - Nursing Actions
      - Monitor the client for symptoms, including acute onset of pain, the client's report of hearing "a pop," internal rotation of the affected extremity, and shortened affected extremity.
      - An abductor pillow or splint is used to prevent adduction, which can cause dislocation of the surgical hip.

CHAPTER 79: MUSCULOSKELETAL SURGICAL PROCEDURES

(A) Application Exercises

1. A 55-year-old client is undergoing a total hip arthroplasty. The nurse is preparing a teaching plan for the client including activity restrictions after the surgery. Which of the following should the nurse include in the teaching plan? (Select all that apply.)

_____ Avoid hip flexion greater than 90°.

_____ Sit in a low recliner.

_____ Avoid external rotation of toes.

_____ Use an abduction pillow while lying on your side in bed.

_____ Continue isometric exercises.

2. Which of the following is a contraindication for total joint arthroplasty surgery?

A. Age greater than 70 years

B. History of cancer

C. Previous joint arthroplasty surgery

D. Recent infection

3. A nurse is admitting a client to the orthopedic unit from the postanesthesia care unit who had a total hip arthroplasty. Which of the following are the appropriate nursing interventions for this client? (Select all that apply.)

_____ Obtain vital signs.

_____ Assess pulses in the surgical extremity.

_____ Assess pain.

_____ Remove surgical drains.

_____ Apply heat to postoperative hip.

_____ Initiate continuous passive motion machine.

4. Develop a discharge teaching plan for a client who is going home after having total hip replacement surgery.

CHAPTER 79: MUSCULOSKELETAL SURGICAL PROCEDURES

 Application Exercises Answer Key

1. A 55-year-old client is undergoing a total hip arthroplasty. The nurse is preparing a teaching plan for the client including activity restrictions after the surgery. Which of the following should the nurse include in the teaching plan? (Select all that apply.)

__X__ **Avoid hip flexion greater than 90°.**

_____ Sit in a low recliner.

_____ Avoid external rotation of toes.

__X__ **Use an abduction pillow while lying on your side in bed.**

__X__ **Continue isometric exercises.**

Total hip precautions will need to be addressed with the client. The client will need to avoid hip flexion greater than 90°. This could cause hip dislocation. When lying on the unoperated side, the client should use an abduction pillow. The client should continue to use the abduction pillow while in bed to avoid crossing his legs while sleeping. Isometric exercises may be continued along with the exercises prescribed by physical therapy. The client needs to avoid low chairs (which will flex the hip more than 90°), sit in higher chairs with arms, and use an elevated toilet seat. The client should be instructed not to cross his legs or internally rotate the affected hip.

NCLEX® Connection: Reduction of Risk Potential, Potential for Complications from Surgical Procedures and Health Alterations

2. Which of the following is a contraindication for total joint arthroplasty surgery?

A. Age greater than 70 years

B. History of cancer

C. Previous joint arthroplasty surgery

D. Recent infection

Recent infection is a contraindication for total joint arthroplasty surgery. Clients who are greater than 70 years of age, have a history of cancer, or have had previous joint arthroplasty surgery are all potential candidates for joint arthroplasty surgery if indicated.

NCLEX® Connection: Reduction of Risk Potential, Potential for Complications from Surgical Procedures and Health Alterations

3. A nurse is admitting a client to the orthopedic unit from the postanesthesia care unit who had a total hip arthroplasty. Which of the following are the appropriate nursing interventions for this client? (Select all that apply.)

    __X__   **Obtain vital signs.**

    __X__   **Assess pulses in the surgical extremity.**

    __X__   **Assess pain.**

    _____   Remove surgical drains.

    _____   Apply heat to postoperative hip.

    _____   Initiate continuous passive motion machine.

Vital signs should be obtained frequently for a client who is postoperative including neurovascular checks that include peripheral pulses. Pain should be assessed and treated with prescribed medications. Ice not heat, may be applied to the incisional site to reduce pain, swelling, and bleeding. The dressing site should be checked frequently, noting any evidence of bleeding, and drainage from surgical drains should be monitored and recorded. Surgical drains should not be removed, as they have been placed to remove drainage from the surgical site during the postoperative period. A continue passive motion (CPM) machine is often used for passive range of motion following a total knee arthroplasty.

(N) **NCLEX® Connection: Reduction of Risk Potential, Potential for Complications from Surgical Procedures and Health Alterations**

4. Develop a discharge teaching plan for a client who is going home after having total hip replacement surgery.

The client should continue to wear thigh-high stockings until the follow-up visit with the surgeon. The client should continue to take medications (an anticoagulant) as prescribed by the provider. Monitor the client for unexpected bleeding. Early and regular ambulation is needed. Teach the client and family the signs/symptoms of deep vein thrombosis, including redness, pain, induration, and warmth in the calf. Notify the provider if symptoms occur.

(N) **NCLEX® Connection: Reduction of Risk Potential, Therapeutic Procedures**

UNIT 10   NURSING CARE OF CLIENTS WITH MUSCULOSKELETAL DISORDERS
Section   Diagnostic and Therapeutic Procedures
Chapter 80   Amputations

Overview

- Amputation is the removal of a body part, most commonly an extremity.

- Amputations are described in regard to the extremity and whether they are located above or below the designated joint.

- The term disarticulation describes an amputation performed through a joint.

- Upper extremity amputations include above- and below-the-elbow amputations, wrist and shoulder disarticulations, and finger amputations.

- Lower extremity amputations include above- and below-the-knee amputations, hip and knee disarticulations, Syme amputation (removal of foot with ankle saved), midfoot and toe amputations.

- Lower extremity amputations are usually done due to peripheral vascular disease and every effort is made to save as much of the extremity as possible. Even loss of the big toe can significantly affect balance and ambulation. Salvage of the knee with a below-the-knee amputation (BKA) also improves function over an above-the-knee amputation (AKA)

- The higher the level of amputation, the greater the amount of effort that will be required to use a prosthesis.

- Older adult clients are poor candidates for prosthetic training due to the amount of energy required for ambulation.

- Significant changes to a client's body image occur after an amputation and should be addressed during the client's perioperative and rehabilitative phases.

Health Promotion and Disease Prevention

- Clients who are diabetic should monitor blood glucose and maintain within the expected reference range.

- Use safety measures when working with heavy machinery or in areas where there is a risk of electrocution or burns.

- Encourage clients to quit or not start smoking.

- Maintain good foot care and seek early medical attention for nonhealing wounds.

Assessment

- Risk Factors

  - Traumatic injury

  - Thermal injury (frostbite, electrocution, burns)

  - Peripheral vascular disease

  - Malignancy

  - Chronic disease processes

    - Peripheral vascular disease resulting in ischemia/gangrene

    - Diabetes mellitus resulting in peripheral neuropathy and peripheral vascular disease

    - Infection (osteomyelitis)

  - Older adult clients have a higher risk of peripheral vascular disease and diabetes mellitus resulting in decreased tissue perfusion and peripheral neuropathy. Both conditions place older adult clients at risk for lower extremity amputation.

- Subjective Data

  - Clients may or may not report pain.

  - History of injury or disease process precipitating amputation

- Objective Data

  - Peripheral pulses (may need to use Doppler)

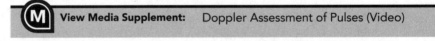

View Media Supplement: Doppler Assessment of Pulses (Video)

  - Temperature of extremities (level of leg at which temperature becomes cool)

  - Color of extremities (black indicates gangrene, cyanosis indicates vascular compromise)

  - Sensation

  - Presence of infection and wounds

- Diagnostic Procedures

  o Several studies are done to determine blood flow at various levels of an extremity.

    - Angiography – allows visualization of peripheral vasculature and areas of impaired circulation

    - Doppler laser and ultrasonography studies – measure speed of blood flow in an extremity

    - Transcutaneous oxygen pressure ($TcPO_2$) – measures oxygen pressures in an extremity

    - Ankle-brachial index – measures difference between ankle and brachial systolic pressures

    - Level of amputation will be determined by level at which adequate blood flow is available for healing.

Collaborative Care

- Surgical Interventions - Surgical Amputation Techniques

  o Closed amputation

    - This is the most common technique used. Skin flap is sutured over end of residual limb, closing site.

  o Open amputation

    - This technique is used when an active infection is present. Skin flap is not sutured over end of residual limb allowing for drainage of infection. Skin flap is closed at a later date.

- Nursing Actions (pre, post)

  o Prevent postoperative complications.

  o Assess surgical site for bleeding. Monitor vital signs frequently.

  o Monitor tissue perfusion of end of residual limb.

    - Palpate residual limb for warmth. Heat may indicate infection.

    - Compare pulse most proximal to incision with pulse in other extremity.

  o Monitor and treat pain.

    - Differentiate between phantom limb and incisional pain.

    - Incisional pain is treated with analgesics.

    - Phantom limb pain may be treated with beta blockers such as propranolol (Inderal) and antiepileptics such as gabapentin (Neurontin).

    - Antispasmodics may be prescribed for muscle spasms.

- o Monitor for signs of infection and/or non-healing of incision.

  - Amputation may not heal if done below level of adequate tissue perfusion.

  - Position the affected extremity in dependent position to promote blood flow/ oxygenation.

  - Administer antibiotics and change dressings as prescribed if open amputation was performed.

  - Record characteristics of drainage, such as amount, color, and odor.

- o Client's perception and feelings regarding amputation of body part

  - Allow for the client/family to grieve for the loss of the body part and change in body image.

  - Feelings may include depression, anger, withdrawal, and grief.

  - The nurse should facilitate supportive environment for both client and family so grief can be processed.

  - Rehabilitation should include adaptation to new body image and integration of prosthetic and adaptive devices into self image.

- o Residual limb preparation and prosthesis fitting

  - Residual limb must be shaped and shrunk in preparation for prosthetic training.

  - Shrinkage interventions include:

    - □ Wrapping the stump, using ace bandages (figure-eight wrap) to prevent restriction of blood flow.

    - □ Utilizing a stump shrinker sock (easier for the client to apply).

    - □ Using an air splint (plastic inflatable device) inflated to 20 to 22 mm Hg for 22 of 24 hr/day.

- o Client Education

  - Explain to the client how to care for and wrap the residual limb and perform limb-strengthening exercises.

  - Demonstrate proper application and care of the prosthesis to the client.

  - Explain to the client how to safely transfer and use mobility devices and adaptive aids.

  - Explain to the client how to manage phantom limb pain.

- Interdisciplinary Care (consultations, referrals)

  o Intensive efforts by the interdisciplinary team will be necessary to facilitate successful rehabilitation.

  o A certified prosthetic orthotist will fit client with prosthesis after wound is healed and stump has shrunk.

  o A physical therapist will train client in the application and care of prosthesis and mobility aids.

  o A psychologist may be needed to help with adjustment to loss of extremity.

- Client Outcomes

  o Client will adapt physically and emotionally to prosthesis.

  o Client will integrate residual limb and prosthesis into body image.

Complications

- Phantom Limb Pain

  o Phantom limb pain is the sensation of pain in the location of the extremity following the amputation. This is related to severed nerve pathways and is a frequent complication in clients who experience chronic limb pain before the amputation. Phantom limb pain occurs less frequently following traumatic amputation. It also tends to lessen with time but some clients experience phantom limb pain or sensation indefinitely.

  o Nursing Actions

    ▪ The nurse should recognize the pain is real and manage it accordingly.

    ▪ It may be described as deep and burning, cramping, shooting, or aching. Symptoms may be managed with various medications (opioids, antispasmodics, antiepileptics, beta blockers).

- Flexion Contractures

  o Flexion contractures can occur in the hip or knee joint following amputation due to improper positioning.

  o Nursing Actions

    ▪ Prevention includes range-of-motion (ROM) exercises and proper positioning

    ▪ Avoid elevating the stump on a pillow after the first 24 hr.

    ▪ Have the client lie prone several times a day.

    ▪ Discourage prolonged sitting.

  o Client Education

    ▪ Have physical therapist teach client some exercises that will prevent contractures.

    ▪ Have the client stand using good posture with residual limb in extension. This will also aid in balance.

CHAPTER 80: AMPUTATIONS

 Application Exercises

Scenario: A nurse is caring for a young adult client who is 24 hr postoperative following a below-the-knee amputation of his right leg as treatment for osteogenic sarcoma. The gauze and elastic dressings are dry and intact. His vital signs are stable and he is prescribed morphine sulfate via PCA.

1. What postoperative measures should the nurse provide to the client to avoid hip or knee flexion contractures?

    A. Elevate residual limb on pillow.

    B. Have the client lie in a prone position.

    C. Wrap stump using a figure-eight pattern.

    D. Encourage use of over bed trapeze.

2. Which of the following postoperative assessments should the nurse perform over for the next few days? (Select all that apply.)

    _____ Presence and amount of drainage (especially bloody drainage)

    _____ Indications of infection (foul odor, purulent drainage, increased pain, fever)

    _____ Measurement for prosthesis

    _____ Presence of stump swelling

    _____ Assessment of type of pain

3. The client reports that he is experiencing pain in the foot that is no longer there. How can the nurse best explain this phenomenon to the client? Explain that he is experiencing

    A. incisional pain coming from the amputated limb.

    B. phantom limb pain, which is common after amputations.

    C. referred pain from the bone that was cut.

    D. imaginary pain because the limb is no longer there.

CHAPTER 80: AMPUTATIONS

 Application Exercises Answer Key

Scenario: A nurse is caring for a young adult client who is 24 hr postoperative following a below-the-knee amputation of his right leg as treatment for osteogenic sarcoma. The gauze and elastic dressings are dry and intact. His vital signs are stable and he is prescribed morphine sulfate via PCA.

1. What postoperative measures should the nurse provide to the client to avoid hip or knee flexion contractures?

   A. Elevate residual limb on pillow.

   B. Have the client lie in a prone position.

   C. Wrap stump using a figure-eight pattern.

   D. Encourage use of over bed trapeze.

   The client should be placed in the prone position several times a day to prevent hip flexion contraction contractions. Elevating the residual limb on a pillow may increase the risk for hip flexion contracture. Wrapping the stump will decrease swelling, but this will not prevent contractures. Lastly, use of the over-bed trapeze by the client will promote independence and mobility, but it will not prevent contractures.

   NCLEX® Connection: Potential for Complications from Surgical Procedures and Health Alterations

2. Which of the following postoperative assessments should the nurse perform over for the next few days? (Select all that apply.)

X	**Presence and amount of drainage (especially bloody drainage)**
X	**Indications of infection (foul odor, purulent drainage, increased pain, fever)**
	Measurement for prosthesis
X	**Presence of stump swelling**
X	**Assessment of type of pain**

   The client's incision and residual limb should be monitored closely for drainage, infection, and swelling. The type of pain experienced is important to assess so it can be appropriately managed (incisional versus phantom limb pain). Measurement for a prosthesis does not occur until the wound has healed and the residual limb has shrunk.

   NCLEX® Connection: Potential for Complications from Surgical Procedures and Health Alterations

3. The client reports that he is experiencing pain in the foot that is no longer there. How can the nurse best explain this phenomenon to the client? Explain that he is experiencing

    A. incisional pain coming from the amputated limb.

    B. phantom limb pain, which is common after amputations.

    C. referred pain from the bone that was cut.

    D. imaginary pain because the limb is no longer there.

Phantom limb pain is real pain that is experienced by clients who have undergone amputations. Its exact cause is unknown. Incisional pain would be experienced at the incisional site, not in the amputated foot. Referred pain is not a complication after amputation of a limb.

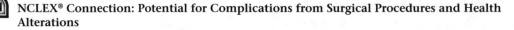 **NCLEX® Connection: Potential for Complications from Surgical Procedures and Health Alterations**

UNIT 10	NURSING CARE OF CLIENTS WITH MUSCULOSKELETAL DISORDERS
Section	Musculoskeletal Disorders
Chapter 81	Osteoporosis

 Overview

- Osteoporosis is the most common metabolic bone disorder resulting in low bone density. Osteoporosis occurs when the rate of bone resorption (osteoclast cells) exceeds the rate of bone formation (osteoblast cells) resulting in fragile bone tissue and subsequent fractures.

- Osteopenia, the precursor to osteoporosis, refers to low bone mineral density for what is expected for the client's age and sex.

- Peak bone mineral density occurs between the ages of 30 and 35. After peak years, bone density decreases, with a significant increase in the rate of loss in postmenopausal women due to estrogen loss.

- Fragile, thin bone tissue is susceptible to fracture.

Health Promotion and Disease Prevention

- Ensure the client's diet includes adequate amounts of calcium and vitamin D, especially before age 35.

- Encourage the client to take a calcium supplement with vitamin D if dietary intake is inadequate (lactose intolerant).

- Encourage the client to expose areas of skin to sun 5 to 30 min twice a week.

- Encourage the client to discuss the pros and cons of hormone replacement therapy post-menopausally with her provider.

- Encourage the client to engage in weight-bearing exercises.

Assessment

- Risk Factors

  o Female

  o Age over 60 (over 75, if male)

  o Postmenopausal estrogen deficiency

  o Family history

  o Thin, lean body build

  o History of low calcium intake with suboptimal levels of vitamin D

  o History of smoking

  o History of high alcohol intake

  o Lack of physical activity/prolonged immobility

  o Secondary osteoporosis results from medical conditions including:

    ▪ Hyperparathyroidism.

    ▪ Long-term corticosteroid use (asthma, systemic lupus erythematosus).

    ▪ Long-term lack of weight-bearing (spinal cord injury).

  o Primary osteoporosis most frequently occurs in postmenopausal women.

  o Older adult clients have an increased risk of falls related to impaired balance, generalized weakness, gait changes, and impaired vision and hearing. Medication side effects can cause orthostatic hypotension, urinary frequency, or confusion, which can also raise the client's risk for falls.

- Subjective Data (symptoms)

  o Reduced height (postmenopausal)

  o Acute back pain after lifting or bending (worse with activity, relieved by rest)

  o Restriction in movement

  o History of fractures

- Objective Data

  o Thoracic (kyphosis)

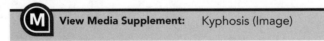
View Media Supplement: Kyphosis (Image)

  o Pain upon palpation over affected area

  o Laboratory Tests

    ▪ Serum calcium, vitamin D, phosphorus, and alkaline phosphatase levels are drawn to rule out other metabolic bone diseases (Paget's disease or osteomalacia).

- o Diagnostic Procedures
  - ■ Radiographs
    - □ Radiographs of the spine and long bones reveal low bone density and fractures.
  - ■ Dual energy x-ray absorptiometry (DEXA)
    - □ Dual energy x-ray absorptiometry (DEXA) is used to screen for early changes in bone density. This painless test measures bone mineral density in the wrist, hip, and vertebral column.
  - ■ Quantitative ultrasound (QUS)
    - □ An ultrasound, usually of the heel. QUS is an inexpensive, portable, and low-risk method to determine osteoporosis and assessing for risk of fracture.

Collaborative Care

- • Nursing Care
  - o Administer medications as prescribed.
  - o Instruct the client and family regarding dietary calcium food sources.
  - o Provide information regarding calcium supplementation (take with food).
  - o Instruct the client of the need for adequate amounts of protein, magnesium, vitamin K, and other trace minerals needed for bone formation.
  - o Reinforce the need for exposure to vitamin D (sunlight, fortified milk).
  - o Encourage weight-bearing exercises to improve strength and reduce bone loss.
  - o Assess the home environment for safety (remove throw rugs, provide adequate lighting, clear walkways).
  - o Reinforce the use of safety equipment and assistive devices.
  - o Instruct the client to avoid inclement weather (ice, slippery surfaces).
  - o Clearly mark thresholds, doorways, and steps.
- • Medications
  - o Several medications can be taken to slow the development of osteoporosis. A combination of several of these medications may be used in place of just one.

CLASSIFICATION/MEDICATION	THERAPEUTIC INTENT	NURSING CONSIDERATIONS
Estrogen Hormone Supplement • Estrogen (Premarin), • Estrogen and medroxyprogesterone (Prempro)	• Replaces estrogen lost due to menopause or surgical removal of ovaries	• Instruct client on potential complications, including breast and endometrial cancers and deep vein thrombosis (DVT). • Reinforce monthly breast self-examinations. Estrogen should be given along with progesterone in women who still have their uterus.
Selective Estrogen Receptor Modulators • Raloxifene hydrochloride (Evista)	• Decreases osteoclast activity, subsequently decreasing bone resorption • Treats postmenopausal osteoporosis as well as breast cancer	• Avoid for clients with a history of DVT. • Monitor liver function tests.
Calcium Supplement • Calcium-carbonate (Os-Cal, Caltrate-600) • Calcium-citrate (Citracal)	• Supplements calcium that is consumed in food products	• Give with food in divided doses with 6 to 8 oz of water. • Calcium supplements may cause GI upset. • Monitor for kidney stones.
Vitamin D Supplement	• Increases absorption of calcium from the intestinal tract and availability of calcium in the serum needed for remineralization of bone • Needed by individuals who are not exposed to adequate amounts of sunlight or who do not meet its daily requirements	• Vitamin D is a fat-soluble vitamin, so toxicity can occur. Symptoms of toxicity include nausea, constipation, and kidney stones.
Bisphosphonates (inhibit bone resorption) • Alendronate sodium (Fosamax) • Ibandronate sodium (Boniva) • Risedronate (Actonel)	• Decreases number and actions of osteoclasts, subsequently inhibiting bone resorption	• Risk for esophagitis. Report early signs of indigestion, chest pain, difficulty swallowing, or bloody emesis to provider immediately. • Take with 8 oz of water in the early morning before eating. • Remain upright for 30 min.
Thyroid Hormone • Calcitonin (Miacalcin)	• Decreases bone resorption by inhibiting osteoclast activity.	• Can be taken IM/SC or nasally; alternate nostrils

- Interdisciplinary Care (consultations, referrals)

    ○ Physical therapy may be used to establish an exercise regimen.

    ○ Clients may need rehabilitation if fractures cause immobilization or disability.

    ○ Most hip fractures are due to osteoporosis. Joint repair or joint arthroplasty requires physical therapy for a full recovery.

- Therapeutic Procedures

    ○ Orthotic devices are available for immobilization of the spine immediately after a compression fracture of the spine.

        ■ Provides support and decreases pain

        ■ A physical therapist fits the device for the client and teaches him how to apply it.

        ■ Nursing Actions

            □ Teach the client how to check for skin breakdown under the orthotic device.

- Surgical Interventions

    ○ Joint repair or joint arthroplasty may be necessary to repair or replace a joint weakened by osteoporosis. This is most often the hip joint.

Complications

- Fractures are the leading complication of osteoporosis. Early recognition and treatment is essential.

    ○ Nursing Actions

        ■ The nurse should review risk factors for osteoporosis and falls, assess the client's dietary intake of calcium, reinforce daily exercise including weight-bearing activities, and ensure proper screening with a DEXA scan.

CHAPTER 81: OSTEOPOROSIS

 Application Exercises

1. An older adult client is admitted to the emergency department with a chief report of back pain. She is unable to recall any trauma or fall. She describes the pain as becoming progressively worse to where she feels completely immobilized due to the pain, and is unable to ambulate even to the bathroom. The nurse suspects that the client has osteoporosis. Which of the following findings support this diagnosis? (Select all that apply.)

_____ History of drinking one glass of wine with dinner daily

_____ Change in height from 65 inches to 62 inches since menopause

_____ Body Mass Index (BMI) of 21

_____ Kyphotic curve at upper thoracic spine

_____ History of taking medroxyprogesterone (Prempro) for the past 8 years

_____ Lactose intolerance

2. Which of the following clients are at risk for osteoporosis? (Select all that apply.)

_____ A 40-year-old male who takes prednisone (Deltasone) daily for severe asthma

_____ A 30-year-old female who jogs daily

_____ A 65-year-old female who is sedentary

_____ A 70-year-old male who smokes

_____ An 80-year-old male who walks daily

3. In providing dietary instructions to a client to minimize the risk of osteoporosis, the nurse should recommend which of the following foods?

A. Bread

B. Yogurt

C. Chicken

D. Rice

CHAPTER 81: OSTEOPOROSIS

 Application Exercises Answer Key

1. An older adult client is admitted to the emergency department with a chief report of back pain. She is unable to recall any trauma or fall. She describes the pain as becoming progressively worse to where she feels completely immobilized due to the pain, and is unable to ambulate even to the bathroom. The nurse suspects that the client has osteoporosis. Which of the following findings support this diagnosis? (Select all that apply.)

_____	History of drinking one glass of wine with dinner daily
__X__	**Change in height from 65 inches to 62 inches since menopause**
__X__	**Body Mass Index (BMI) of 21**
__X__	**Kyphotic curve at upper thoracic spine**
_____	History of taking medroxyprogesterone (Prempro) for the past 8 years
__X__	**Lactose intolerance**

Findings consistent with osteoporosis are loss of height; small, thin frame as evidenced by a BMI of 21; kyphotic curve in upper back; and lactose intolerance. One glass of wine daily is not considered "excessive" drinking; and Prempro is a medication given to prevent osteoporosis.

N NCLEX® Connection: Physiological Adaptation: Pathophysiology

2. Which of the following clients are at risk for osteoporosis? (Select all that apply.)

__X__	**A 40-year-old male who takes prednisone (Deltasone) daily for severe asthma**
_____	A 30-year-old female who jogs daily
__X__	**A 65-year-old female who is sedentary**
__X__	**A 70-year-old male who smokes**
__X__	**An 80-year-old male who walks daily**

Age (female over 60 and males over 75), female gender, corticosteroid therapy, such as prednisone, smoking, and lack of weight-bearing exercise are all risk factors. Jogging will help prevent the occurrence of osteoporosis.

N NCLEX® Connection: Physiological Adaptation: Pathophysiology

3. In providing dietary instructions to a client to minimize the risk of osteoporosis, the nurse should recommend which of the following foods?

    A. Bread

    B. Yogurt

    C. Chicken

    D. Rice

Dairy products are high in calcium, and yogurt is a dairy product. Bread, chicken, and rice do not provide high sources of calcium.

Ⓝ **NCLEX® Connection: Basic Care and Comfort: Nutrition and Oral Hydration**

UNIT 10	NURSING CARE OF CLIENTS WITH MUSCULOSKELETAL DISORDERS
Section	Musculoskeletal Disorders
Chapter 82	Fractures

Overview

- A fracture is a break in a bone secondary to trauma or a pathological condition.

- Fractures caused by trauma are the most common type of fracture.

- Pathological fractures may be caused by metastatic cancer, osteoporosis, or Paget's disease.

- Bone is continually going through a process of remodeling as osteoclasts release calcium from the bone and osteoblasts build up the bone.

- This process occurs at equal rates until an individual reaches their thirties. From this age on, the activity of the osteoclasts outpace the osteoblasts, increasing an individual's risk of osteoporosis as he ages. In women, this process significantly increases post-menopausal. Subsequently, women experience fractures secondary to osteoporosis a decade or so earlier than men.

Health Promotion and Disease Prevention

- Ensure recommended intake of calcium for developmental stage in life.

- Ensure adequate intake of vitamin D and/or exposure to sunlight.

- Teach postmenopausal women the importance of regular bone scans to monitor for development of osteoporosis.

- Engage in weight-bearing exercise on a regular basis.

- Take a bisphosphonate if prescribed by provider.

- Use caution to prevent falls or accidents.

- Prevent injury with the use of seat belts and helmets.

FRACTURES

Overview

- A closed fracture does not break through the skin surface. An open, or compound, fracture disrupts the skin integrity, causing an open wound with a risk of infection.

- Open fractures are graded based upon the extent of tissue injury.

    o Grade I – minimal skin damage

    o Grade II – damage includes skin and muscle contusions

    o Grade III – damage to skin, muscles, nerves, and blood vessels

- A complete fracture goes through the entire bone, dividing it into two parts. An incomplete fracture goes through part of the bone.

- A simple fracture has one fracture line, while a comminuted fracture has multiple fracture lines splitting the bone into multiple pieces.

- A displaced fracture has bone fragments that are not in alignment, and a non-displaced fracture has bone fragments that remain in alignment.

- Common Types of Fractures

    o Comminuted: Bone is fragmented

    o Oblique: Fracture occurs at oblique angle

    o Spiral: Fracture occurs from twisting motion (common with physical abuse)

    o Impacted: Fractured bone is wedged inside opposite fractured fragment

    o Greenstick: Fracture that occurs on one side (cortex), but does not extend completely through the bone. Occurs most often in children.

- Hip fractures are the most common injury in older adults.

(M) View Media Supplement: X-ray of Leg Fracture (Image)

Assessment

- Risk Factors

    o Osteoporosis

        ▪ Women who do not use estrogen replacement therapy after menopause lose estrogen and are unable to form strong new bone.

        ▪ Clients on long-term corticosteroid therapy lose calcium from their bones due to direct inhibition of osteoblast function, inhibition of gastrointestinal calcium absorption, and enhancement of bone resorption.

    o Falls

    o Motor vehicle crashes

    o Substance abuse

- ○ Diseases (bone cancer, Paget's disease)

- ○ Contact sports and hazardous recreational activities (football, skiing)

- ○ Physical abuse

- ○ Lactose intolerance

- ⓖ ○ Age, as bone becomes less dense with advancing age

- Subjective Data

  - ○ Obtain history of trauma, metabolic bone disorders, chronic conditions, and possible use of corticosteroid therapy.

  - ○ Pain and/or reduced movement at the area of fracture or the area distal to the fracture.

- Objective Data

  - ○ Physical Assessment Findings

    - Crepitus: A grating sound created by the rubbing of bone fragments

    - Deformity: May observe internal rotation of extremity, shortened extremity, visible bone with open fracture

    - Muscle spasms: Occur from the pulling forces of the bone when not aligned

    - Edema: Swelling from trauma

    - Ecchymosis: Bleeding into underlying soft tissues from trauma

  - ○ Diagnostic Procedures

    - Standard radiographs, computed tomography (CT) imaging scan, and/or magnetic resonance imagery (MRI)

      - □ Identify the type of fracture and location.

      - □ Indicate pathological fracture resulting from tumor or mass.

      - □ Determine soft tissue damage.

    - A bone scan is used to determine fracture complications/delayed healing.

Collaborative Care

- Nursing Care

  - ○ Provide emergency care at time of injury.

  - ○ Maintain ABCs.

  - ○ Monitor the client's vital signs and neurological status.

  - ○ Assess neurovascular status of injured extremity.

  - ○ Place the client in supine position.

  - ○ Stabilize the injured area including the joints above and below the fracture, avoiding unnecessary movement.

- o Elevate the limb and apply ice.

- o Assess for bleeding and apply pressure, if needed.

- o Cover open wounds with a sterile dressing.

- o Remove clothing and jewelry near injury.

- o Keep the client warm.

- o In the emergency department or an urgent care clinic:

  - ▪ Frequently assess pain and follow pain management protocols, both pharmacologic and nonpharmacologic.

  - ▪ Initiate and continue neurovascular checks on a regular schedule. Immediately report any change in status.

  - ▪ Maintain proper alignment.

  - ▪ Prepare the client for immobilization procedure appropriate for fracture.

IMMOBILIZING INTERVENTIONS: CASTS, SPLINTS, AND TRACTION

Overview

- Immobilization secures the injured extremity in order to:

  - o Prevent further injury.

  - o Promote healing/circulation.

  - o Reduce pain.

  - o Correct a deformity.

- Types of immobilization devices include:

  - o Casts.

  - o Splints/immobilizers.

  - o Traction.

  - o External fixation.

  - o Internal fixation.

- Closed reduction is when a pulling force (traction) is applied manually to realign the displaced fractured bone fragments. Once the fracture is reduced, immobilization is used to allow the bone to heal.

- Open reduction is when a surgical incision is made and the bone is manually aligned and kept in place with plates and screws. This is known as an open reduction and internal fixation (ORIF) procedure.

Collaborative Care

- Nursing Care

  - Neurovascular assessment is essential throughout immobilization. Assessments are performed frequently following initial trauma to prevent neurovascular compromise related to edema and/or immobilization device. Neurovascular assessment includes the assessment of:

    - Pain. Assess the client's pain level, location, and frequency. Assess pain using a 0 to 10 pain rating scale and have the client describe the pain.

    - Sensation. Assess the client for numbness or tingling sensation of extremity. Loss of sensation may indicate nerve damage.

    - Skin temperature. Check the temperature of the affected extremity. The extremity should be warm, not cool, to touch.

    - Capillary refill. Press nail beds of affected extremity until blanching occurs. Blood return should be within 3 seconds.

    - Pulses. Pulses should be palpable and strong. Pulses should be equal to unaffected extremity.

    - Movement. Client should be able to move affected extremity in passive motion.

  - Casts

    - Casts are more effective than splints or immobilizers because they cannot be removed by the client.

    - Types of casts include:

      - Short and long arm and leg casts

      - Spica casts, which refer to a portion of the trunk and one or two extremities. Typically used on children with congenital hip dysplasia

      - Body casts, which encircle the trunk of the body

    - Casting materials

      - Plaster of Paris casts are heavy, not water resistant, and can take 24 to 48 hr to dry

      - Synthetic fiberglass casts are light, water resistant, and dry very quickly (in 30 min)

    - Casts, as circumferential immobilizers, are applied once the swelling has subsided (to avoid compartment syndrome). If the swelling continues after cast application and causes unrelieved pain, the cast can be split on one side (univalved) or on both sides (bivalved).

    - A window can be placed in an area of the cast to allow for skin inspection (e.g., the client has a wound under the cast).

    - Moleskin is used over any rough area of the cast that may rub against the client's skin.

- Nursing Actions

  □ Prior to casting, the area is cleaned and dried. Tubular cotton web roll is placed over the affected area to maintain skin integrity. The casting material is then applied.

  □ After cast application, position the client so that warm, dry air circulates around and under the cast (support the casted area without pressure under or directly on the cast) for faster drying and to prevent pressure from changing the shape of the cast. Use gloves to touch the cast until the cast is completely dry.

  □ Elevate cast above the level of the heart during the first 24 to 48 hr to prevent swelling.

  □ If any drainage is seen on the cast, it should be outlined, dated, and timed, so it can be monitored for any additional drainage.

  ⓖ □ Older adult clients have an increased risk for impaired skin integrity due to the loss of elasticity of the skin and decreased sensation (comorbidities).

- Client Education

  □ Clients are instructed not to place any foreign objects under the cast to avoid trauma to the skin.

  □ Itching under the cast can be relieved by blowing cool air from a hair dryer under the cast.

  □ Plastic coverings over the cast can be used to avoid soiling from urine or feces.

  □ Demonstrate how plastic bags can be used during baths and showers to keep cast dry.

  o Traction

    - Traction uses a pulling force to promote and maintain alignment to the injured area.

    - Goals of traction include:

      □ Realignment of bone fragments.

      □ Decreasing muscle spasms and pain.

      □ Correcting or preventing further deformities.

    - Traction prescriptions should include the type of traction, amount of weight, and whether traction can be removed for nursing care.

- Types of Traction
  - In straight or running traction, the countertraction is provided by the client's body. Movement of the client's body can alter the traction provided. In balanced suspension traction, the countertraction is produced by devices such as slings or splints. The client's body can be moved vertically without altering the traction.

  - Manual: A pulling force is applied by the hands of the provider for temporary immobilization, usually with sedation or anesthesia, in conjunction with the application of an immobilizing device.

  - Skin: Used intermittently. The pulling force is applied by weights that are attached by rope to the client with tape, straps, boots, or cuffs. Examples include chin halter straps, Bryant's traction (used for congenital hip dislocation in children), and Buck's traction (used for hip fractures preoperatively for immobilization in adult clients).

 View Media Supplement: Buck's Traction (Image)

  - Skeletal: Used continuously. The pulling force is applied directly to the bone by weights attached by rope directly to a rod/screw placed through the bone. Examples include skeletal tongs (Gardner-Wells) and femoral or tibial pins (Steinmann pin). Weights up to 25 pounds can be applied as needed.

 View Media Supplement: Skeletal Traction (Image)

  - Halo: Screws are placed through a halo-type bar that encircles the head into the outer table of the bone of the skull. This halo is attached to either bed traction or rods that are secured to a vest worn by the client. Assure that the wrench to release the rods is attached to the vest when using halo traction in the event CPR is necessary.

- Nursing Actions
  - Maintain body alignment and realign if the client seems uncomfortable or reports pain.

  - Avoid lifting or removing weights.

  - Assure that weights hang freely.

  - If the weights are accidentally displaced, replace the weights. If the problem is not corrected, notify the provider.

  - Assure that pulley ropes are free of knots.

  - Notify the provider if the client experiences severe pain from muscle spasms unrelieved with medications and/or repositioning. Move the client in halo traction as a unit, without applying pressure to the rods. This will prevent loosening of the pins and pain

  - Routinely monitor skin integrity and document.

- o Pin Site Care
  - Pin care is done frequently throughout immobilization (skeletal traction and external fixation methods) to prevent and to monitor for signs of infection including:
    - Drainage (color, amount, odor).
    - Loosening of pins.
    - Tenting of skin at pin site (skin rising up pin).
  - Pin care protocols (chlorhexidine) are based on provider preference and institution policy. A primary concept of pin care is that one cotton-tip swab is designated for each pin to avoid cross-contamination.
  - Pin care is provided three times a day or per facility protocol.
  - Crusting at the pin site should not be removed as this provides a natural barrier from bacteria.

- Medications
  - o Prophylactic antibiotics
    - Prophylactic antibiotics are used to prevent infection when fracture immobilization is achieved, using pins, metal screws, or wires. Typically, a broad-spectrum intravenous antibiotic such as cefazolin (Ancef) is administered for 24 to 48 hr post-injury.
  - o Analgesics
    - Opioid and nonopioid analgesics may be used as needed to control pain.
  - o Muscle relaxants
    - Muscle relaxants may be given to relieve muscle spasms.

- Splints and Immobilizers
  - o Splints are removable and allow for monitoring of skin swelling or integrity.
  - o Splints can be used to support fractured/injured areas until casting can be done or used for post-paralysis injuries to avoid joint contracture.
  - o Immobilizers are prefabricated and typically fasten with Velcro straps.
  - o Client Education
    - Ensure client is aware of application protocol regarding full-time or part-time use.
    - Instruct client to observe for skin breakdown at pressure points.

- Surgical Interventions
  - External Fixation
    - External fixation involves fracture immobilization using percutaneous pins and wires that are attached to a rigid external frame.
    - Used to treat:
      - Comminuted fracture with extensive soft tissue damage.
      - Leg length discrepancies from congenital defects.
      - Bone loss related to tumors or osteomyelitis.
    - Advantages include:
      - Immediate fracture stabilization.
      - Allowing three-plane correction of the injury.
      - Minimal blood loss occurring in comparison with internal fixation.
      - Allowing for early mobilization and ambulation.
      - Maintaining alignment of closed fractures that could not be maintained in cast or splint.
      - Permitting wound care with open fractures.
    - Disadvantages include:
      - Risk of pin tract infection.
      - Potential overwhelming appearance to client.
      - Noncompliance issues.
    - Nursing Actions
      - Pin care
      - Observe for signs of fat and pulmonary embolism.
      - Provide antiembolism stockings and sequential compression device to prevent DVT.
    - Client Education
      - Teach the client pin care.
      - Discuss clothing and other materials that can be used to cover the device.
      - If activity is restricted, advise client to perform deep breathing and leg exercises and other techniques to prevent complications to immobilization, such as pneumonia or thrombus formation.
  - Open Reduction and Internal Fixation (ORIF)
    - Open reduction refers to visualization of a fracture through an incision in the skin, with repair made with plates, screws, pins, rods, and prosthetics as needed.
    - After the bone heals, the hardware may be removed, depending on the location and type of hardware.

- ■ Nursing Actions
  - □ Perform a neurovascular assessment.
  - □ Observe the cast or dressing for postoperative drainage. The cast may have a window cut in it through which the incision can be viewed.
  - □ Observe for signs of fat and pulmonary embolism.
  - □ Provide antiembolism stockings and sequential compression device to prevent DVT.
  - □ Monitor the client's pain level.
    - ▸ Assess on a scale of 0 to 10.
    - ▸ Provide analgesics and/or antispasmodics and assess relief.
    - ▸ Position for comfort.
  - □ Monitor for signs of infection.
    - ▸ Monitor the client's vital signs, watching for fever and tachycardia.
    - ▸ Monitor laboratory values (WBC, ESR).
    - ▸ Provide surgical aseptic wound care.
  - □ Increase physical mobility as appropriate.
    - ▸ Consult physical and occupational therapy for ambulation and activities of daily living (ADLs).
    - ▸ Monitor orthostatic blood pressure when the client gets out of bed for the first time.
    - ▸ Turn and reposition the client every 2 hr.
    - ▸ Have the client get out of bed from the unaffected side.
    - ▸ Position the client for comfort (within restrictions).
  - □ Support nutrition.
    - ▸ Encourage increased calorie intake.
    - ▸ Ensure use of calcium supplements.
    - ▸ Encourage small, frequent meals with snacks.
    - ▸ Monitor for constipation.
- ● Therapeutic Outcomes
  - ○ Client will not develop complications related to a bone fracture or its treatment (compartment syndrome, fat embolism, osteomyelitis).
  - ○ Client will demonstrate proper use of mobility devices such as crutches or walker.

Complications

- Compartment syndrome

  - Compartment syndrome occurs when pressure within one or more of the muscle compartments of the extremity compromises circulation, resulting in an ischemia–edema cycle. Capillaries dilate in an attempt to pull oxygen into the tissue. Increased capillary permeability from the release of histamine leads to edema from plasma proteins leaking into the interstitial fluid space. Increased edema causes pressure on the nerve endings, resulting in pain. Blood flow is further reduced and ischemia persists resulting in compromised neurovascular status.

  - Pressure can result from external sources, such as a tight cast or a constrictive bulky dressing.

  - Internal sources, such as an accumulation of blood or fluid within the muscle compartment, can cause pressure as well.

  - Compartment pressure is monitored with a handheld device or with a catheter connected to a transducer. Normal compartmental pressure is 0 to 8 mm Hg. Clinical manifestations (evolving neurovascular compromise) and compartmental pressure readings greater than 8 mm Hg are used to indicate an emergent need for treatment.

  - Findings include:

    - Increased pain unrelieved with elevation.

    - Intense pain when passively moved.

    - Paresthesia or numbness.

    - Color of tissue is pale (pallor).

  - If untreated, tissue necrosis can result. Neuromuscular damage occurs within 4 to 6 hr.

  - Surgical treatment is a fasciotomy.

    - A surgical incision is made through the subcutaneous tissue and fascia of the affected compartment to relieve the pressure and restore circulation.

    - After the fasciotomy, the open wounds require sterile packings and dressings until secondary closure occurs. Skin grafts may be necessary.

  - Nursing Actions

    - Prevention includes:

      - Cutting the cast on one side (univalve) or both sides (bivalve).

      - Loosening the constrictive dressing or cutting the bandage or tape.

      - Elevating the extremity and applying ice. If compartment syndrome is suspected, the extremity should not be elevated above the level of the heart to ensure adequate perfusion.

- ○ Client Education

    - ■ Instruct the client to report pain not relieved by analgesics or pain that continues to increase in intensity.

    - ■ Client should also be instructed to report numbness, tingling, or a change in color of the extremity.

- Fat embolism

    - ○ Fat embolism can occur, usually within 48 hr following long bone fractures. Fat globules from the bone marrow are released into the vasculature and travel to the small blood vessels, including those in the lungs, resulting in acute respiratory insufficiency. Careful diagnosis should differentiate between fat embolism and pulmonary embolism.

    - ○ Clinical manifestations include:

        - ■ Decreased mental acuity related to low arterial oxygen level (earliest sign).

        - ■ Respiratory distress.

        - ■ Tachycardia.

        - ■ Tachypnea.

        - ■ Fever.

        - ■ Cutaneous petechiae – pinpoint-sized subdermal hemorrhages that occur on the neck, chest, upper arms, and abdomen (from the blockage of the capillaries by the fat globules). This is a discriminating finding from a pulmonary embolism.

    - ○ Nursing Actions

        - ■ Prevention includes immobilization of fractures of the long bones and minimal manipulation during turning if immobilization procedure has not yet been performed.

        - ■ Treatment includes oxygen for respiratory compromise, corticosteroids for cerebral edema, vasopressors, and fluid replacement for shock, as well as pain and antianxiety medications as needed.

- Deep vein thrombosis

    - ○ Deep vein thrombosis is the most common complication following trauma, surgery, or disability related to immobility.

    - ○ Nursing Actions

        - ■ Administer anticoagulants as prescribed.

        - ■ Encourage intake of fluids to prevent hemoconcentration.

        - ■ Instruct client to rotate feet at the ankles and perform other lower extremity exercises as permitted by immobilization device employed.

- Osteomyelitis

  - Osteomyelitis is an inflammation within the bone secondary to penetration by infectious organisms (trauma, surgery).

  - Signs and symptoms

    - Bone pain that is worse with movement

    - Erythema and edema at the site of the infection

    - Fever

    - Leukocytosis and possible elevated sedimentation rate

    - Many of these signs will disappear if the infection becomes chronic.

  - Diagnostic procedures

    - Definitive diagnosis is with a bone biopsy.

    - Cultures are performed for detection of possible aerobic and anaerobic organisms.

    - If septicemia develops, blood cultures will be positive for offending microbes.

  - Treatment

    - Long course (3 months) of IV and oral antibiotic therapy.

    - Surgical debridement may also be indicated. If a significant amount of the bone requires removal, a bone graft may be necessary.

    - Hyperbaric oxygen treatments may be needed to promote healing in chronic cases of osteomyelitis.

    - Unsuccessful treatment can result in amputation.

  - Nursing Actions

    - Administer antibiotics as prescribed to maintain a constant blood level.

    - Administer analgesics as needed.

    - Conduct neurovascular assessments if debridement is done.

    - If wound is left open to heal, standard precautions are adequate and clean technique can be used during dressing changes.

- Avascular necrosis

  - Avascular necrosis results from the circulatory compromise that occurs after a fracture. Blood flow is disrupted to the fracture site and the resulting ischemia leads to tissue (bone) necrosis.

  - Replacement of damaged bone with a bone graft or prosthetic replacement may be necessary.

- Failure of Fracture to Heal
  - A fracture that has not healed within 6 months of injury is considered to be experiencing "delayed union".
  - Malunion: Fracture heals incorrectly
  - Nonunion: Fracture that never heals
    - Electrical bone stimulation and bone grafting can be used to treat nonunion.
    - May occur more frequently in older adults due to impaired healing process.
  - Malunion or nonunion may cause immobilizing deformity of bone involved.

CHAPTER 82: FRACTURES

 Application Exercises

1. Which of the following client statements indicates an understanding of how to safely manage an external fixation device applied to his distal radius and ulna? (Select all that apply.)

_____ "I will clean the pins three times a day."

_____ "I will use one cotton swab on each pin."

_____ "I will report loosening of the pins to the provider."

_____ "I will lift my arm by the middle of the device to reposition it."

_____ "I should remove any crusting that forms around the pin."

2. A nurse is caring for an older adult client who is admitted with a right hip fracture and has surgery scheduled for the next morning. Which of the following immobilization devices should the nurse anticipate will be used for this client preoperatively?

A. Skeletal traction

B. Buck's traction

C. Halo traction

D. Gardner-Wells traction

3. A nurse is caring for a client who has a compound fracture of the right forearm that was recently casted. Which of the following is an early sign of neurovascular compromise?

A. Paresthesia

B. Pulselessness

C. Paralysis

D. Polar

4. A client had an external fixation device applied 2 hr ago for a fractured left tibia and fibula. Which of the following findings indicate the possibility of compartment syndrome? (Select all that apply.)

_____ Toes are cool to the touch bilaterally.

_____ Left toes are slightly edematous compared to right.

_____ Pedal pulse is diminished.

_____ Pain is unrelieved by second dose of oral narcotic.

_____ Left toes will not move.

5. A nurse is caring for a client who has osteomyelitis and had the wound debrided, leaving a non-draining wound. IV antibiotics have been administered for 7 days and the client is being discharged with care continued in the home setting. Which of the following should the nurse include when teaching the client about home care of osteomyelitis?

    A. Antibiotic therapy will need to be continued for at least 3 months.

    B. Relief of pain indicates that the infection has been eradicated.

    C. Contact precautions must be instituted.

    D. Aseptic technique must be used during dressing changes.

CHAPTER 82: FRACTURES

 Application Exercises Answer Key

1. Which of the following client statements indicates an understanding of how to safely manage an external fixation device applied to his distal radius and ulna? (Select all that apply.)

   __X__   **"I will clean the pins three times a day."**

   __X__   **"I will use one cotton swab on each pin."**

   __X__   **"I will report loosening of the pins to the provider."**

   _____   "I will lift my arm by the middle of the device to reposition it."

   _____   "I should remove any crusting that forms around the pin."

Pin care protocols are based on provider preference and institution policy. Every 8 hr is a common parameter for a pin care schedule. A primary concept of pin care is that one cotton-tip swab is used per pin to avoid cross-contamination. Loosening of the pins may indicate infection and should be reported to the provider. The external device should not be used to move or lift the extremity, and crusting around the pin should be allowed to develop as it produces a natural barrier to bacteria.

 NCLEX® Connection: Reduction of Risk Potential: Potential for Complications of Diagnostic Tests/Treatments/Procedures

2. A nurse is caring for an older adult client who is admitted with a right hip fracture and has surgery scheduled for the next morning. Which of the following immobilization devices should the nurse anticipate will be used for this client preoperatively?

   A. Skeletal traction

   B. Buck's traction

   C. Halo traction

   D. Gardner-Wells traction

The nurse should anticipate the use of a Buck's traction, which is a boot applied to the lower part of the affected extremity. This will temporarily immobilize the extremity until surgery can be done. Skeletal traction will not be necessary, since a surgical repair is scheduled for the next day. Halo and Gardner-Wells traction are forms of skeletal traction for cervical injuries.

 NCLEX® Connection: Reduction of Risk Potential: Potential for Complications from Surgical Procedures and Health Alterations

3. A nurse is caring for a client who has a compound fracture of the right forearm that was recently casted. Which of the following is an early sign of neurovascular compromise?

A. Paresthesia

B. Pulselessness

C. Paralysis

D. Polar

An early sign of neurovascular compromise is paresthesia. Pulselessness, paralysis, and polar or coldness of the extremity are late signs of neurovascular compromise.

 NCLEX® Connection: Reduction of Risk Potential: System-Specific Assessment

4. A client had an external fixation device applied 2 hr ago for a fractured left tibia and fibula. Which of the following findings indicate the possibility of compartment syndrome? (Select all that apply.)

_____ Toes are cool to the touch bilaterally.

_____ Left toes are slightly edematous compared to right.

__X__ **Pedal pulse is diminished.**

__X__ **Pain is unrelieved by second dose of oral narcotic.**

__X__ **Left toes will not move.**

The symptoms of compartment syndrome include diminished pedal pulse on the affected limb, pain unrelieved by the second dose of oral narcotic, and the inability to move toes on the affected limb. Toes that are cool bilaterally as well as mild edema of the toes of the affected extremity are expected findings.

 NCLEX® Connection: Reduction of Risk Potential: System-Specific Assessment

5. A nurse is caring for a client who has osteomyelitis and had the wound debrided, leaving a non-draining wound. IV antibiotics have been administered for 7 days and the client is being discharged with care continued in the home setting. Which of the following should the nurse include when teaching the client about home care of osteomyelitis?

A. Antibiotic therapy will need to be continued for at least 3 months.

B. Relief of pain indicates that the infection has been eradicated.

C. Contact precautions must be instituted.

D. Aseptic technique must be used during dressing changes.

Antibiotic therapy will need to continue for at least 3 months. Some clients go home with an IV in place so intravenous antibiotics can continue to be administered. Early discontinuation of prescribed antibiotic can allow infection to continue and become chronic. Pain may disappear prior to the entire infection being eradicated, so this should not be used as an indicator of a cure. Since the wound is already infected, most providers only recommend contact precautions be implemented if the wound is draining and clean technique be used for dressing changes.

 NCLEX® Connection: Safety and Infection Control: Standard/Transmission-Based/Other Precautions

UNIT 10	NURSING CARE OF CLIENTS WITH MUSCULOSKELETAL DISORDERS
Section	Musculoskeletal Disorders

Chapter 83   Osteoarthritis

Overview

- Osteoarthritis (OA) is a disorder characterized by progressive deterioration of the articular cartilage. It is a noninflammatory (unless localized), nonsystemic disease.

- It is no longer thought to be only a wear-and-tear disease associated with aging, but also a process in which new tissue is produced as a result of cartilage destruction within the joint. The destruction outweighs the production. The cartilage and bone beneath the cartilage erode and osteophytes (bone spurs) form, resulting in narrowed joint spaces. The changes within the joint lead to pain, immobility, muscle spasms, and potential inflammation.

- Early in the disease process of OA, it may be difficult to distinguish from rheumatoid arthritis (RA).

CHARACTERISTIC	OSTEOARTHRITIS	RHEUMATOID ARTHRITIS
Disease process	Cartilage destruction with bone spur growth at joint ends; degenerative	Synovial membrane inflammation resulting in cartilage destruction and bone erosion; inflammatory
Symptoms	Pain with activity that improves at rest	Swelling, redness, warmth, pain at rest or after immobility (morning stiffness)
Effusions	Localized inflammatory response	All joints
Body Size	Usually overweight	Usually underweight
Nodes	Heberden's and Bouchard's nodes	Swan neck and boutonnière deformities of hands
Systemic involvement	No; articular	Yes; lungs, heart, skin, and extra-articular
Symmetrical	No	Yes
Diagnostic tests	X-rays	X-rays, and positive rheumatoid factor

 View Media Supplement: Heberden's and Bouchard's Nodes (Images)

Health Promotion and Disease Prevention

- Encourage the client to use joint-saving measures (good body mechanics, labor-saving devices).

- Encourage the client to maintain a healthy weight.

- Encourage the client to avoid or limit repetitive strain on joints (jogging).

Assessment

- Risk Factors

  o Age (a majority of adults over the age of 55 have joint changes on x-ray).

  o Female sex

  o Obesity

  o Possible genetic link

  o History of repetitive stress on joints (manual laborers, professional athletes, marathon runners)

- Subjective Data

  o Joint pain and stiffness that resolves with rest or inactivity

  o History of injury or repetitive stress

  o History of obesity

- Objective Data

  o Pain with joint palpation or range of motion (observe for muscle atrophy, loss of function, limp when walking, and restricted activity due to pain)

  o Crepitus in one or more of the affected joints

  o Enlarged joint related to bone hypertrophy

  o Heberden's nodes enlarged at the distal interphalangeal (DIP) joints

  o Bouchard's nodes located at the proximal interphalangeal (PIP) joints (OA is not a symmetrical disease, but these nodes can occur bilaterally.)

  o Inflammation resulting from secondary synovitis, indicating advanced disease

  o Laboratory Tests

    ▪ Erythrocyte sedimentation rate (ESR) and high-sensitivity C-reactive protein may be increased slightly related to secondary synovitis. Osteoarthritis without synovitis is not an inflammatory disorder.

- o Diagnostic Procedures
  - Radiographs and CT scans can determine structural changes within the joint.
    - □ Decreased joint space
    - □ Bone spurs

Collaborative Care

- Nursing Care
  - o Assess/Monitor
    - Pain – Level (0 to 10), location, characteristics, quality, and severity
    - Degree of functional limitation
    - Levels of fatigue and pain after activity
    - Range of motion
    - Proper functional/joint alignment
    - Home barriers
    - Ability to perform ADLs
  - o Instruct the client about the use of analgesics and NSAIDS prior to activity and around the clock as needed.
  - o Balance rest with activity.
  - o Instruct the client on proper body mechanics.
  - o Encourage the use of thermal applications: heat to alleviate pain and ice for acute inflammation.
  - o Encourage the use of complementary and alternative therapies, including acupuncture, tai chi, hypnosis, magnets, and music therapy.
  - o Encourage the use of splinting for joint protection and the use of larger joints.
  - o Encourage the use of assistive devices to promote safety and independence, including an elevated toilet seat, shower bench, and long-handled reacher and shoe horn.
  - o Encourage the use of a daily schedule of activities that will promote independence (high-energy activities in the morning).
  - o Encourage a well-balanced diet and ideal body weight. Consult a dietitian to provide meal planning for balanced nutrition.

- Medications

  - Analgesic therapy

    - Acetaminophen

      - Does not provide anti-inflammatory benefits, which may not be needed if synovitis is not present

      - Nursing Actions

        ▸ Monitor liver function tests.

    - NSAIDs

      - Analgesics and antiinflammatories that are used to relieve pain and synovitis if present

      - May replace acetaminophen with an NSAID if adequate relief is not obtained

    - Topical analgesics

      - Trolamine salicylate (Aspercreme) – It may provide varying amounts of temporary pain relief, depending on the client response. Apply topically over the area of involvement. It contains salicylate.

      - Capsaicin (Axsain, Capsin) – It may provide varying amounts of temporary pain relief depending on the client response. Apply topically over an area of involvement. It is made from alkaloid that is derived from hot peppers. It is thought to prevent transmission of pain sensations from peripheral neural transmitters.

      - Client Education

        ▸ Instruct the client to wear gloves during application (capsaicin).

        ▸ Explain to the client that a burning sensation of the skin after application is normal and should subside.

        ▸ Instruct the client to apply frequently (up to 4 times a day) for maximum benefit.

    - Glucosamine (rebuilds cartilage)

      - Glucosamine is a naturally occurring chemical involved in the makeup of cartilage. Glucosamine sulfate is believed to aid glycosaminoglycan synthesis and subsequently rebuilds cartilage. Glucosamine is often taken in combination with chondroitin, a glycosaminoglycan also involved in the makeup of articular cartilage.

      - Client Education

        ▸ Consult the provider regarding dosage.

- - Intra-articular injections
    - □ Glucocorticoids – Used to treat localized inflammation
    - □ Hyaluronic acid (Hyalgan, Synvisc) – It is used to replace the body's natural hyaluronic acid, which is destroyed by joint inflammation. It is currently only approved for treatment of knee joints.
    - □ Client Education
      - ▸ Hyaluronic acid – Instruct the client to notify the provider if allergic to birds, feathers, or eggs because this medication is made from combs of chickens.

- Interdisciplinary Care

  - The client may be referred to physical therapy for the application of heat, diathermy (treatment with electrical currents), ultrasonography (treatment with sound waves), or stretching and strengthening exercises.

  - A transcutaneous electrical nerve stimulation (TENS) unit may also be prescribed by the provider and applied by the physical therapist with client instruction on how to use it.

  - A nutritionist may assist the client in diet for weight loss or control in relation to reduced activity level.

- Therapeutic Procedures

  - Conservative therapy

    - Conservative therapy includes balancing rest with activity, using bracing or splints, and applying thermal therapies (heat or cold).

- Surgical Interventions

  - Total joint arthroplasty

    - When all other conservative measures fail, the client may choose to undergo total joint arthroplasty to relieve the pain and improve mobility and quality of life.

- Client outcomes

  - The client will schedule activities and use conservative therapies that allow completion of ADLs.

  - The client will slow or stop progression of the disease by making lifestyle alterations.

CHAPTER 83: OSTEOARTHRITIS

 Application Exercises

1. Identify which of the following client characteristics a nurse should recognize is indicative of osteoarthritis (OA). (Select all that apply.)

_____ Heberden's nodes

_____ Systemic response

_____ Small body frame

_____ Pain with activity

_____ Need for total joint arthroplasty

2. A nurse is caring for a client who reports right knee pain with ambulation. Which of the following should the nurse include during the assessment that may indicate OA? (Select all that apply.)

_____ Pain (type, location, aggravating and alleviating factors)

_____ Joint swelling

_____ Ability to complete ADLs

_____ Family history of OA

_____ Erythrocyte sedimentation rate

_____ History of joint trauma

_____ Body mass index (BMI)

3. A nurse is providing a client teaching about a newly prescribed medication, capsaicin (Axsain, Capsin). Which of the following information is appropriate to include?

A. Apply while wearing gloves.

B. Avoid drinking alcohol.

C. Take the medication in combination with chondroitin.

D. Apply once daily.

CHAPTER 83: OSTEOARTHRITIS

 Application Exercises Answer Key

1. Identify which of the following client characteristics a nurse should recognize is indicative of osteoarthritis (OA). (Select all that apply.)

   X   **Heberden's nodes**

          Systemic response

          Small body frame

   X   **Pain with activity**

   X   **Need for total joint arthroplasty**

OA is a localized disease that can produce Heberden's nodes on the interphalangeal joints, pain that worsens with activity, and degeneration of the joint's cartilage and articular surfaces that may necessitate joint arthroplasty. It is more frequent in individuals who are overweight.

 NCLEX® Connection: Reduction of Risk Potential, System Specific Assessment

2. A nurse is caring for a client who reports right knee pain with ambulation. Which of the following should the nurse include during the assessment that may indicate OA? (Select all that apply.)

   X   **Pain (type, location, aggravating and alleviating factors)**

   X   **Joint swelling**

   X   **Ability to complete ADLs**

   X   **Family history of OA**

          Erythrocyte sedimentation rate

   X   **History of joint trauma**

   X   **Body mass index (BMI)**

The nurse should assess the type, location, and factors that increase or decrease pain; joint swelling; ability to complete ADLs; family history of OA; history of any joint trauma; and BMI to determine obesity. Although the erythrocyte sedimentation rate may be slightly elevated in OA with secondary synovitis, it is not an indicator of OA.

 NCLEX® Connection: Reduction of Risk Potential, System Specific Assessment

3. A nurse is providing a client teaching about a newly prescribed medication, capsaicin (Axsain, Capsin). Which of the following information is appropriate to include?

A. Apply while wearing gloves.

B. Avoid drinking alcohol.

C. Take the medication in combination with chondroitin.

D. Apply once daily.

Capsaicin is made from hot peppers, so gloves should be worn during application. It is not necessary to avoid alcohol. Glucosamine may be taken with chondroitin. Instruct the client to apply frequently (up to 4 times a day) for maximum benefit.

NCLEX® Connection: Physiological Adaptation, Illness Management

UNIT 11: NURSING CARE OF CLIENTS WITH INTEGUMENTARY DISORDERS

- Diagnostic and Therapeutic Procedures
- Integumentary Disorders

NCLEX® CONNECTIONS

When reviewing the chapters in this unit, keep in mind the relevant sections of the NCLEX® outline, in particular:

CLIENT NEEDS: BASIC CARE AND COMFORT	CLIENT NEEDS: REDUCTION OF RISK POTENTIAL	CLIENT NEEDS: PHYSIOLOGICAL ADAPTATION

Relevant topics/tasks include:
- Mobility/Immobility
  ○ Promote circulation.
- Nutrition and Oral Hydration
  ○ Evaluate the impact of disease/illness on the nutritional status of the client.
	Relevant topics/tasks include:
	- Laboratory Values
	  ○ Obtain specimens other than blood for diagnostic testing.
	- Potential for Alterations in Body Systems
	  ○ Identify the client's potential for skin breakdown.
	- System Specific Assessment
	  ○ Identify factors that result in delayed wound healing.
		Relevant topics/tasks include:
		- Alterations in Body Systems
		  ○ Assess the client for signs and symptoms of adverse effects of radiation therapy.
		- Fluid and Electrolyte Imbalances
		  ○ Identify signs and symptoms of the client's fluid and/or electrolyte imbalance.
		- Medical Emergencies
		  ○ Provide emergency care for wound disruption.

Overview

- Integumentary diagnostic procedures involve identification of pathogenic micro-organisms. The most accurate and definitive way to identify micro-organisms and cell characteristics is by examining blood, body fluids, and tissue samples under a microscope.

- Integumentary diagnostic procedures that nurses should be knowledgeable about:

  o Culture and sensitivity

  o Biopsy

Culture and Sensitivity

  o Culture refers to isolation of the pathogen on culture media.

  o Sensitivity refers to the effect that antimicrobial agents have on the micro-organism.

   ▪ If the micro-organism is killed by the antimicrobial, the microbe is considered to be sensitive to that medication.

   ▪ If tolerable levels of the medication are unable to kill the microbe, the microbe is considered to be resistant to that medication.

  o A culture and sensitivity can be done on a sample of purulent drainage, urine, sputum, and other body fluids.

  o Cultures should be done prior to initiating antimicrobial therapy.

- Indications

  o Evidence of an infection may include an area that is raised, reddened, edematous, and/or warm. There may be purulent drainage and/or fever.

- Interpretation of Findings

  o The microbe responsible for the infection is identified in the culture, and the antimicrobials that are sensitive to that microbe are listed.

  o Heavy growth of greater than 100,000 colonies definitively diagnoses an infection. Negative results are less than 10,000 colonies.

- ○ Indeterminate results are 10,000 to 100,000 colonies.

- ○ Appropriate medications are those with 3 to 4 degrees of sensitivity.

- Preprocedure

  - ○ Nursing Actions

    - Use standard precautions when collecting and handling specimens.

    - Most specimens will be collected by the nurse.

  - ○ Client Education

    - Encourage the client to wash hands frequently.

    - The client should notify the nurse when a sample is available for collection, such as a urinalysis.

- Intraprocedure

  - ○ Nursing Actions

    - A sufficient quantity of a specimen should be collected and placed in a sterile container. Culturette tubes are also available and contain a sterile cotton-tipped applicator and a fixative that is released after the infectious exudate is applied to the applicator and inserted in the tube.

    - The specimen must be properly labeled and delivered to the laboratory promptly for appropriate storage and analysis. Check facility protocol regarding the timeframe in which cultures should be delivered to the laboratory.

- Postprocedure

  - ○ Nursing Actions

    - Results of culture and sensitivity tests are usually available preliminarily within 24 to 48 hr with final results in 72 hr.

    - If culture and sensitivity results reveal that the cultured organism is not sensitive to prescribed antimicrobial agents, it is the nurse's responsibility to report the results to the provider before administering subsequent doses of an ineffective antimicrobial.

      - □ Ideally, antimicrobial therapy should not begin until after the specimen for culture and sensitivity has been collected.

Biopsy

- Biopsy is the removal of a sample of tissue by excision or needle aspiration for cytological (histological) examination.

  - ○ A biopsy is the extraction of a very small amount of tissue, such as bone marrow, cervical, endometrial, brain, liver, lung, pleural, renal, skin, and lymph node tissue, to definitively diagnose cell type and to confirm or rule out malignancy. Biopsies can be performed with local anesthesia or moderate sedation in an ambulatory setting, intraoperatively, and/or during scope procedures.

- Indications

  ○ Evidence of skin lesion, which may include an area of discoloration that is thickened, thinned, raised, flat, rough, painful, open, dry and/or itchy.

  ○ A biopsy is commonly performed to diagnose or to rule out diseases such as cancer.

- Interpretation of Findings

  ○ After a biopsy is completed, the tissue sample is sent to pathology for interpretation.

- Preprocedure

  ○ Nursing Actions

    ■ Ensure that the client has signed the informed consent form.

    ■ Explain the procedure to the client.

  ○ Client Education

    ■ Inform the client about what to expect in regard to the formation of a scar.

    ■ Teach the client about what to expect about the test/procedure.

- Intraprocedure

  ○ Nursing Actions

    ■ Assist the provider with the test/procedure as needed.

    ■ As appropriate, apply pressure to the biopsy site to control bleeding.

    ■ As appropriate, place a sterile dressing over the biopsy site.

- Postprocedure

  ○ Nursing Actions

    ■ Monitor the client for evidence of infection (fever, increased WBC count, pain) and/or bleeding.

    ■ As appropriate, monitor the biopsy site.

    ■ Postbiopsy discomfort is usually relieved by mild analgesics.

    ■ Older adults are at a greater risk for complications associated with sedation for biopsy procedures due to chronic illnesses.

  ○ Client Education

    ■ Teach the client to report excessive bleeding and/or signs of infection to the provider.

    ■ Teach the client to check the incision daily. The incision should be clean, dry and intact.

    ■ If sutures are in place, remind the client to return in 7 to 10 days to have them removed.

- Complications
  - ○ Infection
    - Infection may occur after a biopsy.
- Nursing Actions
  - □ Monitor the biopsy site for signs of infection, such as increased redness, swelling, and purulent drainage. Other indications may include fever and increase in WBC count.
  - □ Apply an antibacterial ointment.
  - □ Keep the incisional site clean and dry.
  - ○ Bleeding
    - Bleeding can occur from the site and needs to be reported to the primary care provider immediately.

CHAPTER 84: INTEGUMENTARY DIAGNOSTIC PROCEDURES

(A) Application Exercises

1. A nurse is reading a culture and sensitivity report on her client, who she suspects has a wound infection. Which of the following findings indicates that the client has an infection?

    A. Colony growth of 12,000

    B. Colony growth of less than 9,000

    C. Colony growth of more than 20,000

    D. Colony growth of more than 120,000

2. A nurse is providing discharge instructions for a client who had a skin biopsy and has sutures in place. Which of the following statements by the client indicates a need for further teaching?

    A. "I can expect redness around the biopsy site for the first 3 days."

    B. "I should call my doctor if I have a fever."

    C. "I should apply an antibiotic ointment to the area of the biopsy."

    D. "I can return to the doctor's office in 7 days to have my sutures removed."

3. A nurse in a long-term care setting has just admitted an older adult client who has an open wound on his heel. Which of the following findings should alert the nurse that the wound may be infected? (Select all that apply.)

    _____ The client has a low grade fever.

    _____ The client's WBC count is elevated.

    _____ The wound is draining yellow fluid.

    _____ The client reports that he has reduced sensation in his foot.

    _____ The area around the wound is warm to touch.

CHAPTER 84: INTEGUMENTARY DIAGNOSTIC PROCEDURES

 Application Exercises Answer Key

1. A nurse is reading a culture and sensitivity report on her client, who she suspects has a wound infection. Which of the following findings indicates that the client has an infection?

> A. Colony growth of 12,000
>
> B. Colony growth of less than 9,000
>
> C. Colony growth of more than 20,000
>
> **D. Colony growth of more than 120,000**

> **Colony growth of more than 100,000 indicates an infection that needs treatment. Colony growths of 12,000 and 20,000 are indeterminate results. Colony growth of less than 10,000 is a negative result.**

 NCLEX® Connection: Reduction of Risk Potential, Laboratory Values

2. A nurse is providing discharge instructions for a client who had a skin biopsy and has sutures in place. Which of the following statements by the client indicates a need for further teaching?

> **A. "I can expect redness around the biopsy site for the first 3 days."**
>
> B. "I should call my doctor if I have a fever."
>
> C. "I should apply an antibiotic ointment to the area of the biopsy."
>
> D. "I can return to the doctor's office in 7 days to have my sutures removed."

> **An area of redness indicates the possibility of infection, and the client should notify the provider. Fever is also a sign of infection and should be reported to the provider. An antibiotic ointment may be prescribed to prevent infection. Sutures are removed about 1 week after the procedure.**

 NCLEX® Connection: Safety and Infection Control, Standard Precautions/Transmission-Based Precautions/Surgical Asepsis

3. A nurse in a long-term care setting has just admitted an older adult client who has an open wound on his heel. Which of the following findings should alert the nurse that the wound may be infected? (Select all that apply.)

   X   **The client has a low grade fever.**

   X   **The client's WBC count is elevated.**

   X   **The wound is draining yellow fluid.**

           The client reports that he has reduced sensation in his foot.

   X   **The area around the wound is warm to touch.**

Signs of a wound infection include fever and elevated WBC count. Drainage from the wound may be yellow, green or have a blue tinge. The area around the wound may also be warm to the touch. Reduced tactile sensation is a normal finding in an older adult and is not an indication that the wound is infected.

NCLEX® Connection: Reduction of Risk Potential, Diagnostic Tests

Overview

- Psoriasis is a skin disorder that is characterized by scaly, dermal patches and is caused by an overproduction of keratin. This overproduction can occur at a rate up to nine times the rate of normal cells. It is thought to be an autoimmune disorder and has periods of exacerbations and remissions.

- In some clients, psoriasis can also affect the joints, causing arthritis-type changes and pain.

View Media Supplement: Psoriasis (Image)

- Seborrheic dermatitis is a skin disorder caused by inflammation of areas of the skin that contain a high number of sebaceous glands. It is characterized by papulopustules (oily form) or flaky plaques (dry form) that form on the surface of the skin. Dandruff is a type of seborrheic dermatitis.

- Seborrheic dermatitis also occurs for periods of time interspersed with symptom-free periods.

PSORIASIS

Assessment

- Risk Factors

  ○ Genetics

  ○ Stress

  ○ Seasons

  ○ Hormones

- Subjective Data

  ○ Exacerbation and remission of pruritic lesions

- Objective Data
  - Physical Assessment Findings
    - Scaly patches
    - Bleeding stimulated by removal of scales
    - Skin lesions primarily on the scalp, elbows and knees, and genitals
    - Pitting, crumbling nails

Collaborative Care

- Medications
  - Topical Corticosteroids – Triamcinolone acetonide (Kenalog)
    - Reduces secondary inflammatory response of lesions
    - Nursing Actions
      - Observe skin for thinning, striae with high-potency corticosteroids.
    - Client Education
      - Instruct the client to apply high-potency corticosteroids as prescribed to prevent side effects (avoid use on face or in skin folds, and take periodic medication vacations).
      - The provider may instruct the client to use occlusive dressings on smaller areas and gloves on the hands to increase absorption.
  - Tar Preparations – Coal Tar (Balnetar)
    - Represses cell division and decreases inflammation and itching
    - May stain skin and hair.
    - May stimulate growth of skin cancers
    - Nursing Actions
      - Instruct the client on proper application.
      - Instruct the client on how to assess for cancerous lesions.
    - Client Education
      - Due to odor and staining, the client should apply this product at night and cover areas of body with old pajamas, gloves, and socks.
  - Topical epidermopoiesis suppressive medications – Calcipotriene (Dovonex), tazarotene (Tazorac)
    - Reduces accelerated development of epidermal cells
    - Not recommended for older adults
    - Tazarotene (Tazorac) may cause birth defects. Women should be advised to use birth control during use.

- ■ Nursing Actions
    - □ Calcipotriene (Dovonex) – Monitor for symptoms of hypercalcemia (elevated serum calcium, muscle weakness, fatigue, anorexia).
- ■ Client Education
    - □ Instruct the client to avoid using the product on the face or in skin folds.
    - □ Instruct the client that burning and stinging can occur upon application.
    - □ Instruct the client to not use the product concurrently with corticosteroids.
    - □ Tazarotene (Tazorac) – Advise the client to use sunscreen and avoid sun exposure.
- ○ Cytotoxic medications (severe, intractable cases) – Methotrexate (Mexate), azathioprine (Imuran), cyclosporine (Neoral)
    - □ Reduces turnover of epidermal cells
    - □ Contraindicated in pregnant women
    - ■ Nursing Actions
        - □ Monitor laboratory tests for organ toxicity and bone marrow suppression.
    - ■ Client Education
        - □ Instruct the client to avoid alcohol while taking this medication.
        - □ Advise the client to monitor for fever, sore throat, increased bleeding or bruising, and fatigue.
- • Therapeutic Procedures
    - ○ PUVA - Psoralen (photosensitizing medication) and ultraviolet light
        - □ Psoralen is given 2 hr before light treatments.
        - □ Treatments are given 2 to 3 times per week, avoiding consecutive days.
        - ■ Nursing Actions
            - □ Monitor the skin's response to light.
            - □ Ensure that the client wears eye protection during treatment.
        - ■ Client Education
            - □ Notify the provider of extreme redness, swelling, and discomfort.
    - ○ Oil or coal tar baths
        - □ Removal of scales can be done using oil or coal tar bath.
        - □ Treatments are done on a regular basis.
        - ■ Client Education
            - □ Teach the client how to add oil/tar to water and remove scales using a soft brush after soaking followed by acid based emollient.

- Client Outcomes
  - The client will see a decrease in the number and size of the lesions.
  - The client will verbalize increased coping with chronic condition.
  - The client will have extended periods of remission from disease.

SEBORRHEIC DERMATITIS

Health Promotion and Disease Prevention

- Keep skin dry. Avoid overheating and perspiring.
- Do not scratch pruritic lesions.

Assessment

- Risk Factors
  - Genetics
  - Stress
  - Hormones
  - Older adults can develop seborrheic keratoses, which are more plaque-like in appearance.

    (M) View Media Supplement: Seborrheic Keratoses (Image)

- Subjective Data
  - Report of periods of exacerbations and remissions
  - Pruritic lesions
- Objective Data
  - Physical Assessment Findings
    - Waxy or flaky appearing plaques and/or scales
    - Skin lesions primarily on the oily areas of the body (scalp, forehead, nose, axilla, groin)
    - Seborrheic keratoses lesions may be pigmented tan, brown, or black.

Collaborative Care

- Medications
  - ○ Topical corticosteroids
    - □ Reduces secondary inflammatory response of lesions
    - ■ Client Education
      - □ Instruct the client to avoid getting medication in the eyes or skin folds.
  - ○ Antiseborrheic shampoos
    - □ Contain selenium sulfide, sulfur, or salicylic acid
    - ■ Client education
      - □ The client should use at least three times per week.
      - □ The client should leave shampoo on for 3 to 5 min.
- Client Outcomes
  - ○ The client will report decreased pruritus of affected areas.
  - ○ The client will report increased periods of remissions.

CHAPTER 85: CHRONIC SKIN CONDITIONS

 Application Exercises

1. A nurse is caring for a client who has a long history of psoriasis and has consented to PUVA treatment. Which of the following should the nurse include in the teaching about this type of therapy?

    A. NSAIDs will need to be avoided during treatment.

    B. A medication will be given to enhance photosensitivity.

    C. PUVA will need to be done every night.

    D. Gentle removal of scales should be done after each treatment.

2. A nurse is assessing a client's skin lesions. The lesions' characteristics include waxy-looking, flat, brown papules that are located on the client's forehead and nose. The nurse should determine that the lesions are more characteristic of which of the following?

    A. Actinic keratoses

    B. Seborrheic keratoses

    C. Psoriasis

    D. Melanoma

3. A nurse is caring for a client who has been prescribed topical corticosteroids. Which of the following should the nurse instruct the client to do to enhance the efficacy of the medication? (Select all that apply.)

    _____ Apply an occlusive dressing after application.

    _____ Apply three to four times per day.

    _____ Wear gloves after application for lesions on the hands.

    _____ Avoid using the medication in the skin folds.

    _____ Use the medication continuously over a period of several months.

CHAPTER 85: CHRONIC SKIN CONDITIONS

 Application Exercises Answer Key

1. A nurse is caring for a client who has a long history of psoriasis and has consented to PUVA treatment. Which of the following should the nurse include in the teaching about this type of therapy?

   A. NSAIDs will need to be avoided during treatment.

   B. A medication will be given to enhance photosensitivity.

   C. PUVA will need to be done every night.

   D. Gentle removal of scales should be done after each treatment.

   PUVA treatments involve taking a medication, such as a psoralen, to enhance photosensitivity. It is given 2 hr prior to phototherapy with UVA lights. UVA light treatment decreases cellular proliferation. NSAIDs do not need to be avoided during treatment. Treatments are given two to three times per week, avoiding consecutive days; scales should not be removed after each treatment.

   Ⓝ NCLEX® Connection: Pharmacological and Parenteral Therapies Expected Actions/Outcomes

2. A nurse is assessing a client's skin lesions. The lesions' characteristics include waxy-looking, flat, brown papules that are located on the client's forehead and nose. The nurse should determine that the lesions are more characteristic of which of the following?

   A. Actinic keratoses

   B. Seborrheic keratoses

   C. Psoriasis

   D. Melanoma

   Seborrheic keratoses are waxy papules that may or may not be pigmented and typically occur in areas of the body that have sebaceous glands, such as the forehead and nose.

   Ⓝ NCLEX® Connection: Reduction of Risk Potential, System Specific Assessment

3. A nurse is caring for a client who has been prescribed topical corticosteroids. Which of the following should the nurse instruct the client to do to enhance the efficacy of the medication? (Select all that apply.)

   __X__   **Apply an occlusive dressing after application.**

   _____   Apply three to four times per day.

   __X__   **Wear gloves after application for lesions on the hands.**

   __X__   **Avoid using the medication in the skin folds.**

   _____   Use the medication continuously over a period of several months.

The efficacy of topical corticosteroids can be enhanced by using occlusive dressings that enhance the exposure of the lesions to the medication. If the lesions are on the hands, gloves should be worn after application. Corticosteroids should not be applied close to the eyes due to risk of cataracts, or skin folds due to risk of yeast infections. Topical corticosteroids should only be applied two times per day and should be periodically stopped to prevent development of local and systemic side effects.

Ⓝ NCLEX® Connection: Pharmacological and Parenteral Therapies, Expected Actions/ Outcomes

UNIT 11	NURSING CARE OF CLIENTS WITH INTEGUMENTARY DISORDERS
Section	Integumentary Disorders
Chapter 86	**Pressure Ulcers, Wounds, and Wound Management**

 Overview

- A wound is a result of injury to the skin. Although there are many different types and degrees of injury, the basic phases of healing are essentially the same for most wounds.

- A pressure ulcer (formerly called a decubitus ulcer) is a specific type of tissue injury caused by unrelieved pressure that results in ischemia and damage to the underlying tissue.

- Pressure ulcers are classified according to a staging system developed by the National Pressure Ulcer Advisory Panel. The stages are:

  ○ Suspected deep tissue injury – Discolored but intact skin caused by damage to underlying tissue

  ○ Stage I – Intact skin with an area of persistent, nonblanchable redness, typically over a bony prominence, which may feel warm or cool to touch. The tissue is swollen and congested, with possible discomfort at the site. With darker skin tones, the ulcer may appear blue or purple.

  ○ Stage II – Partial-thickness skin loss involving the epidermis and the dermis. The ulcer is visible and superficial and may appear as an abrasion, blister, or shallow cavity. Edema persists, and the ulcer may become infected, possibly with pain and scant drainage.

  ○ Stage III – Full-thickness tissue loss with damage to or necrosis of subcutaneous tissue. The ulcer may reach, but not extend thorough the fascia below. The ulcer appears as a deep crater with or without undermining of adjacent tissue and without exposed muscle or bone. Drainage and infection are common.

  ○ Stage IV – Full-thickness tissue loss with destruction, tissue necrosis, or damage to muscle, bone, or supporting structures. There may be sinus tracts, deep pockets of infection, tunneling, undermining, eschar (black scab-like material), or slough (tan, yellow, or green scab-like material).

  ○ Unstageable – Ulcers whose stages cannot be determined because eschar or slough obscures the wound.

(M) View Media Supplement: Pressure Ulcer Staging (Image)

WOUND HEALING AND MANAGEMENT

Overview

- General Principles of Wound Management

  o Wounds impair skin integrity.

  o Inflammation is a localized protective response triggered by injury or destruction of tissue.

  o Wounds heal by various processes and in stages.

  o Wounds may become infected by the invasion of pathogenic microorganisms.

  o Principles of wound care include assessment, cleansing, and protection.

  o Wound care is a nursing responsibility that has a significant impact on wound healing.

- Stages of Wound Healing

  o The inflammatory stage occurs in the first 3 days after the initial trauma. Attempts are made at the site to:

    - Control bleeding with clot formation.

    - Deliver oxygen, WBC, and nutrients to the area via the blood supply.

  o The proliferative stage lasts the next 3 to 24 days. Effects to the wound include:

    - Replacing lost tissue with connective or granulated tissue.

    - Contraction of the wound's edges.

    - Resurfacing of new epithelial cells.

  o The maturation or remodeling stage involves the strengthening of the collagen scar and the restoration of a more normal appearance. It can take more than 1 year to complete, depending on the extent of the original wound.

- Healing Process

TYPE OF HEALING	CHARACTERISTICS	WOUND TYPE
Primary intention	• Little or no tissue loss • Edges are approximated, as with a surgical incision	• Heals rapidly • Low risk of infection • Minimal or no scarring
Secondary intention	• Loss of tissue • Wound edges widely separated, as with pressure ulcers and stab wounds	• Increased risk of infection • Scarring
Tertiary intention	• Widely separated • Deep • Spontaneous opening of a previously closed wound • Risk of infection	• Extensive drainage and tissue debris • Closes later • Long healing time

Health Promotion and Disease Prevention

- Maintain clean, dry skin and wrinkle-free linens.

  o Appropriately use pressure-reducing surfaces and pressure-relieving devices.

  o Inspect the skin frequently and document the client's risk using a tool such as the Braden scale.

  o Clean and dry the skin immediately following urine or stool incontinence.

  o Apply moisture barrier creams to the skin of clients who are incontinent.

  o Use tepid water (not hot), use minimal scrubbing, and pat the skin dry.

  o Encourage clients to consume diets high in protein and vegetables.

  o Encourage clients to take vitamins and supplements.

Assessment

- Risk Factors

  o Increased age delays healing because of:

    ■ Loss of skin turgor

    ■ Skin fragility

    ■ Decreased peripheral circulation and oxygenation

    ■ Slower tissue regeneration

    ■ Decreased absorption of nutrients

    ■ Decreased collagen

    ■ Impaired function of the immune system

  o Overall wellness – A compound fracture of the femur in a client who has a head injury will present more healing problems.

  o Immune function is the body's ability to fight infection by destroying invading pathogens.

  o Medications may interfere with the body's ability to respond to and/or prevent infection.

  o Nutrition provides energy and elements required for wound healing.

  o Tissue perfusion provides circulation that delivers the required elements for tissue repair and infection control.

  o Obesity – Fatty tissue lacks blood supply.

  o Chronic diseases, such as diabetes mellitus, place additional stress on the body's healing mechanisms.

  o Chronic stress further impedes healing.

- o Smoking impairs oxygenation and clotting.

- o Wound stress, such as from vomiting or coughing, puts pressure on the suture line and disrupts the wound healing process.

- • Subjective and Objective Data

  - o Appearance

    - ▪ Note the color of open wounds. The following colors reflect a wound's condition:

      - □ Red – Healthy regeneration of tissue

      - □ Yellow – Presence of purulent drainage and slough

      - □ Black – Presence of eschar that hinders healing and must be removed

    - ▪ Closed wounds – Skin edges should be well-approximated.

  - o Drainage is a normal result of the healing process and occurs during the inflammatory and proliferative phases of healing.

    - ▪ Note the amount of drainage from a drain or a dressing.

    - ▪ With each cleansing, observe the skin around a drain for irritation and breakdown.

    - ▪ The character of drainage is distinguished by consistency, color, and odor.

      - □ Serous drainage is the portion of the blood (serum) that is watery and clear or slightly yellow in appearance.

      - □ Sanguineous drainage contains serum and red blood cells. It is thick and appears reddish.

      - □ Serosanguineous drainage contains both serum and blood. It is watery and appears blood streaked or blood tinged.

      - □ Purulent drainage is the result of infection. It is thick and contains white blood cells, tissue debris, and bacteria. It may have a foul odor, and its color reflects the type of organism present (green may indicate a pseudomonas infection).

  - o Wound closure (staples, sutures, wound closure strips [Steri-strips])

Collaborative Care

- • Nursing Care

  - o Provide adequate hydration and meet protein and calorie needs.

    - ▪ Encourage an intake of 2,000 to 3,000 mL of water/day if not contraindicated (due to heart failure or renal failure).

    - ▪ Provide education about good sources of protein (meat, fish, poultry, eggs, dairy products, beans, nuts, whole grains).

    - ▪ Note if serum albumin levels are low (below 3.5 g/dL), because a lack of protein puts the client at greater risk for delayed wound healing and infection.

    - ▪ Provide nutritional support as indicated (vitamin and mineral supplements, nutritional supplements, enteral nutrition, parenteral nutrition).

○ Perform wound cleansing.

▪ Cleanse in a direction from the least contaminated toward the most contaminated.

▪ Use gentle friction when cleansing or applying solutions to the skin to avoid bleeding or further injury to the wound.

▪ While other mild cleansing agents may be prescribed, isotonic solutions remain the preferred cleansing agents.

▪ Never use the same gauze to cleanse across an incision or wound more than once.

▪ Irrigation with a solution-filled syringe held 2.5 cm (1 in) above the wound may be used.

(M) View Media Supplement: Wound Irrigation with Packing and Dry Dressing

○ For wound dressings, use:

▪ Woven gauze (sponges) – Absorb exudate from the wound

▪ Nonadherent material – Does not adhere to the wound bed

▪ Self-adhesive, transparent film – A temporary "second skin" ideal for small, superficial wounds

▪ Hydrocolloid – An occlusive dressing that swells in the presence of exudate

□ Used to maintain a granulating wound bed

□ May be left in place up to 5 days

▪ Hydrogel (Aquasorb)

□ May be used on infected, deep wounds

□ Provides a moist wound bed

○ Use the negative pressure of a wound vacuum-assisted closure if prescribed.

○ Remove sutures/staples as prescribed.

○ Assess onset, quality, duration, and severity of the pain.

○ Administer analgesics as prescribed.

○ Administer antimicrobials (topical and/or systemic) as prescribed.

○ Document the location and type of wound/incision, the status of the wound and the type of drainage, the type of dressing and materials used, the client teaching provided, and how the client tolerated the procedure.

- Medications

  - Antimicrobial Therapy

    - Antimicrobial therapy kills or inhibits the growth of microorganisms such as bacteria, fungi, viruses, and protozoans. Antimicrobial medications either kill pathogens or prevent their growth.

    - Nursing Considerations

      - Administer antimicrobial therapy as prescribed.

      - Monitor for medication effectiveness (reduced fever, increased level of comfort, decreasing white blood cell count).

      - Maintain medication schedule to assure consistent blood levels of antibiotic.

  - Antipyretics (acetaminophen, aspirin) are used for fever and discomfort as prescribed.

    - Nursing Considerations

      - Monitor fever to determine effectiveness.

      - Graph client's temperature fluctuations on medical record.

  - Analgesics Therapy

      - Analgesics (hydrocodone [Vicodin] and morphine [Sulfate]) are used for pain in the wound as prescribed.

      - Nursing Considerations

        - Administer analgesics therapy as prescribed.

        - Monitor effectiveness of medication related to pain.

        - Monitor level of consciousness, especially respiratory distress with morphine.

- Interdisciplinary Care

  - Nutritional services may be consulted for meal choices to promote wound healing.

  - Pain management services may be consulted if pain persists and/or is uncontrolled.

  - Rehabilitation care may be consulted if client has prolonged weakness and needs assistance with increasing level of activity.

  - Wound care consultant may be notified for management of wound care and dressing changes.

- Care After Discharge

  - Set-up referral services, such as home health, pharmacy services, or wound care consultants, to provide items such as wound dressing materials.

  - Contact community outreach programs, such as Meals on Wheels, or a nutritionist to provide meals high in protein and vegetables to promote wound healing.

  - For a client who has a chronic wound, a long-term care facility may be indicated.

RN ADULT MEDICAL SURGICAL NURSING

- ○ Client Education
  - Have the client demonstrate a dressing change before discharge.
  - Encourage the client to eat a diet high in protein and vegetables to promote wound healing.
  - Encourage the client to take vitamins and supplements to promote wound healing.
  - Remind the client to keep skin clean and dry.
  - Remind the client to report any signs of infection or further skin breakdown.
- Client Outcomes
  - ○ The client will have improved skin integrity.
  - ○ The client will be free of infection.
  - ○ The client will be free of pain.

Complications

- Dehiscence is a partial or total rupture (separation) of a sutured wound, usually with separation of underlying skin layers. Evisceration is a dehiscence that involves the protrusion of visceral organs through a wound opening. It is usually caused by the increased flow of serosanguineous fluid about 3 to 11 days postoperatively.
  - ○ Signs/symptoms of dehiscence include:
    - A significant increase in the flow of serosanguineous fluid on the wound dressings
    - Immediate history of sudden straining (coughing, sneezing, vomiting)
    - The client reporting a change or "popping" or "giving way" in the wound area
    - Visualization of viscera
  - ○ Risk factors include:
    - Chronic disease
    - Advanced age
    - Obesity
    - Invasive abdominal cancer
    - Vomiting
    - Dehydration/malnutrition
    - Ineffective suturing
    - Abdominal surgery
  - ○ Evisceration/dehiscence requires emergency treatment.

- o Nursing Actions

  - ▪ Call for help.

  - ▪ Stay with the client.

  - ▪ Cover the wound and any protruding organs with sterile towels or dressings that have been soaked in a sterile 0.9% sodium chloride solution. Do not attempt to reinsert the organs.

  - ▪ Position the client supine with the hips and knees bent.

  - ▪ Observe the client for signs of shock.

  - ▪ Maintain a calm environment.

    (M) **View Media Supplement:** Dehiscence & Evisceration (Image)

- • Infection

  - o Risk factors

    - ▪ Extremes in age (immature immune system, decreased immune function)

    - ▪ Impaired circulation and oxygenation (COPD, peripheral vascular disease)

    - ▪ Wound condition/nature (gunshot wound vs. surgical incision)

    - ▪ Impaired/suppressed immune system

    - ▪ Malnutrition, such as with alcoholism

    - ▪ Chronic disease

    - ▪ Poor wound care, such as breaches in technique

  - o Signs and symptoms are usually apparent within 2 to 7 days of injury/surgery.

    - ▪ Purulent drainage

    - ▪ Pain

    - ▪ Redness and edema (in and around the wound)

    - ▪ Fever

    - ▪ Chills

    - ▪ Increased pulse and respiratory rate

    - ▪ Increase in WBC

  - o Nursing Actions

    - ▪ Prevent infection by using appropriate asepsis when performing dressing changes.

    - ▪ Provide optimal nutrition to promote the immune response.

    - ▪ Provide for adequate rest to promote healing.

    - ▪ Administer antibiotic therapy as prescribed.

PRESSURE ULCERS

Overview

- Pressure ulcers range from nonblanchable tissue redness to full thickness skin loss with damage to underlying muscle and bone.

- Excellent nursing care is the primary factor in the prevention of pressure ulcers.

- The primary focus of prevention and treatment is to relieve the pressure and provide optimal nutrition and hydration.

- All clients must be assessed regularly for skin-integrity status and evaluated regularly for risk factors that contribute to impaired skin integrity.

- Pressure ulcers are a significant source of morbidity and mortality among older adults and those who have limited mobility.

Assessment

- Risk Factors

    o   Skin changes related to aging

    o   Immobility

    o   Incontinence or excessive moisture

    o   Skin friction and shearing

    o   Vascular disorders

    o   Obesity

    o   Inadequate nutrition and/or hydration

    o   Anemia

    o   Fever

    o   Impaired circulation

    o   Edema

    o   Sensory deficits

    o   Impaired cognitive functioning, neurological disorders

    o   Chronic diseases (diabetes mellitus, chronic renal failure, congestive heart disease, chronic lung disease)

    o   Sedation that impairs spontaneous repositioning

Collaborative Care

- Nursing Care

  - Reposition the client in bed at least every 2 hr and every 1 hr in a chair. Document position changes.

    - Place pillows strategically between bony surfaces.

    - Maintain the head of the bed at or below a 30° angle, unless contraindicated, to relieve pressure on the sacrum, buttocks, and heels.

    - Keep the client from sliding down in bed, as this increases shearing forces that pull tissue layers apart and cause damage.

    - Lift, rather than pull, the client up in bed or in a chair, because pulling creates friction that can damage the outer layer of the skin (epidermis).

    - Raise the client's heels off of the bed to prevent pressure on the heels.

    - Ambulate the client as soon as possible and as often as possible.

    - Implement active/passive exercises for immobile clients.

    - Do not massage bony prominences.

  - Provide adequate hydration (2,000 to 3,000 mL/day) (unless contraindicated) and meet protein and calorie needs.

    - Note if serum albumin levels are low (below 3.5 g/dL), because a lack of protein puts the client at greater risk for skin breakdown, slowed healing, and infection.

    - Provide nutritional support, such as vitamin and mineral supplements, nutritional supplements, enteral nutrition, and parenteral nutrition, as indicated.

  - Treatment

STAGES	INTERVENTIONS
Suspected deep tissue injury and Stage I	• Relieve pressure. • Encourage frequent turning/repositioning. • Use pressure-relieving devices (air-fluidized beds). • Implement pressure-reduction surfaces (air mattress, foam mattress). • Keep the client dry, clean, well-nourished, and hydrated.
Stage II	• Maintain a moist healing environment (saline or occlusive dressing). • Promote natural healing while preventing the formation of scar tissue. • Provide nutritional supplements as prescribed. • Administer analgesics as prescribed.

STAGES	INTERVENTIONS

Stage III	• Clean and/or debride:
	  ○ Prescribed dressing
	  ○ Surgical intervention
	  ○ Proteolytic enzymes
	• Provide nutritional supplements as prescribed.
	• Administer analgesics as needed.
	• Administer antimicrobials (topical and/or systemic) as prescribed.

Stage IV	• Clean and/or debride:
	  ○ Prescribed dressing
	  ○ Surgical intervention
	  ○ Proteolytic enzymes
	• Perform nonadherent dressing changes every 12 hr.
	• Treatment may include skin grafts.
	• Provide nutritional supplements as prescribed.
	• Administer analgesics as prescribed.
	• Administer antimicrobials (topical and/or systemic) as prescribed.

Unstageable	• Eschar should cover wound as protective barrier. • Provide nutritional supplements as prescribed. • Administer analgesics as prescribed. • Administer antimicrobials (topical and/or systemic) as prescribed.

- Assess onset, quality, duration, and severity of the pain.

- Administer analgesics as prescribed.

- Administer antimicrobials (topical and/or systemic) as prescribed.

- Medications

  - Antimicrobial Therapy

    - Antimicrobial therapy kills or inhibits the growth of micro-organisms, such as bacteria, fungi, viruses, and protozoans. Antimicrobial medications either kill pathogens or prevent their growth.

    - Nursing Considerations

      - Administer antimicrobial therapy as prescribed.

      - Monitor for medication effectiveness (reduced fever, increased level of comfort, decreasing WBC count).

      - Maintain medication schedule to assure consistent blood levels of antibiotic.

- o Antipyretics (acetaminophen, aspirin) are used for fever and discomfort as prescribed.
  - ■ Nursing Considerations
    - □ Monitor fever to determine effectiveness.
    - □ Graph client's temperature fluctuations on medical record.
- o Analgesics Therapy
  - ■ Analgesics (hydrocodone [Vicodin] morphine) are used for pain in the wound as prescribed.
  - ■ Nursing Considerations
    - □ Administer analgesic therapy as prescribed.
    - □ Monitor effectiveness of medication related to pain.
    - □ Monitor level of consciousness, especially respiratory distress with morphine.

- Interdisciplinary Care
  - o Nutritional services may be consulted for meal choices to promote wound healing.
  - o Pain management services may be consulted if pain is persists and/or is uncontrolled.
  - o Rehabilitation care may be consulted if the client has prolonged weakness and needs assistance with increasing level of activity.
  - o Wound care consultants may be notified for management of wound care and dressing changes.

- Care After Discharge
  - o Set up referral services, such as home health, pharmacy services, or wound care consultants to provide items such as wound dressing materials.
  - o Contact community outreach programs, such as Meals on Wheels, or a nutritionist to provide meals high in protein and vegetables to promote wound healing.
  - o For a client who has a chronic wound, a long-term care facility may be indicated.
  - o Client Education
    - ■ Have client demonstrate dressing change before discharge.
    - ■ Encourage client to eat a diet high in protein and vegetables to promote wound healing.
    - ■ Encourage client to take vitamins and supplements to promote wound healing.
    - ■ Remind client to keep skin clean and dry.
    - ■ Remind client to report any signs of infection or further skin breakdown.

- Client Outcomes
  - o The client will have improved skin integrity.
  - o The client will be free of infection.
  - o The client will be free of pain.

Complications

- Deterioration to a Higher Stage Ulceration and/or Infection

  o Nursing Actions

    ▪ Assess/monitor the ulcer frequently and report increases in the size or depth of the lesion, changes in granulation tissue (color, texture), and changes in exudate (color, quantity, odor).

    ▪ Follow the facility's protocol for ulcer treatment.

- Systemic Infection

  o Nursing Actions

    ▪ Assess/monitor the client for signs of sepsis (changes in level of consciousness, persistent recurrent fever, tachycardia, tachypnea, hypotension, oliguria, increased WBC).

    ▪ Prevent infection by using appropriate asepsis when performing ulcer treatment and dressing changes.

    ▪ Provide optimal nutrition to promote the immune response.

    ▪ Provide for adequate rest to promote healing.

    ▪ Administer antibiotic therapy as prescribed.

CHAPTER 86: PRESSURE ULCERS, WOUNDS, AND WOUND MANAGEMENT

Ⓐ Application Exercises

1. An adolescent client who has diabetes mellitus is recovering from an appendectomy. This is the third postoperative day. The client has been prescribed a regular diet and is tolerating it well. He has ambulated successfully around the unit with the help of his parents and is requesting pain medication every 6 to 8 hr while reporting pain at a 2 on a scale of 0 to 10 after medication is given. His incision is approximated and free of redness with scant serous drainage noted on the dressing. What type of healing process should the nurse expect this wound to be undergoing? Explain.

2. Which of the following diagnostic tests is relevant for assessing the risk of developing a pressure ulcer for an older adult client who has no major health issues?

    A. Serum albumin

    B. WBCs

    C. RBCs

    D. Serum potassium

3. Which of the following findings may negatively impact wound healing? (Select all that apply.)

    _____ Family history of pressure ulcers

    _____ Type 2 diabetes mellitus

    _____ Strict vegetarian

    _____ Cigarette smoker

    _____ Long-term use of glucocorticosteroids

4. Which of the following term describes wound drainage that is thick and yellow?

    A. Serous

    B. Sanguineous

    C. Serosanguineous

    D. Purulent

Scenario: An older adult woman who has type 2 diabetes mellitus has undergone surgery for a bowel obstruction 6 days ago. Prior to surgery, she experienced nausea and vomiting for 3 days. She has been NPO since the surgery and is receiving IV fluids. During the last 24 hr, she has reported nausea, and she has vomited small amounts of clear liquid three times in the last 8 hr. Her vital signs are stable. The client weighs 81.6 kg (180 lb), is 157.5 cm (5 ft 2 in) tall, and smokes two packs of cigarettes per day. Currently, her incision is well approximated and free of redness, tenderness, or swelling.

5. List the signs and symptoms the nurse should watch for that indicate development of a wound infection.

6. What risk factors for poor healing does this client exhibit?

7. Later that day, the client becomes confused and pulls off her surgical dressing. The nurse enters the room and finds the client with an extensive dehiscence. Which of the following nursing interventions are appropriate? (Select all that apply.)

_____ Repack the wound.

_____ Call for help.

_____ Assist the client to a chair.

_____ Cover the wound with a sterile dressing moistened with normal saline.

_____ Stay with the client.

8. What placed this client at risk for a wound dehiscence/evisceration?

CHAPTER 86: PRESSURE ULCERS, WOUNDS, AND WOUND MANAGEMENT

 Application Exercises Answer Key

1. An adolescent client who has diabetes mellitus is recovering from an appendectomy. This is the third postoperative day. The client has been prescribed a regular diet and is tolerating it well. He has ambulated successfully around the unit with the help of his parents and is requesting pain medication every 6 to 8 hr while reporting pain at a 2 on a scale of 0 to 10 after medication is given. His incision is approximated and free of redness with scant serous drainage noted on the dressing. What type of healing process should the nurse expect this wound to be undergoing? Explain.

   This wound is healing by primary intentions because it is a surgical incision.

    NCLEX® Connection: Physiological Adaptation: Alterations in Body Systems

2. Which of the following diagnostic tests is relevant for assessing the risk of developing a pressure ulcer for an older adult client who has no major health issues?

   A. Serum albumin

   B. WBCs

   C. RBCs

   D. Serum potassium

   Serum albumin would provide information regarding the adequacy of protein intake. Inadequate protein poses a great risk for altered skin integrity and ineffective healing. The other options are not indicative of this finding.

    NCLEX® Connection: Reduction of Risk Potential: Diagnostic Tests

3. Which of the following findings may negatively impact wound healing? (Select all that apply.)

_____	Family history of pressure ulcers
X	**Type 2 diabetes mellitus**
X	**Strict vegetarian**
X	**Cigarette smoker**
X	**Long-term use of glucocorticosteroids**

   Diabetes mellitus negatively impacts the immune response. A strict vegetarian may not have adequate protein intake, which would negatively impact wound healing, as would smoking (because it impairs oxygenation) and the use of glucocorticosteroids (because they depress the immune response). A family history is not indicative of developing pressure ulcers.

    NCLEX® Connection: Physiological Adaptation: Alterations in Body Systems

4. Which of the following term describes wound drainage that is thick and yellow?

    A. Serous

    B. Sanguineous

    C. Serosanguineous

    D. Purulent

Wound exudate depends on the presence or absence of infection – Uninfected wounds have serous (clear, thin, maybe slightly yellow) or serosanguineous exudate (thin, blood tinged), and infected wounds have purulent exudate. Purulent drainage is thick and contains white blood cells, tissue debris, and bacteria. The color varies among infective organisms (yellow with Staphylococcus and green with Pseudomonas).

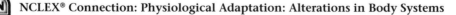 NCLEX® Connection: Physiological Adaptation: Alterations in Body Systems

Scenario: An older adult woman who has type 2 diabetes mellitus has undergone surgery for a bowel obstruction 6 days ago. Prior to surgery, she experienced nausea and vomiting for 3 days. She has been NPO since the surgery and is receiving IV fluids. During the last 24 hr, she has reported nausea, and she has vomited small amounts of clear liquid three times in the last 8 hr. Her vital signs are stable. The client weighs 81.6 kg (180 lb), is 157.5 cm (5 ft 2 in) tall, and smokes two packs of cigarettes per day. Currently, her incision is well approximated and free of redness, tenderness, or swelling.

5. List the signs and symptoms the nurse should watch for that indicate development of a wound infection.

    Purulent drainage

    Pain

    Redness and edema (in and around the wound)

    Fever

    Chills

    Increased pulse and respiratory rate

    Increased white blood cell count

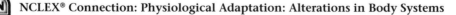 NCLEX® Connection: Physiological Adaptation: Alterations in Body Systems

6. What risk factors for poor healing does this client exhibit?

    The client is obese, has diabetes mellitus, smokes, and adequate nutritional intake is impaired.

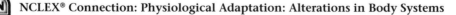 NCLEX® Connection: Physiological Adaptation: Alterations in Body Systems

7. Later that day, the client becomes confused and pulls off her surgical dressing. The nurse enters the room and finds the client with an extensive dehiscence. Which of the following nursing interventions are appropriate? (Select all that apply.)

          Repack the wound.

  X   **Call for help.**

          Assist the client to a chair.

  X   **Cover the wound with a sterile dressing moistened with normal sterile saline.**

  X   **Stay with the client.**

It is appropriate for the nurse to call for help, stay with the client, and cover the wound with a sterile dressing that is moistened with normal sterile saline. The nurse should not attempt to reinsert the organs and repack the wound. The client should be placed in the supine position with hips and knees bent.

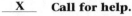 NCLEX® Connection: Physiological Adaptation: Alterations in Body Systems

8. What placed this client at risk for a wound dehiscence/evisceration?

Age

Obesity

Abdominal surgery 6 days ago

Recent vomiting

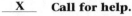 NCLEX® Connection: Physiological Adaptation: Alterations in Body Systems

UNIT 11	NURSING CARE OF CLIENTS WITH INTEGUMENTARY DISORDERS
Section	Integumentary Disorders
Chapter 87	Burns

 Overview

- Thermal, chemical, electrical, and radioactive agents can cause burns, which result in cellular destruction of the skin layers and underlying tissue. The type of burn and the severity of the burn impact the treatment plan.

  - Thermal burns occur when there is exposure to flames, steam, or hot liquids. This type of burn occurs most frequently, especially in older adults and children.

  - Chemical burns occur when there is exposure to a caustic agent. Cleaning agents used in the home (drain cleaner, bleach) and agents used in the industrial setting (caustic soda, sulfuric acid) cause chemical burns.

  - Electrical burns occur when an electrical current passes through the body and can result in severe damage, including loss of organ function, tissue destruction with subsequent need for amputation of a limb, and cardiac and/or respiratory arrest.

  - Radiation burns most frequently occur as a result of therapeutic treatment for cancer or from sunburn.

- In addition to destruction of body tissue, a burn injury results in the loss of:

  - Temperature regulation

  - Sweat and sebaceous gland function

  - Sensory function

  - Metabolism increases to maintain body heat

- The severity of the burn is based on the:

  - Percentage of total body surface area (TBSA) – Standardized charts for age groups are used to identify the extent of the injury.

  - Depth of the burn – Burns are classified in regard to the layers of skin and tissue involved.

  - Body location of the burn – In areas where the skin is thinner, there is more damage to underlying tissue (any part of the face, hand, perineum, feet).

(G)

    o   Age of the client – Young clients and older adult clients have less reserve capacity to deal with a burn injury. For the older adult client, the skin is thinner. Thus, more damage to underlying tissue may occur.

    o   Causative agent – Thermal, chemical, electrical, or radioactive.

    o   Presence of other injuries – The presence of fractures or other injuries increases the risk of complications.

    o   Involvement of the respiratory system – Inhalation of deadly fumes, smoke, steam, and heated air can cause respiratory failure or airway edema; carbon monoxide poisoning can also occur, especially if the injury took place in an enclosed area.

    o   Overall health of the client – A client who has a chronic illness has a greater risk of complications and a more serious prognosis.

- Three Phases of Burn Care

    o   Emergent (Resuscitative phase)

        ■ First 24 to 48 hr after the burn occurs

    o   Acute

        ■ Begins when fluid resuscitation is finished

        ■ Ends when the wound is covered by tissue

    o   Rehabilitative

        ■ Begins when most of the burn area is healed

        ■ Ends when reconstructive and corrective procedures are complete (may last for years)

Health Promotion and Disease Prevention

- Ensure that the number and placement of fire extinguishers and smoke alarms in the home is adequate and that they are operable.

- Keep emergency numbers near the phone.

- Have a family exit and meeting plan for fires.

- Review with clients of all ages that in the event that the client's clothing or skin is on fire, the client should "Stop, drop, and roll" to extinguish the fire.

- Store matches and lighters out of reach and out of sight of children and adults who lack the ability to protect themselves.

- Reduce setting on water heater to no higher than 120° F.

- Teach clients to avoid sun exposure between 1000 and 1600 hr, use sun block, and protective clothing.

- Teach clients to avoid using tanning beds.

- Avoid smoking in bed and smoking when under the influence of alcohol or sedating medications.

Assessment

- Risk Factors
  - Risk for Death from Burns
    - Age > 60 years
    - Burn involves > 40% total body surface area
    - Inhalation injury
  - Older adults are at higher risk for damage to subcutaneous tissue, muscle, connective tissue, and bone because their skin is thinner.
  - Older adults have a higher risk for complications from burns because of chronic illnesses (e.g., diabetes mellitus, cardiovascular disease).
- Subjective Data
  - To evaluate the extent of damage when assessing burns, it is important to know:
    - The type of burning agent (dry heat, moist heat, chemical, electrical, ionizing radiation)
    - The duration of contact
    - The area of the body in which the burn occurred

- Objective Data

  o Physical Assessment Findings

    ■ Assess depth of injury:

DEPTH	AREA INVOLVED/ APPEARANCE	SENSATION/HEALING	EXAMPLE
Superficial – damage to epidermis	• Pink to red, tender, no blisters, mild edema, and no eschar	• Painful • Heals within 5 to 10 days • No scarring	• Sunburn
Superficial partial thickness – damage to the entire epidermis and some parts of the dermis	• Pink to red, blisters, mild to moderate edema, and no eschar,	• Painful • Heals within 14 days • No scarring	• Flame or burn scalds
Deep partial thickness – damage to entire epidermis and deep into the dermis	• Red to white, with moderate edema, free of blisters, and soft and dry eschar.	• Painful and sensitive to touch • Heals within 14 to 36 days • Scarring likely • Possible grafting involved	• Flame and burn scalds • Grease, tar, or chemical burns • Exposure to hot objects for prolonged time
Full thickness – damage to the entire epidermis and dermis, and may extend into the subcutaneous tissue. Nerve damage also occurs	• Red to tan, black, brown, or white, • Free from blisters, severe edema, and hard and inelastic eschar.	• Pain may or may not be present. • As burn heals, painful sensations return and severity of pain increases. • Heals within weeks to months • Scarring • Grafting required	• Burn scalds • Grease, tar, chemical, or electrical burns • Exposure to hot objects for prolonged time
Deep full thickness – damage to all layers of skin and extends to muscle, tendons and bones.	• Black, no edema	• Heals within weeks to months • Scarring • Grafting required	• Chemical burns

Ⓜ View Media Supplement: Burn Staging (Images)

- o Levels of Care
  - Inhalation damage findings may include singed nasal hair, eye brows, and eye lashes; a sooty appearance to sputum; hoarseness; and wheezing. Clinical manifestations may not be evident for 24 to 48 hr and are seen as wheezing, hoarseness, and increased respiratory secretions.
  - Carbon monoxide inhalation (suspected if the injury took place in an enclosed area) findings include erythema (pink or cherry red color of skin) and upper airway edema, followed by sloughing of the respiratory tract mucosa.
  - Hypovolemia and shock may result when injury to at least 20% to 30% TBSA occurs. Fluid shifts from the intercellular and intravascular space to the interstitial space.
    - □ Additional findings include hypotension, tachycardia, and decreased cardiac output.
- o Laboratory Tests
  - Laboratory values that should be evaluated include – CBC, serum electrolytes, BUN, ABGs, fasting blood glucose, liver enzymes, urinalysis, and clotting studies.
    - □ Initial fluid shift (first 24 hr after injury)
      - ▸ Hct and Hgb – Elevated due to loss of fluid volume and fluid shifts into interstitial spacing (third spacing)
      - ▸ Sodium – Decreased due to third spacing (Hyponatremia)
      - ▸ Potassium – Increased due to cell destruction (Hyperkalemia)
  - Fluid mobilization (48 to 72 hr after injury)
    - □ Hgb and Hct – Decreased due to fluid shift from interstitial back into vascular fluid
    - □ Sodium – Remains decreased due to renal and wound loss
    - □ Potassium – Decreased due to renal loss and movement back into cells (Hypokalemia)
  - WBC count – Initial increase then decrease with left shift
  - Blood glucose – Elevated due to stress response
  - ABGs – Slight hypoxemia and metabolic acidosis
  - Total protein and albumin – Low due to fluid loss

Collaborative Care

- Nursing Care
  - Minor Burns
    - Stop the burning process.
      - Remove clothing or jewelry that might conduct heat.
      - Apply cool water soaks or run cool water over injury; do not use ice.
      - Flush chemical burns with large amounts of water.
      - Cover the burn with clean cloth to prevent contamination and hypothermia.
      - Provide warmth.
      - If necessary, have client go to a health care facility for medical care.
    - Provide analgesia.
    - Cleanse with mild soap and tepid water (avoid excess friction).
    - Use antimicrobial ointment.
    - Apply dressing (nonadherent, hydrocolloid) if the burn area is irritated by clothing.
    - Educate the family to avoid using greasy lotions or butter on burn.
    - Educate family to monitor for signs of infection.
    - Check immunization status for tetanus and determine need for immunization.
  - Moderate and Major Burns
    - Maintain airway and ventilation.
    - Provide humidified supplemental oxygen as ordered.
    - Monitor vital signs.
    - Maintain cardiac output.
      - Initiate intravenous access. If a large area of the body is burned, a central venous catheter is inserted.
      - Fluid replacement is important during the first 24 hr.
        - ‣ Rapid fluid replacement is needed during the emergent phase to maintain tissue perfusion and prevent hypovolemic (burn) shock.
        - ‣ Fluid resuscitation is based on individual client needs (evaluation of urine output, cardiac output, blood pressure, status of electrolytes).
        - ‣ Isotonic crystalloid solutions, such as 0.9% sodium chloride, or lactated Ringer's solution, are used during the early stage of burn recovery.

- ▸ Colloid solutions, such as albumin, or synthetic plasma expanders (Hespan) Plasma-Lyte, may be used after the first 24 hr of burn recovery.
- ▸ Maintain urine output of 30 mL/hr (0.5 to 1.0 mL/kg/hr).
- ▸ Be prepared to administer blood products as needed.
  - ☐ Monitor for manifestations of shock.
    - ▸ Alterations in sensorium (confusion)
    - ▸ Increased capillary refill time
    - ▸ Urine output less than 30 mL/hr
    - ▸ Spiking fever
    - ▸ Decreased bowel sounds
    - ▸ Blood pressure may remain normotensive, even in hypovolemia.
- ○ Pain Management
  - ■ Establish ongoing monitoring of pain and effectiveness of pain treatment.
  - ■ Avoid IM or subcutaneous injections.
  - ■ Use intravenous opioid analgesics such as morphine sulfate, hydromorphone (Dilaudid), and fentanyl (Sublimaze). Anesthetics such as ketamine (Ketalar), pentobarbital sodium (Nembutal), and nitrous oxide may also be used.

  - ■ Monitor for respiratory depression when using opioid analgesics.
  - ■ The use of patient-controlled analgesia is appropriate for some clients. They help decrease pain level, and the client benefits from having a sense of control.
  - ■ Administer pain medication prior to dressing changes or procedures.
  - ■ Use nonpharmacologic methods for pain control, such as guided imagery, music therapy, and therapeutic touch, to enhance the effects of analgesic medications and lead to more effective pain management.
- ○ Prevent Infection
  - ■ Follow standard precautions when performing wound care.
  - ■ Restrict plants and flowers due to the risk of contact with pseudomonas.
  - ■ Restrict consumption of fresh fruits and vegetables.
  - ■ Limit visitors.
  - ■ Use reverse isolation if prescribed.
  - ■ Monitor for signs and symptoms of infection and report to provider.
  - ■ Use client-designated equipment such as BP cuffs, thermometers.
  - ■ Administer tetanus toxoid if indicated.
  - ■ Administer antibiotics if infection present.

- o Nutritional Support

    - The client who has a large area of burn injury will be in a hypermetabolic and hypercatabolic state. The client may need 5,000 calories per day.

    - Increase caloric intake to meet increased metabolic demands and prevent hypoglycemia.

    - Increase protein intake to prevent tissue breakdown and to promote healing.

    - Enteral therapy or total parenteral nutrition (TPN) may be necessary due to decreased gastrointestinal motility and increased caloric needs.

- o Restoration of Mobility

    - Maintain correct body alignment, splint extremities, and facilitate position changes to prevent contractures.

    - Maintain active and passive range of motion.

    - Assist with ambulation as soon as the client is stable.

    - Apply pressure dressings to prevent contractures and scarring.

    - Closely monitor areas at high risk for pressure sores (heels, sacrum, back of head).

- o Psychological Support

    - Provide emotional support.

    - Assist with coping.

- Medications

    - o Topical Agents

ANTIMICROBIAL CREAM	USES AND ADVANTAGES	DISADVANTAGES
Silver nitrate 0.5%	• Use on wounds exposed to air, or with modified or occlusive dressing. • May affect joint movement • Reduces fluid evaporation • Bacteriostatic against pseudomonas and staphylococcus • Inexpensive	• Does not penetrate eschar • Stains clothing and linen • Discolors wound, making assessment difficult • Painful on application
Silver sulfadiazine 1% (Silvadene)	• Use with occlusive dressings. • Maintains joint mobility • Effective against gram-negative bacteria, gram-positive bacteria, and yeast	• May cause transient neutropenia • Contraindicated with allergies to sulfa • Does not penetrate eschar • Painful to remove from wound • Decreases granulocyte formation

ANTIMICROBIAL CREAM	USES AND ADVANTAGES	DISADVANTAGES
Mafenide acetate (Sulfamylon)	• Use on wounds exposed to air. • Use as a solution for occlusive dressings to keep the dressing moist. • Penetrates eschar and goes into underlying tissues • Effective with electrical and infected wounds • Biostatic against gram-negative and gram-positive bacteria	• Painful to apply and remove • May cause metabolic acidosis or hyperpnea • Inhibits wound healing • Hypersensitivity may develop
Bacitracin	• Use on wounds exposed to air or with modified dressings. • Maintains joint mobility • Bacteriostatic against gram-positive organisms • Painless and easy to apply	• Limited effectiveness on gram-negative organisms

- Interdisciplinary Care

  o Initiate referral to a registered dietitian, social worker, psychological counselor, or occupational/physical therapist if indicated.

  o Respiratory therapy to improve pulmonary function may also be needed.

- Therapeutic Procedures

  o Wound Care

    ▪ Nonsurgical management

    ▪ Nursing Actions

      □ Premedicate the client with analgesic as prescribed prior to all wound care.

      □ Remove all previous dressings.

      □ Assess for odors, drainage, and discharge.

      □ Cleanse the wound as prescribed, removing all previous ointments (it is important to cleanse the wound thoroughly).

- Assist with debridement.
  - ▸ Mechanical – Use scissors and forceps to cut away the dead tissue during the hydrotherapy treatment
  - ▸ Hydrotherapy (place the client in a warm tub of water or use warm running water, as if to shower) to cleanse the wound.
    - ▹ Use mild soap or detergent to gently wash burns and then rinse with room-temperature water.
    - ▹ Encourage the client to exercise his joints during the hydrotherapy treatment.
  - ▸ Enzymatic – Apply a topical enzyme to break down and remove dead tissue.
- Ensure that the client does not become hypothermic during the treatment.
- Apply a thin layer of topical antibiotic ointment as prescribed and cover with dressing, using surgical aseptic technique.

○ Skin Coverings

- Biologic skin coverings are temporarily used to promote healing of large burns. Additionally, biologic skin coverings promote the retention of water and protein and provide coverage of nerve endings, thus reducing the amount of pain experienced by the client. The provider stipulates whether they are to be covered or left uncovered.
  - Allograft (homograft) – Skin is donated from human cadavers that is used for partial- and full-thickness burn wounds.
  - Xenograft (heterograft) – Obtained from animals, such as pigs, for partial-thickness burn wounds
  - Amnion – Obtained from human placenta; requires frequent changes
  - Synthetic skin coverings – Used for partial-thickness burn wounds.
    - ▸ Many of the synthetic skin coverings are made of materials that are clear enough to see through so that the wound can be visualized without removing the dressing.
- Permanent skin coverings may be the treatment of choice for burns covering large areas of the body.
  - Autografts
    - ▸ Sheet graft – Sheet of skin used to cover wound
    - ▸ Mesh graft – Sheet of skin placed in mesher so skin graft has small slits in it; allows graft to cover larger areas of the burn wound
  - Artificial skin – Synthetic product that is used for partial- and full-thickness burn wounds (healing is faster)
  - Cultured epithelium – Epithelia cells cultured for use when grafting sites are limited

- ■ Nursing Actions
  - □ Maintain immobilization of graft site.
  - □ Elevate extremity.
  - □ Provide wound care to the donor site.
  - □ Administer pain medication.
  - □ Monitor for signs of infection before and after skin coverings or grafts are applied.
    - ▸ Discoloration of unburned skin surrounding burn wound
    - ▸ Green color to subcutaneous fat
    - ▸ Degeneration of granulation tissue
    - ▸ Development of subeschar hemorrhage
    - ▸ Hyperventilation indicating systemic involvement of infection
    - ▸ Unstable body temperature
- ■ Client Education
  - □ Instruct the client to keep extremity elevated.
  - □ Instruct the client to report signs and symptoms of infection.
  - □ Determine the client's level of pain and provide addition measures to control donor site pain.

- Care After Discharge
  - ○ Initiate referral for home health nursing care.
  - ○ Initiate referral to occupational therapy for evaluation of the home environment and assistance to relearn how to perform ADLs.
  - ○ Initiate referral to social services for community support services.
- Client Education
  - ■ Instruct the client to continue to perform range-of-motion exercises and to work with a physical therapist to prevent contractures.
  - ■ Provide client instruction on how to assess the wound for infection and how to perform wound care.
- Client Outcomes
  - ○ The client remains free of complications.
  - ○ The client is able to perform ADLs.
  - ○ The client verbalizes an understanding of self care.

Complications

- Airway Injury

    o Thermal injuries to the airway may result from steam or chemical inhalation, aspiration of scalding liquid, and explosion while breathing. If the injury took place in an enclosed space, carbon monoxide poisoning should be suspected.

    o Clinical manifestations may be delayed for 24 to 48 hr.

    o Signs and symptoms include progressive hoarseness, brassy cough, difficulty swallowing, drooling, increased secretions, adventitious breath sounds, and expiratory sounds that include audible wheezes, crowing, and stridor.

    o Nursing Actions

    ▪ Maintain airway and ventilation, and provide oxygen as prescribed.

    o Client Education

    ▪ Educate the client and family about airway management, such as deep breathing, coughing, and elevating the head of the bed.

- Fluid and Electrolyte Imbalances

    o Nursing Actions

    ▪ Assess fluid volume status.

    □ Daily weights

    □ Meticulous I&O

    ▪ Monitor laboratory results and compare to previous data.

    ▪ Administer IV fluids and electrolytes.

    o Client Education

    ▪ Educate the client and family about signs and symptoms of electrolyte imbalances and the need to alert the provider immediately.

- Wound Infections

    o Nursing Actions

    ▪ Assess for discoloration, edema, odor, and drainage.

    ▪ Assess for fluctuations in temperature and heart rate.

    ▪ Obtain wound culture.

    ▪ Administer antibiotics as prescribed.

    ▪ Monitor laboratory results, observing for anemia and infection.

    ▪ Maintain surgical aseptic technique with dressing changes.

    o Client Education

    ▪ Educate the client and family on the importance of infection control.

CHAPTER 87: BURNS

 Application Exercises

1. A nurse in a provider's office is collecting data from a client who has a severe sunburn. Which of the following is the proper classification of this burn?

   A. Superficial

   B. Superficial partial-thickness

   C. Deep partial-thickness

   D. Full-thickness

2. A nurse is caring for a client who sustained burns to 35% of his total body surface area. Of the burns, 20% are full-thickness. The burns are on the client's arms, face, neck, and shoulders. The client's voice seems hoarse and he has a brassy cough. The nurse recognizes that these findings are indicative of which of the following?

   A. Pulmonary edema

   B. Bacterial pneumonia

   C. Inhalation injury

   D. Carbon monoxide poisoning

3. A nurse is caring for a client who was admitted 24 hr ago with deep partial-thickness and full-thickness burns to 40% of his body. Which of the following are expected findings for this client? (Select all that apply.)

   _____ Hypertension

   _____ Bradycardia

   _____ Hyperkalemia

   _____ Hyponatremia

   _____ Decreased hematocrit

4. A nurse is preparing to administer fentanyl (Sublimaze) to a client who was admitted to the hospital 24 hr ago with deep partial-thickness and full-thickness burns over 60% of his body. The nurse should plan to use which of the following routes to administer the medication?

   A. Subcutaneous

   B. Intramuscular

   C. Intravenous

   D. Transdermal

CHAPTER 87: BURNS

 Application Exercises Answer Key

1. A nurse in a provider's office is collecting data from a client who has a severe sunburn. Which of the following is the proper classification of this burn?

   A. Superficial

   B. Superficial partial-thickness

   C. Deep partial-thickness

   D. Full-thickness

   A sunburn is a superficial burn. A superficial partial-thickness burn may be caused by a flame or burn scald; a deep partial-thickness or full-thickness burn may be caused by grease or tar.

    NCLEX® Connection: Physiological Adaptation: Pathophysiology

2. A nurse is caring for a client who sustained burns to 35% of his total body surface area. Of the burns, 20% are full-thickness. The burns are on the client's arms, face, neck, and shoulders. The client's voice seems hoarse and he has a brassy cough. The nurse recognizes that these findings are indicative of which of the following?

   A. Pulmonary edema

   B. Bacterial pneumonia

   C. Inhalation injury

   D. Carbon monoxide poisoning

   Wheezing and hoarseness are indicative of inhalation injury and this finding requires immediate attention by the nurse. These findings are not indicative of pulmonary edema, bacterial pneumonia, or carbon monoxide poisoning.

    NCLEX® Connection: Reduction of Risk Potential: System Specific Assessment

3. A nurse is caring for a client who was admitted 24 hr ago with deep partial-thickness and full-thickness burns to 40% of his body. Which of the following are expected findings for this client? (Select all that apply.)

   _____   Hypertension

   _____   Bradycardia

   X   **Hyperkalemia**

   X   **Hyponatremia**

   _____   Decreased hematocrit

A client who has partial-thickness and full-thickness burns to 40% of his body may experience shock. Immediately after the burn injury, fluids shift from the intracellular space into the interstitial space. Fluid leaks from the capillaries at the site of the burn and throughout the body. Due to the loss of fluids in the intracellular space and the intravascular space, the client experiences hypovolemia. In response to shock, the client develops hypotension and tachycardia. Leakage of fluid from the intracellular space causes hyperkalemia. Sodium is retained in the interstitial space, leading to hyponatremia. Due to hypovolemia, hematocrit is elevated.

(N) NCLEX® Connection: Physiological Adaptation: Fluid and Electrolyte Imbalances

4. A nurse is preparing to administer fentanyl (Sublimaze) to a client who was admitted to the hospital 24 hr ago with deep partial-thickness and full-thickness burns over 60% of his body. The nurse should plan to use which of the following routes to administer the medication?

   A. Subcutaneous

   B. Intramuscular

   C. Intravenous

   D. Transdermal

The intravenous route is used to administer pain medication to a client who has a major burn during the emergent phase. Once IV access is established, it will provide the most rapid relief. Injections should be avoided due to risk of infection and transdermal medications may be ineffective due to tissue damage.

(N) NCLEX® Connection: Pharmacological and Parenteral Therapies Pharmacological Pain Management

UNIT 11	NURSING CARE OF CLIENTS WITH INTEGUMENTARY DISORDERS
Section	Integumentary Disorders
Chapter 88	Skin Cancer

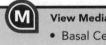 Overview

- Sunlight exposure is the leading cause of skin cancer. The most effective strategy for prevention of skin cancer is avoidance or reduction of skin exposure to sunlight.

- Precancerous skin lesions, called actinic keratoses, are common in people with chronically sun-damaged skin, such as older adults.

- There are three types of skin cancer.

  o Squamous cell carcinoma is a cancer of the epidermis that can be localized, but it may metastasize to other tissue and organs.

  o Basal cell carcinoma is a cancer of the basal cell layer of the epidermis, that can damage surrounding tissue and can advance to include underlying structures. This type of cancer is not usually metastatic, but the rate of recurrence is very high.

  o Malignant melanoma is an aggressive, metastatic cancer that originates in the melanin-producing cells of the epidermis.

View Media Supplement:
- Basal Cell Cancer (Image)
- Squamous Cell Cancer (Image)

Health Promotion and Disease Prevention

  o Advise the client to:

  o Limit exposure to sunlight, especially between 1000 and 1500 hr.

  o Use sunblock that has an SPF of at least 15, with both UVA and UVB protection. Sunblock should be reapplied at least every 2 hr.

  o Wear protective clothing, hats, sunglasses, and lip balm that has an SPF of at least 15.

  o Stay away from tanning booths.

  o Examine body monthly for suspicious lesions and develop a body map (diagram of skin scars or lesions) to monitor for changes.

Assessment

- Risk Factors

  - Exposure to ultraviolet light (such as natural light or tanning booths) over long periods of time

  - Chronic skin irritation and burn scars

  - Fair complexion (blonde or red hair, fair skin, freckles, blue eyes) with a tendency to burn easily

  - Presence of several large or many small moles

  - Family or personal history of melanoma

  - Location in upper elevations or close proximity to equator (thinner layer of ozone)

- Subjective Data

  - Report of change in appearance of mole or lesion

- Objective Data

  - Physical Assessment Findings

    - Basal and squamous cell carcinomas

      - Small, waxy nodule with small, superficial blood vessels (basal cell)

      - Rough, scaly lesion that may bleed and has a central area of ulceration or crusting (squamous cell)

      - Size varies in relation to duration of lesion

    - Melanoma

      - Assess for suspicious lesions in the: face and scalp, the shoulders and back, legs, feet, and between the toes. Lesions may occur on the palms and soles of individuals who have dark skin. Satellite lesions may also be present.

      - The ABCDs of suspicious lesions

        - **Asymmetry** – One side does not match the other

        - **Borders** – Ragged, notched, irregular, or blurred edges

        - **Color** – Lack of uniformity in pigmentation (shades of tan, brown, or black)

        - **Diameter** – Width greater than 6 mm, or about the size of a pencil eraser or a pea

 View Media Supplement: Melanomas (Images)

      - Palpate regional lymph nodes for enlargement.

      - Because of the cumulative effects of sun damage over the lifespan, screening for suspicious lesions is an essential part of the routine physical assessment of older adult clients.

- ○ Laboratory Tests
  - ■ No test is available to help diagnose skin cancer. If melanoma is diagnosed, blood tests will be ordered (CBC, liver) to check for organ involvement.
  - ■ Diagnostic Procedures
    - □ Biopsy (of suspicious lesions) – Definitive

	INSTRUMENT	PROCEDURE
Punch	A 2 to 6 mm, Circular instrument (punch) that is 2 to 6 millimeter in diameter	• A small circle of tissue is removed to the depth of subcutaneous fat. • The area may be sutured.
Shave	Scalpel or razor blade	• The skin elevated above the surrounding tissue by an injection of a local anesthetic is shaved off. • This is used for superficial or raised lesions
Excision	Scalpel	• A deep incision is made and then sutured after the entire lesion is removed. • This is used for large or deep lesions.

- ▸ Nursing Actions
  - ▹ Prepare the client by offering a brief explanation of what to expect.
  - ▹ Establish a sterile field and assemble supplies and instruments, including local anesthetic, specimen containers, and dressings.
  - ▹ Ensure that informed consent has been obtained.
  - ▹ Provide wound care following excision.
  - ▹ Schedule a follow-up appointment and provide home care instructions.
- ▸ Client Education
  - ▹ Ensure that the client is knowledgeable about how to assess for suspicious lesions on a regular basis.

Collaborative Care

- • Therapeutic Procedures
  - ○ Cryosurgery
    - ■ Freeze tissue by applying of liquid nitrogen (-200° C).
    - ■ Client Education
      - □ Teach the client to cleanse with hydrogen peroxide and apply a topical antimicrobial until healed.

- o Topical chemotherapy
  - ▪ Topical chemotherapy with 5-flourouracil cream for treatment of actinic keratoses
  - ▪ Client Education
    - ▫ Prepare the client for extended treatment that will cause the lesion to weep, crust, and erode.
    - ▫ Reassure the client that the appearance will improve after treatment.
- o Interferon
  - ▪ Used for postoperative treatment of stage III or greater melanomas
  - ▪ Nursing Actions
    - ▫ Report and provide relief for side effects or toxic effects of chemotherapy.
    - ▫ Encourage adequate nutrition and fluid intake.

- Surgical Interventions
  - o Excision
    - ▪ The extent of excision is based on the size and depth of the invasion.
    - ▪ Sentinel lymph node may also be biopsied to assess for metastasis.
    - ▪ The incision will be closed with sutures if possible. A skin graft may be necessary for large areas.
    - ▪ Client Education
      - ▫ Advise the client about postoperative wound care and care of the skin graft if used.

- Client Outcomes
  - o The client will identify suspicious lesions during the early stage and notify the provider.
  - o The client will take precautions to prevent unnecessary exposure to ultraviolet light and direct sunlight.

CHAPTER 88: SKIN CANCER

Ⓐ Application Exercises

Scenario: A nurse is caring for a man who came to his health care provider for removal of a large mole from his right shoulder. The client reports that the mole has bothered him for a couple of weeks. He was scraped on the shoulder by a wooden pallet, and the mole has been crusting and oozing since.

1. When conducting an initial interview, which of the following are important questions for the nurse to ask the client to determine risk factors for malignant melanoma. (Select all that apply.)

_____ Recent changes in size, color, or shape of the lesion

_____ Geographic location where the client previously and currently resides

_____ History of colon cancer

_____ Occupation

_____ Recreational activities

_____ Use of oral corticosteroids

_____ Occupational exposure to chemicals

2. What are characteristics of this client's mole that might suggest a malignancy?

3. A nurse working in a skin clinic knows that which of the following has the highest risk for metastases?

    A. Melanoma

    B. Basal cell carcinoma

    C. Squamous cell carcinoma

    D. Actinic keratosis

4. A nurse is caring for a client who has multiple types of skin lesions. Which of the following skin lesions are suggestive of a malignant melanoma? (Select all that apply.)

_____ An irregularly colored mole

_____ A lesion with asymmetric borders

_____ A rough, scaly patch

_____ A uniformly colored papule

_____ Diffuse vesicles

CHAPTER 88: SKIN CANCER

 Application Exercises Answer Key

Scenario: A nurse is caring for a man who came to his health care provider for removal of a large mole from his right shoulder. The client reports that the mole has bothered him for a couple of weeks. He was scraped on the shoulder by a wooden pallet, and the mole has been crusting and oozing since.

1. When conducting an initial interview, which of the following are important questions for the nurse to ask the client to determine risk factors for malignant melanoma. (Select all that apply.)

__X__	**Recent changes in size, color, or shape of the lesion**
__X__	**Geographic location where the client previously and currently resides**
_____	History of colon cancer
__X__	**Occupation**
__X__	**Recreational activities**
_____	Use of oral corticosteroids
__X__	**Occupational exposure to chemicals**

Recent changes in size, color, or shape of the lesion; geographic location where the client previously and currently resides; occupation; recreational activities; and occupational exposure to chemicals are important questions to ask because they are risk factors for malignant melanoma. History of colon cancer and use of oral corticosteroids are not risk factors for developing malignant melanoma.

NCLEX® Connection: Reduction of Risk Potential: System-Specific Assessment

2. What are characteristics of this client's mole that might suggest a malignancy?

Injury to a lesion located on a part of the body prone to chronic sun exposure and irritation

Oozing, bleeding, and crusting of the lesion

NCLEX® Connection: Physiological Adaptation: Pathophysiology

3. A nurse working in a skin clinic knows that which of the following has the highest risk for metastases?

A. Melanoma

B. Basal cell carcinoma

C. Squamous cell carcinoma

D. Actinic keratosis

A melanoma has the highest risk of metastasis. Basal cell carcinoma rarely metastasizes. Squamous cell carcinomas can metastasize, but it occurs much less quickly than a melanoma. Actinic keratosis is a precancerous lesion.

NCLEX® Connection: Physiological Adaptation: Pathophysiology

4. A nurse is caring for a client who has multiple types of skin lesions. Which of the following skin lesions are suggestive of a malignant melanoma? (Select all that apply.)

   X   **An irregularly colored mole**

   X   **A lesion with asymmetric borders**

_____ A rough, scaly patch

_____ A uniformly colored papule

_____ Diffuse vesicles

An irregularly colored or shaped mole and a lesion with asymmetric borders are suggestive of malignant melanoma. The other skin lesions are not.

Ⓝ NCLEX® Connection: Reduction of Risk Potential: System Specific Assessment

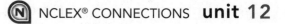

UNIT 12: NURSING CARE OF CLIENTS WITH ENDOCRINE DISORDERS

- Diagnostic and Therapeutic Procedures
- Pituitary Disorders
- Thyroid Disorders
- Adrenal Disorders
- Diabetes Mellitus

NCLEX® CONNECTIONS

When reviewing the chapters in this unit, keep in mind the relevant sections of the NCLEX® outline, in particular:

CLIENT NEEDS: PHARMACOLOGICAL AND PARENTERAL THERAPIES	CLIENT NEEDS: REDUCTION OF RISK POTENTIAL	CLIENT NEEDS: PHYSIOLOGICAL ADAPTATION
Relevant topics/tasks include:	Relevant topics/tasks include:	Relevant topics/tasks include:

• Adverse Effects/ Contraindications/Side Effects/Interactions
  ○ Manage the client experiencing side effects and adverse reactions of medication.
• Dosage Calculation
  ○ Use clinical decision making/critical thinking when calculating dosages.
• Medication Administration
  ○ Titrate dosage of medication based on assessment and ordered parameters.
	• Diagnostic Tests
	  ○ Apply knowledge of related nursing procedures and psychomotor skills when caring for clients undergoing diagnostic testing.
	• Laboratory Values
	  ○ Notify the provider about laboratory test results.
	• Therapeutic Procedures
	  ○ Educate the client about treatments and procedures.
		• Fluid and Electrolyte Imbalances
		  ○ Apply knowledge of pathophysiology when caring for the client with fluid and electrolyte imbalances.
		• Illness Management
		  ○ Educate the client about managing illness.
		• Pathophysiology
		  ○ Identify pathophysiology related to an acute or chronic condition.

UNIT 12	NURSING CARE OF CLIENTS WITH ENDOCRINE DISORDERS
Section	Diagnostic and Therapeutic Procedures
Chapter 89	Endocrine Diagnostic Procedures

Overview

- The function of the endocrine system is evaluated primarily by using laboratory tests. These tests vary according to the organ or system under analysis.

- Many of these tests are blood tests used to determine an excess or lack of a particular hormone in the body. Some of these tests are used to stimulate a reaction in the body that will facilitate diagnosis of a particular disorder.

- Endocrine diagnostic procedures that nurses should be knowledgeable about include those used to diagnose disorders of the:

  - Posterior pituitary gland.

  - Adrenal cortex.

  - Adrenal medulla.

  - Metabolism of carbohydrates.

  - Thyroid and anterior pituitary glands.

Posterior Pituitary Gland

- The posterior pituitary gland secretes the hormone vasopressin (antidiuretic hormone [ADH]). ADH increases permeability of the renal distal tubules, causing the kidneys to reabsorb water.

  - A deficiency of ADH causes diabetes insipidus, which is characterized by the excretion of a large quantity of diluted urine.

  - Excessive secretion of ADH causes the syndrome of inappropriate antidiuretic hormone (SIADH). In SIADH, the kidneys retain water, urine becomes concentrated, output drops, and extracellular fluid volume is increased.

  - Diagnostic tests for the posterior pituitary gland include the water deprivation test, serum ADH, serum and urine electrolytes and osmolality, and urine-specific gravity.

- Water deprivation test

  ○ The water deprivation test measures the kidneys' ability to concentrate urine in light of an increased plasma osmolality and a low plasma vasopressin level. It is a specialized test that must be performed in a controlled setting, and the client should be observed constantly throughout the test.

  ○ Indications

    ▪ This test is performed for clients who have a diagnosis of diabetes insipidus.

    ▪ It should only be conducted if the client's baseline serum sodium level is within the expected reference range and the osmolality of the urine is below 300 mOsm/kg H_2O.

    ▪ This test should not be performed on clients who have renal insufficiency, uncontrolled diabetes mellitus, hypovolemia of any etiology, or untreated adrenal or thyroid hormone deficiency.

  ○ Interpretation of Findings

    ▪ The test is positive for diabetes insipidus if the kidneys are unable to concentrate urine despite increased plasma osmolality.

  ○ Preprocedure

    ▪ Nursing Actions

      □ Begin the test between 0700 and 0900 and ensure that someone has the ability to remain with the client throughout the test.

      □ Obtain IV access.

  ○ Intraprocedure

    ▪ Nursing Actions

      □ Place the client in a recumbent position for 30 min, during which the following steps can be performed (The client may sit or stand during voiding and weight determination.)

        ‣ Obtain 7 to 10 mL of heparinized blood in an iced tube and send to the laboratory for immediate processing to determine sodium level.

        ‣ Ask the client to empty his bladder, record the amount, and send the specimen to the laboratory for immediate processing to determine osmolality.

        ‣ Weigh the client to nearest 0.1 kg. Record weight and obtain and record blood pressure and pulse.

      □ Initiate a complete fluid restriction and have the client maintain a semi-recumbent position except to void if necessary.

      □ Repeat the three steps hourly and record the client's symptoms, if there are any.

      □ Continue the steps until the serum sodium concentration or osmolality rises above the upper limit of the expected reference range.

- ○ Complications
  - ▪ Dehydration
    - ☐ Dehydration can occur due to a decrease in vascular volume.
    - ☐ Nursing Actions
      - ▸ Monitor the client closely.
      - ▸ Early indications of dehydration include postural hypotension, tachycardia, and dizziness.
- Serum ADH, serum and urine electrolytes and osmolality, and urine-specific gravity
  - ○ These tests are performed to diagnose SIADH.

TEST	NORMAL REFERENCE RANGE	INTERPRETATION OF FINDINGS	NURSING ACTIONS
Serum ADH	• 0 to 4.7 pg/mL	• Increased serum ADH is indicative of SIADH.	• The client should fast and avoid stress for 12 hr prior to the test. • Some medications may interfere with the test. Review medications with the provider. • Blood is drawn and then transported to the laboratory within 10 min.
Serum electrolytes	• Sodium – 136 to 145 mEq/L • Potassium – 3.5 to 5.0 mEq/L • Chloride – 98 to 106 mEq/L • Magnesium – 1.3 to 2.1 mEq/L	• Low serum sodium and high urine sodium content are expected with SIADH. • Decreased serum osmolality and increased urine osmolality are indicative of SIADH.	• No pre- or postprocedure care required – serum samples of blood and urine are analyzed for electrolyte components.
Urine electrolytes and osmolality	• Urine sodium – 75 to 200 mEq/day • Urine potassium – 26 to123 mEq/day (intake dependent) • Urine chloride – 110 to 250 mEq/24 hr • Urine osmolality – 250 to 900 mOsm/kg		

TEST	NORMAL REFERENCE RANGE	INTERPRETATION OF FINDINGS	NURSING ACTIONS
Urine-specific gravity	• 1.003 to 1.030	• The urine sample is analyzed for specific gravity. • A decrease in urine output and an increase in urine-specific gravity occur as a result of excess production of ADH.	• This test is usually performed in a laboratory but can be done in the clinical unit using a calibrated hydrometer or a temperature-compensated refractometer.

Adrenal Cortex

- Cushing's disease and Cushing's syndrome (hypercortisolism) are characterized by a hyperfunctioning adrenal cortex and an excess production of cortisol. Addison's disease is characterized by hypofunctioning of the adrenal cortex and a consequent lack of adequate amounts of serum cortisol.

  - Diagnostic tests for the adrenal cortex include the dexamethasone (Decadron) suppression test, plasma and salivary cortisol, 24-hr urine for cortisol, serum adrenocorticotropic hormone (ACTH), and ACTH stimulation tests.

  - A CT scan and/or an MRI may be performed to determine if there is atrophy of the adrenal glands causing hypofunction.

- Dexamethasone suppression test

  - This test is performed to determine if dexamethasone, which is a steroid similar to cortisol, has an effect on cortisol levels. Typically, the client takes a low or high dose of dexamethasone by mouth, and blood is drawn the next morning to determine if cortisol is present.

    - A low dose of dexamethasone is given to screen a client for Cushing's disease; high doses are given to determine the cause of the disease.

    - Some medications are withheld and stress is reduced prior to and during testing, as these can affect the outcome of the test results.

  - Indications

    - Cushing's disease

  - Interpretation of Findings

    - When decreased amounts of ACTH are produced by the pituitary gland, decreased amounts of cortisol are released by the adrenal glands.

    - When dexamethasone is given to clients who have Cushing's disease, there is no decrease in the production of ACTH and cortisol.

- Plasma and salivary cortisol, 24-hr urine for cortisol, serum ACTH, and ACTH stimulation tests

- Plasma and salivary cortisol, 24-hr urine for cortisol, serum ACTH, and ACTH stimulation tests

TEST	NORMAL REFERENCE RANGE	INTERPRETATION OF FINDINGS	NURSING ACTIONS
Plasma cortisol	This test varies according to the time of day. Since it has a diurnal pattern, higher levels are present in the early morning, and the lowest levels occur around midnight, or 3 to 5 hr after the onset of sleep.	Diurnal variations are not seen in a client who has Cushing's syndrome.	• Plasma cortisol is usually collected at midnight.
Salivary cortisol	A typical salivary cortisol value at midnight is < 2.0 ng/mL.	Higher levels indicate hypercortisolism.	• Salivary cortisol is usually collected at midnight. • A sample of saliva is obtained by placing a salivary cushion pad inside the client's cheek, directly over the salivary gland.
Urinary cortisol	10 to 100 mcg/day	Higher levels indicate hypercortisolism.	• Urinary cortisol is measured during 24-hr urine collection. ○ The client empties his bladder and then collects all urine excreted during the next 24-hr period. ○ The urine must be kept in a jug with boric acid added and kept on ice. ○ If the client is receiving spironolactone, this should be held for 7 days prior to the test.
Serum ACTH	Typical early morning values are from 25 to 200 pg/mL, and early evening values are usually from 0 to 50 pg/mL.	ACTH may be elevated with Addison's disease or decreased with Cushing's disease.	• Serum ACTH is most accurate if performed in the morning.

TEST	NORMAL REFERENCE RANGE	INTERPRETATION OF FINDINGS	NURSING ACTIONS
ACTH stimulation test	If no increase in cortisol occurs after administration of ACTH, the test is positive for Addison's disease or hypocortisolism.	ACTH stimulation test determines the functioning of the pituitary gland in relation to stimulating the secretion of adrenal hormones of cortisol.	• Two consecutive collections of 24-hr urine are used, one prior to and one after the administration of ACTH.

Adrenal Medulla

- Disorders of the adrenal medulla may result in the hypersecretion of catecholamines, resulting in stimulation of a sympathetic response, such as tachycardia, hypertension, and diaphoresis.

  ○ Diagnostic tests for the adrenal medulla include vanillylmandelic acid (VMA) testing, the clonidine suppression test, and the phentolamine blocking test.

- VMA testing

  ○ VMA testing is a 24-hr urine collection for vanillylmandelic acid (VMA), a breakdown product of catecholamines. Analysis of other urinary catecholamines may also be measured, such as dopamine and normetanephrine.

  ○ Indications

    ▪ Diagnosis of pheochromocytoma

  ○ Interpretation of Findings

    ▪ Normal VMA is 2 to 7 mg/24 hr.

    ▪ High VMA levels at rest indicate pheochromocytoma.

  ○ Preprocedure

    ▪ Nursing Actions

      □ Monitor/instruct the client regarding 24-hr urine collection. Urine is collected for 24 hr (in a container with a preservative) beginning with an empty bladder.

    ▪ Client Education

      □ Caffeine, vanilla, bananas, and chocolate may be restricted for 2 to 3 days before the test. The client may also be asked to hold aspirin and antihypertensive medications.

      □ Instruct the client to maintain a moderate level of activity.

- Clonidine suppression test

  - The client's plasma catecholamines levels are taken prior to and 3 hr after administration of clonidine (Catapres).

  - Indications

    - Diagnosis of pheochromocytoma

  - Interpretation of Findings

    - If a client does not have a pheochromocytoma, clonidine suppresses catecholamine release and decreases the serum level of catecholamines (decreases blood pressure).

    - If the client does have a pheochromocytoma, the clonidine has no effect (no decreased blood pressure).

  - Pre/intraprocedure

    - Nursing Actions

      - Inform the client about the test.

      - Monitor the client for hypotension.

  - Postprocedure

    - Client Education

      - Inform the client that tiredness may be a side effect after the test.

- Phentolamine blocking test

  - Phentolamine (Regitine), an alpha blocker, is administered to the client.

  - Indications

    - Diagnosis of pheochromocytoma

  - Interpretation of Findings

    - A rapid decrease in systolic blood pressure of $\geq$ 35 mm Hg and diastolic blood pressure of $\geq$ 25 mm Hg with the administration of phentolamine is diagnostic for pheochromocytoma.

  - Intraprocedure

    - Nursing Actions

      - Monitor the client's blood pressure

Carbohydrate Metabolism

- Dysfunction of carbohydrate metabolism may be caused by insulin deficiency, as in type 1 diabetes mellitus, or insulin resistance, as in type 2 diabetes mellitus, resulting in hyperglycemia.

  - Diagnostic tests to evaluate carbohydrate metabolism include fasting blood glucose, oral glucose tolerance testing, and glycosylated hemoglobin (HbA1c).

TEST	NORMAL REFERENCE RANGE	INTERPRETATION OF FINDINGS	NURSING ACTIONS
Fasting blood glucose	<110 mg/dL	• This test is done to determine the client's blood glucose when no foods or fluids (other than water) have been consumed for the past 8 hr.	• Ensure that the client has fasted (no food or drink other than water) for the 8 hr prior to the blood draw. • Antidiabetic medications should be postponed until after the level is drawn.
Oral glucose tolerance test	<140 mg/dL	• This test is done to determine the client's ability to metabolize a standard amount of glucose.	• Instruct the client to consume a balanced diet for the 3 days prior to the test and fast for the 10 to 12 hr prior to the test. • A fasting blood glucose level is drawn at start of the test. • The client is then instructed to consume a specified amount of glucose. • Blood glucose levels are drawn every 30 min for 2 hr. Clients must be assessed for hypoglycemia throughout the procedure.
Glycosylated hemoglobin (HbA1c)	Guidelines - an HbA1c of 5% or less indicates the absence of diabetes mellitus; an HbA1c of 5.7% to 6.4% indicates prediabetes mellitus, and an HbA1c of 6.5% or higher indicates diabetes mellitus.	• HbA1c is the best indicator of an average blood glucose level for the past 120 days. • This test assists in evaluating treatment effectiveness and compliance with the diet plan, medication regimen, and exercise schedule.	• No pre- or postprocedure care is required. The test requires a laboratory draw of a random blood sample.

Thyroid and Anterior Pituitary Gland

- Hyperthyroidism and hypothyroidism are conditions in which there are inappropriate amounts of the thyroid hormones triiodothyronine (T_3) and thyroxine (T_4) circulating. These inappropriate amounts of T_3 and T_4 cause an increase or decrease in metabolic rate that affects all body systems.

- The anterior pituitary gland secretes thyroid stimulating hormone (TSH). Hyposecretion of TSH may lead to secondary hypothyroidism, and hypersecretion of TSH may cause secondary hyperthyroidism.

  - Diagnostic tests to evaluate the function of the thyroid and anterior pituitary glands include serum triiodothyronine (T_3), serum thyroxine (T_4), serum thyroid stimulating hormone (TSH), serum thyrotropin-releasing hormone (TRH) stimulation test, and radioactive iodine uptake (RAIU).

  - Ultrasounds or scans may also be performed to determine the size, shape, and presence of nodules and masses on these glands.

TEST	NORMAL REFERENCE RANGE	INTERPRETATION OF FINDINGS	NURSING ACTIONS
T_3 T_4	70 to 205 ng/dL 4.0 to 12.0 mcg/dL	• Low and high levels of each indicate hypothyroidism and hyperthyroidism respectively; a high level of T_3 is more diagnostic of hyperthyroidism than is T_4.	• No pre- or postprocedure care is required for either test; the laboratory requires a random blood sample.
TSH	0.4 to 6.15 microunits/mL	• It stimulates the release of thyroid hormone by the anterior pituitary gland. • TSH may be elevated or decreased, depending on the cause. An increased value indicates primary hypothyroidism or secondary hyperthyroidism. A decreased value indicates primary hyperthyroidism (Grave's disease) or secondary hypothyroidism.	• No pre- or postprocedure care is required; the laboratory requires a random blood sample.
TRH	Relative to baseline	• It is normal for the TSH to double the baseline value shortly after administration. • If the TSH increases two fold or more above baseline, this finding is indicative of hypothyroidism.	• The TRH is assessed by giving a bolus of thyrotropin-releasing hormone, and serum concentrations of TSH are assessed at intervals.

TEST	NORMAL REFERENCE RANGE	INTERPRETATION OF FINDINGS	NURSING ACTIONS
RAIU	< 35% of injected amount of radioactive iodine (^{123}I)	• It measures the amount of ^{123}I that is absorbed by the thyroid gland. • Clients who have hyperthyroidism absorb high amounts (> 35%) of ^{123}I.	• The client is administered an oral radioactive dose of ^{123}I, and the amount absorbed is measured by a scintillation counter. • This test cannot be done if the client is pregnant or has had another test done that used an iodine-containing dye.

CHAPTER 89: ENDOCRINE DIAGNOSTIC PROCEDURES

 Application Exercises

1. A client asks the nurse why the provider bases the medication regimen on the HbA1c instead of the log of morning fasting blood glucose levels. Which of the following is an appropriate response by the nurse?

    A. "It measures how well your insulin is regulating your blood glucose between meals."

    B. "It indicates how well your blood glucose has been regulated over the past 3 to 4 months."

    C. "It is the first blood test that should be done to diagnose if an individual has diabetes."

    D. "It will determine if an individual's dose of Regular insulin needs to be adjusted."

2. A nurse is reviewing the laboratory tests for a client who has suspected hyperthyroidism. An elevation of which of the following values is the most accurate diagnostic indicator that the client is experiencing a hyperthyroid state?

    A. T_3

    B. VMA

    C. TSH

    D. TRH

3. Which of the following laboratory values should the nurse expect for a client who is producing too much antidiuretic hormone? (Select all that apply.)

    _____ Low serum sodium

    _____ High serum potassium

    _____ Low urine creatinine

    _____ High urine sodium

    _____ Decreased urine osmolality

    _____ Increased serum osmolality

    _____ Increased urine-specific gravity

4. A client is suspected of having primary adrenal insufficiency. Which of the following responses should the nurse anticipate after an intravenous injection of 1.0 mg of ACTH?

    A. Little or no increase in plasma cortisol

    B. Significant increase in plasma cortisol

    C. Decrease in plasma cortisol

    D. Delayed increase in plasma cortisol

CHAPTER 89: ENDOCRINE DIAGNOSTIC PROCEDURES

 Application Exercises Answer Key

1. A client asks the nurse why the provider bases the medication regimen on the HbA1c instead of the log of morning fasting blood glucose levels. Which of the following is an appropriate response by the nurse?

    A. "It measures how well your insulin is regulating your blood glucose between meals."

    B. "It indicates how well your blood glucose has been regulated over the past 3 to 4 months."

    C. "It is the first blood test that should be done to diagnose if an individual has diabetes."

    D. "It will determine if an individual's dose of Regular insulin needs to be adjusted."

HbA1c measures the client's blood glucose control over the past 120 days, or 3 to 4 months. It is the best indicator of blood glucose over an extended period of time instead of a short period of time, such as between insulin injections.

 NCLEX® Connection: Reduction of Risk Potential, Laboratory Values

2. A nurse is reviewing the laboratory tests for a client who has suspected hyperthyroidism. An elevation of which of the following values is the most accurate diagnostic indicator that the client is experiencing a hyperthyroid state?

    A. T_3

    B. VMA

    C. TSH

    D. TRH

A client's T_3 increases in a hyperthyroid state, making it a stronger marker for diagnosing hyperthyroidism. TSH and TRH decrease during a hyperthyroid state due to the negative feedback imposed by the hypothalamus when levels of T_3 and T_4 are high. VMA is a test for pheochromocytoma and reflects the amount of catecholamine byproducts.

 NCLEX® Connection: Reduction of Risk Potential, Laboratory Values

3. Which of the following laboratory values should the nurse expect for a client who is producing too much antidiuretic hormone? (Select all that apply.)

   X   **Low serum sodium**

        High serum potassium

        Low urine creatinine

   X   **High urine sodium**

        Decreased urine osmolality

        Increased serum osmolality

   X   **Increased urine-specific gravity**

SIADH causes a client to retain water, creating dilutional hyponatremia with concurrent urinary excretion of sodium. This will be manifested by a low serum sodium, high urine sodium, and increased urine-specific gravity. Serum potassium and urine creatinine should be unaffected.

 NCLEX® Connection: Reduction of Risk Potential, Laboratory Values

4. A client is suspected of having primary adrenal insufficiency. Which of the following responses should the nurse anticipate after an intravenous injection of 1.0 mg of ACTH?

   A. Little or no increase in plasma cortisol

   B. Significant increase in plasma cortisol

   C. Decrease in plasma cortisol

   D. Delayed increase in plasma cortisol

A client who has primary adrenal insufficiency does not produce enough aldosterone and cortisol. Therefore, during an ACTH stimulation test, the expected response would be little or no increase in plasma cortisol. A decrease in baseline cortisol level would not be expected, nor would an increase, either immediate or delayed.

 NCLEX® Connection: Reduction of Risk Potential, Laboratory Values

UNIT 12	NURSING CARE OF CLIENTS WITH ENDOCRINE DISORDERS

Section   Pituitary Disorders

Chapter 90   Posterior Pituitary Disorders

Overview

- The posterior pituitary gland secretes the hormone vasopressin, or antidiuretic hormone (ADH).

  o Vasopressin increases permeability of the renal distal tubules, causing the kidneys to reabsorb water.

  o A deficiency of ADH causes diabetes insipidus (DI).

  ▪ DI is characterized by the excretion of a large quantity of diluted urine.

  o Excessive secretion of ADH causes the syndrome of inappropriate antidiuretic hormone (SIADH).

  ▪ In SIADH, the kidneys retain water, urine output drops, and extracellular fluid volume is increased.

- Posterior pituitary disorders result in fluid and electrolyte imbalances.

DIABETES INSIPIDUS

Overview

- Diabetes insipidus results from a deficiency of ADH, which is secreted by the posterior lobe of the pituitary gland (neurohypophysis).

- Decreased ADH reduces the ability of collecting and distal renal tubules in the kidneys to concentrate urine, resulting in excessive diluted urination, excessive thirst, and excessive fluid intake.

- Types of diabetes insipidus:

  o Neurogenic (also known as central or primary) – Caused by damage to the hypothalamus or pituitary gland from trauma, irradiation, or cranial surgery

  o Nephrogenic – Inherited; renal tubules do not react to ADH

  o Drug-induced – Lithium carbonate (Lithobid) or demeclocycline (Declomycin) may alter the way the kidneys respond to ADH.

Assessment

- Risk Factors

    o Clients who have a head injury, a tumor or lesion, surgery near or around the pituitary gland, or an infection, (meningitis, encephalitis)

    o Clients who are taking lithium carbonate (Lithobid) or demeclocycline (Declomycin)

    o Older adult clients are at higher risk for dehydration due to lower water content of the body, decreased thirst response, decreased ability of the kidneys to concentrate urine, increased use of diuretics, and swallowing difficulties or poor food intake.

- Subjective Data

    o Polyuria (abrupt onset of excessive urination, urinary output of 5 to 20 L/day of dilute urine)

    o Polydipsia (excessive thirst, consumption of 4 to 30 L/day)

    o Nocturia

    o Fatigue

    o Dehydration, as evidenced by extreme thirst, weight loss, muscle weakness, headache, tachycardia, hypotension, poor skin turgor, dry mucous membranes, constipation, and dizziness

- Objective Data

    o Physical Assessment Findings

    o Laboratory Tests

    - Urine chemistry – Think DILUTE.

        □ Decreased urine specific gravity (less than 1.005)

        □ Decreased urine osmolality (less than 300 mOsm/L)

        □ Decreased urine pH

        □ Decreased urine sodium

        □ Decreased urine potassium

        □ As urine volume increases, urine osmolality decreases.

    - Serum chemistry – Think CONCENTRATED.

        □ Increased serum osmolality (greater than 300 mOsm/L)

        □ Increased serum sodium

        □ Increased serum potassium

        □ As serum volume decreases, the serum osmolality increases.

    - Radioimmunoassay – Decreased ADH

- ○ Diagnostic Procedures
  - ▪ Water deprivation test
    - □ This is an easy and reliable diagnostic test. Dehydration is induced by withholding fluids. Urine output is measured and tested hourly.
    - □ The test is positive for diabetes insipidus if the kidneys are unable to concentrate urine despite increased plasma osmolarity.
    - □ Nursing Actions
      - ▸ Begin by obtaining baseline weight, vital signs, serum electrolytes and osmolarity, and urine specific gravity and osmolarity.
      - ▸ Monitor hourly vital signs and hourly urine specific gravity and osmolarity.
      - ▸ Monitor for severe dehydration.
        - ▹ Early indications may be postural hypotension, tachycardia and dizziness. The nurse should be prepared to discontinue the test if these indicators develop.
    - □ Client Education
      - ▸ Explain the test procedure to the client.
      - ▸ Advise the client to notify the nurse of any dizziness, headache, or nausea.
  - ▪ Vasopressin test
    - □ A subcutaneous injection of vasopressin produces a urine output with an increased specific gravity if the client has central diabetes insipidus. This helps differentiate central from nephrogenic diabetes insipidus.
    - □ Nursing Actions
      - ▸ Monitor vital signs and urine specific gravity and osmolarity hourly.
    - □ Client Education
      - ▸ Explain the test procedure to the client. Advise the client to notify the nurse of any dizziness, headache, or nausea.

Collaborative Care

- • Nursing Care
  - ○ Monitor vital signs, urinary output, central venous pressure, intake and output, specific gravity, and laboratory studies (potassium, sodium, BUN, creatinine, specific gravity, osmolarity).
  - ○ Weigh the client daily.
  - ○ Promote the prescribed diet (regular diet with restriction of foods that exert a diuretic effect, such as caffeine).

- IV therapy – Hydration (intake and output must be matched to prevent dehydration), and electrolyte replacement

- Promote safety – Keep bedside rails up and provide assistance with walking if the client is dizzy or has muscle weakness. Make sure the client has easy access to a bathroom or bedpan and answer the call lights promptly.

- Add bulk foods and fruit juices to the diet if constipation develops. The client may require a mild laxative.

- Assess skin turgor and mucous membranes.

- Provide meticulous skin and mouth care and apply a lubricant to cracked or sore lips. Use a soft toothbrush and mild mouthwash to avoid trauma to the oral mucosa. Use alcohol-free skin care products and apply emollient lotion after baths.

- Encourage the client to drink fluids in response to thirst.

- Administer medications as prescribed.

- Medications

  - ADH replacement agents – Desmopressin acetate (DDAVP) or aqueous vasopressin (Pitressin) administered intranasally, orally, or parenterally

    - Used as a synthetic posterior pituitary hormone that causes an increase in water absorption from kidneys and a decrease in urine output

    - Nursing Considerations

      - Monitor vital signs, urinary output, central venous pressure, intake and output, specific gravity, and laboratory studies (potassium, sodium, BUN, creatinine, specific gravity, osmolarity).

      - Monitor blood pressure.

      - Dose may need to be adjusted to urine output.

    - Client Education

      - For an intranasal dose, teach the client to clear nasal passage and sit upright prior to nasal inhalation.

      - Instruct the client to monitor weight and notify the provider of a gain greater than 2 lb in 24 hr.

      - Instruct the client to restrict fluids if directed and notify the health care provider of headache or confusion.

  - ADH stimulants – Carbamazepine (Tegretol)

    - Anticonvulsants stimulate release of ADH. They may be effective in partial central diabetes insipidus.

    - Nursing Considerations

      - Monitor vital signs, urinary output, central venous pressure, intake and output, specific gravity, and laboratory studies (potassium, sodium, BUN, creatinine, specific gravity, osmolarity).

- □ Monitor blood pressure.

- □ Monitor for dizziness or drowsiness related to the medication.

- □ Monitor for signs of thrombocytopenia, (sore throat, bruising, fever).

  - ■ Client Education

    - □ Advise the client to:

      - ▸ Take the medication with food to reduce gastric distress.

      - ▸ Use caution driving or operating heavy machinery until effects of the medication are established.

      - ▸ Notify the provider of sore throat, fever, or bleeding.

  - ○ Vasopressin (Pitressin)

    - ■ Posterior pituitary hormone that causes an increase in water absorption from kidneys and a decrease in urine output

    - ■ Nursing Considerations

      - □ Give vasopressin cautiously to clients who have coronary artery disease because the medication may cause vasoconstriction.

      - □ Monitor vital signs, urinary output, central venous pressure, intake and output, specific gravity, and laboratory studies (potassium, sodium, BUN, creatinine, specific gravity, osmolarity).

      - □ Monitor blood pressure.

      - □ Monitor for headache, confusion, or other signs of water intoxication.

    - ■ Client Education

      - □ Educate the client regarding lifelong vasopressin therapy, daily weights, and the importance of reporting weight gain, polyuria, and polydipsia to the health care provider.

      - □ Instruct the client to restrict fluids if directed, and notify the health care provider of headache or confusion.

- • Interdisciplinary Care

  - ○ Home assistance for fluid, medication, and dietary management may be required.

- • Care After Discharge

  - ○ Client Education

    - ■ Discharge instructions should include information about medications in discharge instructions.

    - ■ Instruct the client to weigh himself daily, eat a diet that is high in fiber, wear a medical alert wristband, and monitor fluid intake.

- Teach the client to monitor for signs of dehydration, (weight loss; dry, cracked lips; confusion; weakness).

- Advise the client to restrict fluids if instructed to prevent water intoxication, and avoid consumption of alcohol.

- Client Outcomes

  ○ The client will establish and maintain fluid and electrolyte balance through medication and fluid management.

Complications

- Untreated diabetes insipidus can produce hypovolemia, hyperosmolarity, hypernatremia, circulatory collapse, unconsciousness, central nervous system damage, and seizures.

  ○ Excessive urine output causing severe dehydration can lead to these complications.

  ○ Nursing Actions

    - Monitor fluid balance and prevent dehydration with providing proper fluid intake.

  ○ Client Education

    - Advise the client to seek early medical attention for any sign of diabetes insipidus and follow care instructions.

SYNDROME OF INAPPROPRIATE ANTIDIURETIC HORMONE (SIADH)

Overview

- Syndrome of inappropriate antidiuretic hormone (SIADH) is an excessive release of antidiuretic hormone (ADH), also known as vasopressin, secreted by the posterior lobe of the pituitary gland (neurohypophysis).

- Excess ADH leads to renal reabsorption of water and suppression of renin-angiotensin mechanism, causing renal excretion of sodium leading to water intoxication, cellular edema, and dilutional hyponatremia. Fluid shifts within compartments cause decreased serum osmolarity.

Assessment

- Risk Factors

  ○ Conditions that stimulate the hypothalamus to hypersecrete ADH include malignant tumors (the most common cause is oat-cell lung cancer), increasing intrathoracic pressure (such as with positive pressure ventilation), head injury, meningitis, cardiovascular accident, medications (alcohol, lithium carbonate, phenytoin), trauma, pain, and stress.

  ○ Diuretics are sometimes used to treat conditions such as heart failure. Sodium losses due to diuretic use can further contribute to the problems caused by SIADH. A careful client history and medication review may help alert nurses to the possibility of SIADH.

- Subjective Data

  - Early symptoms of SIADH include headache, weakness, anorexia, muscle cramps, and weight gain (without edema because water, not sodium, is retained).

  - As the serum sodium level decreases, the client experiences personality changes, hostility, sluggish deep tendon reflexes, nausea, vomiting, diarrhea, and oliguria.

- Objective Data

  - Physical Assessment Findings

    - Confusion, lethargy, and Cheyne-Stokes respirations herald impending crisis. When the serum sodium level drops further, seizures, coma, and death may occur.

    - Manifestations of fluid volume excess include tachycardia, possibly hypertension, crackles in lungs, distended neck veins, and taut skin. Intake is greater than output.

  - Laboratory Tests

    - Urine chemistry – Think CONCENTRATED.

      - Increased urine sodium

      - Increased urine osmolarity

      - As urine volume decreases, urine osmolarity increases.

    - Blood chemistry – Think DILUTE.

      - Decreased serum sodium

      - Decreased serum osmolarity (less than 270 mEq/L)

      - As serum volume increases, serum osmolarity decreases.

      - Radioimmunoassay – Increased ADH

Collaborative Care

- Nursing Care

  - Restrict oral fluids to 500 to 1,000 mL/day to prevent further hemodilution (first priority). During fluid restriction, provide comfort measures for thirst, including mouth care, ice chips, lozenges, and staggered water intake.

  - Flush all enteral and gastric tubes with 0.9% sodium chloride, instead of water to replace sodium and prevent further hemodilution.

  - Monitor intake and output accurately. Report decreased urine output.

  - Monitor vital signs for increased blood pressure, tachycardia, and hypothermia.

  - Monitor for decreased serum sodium/osmolarity and elevated urine sodium/osmolarity.

  - Weigh daily. A weight gain of 0.9 kg (2 lb) indicates a gain of 1 L of fluid.

- ○ Report altered mental status (headache, confusion, lethargy, seizures, coma).

- ○ Reduce environmental stimuli and position the client as needed.

- ○ Provide a safe environment for clients who have altered levels of consciousness. Take seizure precautions.

- ○ Monitor the client for signs and symptoms of heart failure, which can occur from fluid overload. Use of a loop diuretic may be indicated.

- Medications

    - ○ Demeclocycline (Declomycin)

        - ■ Tetracycline derivative

        - ■ May cause drug-induced diabetes insipidus

        - ■ Nursing Considerations

            - □ Monitor for effective treatment, such as increased serum sodium/osmolarity and decreased urine sodium osmolarity.

        - ■ Client Education

            - □ Advise the client that it may take a week to see results.

            - □ Advise the client to monitor for signs of a yeast infection, such as a white, cheese-like film inside the mouth.

            - □ Have the client her rinse toothbrush with a diluted bleach solution (10%) and increase consumption of yogurt.

    - ○ Lithium (Lithium Carbonate)

        - ■ Used to block the renal response to ADH

        - ■ May induce diabetes insipidus

        - ■ Nursing Considerations

            - □ Monitor for adverse effects (lithium toxicity, nausea, diarrhea, tremors ataxia).

            - □ Monitor glucose levels.

            - □ Monitor ECG for dysrhythmias.

            - □ Monitor for effective treatment, (increased serum sodium/osmolarity, decreased urine sodium/osmolarity).

        - ■ Client Education

            - □ Advise the client to monitor for symptoms of lithium toxicity.

            - □ Advise the client to take the medication food.

            - □ Advise the client to allow 1 to 3 weeks to see effects.

- ○ Furosemide (Lasix)
  - ▪ A loop diuretic used to increase water excretion from kidneys
  - ▪ Nursing Considerations
    - □ Use with caution.
    - □ Loop diuretics cause sodium excretion and may worsen hyponatremia.
  - ▪ Client Education
    - □ Advise the client to change positions slowly in case of postural hypotension.
    - □ Advise the client to notify the health care provider of signs of hyponatremia, such as nausea, decreased appetite, and vomiting.

- • Interdisciplinary Care
  - ○ Home care for may be required for fluid, medication, and dietary management.

- • Therapeutic Procedures
  - ○ Hypertonic IV fluid
    - ▪ The goal of hypertonic saline therapy is to elevate the sodium level enough to alleviate signs of neurologic compromise/not to raise the level to normal.
    - ▪ Nursing Actions
      - □ In severe hyponatremia/water intoxication, administration of 200 to 300 mL of hypertonic IV fluid (3% to 5% sodium chloride).
      - □ Monitor for fluid overload and heart failure (distended neck veins, crackles in lungs).
    - ▪ Client Education
      - □ Explain the procedure to the client.
      - □ Advise the client to notify the nurse of difficulty breathing or shortness of breath, which may indicate heart failure.
      - □ Include information about medications with discharge instructions.
      - □ Instruct the client to obtain daily weights, wear a medical alert wristband, and restrict fluid intake.
      - □ Advise the client to monitor for signs of hypervolemia, (weight gain, difficulty breathing) and any neurological changes (tremors, disorientation), which may lead to seizures.
      - □ Advise the client to notify the health care provider of signs of hyponatremia, such as nausea, decreased appetite, and vomiting.
      - □ Advise the client to avoid consumption of alcohol.

- • Client Outcomes
  - ○ The client will establish and maintain fluid and electrolyte balance through medication and fluid management.

Complications

- Water intoxication, cerebral edema, and severe hyponatremia

    o Without prompt treatment, SIADH may lead to these complications with resultant coma and death.

    o Nursing Actions

        ■ Monitor for early signs of water intoxication, such as lung crackles, distended neck veins, and changes in neurological state, (twitching, disorientation).

        ■ Monitor and document neurologic status frequently.

        ■ Institute seizure precautions.

        ■ Medicate the client as prescribed.

        ■ Monitor serum sodium level.

    o Client Education

        ■ Instruct the client and family about fluid restrictions and offer information about the condition and treatment.

        ■ Provide support to ease the client's fear about the disease.

- Central pontine myelinolysis (CPM)

    o Treatment for SIADH may result in central pontine myelinolysis (CPM), a condition characterized by nerve damage that is caused by the destruction of the myelin sheath in the brainstem (pons). The most common cause is a rapid change in sodium levels in the body. This most commonly occurs when a client is being treated for hyponatremia and the levels rise too fast.

    o Nursing Actions

        ■ During treatment with hypertonic saline or loop diuretics, plasma osmolarity and serum sodium should be monitored every 2 to 4 hr. Any deterioration in neurologic status should be reported immediately.

    o Client Education

        ■ Inform the client and family about the condition.

        ■ Explain all procedures and information about medication and treatment.

CHAPTER 90: POSTERIOR PITUITARY DISORDERS

(A) Application Exercises

1. A nurse is caring for a client who has primary diabetes insipidus. Which of the following manifestations should the nurse expect to find? (Select all that apply.)

_____ Serum sodium of 155 mEq/L

_____ Fatigue

_____ Serum osmolarity of 250 mOsm/L

_____ Polyuria

_____ Increased thirst

_____ Nocturia

2. A nurse is caring for a client who has diabetes insipidus. Which of the following tests should the nurse use to assess the client's urine for diabetes insipidus?

A. Glucose

B. Specific gravity

C. Ketones

D. RBCs

3. A nurse is caring for a client who has syndrome of inappropriate antidiuretic hormone (SIADH). Which of the following manifestations should the nurse expect to find? (Select all that apply.)

_____ Serum sodium less than 120 mEq/L

_____ Urine specific gravity 1.001

_____ Serum osmolarity 230 mOsm/L

_____ Polyuria

_____ Increased thirst

_____ Urine osmolarity greater than 1,500 mOsm/L

4. A nurse is assessing a client who has SIADH. Which of the following assessment findings indicate a dangerous complication of SIADH?

A. Decreased central venous pressure (CVP)

B. Increased urine output

C. Distended neck veins

D. Extreme thirst

CHAPTER 90: POSTERIOR PITUITARY DISORDERS

 Application Exercises Answer Key

1. A nurse is caring for a client who has primary diabetes insipidus. Which of the following manifestations should the nurse expect to find? (Select all that apply.)

  __X__   **Serum sodium of 155 mEq/L**

  __X__   **Fatigue**

  _____   Serum osmolarity of 250 mOsm/L

  __X__   **Polyuria**

  __X__   **Increased thirst**

  __X__   **Nocturia**

Primary diabetes insipidus is caused by a reduction in the secretion of ADH. Manifestations include increased serum sodium, fatigue, excessive urination, increased thirst, and nocturia. Serum osmolarity will be greater than 300 mOsm/L.

NCLEX® Connection: Reduction of Risk Potential, System Specific Assessment

2. A nurse is caring for a client who has diabetes insipidus. Which of the following tests should the nurse use to assess the client's urine for diabetes insipidus?

A. Glucose

B. Specific gravity

C. Ketones

D. RBCs

The urine of a client who has diabetes insipidus should be checked frequently for specific gravity. Urine will be dilute with a urine specific gravity of less than 1.005.

NCLEX® Connection: Reduction of Risk Potential, System Specific Assessment

3. A nurse is caring for a client who has SIADH. Which of the following manifestations should the nurse expect to find? (Select all that apply.)

   X   **Serum sodium less than 120 mEq/L**

         Urine specific gravity 1.001

   X   **Serum osmolarity 230 mOsm/L**

         Polyuria

         Increased thirst

   X   **Urine osmolarity greater than 1,500 mOsm/L**

SIADH is caused by an increase in the secretion of ADH. SIADH causes hypervolemia as indicated by dilutional hyponatremia and decreased serum osmolarity. Urine will be concentrated with osmolarity greater than 900 mOsm/L. Other findings of SIADH may include concentrated urine (specific gravity greater than 1.030) and reduced urine output. Increased thirst is a finding consistent with diabetes insipidus.

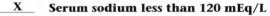 NCLEX® Connection: Reduction of Risk Potential, System Specific Assessment

4. A nurse is assessing a client who has syndrome of inappropriate antidiuretic hormone (SIADH). Which of the following assessment findings indicate a dangerous complication of SIADH?

    A. Decreased central venous pressure (CVP)

    B. Increased urine output

    C. Distended neck veins

    D. Extreme thirst

Distended neck veins, shortness of breath, and crackles heard with breath sounds are signs of fluid overload that may lead to pulmonary edema or heart failure. Decreased CVP, increased urine output, and extreme thirst are not findings associated with SIADH.

NCLEX® Connection: Physiological Adaptation, Illness Management

Overview

- The thyroid gland produces three hormones: thyroxine (T_4), triiodothyronine (T_3), and thyrocalcitonin (calcitonin). Secretion of T_3 and T_4 is regulated by the anterior pituitary gland through a negative feedback mechanism.

- When serum T_3 and T_4 levels decrease, thyroid-stimulating hormone (TSH) is released by the anterior pituitary. This stimulates the thyroid gland to secrete more hormones until normal levels are reached.

- T_3 and T_4 affect all body systems by regulating overall body metabolism, energy production, and fluid and electrolyte balance and controlling tissue use of fats, proteins, and carbohydrates.

- Calcitonin inhibits mobilization of calcium from bone and reduces blood calcium levels.

- Hyperthyroidism is a clinical syndrome caused by excessive circulating thyroid hormones. Because thyroid activity affects all body systems, excessive thyroid hormone exaggerates normal body functions and produces a hypermetabolic state.

Health Promotion and Disease Prevention

- Client Education

  - Advise the client to:

    - Take all medications as directed.

    - Check with the health care provider prior to taking over-the-counter medications.

    - Keep all follow-up appointments.

    - Adjust diet to increased metabolism when needed.

    - Try to avoid stress and get rest as needed.

    - Notify the health care provider of fever, increased restlessness, palpitations, or chest pain.

Assessment

- Risk Factors

  - Causes of hyperthyroidism – Action of immunoglobulins on the thyroid gland

    - Graves' disease is the most common cause. Autoimmune antibodies apparently mimic TSH, thus leading to hypersecretion of thyroid hormones.

- Subjective Data

  - Nervousness, irritability, hyperactivity, emotional lability, and decreased attention span

  - Weakness, easy fatigability, and exercise intolerance

  - Heat intolerance

  - Weight change (usually loss) and increased appetite

  - Insomnia and interrupted sleep

  - Frequent stools and diarrhea

  - Menstrual irregularities and decreased libido

  - Warm, sweaty, flushed skin with velvety-smooth texture

  - Tremor, hyperkinesias and hyperreflexia

  - Vision changes, exophthalmos, retracted eye lids, and staring gaze

    > **(M) View Media Supplement:** Exophthalmos (Image)

  - Hair loss

  - Goiter

- Objective Data

  - Physical Assessment Findings

    - Bruit over the thyroid gland

    - Elevated systolic blood pressure, widened pulse pressure, and S_3 heart sound

    - Tachycardia and dysrhythmias

    - Findings in older adult clients are often more subtle than those in younger clients.

    - Occasionally an older adult client with hyperthyroidism will demonstrate apathy or withdrawal instead of the more typical hypermetabolic state.

    - Older adult clients with hyperthyroidism often present with heart failure and atrial fibrillation.

- o Laboratory Tests

  - Serum TSH test – Decreased in the presence of Graves' disease (may be elevated in secondary or tertiary hyperthyroidism)

  - Free thyroxine index (FTI) and T_3 – Elevated in the presence of disease

  - Thyrotropin-releasing hormone (TRH) stimulation test – Failure of expected rise in TSH

- o Diagnostic Procedures

  - Radioiodine (^{123} I) uptake and thyroid scan

    - □ Clarifies size of gland and detects presence of hot or cold nodules

  - Nursing Actions

    - □ Confirm that the client is not pregnant prior to the scan.

    - □ Take a medication history to determine the use of iodides.

    - □ Recent use of contrast media and oral contraceptives may cause falsely elevated serum thyroid hormone levels.

    - □ Severe illness; malnutrition; and the use of aspirin, corticosteroids, and phenytoin sodium may cause a false decrease in serum thyroid hormone levels.

    - □ Inform the health care provider if the client received any iodine contrast within 4 weeks of test.

  - Client Education

    - □ Advise the client to avoid foods high in iodine for 1 week prior to the test.

    - □ Suggest that the client use noniodized salt, avoid fish and shellfish, reduce milk intake, and avoid canned fruits and vegetables.

Collaborative Care

- • Nursing Care

  - o Minimize the client's energy expenditure by assisting with activities as necessary and by encouraging the client to alternate periods of activity with rest.

  - o Promote a calm environment.

  - o Assess the client's mental status and decision-making ability. Intervene as needed to ensure safety.

  - o Monitor the client's nutritional status. Provide increased calories, protein, and other nutritional support as necessary.

  - o Provide eye protection (patches, eye lubricant, tape to close eyelids) for a client with exophthalmos.

  - o Monitor vital signs and hemodynamic parameters (for a client who is actually ill) for signs of heart failure.

- o Monitor ECG for dysrhythmias and temperature for elevation.

- o Assure the family that any abrupt changes in the client's behavior are likely disease related and should subside with antithyroid therapy.

- o Administer antithyroid medications as prescribed.

- o Prepare the client for a total/subtotal thyroidectomy if the client is unresponsive to antithyroid medications or has an airway-obstructing goiter.

- Medications

  - o Propylthiouracil (PTU) or methimazole (Tapazole)

    - Antihyperthyroid medications that act by blocking thyroid hormone synthesis and reducing thyroid hormone level

    - Nursing Considerations

      - □ Monitor for signs of hypothyroidism, such as intolerance to cold, edema, bradycardia, increase in weight, or depression.

      - □ Monitor CBC for leukopenia or thrombocytopenia.

    - Client Education

      - □ Instruct the client to take the medication with meals.

      - □ Advise the client to take the medication in divided doses at regular intervals to maintain an even therapeutic drug level.

      - □ Advise client to report fever, sore throat, or bruising to primary care provider.

      - □ Advise the client to report any sign of jaundice (yellowing of skin or eyes, darkening of urine).

      - □ Advise the client to follow the health care provider's instructions about dietary intake of iodine.

  - o Propranolol (Inderal)

    - Beta-adrenergic blocker – Treats sympathetic nervous system effects (tachycardia, palpitations)

    - Nursing Considerations

      - □ Monitor blood pressure, heart rate, and ECG.

    - Client Education

      - □ Advise the client to take the dose with meals to increase absorption.

      - □ Teach the client to check apical pulse prior to each dosage.

      - □ Advise the client to notify the health care provider of significant changes.

- o Saturated solution of potassium iodide (SSKI)

  - ■ Iodine-containing medications – Inhibit the release of stored thyroid hormone and retard hormone synthesis

  - ■ Nursing Considerations

    - □ These medications are for short-term use only.

    - □ Give 1 hr after an antithyroid medication.

    - □ Use of these medications is contraindicated in pregnancy.

  - ■ Client Education

    - □ Instruct the client to notify the health care provider of fever, sore throat, or mouth ulcers.

- Interdisciplinary Care

  - o Interdisciplinary care may involve an endocrinologist and a radiologist.

- Therapeutic Procedures

  - o Radioactive iodine therapy – Radioactive iodine is taken up by the thyroid and destroys some of the hormone-producing cells.

    - ■ Nursing Actions

      - □ Radioactive iodine therapy is contraindicated in women who are pregnant.

      - □ Monitor for symptoms of hypothyroidism, such as edema intolerance to cold, bradycardia, increase in weight, or depression.

    - ■ Client Education

      - □ Advise the client that the effects of therapy may not be evident for 6 to 8 weeks.

      - □ Advise the client to continue to take the medication as directed.

      - □ Advise the client to stay away from infants or small children for 2 to 4 days and to avoid becoming pregnant for 6 months following therapy.

- Surgical Interventions

  - o Total or subtotal thyroidectomy

    - ■ A thyroidectomy is the surgical removal of part or all of the thyroid gland.

      - □ A subtotal thyroidectomy may be performed for the treatment of hyperthyroidism when medication therapy fails or radiation therapy is contraindicated. It may also be used to correct diffuse goiter and thyroid cancer. After surgery, the remaining thyroid tissue usually supplies enough thyroid hormone for normal function.

      - □ A total thyroidectomy may be performed for certain types of thyroid cancers. Lifelong thyroid replacement therapy is required for clients who have total thyroidectomies.

- Nursing Actions
  - Preprocedure
    - Explain the purpose of the thyroidectomy to the client. Tell the client that there will be an incision in the neck, a dressing, and possibly a drain in place. Tell the client that some hoarseness and a sore throat from intubation and anesthesia may be experienced.
    - The client is usually prescribed propylthiouracil or methimazole 4 to 6 weeks before surgery.
    - The client should also receive iodine for 10 to 14 days before surgery. This helps reduce the gland's size and prevents excess bleeding.
    - Propranolol (Inderal) may also be given to block adrenergic effects.
    - Notify the provider immediately if the client fails to follow the medication regimen.
  - Postprocedure
    - Keep the client in a high-Fowler's position to promote venous return from the head and neck and to decrease oozing into the incision.
    - Check for laryngeal nerve damage by asking the client to speak as soon as she awakens from anesthesia.
    - Administer a mild analgesic as prescribed to relieve a sore neck or throat. Reassure the client that her discomfort will resolve within a few days.
    - If no drain is in place, prepare the client for discharge the day following surgery as indicated. However, if a drain is in place, the health care provider will usually remove it, along with half of the surgical clips, on the second day after surgery. The remaining clips are removed the following day before discharge.
- Client Education
  - Instruct the client to cough and breathe deeply while stabilizing her neck.
  - Show the client how to change positions, while supporting the back of the client's neck.
  - Remind the client to be careful of the incisional drain if applicable.
  - Advise the client that her voice will be hoarse and to expect some pain.
  - Advise the client to notify the nurse of any tingling sensation of the mouth, tingling of the distal extremities, or muscle twitching.
  - Remind the client that she will be asked to try to talk at intervals to check for nerve damage.
  - Instruct the client to notify the health care provider of incisional drainage, swelling, or redness that may indicate infection.
  - Advise the client and family to monitor for signs of hyperthyroidism, such as tachycardia, irritability, increased warmth, and insomnia.

     ☐ Advise the client and family to monitor for signs of hyperthyroidism, such as tachycardia, irritability, increased warmth, and insomnia.

     ☐ Advise the client and family to monitor for signs of hypothyroidism, such as hypothermia, lethargy, and weight gain.

     ☐ Instruct the client to take all medications as directed.

     ☐ Instruct clients who have had a total thyroidectomy that lifelong thyroid replacement medications will be required.

     ☐ Advise the client to check with the health care provider prior to taking over-the-counter medications.

     ☐ Instruct the client to keep all follow-up appointments.

       ▸ Advise the client to notify the health care provider of fever, increased restlessness, palpitations, or chest pain.

- Medications
  - Calcium gluconate and calcium chloride
    - Calcium supplement for emergency treatment of hypocalcemia due to damage of the parathyroid
    - Nursing Considerations
      - ☐ Keep emergency equipment near the bedside.
      - ☐ Monitor the client for signs of hypocalcemia, such as tingling, muscle twitching, and numbness of mouth or distal extremities.
    - Client Education
      - ☐ Advise the client to notify the nurse of any muscle twitching or tingling sensation of the mouth or distal extremities.
  - Prednisone (Deltasone)
    - Corticosteroid used to reduce postoperative edema
    - Nursing Considerations
      - ☐ Monitor for swelling.
      - ☐ Monitor the airway.
      - ☐ Provide humidity to reduce swelling.
      - ☐ Monitor blood pressure and serum glucose.
      - ☐ Reduce dosage gradually.
    - Client Education
      - ☐ Advise the client to take the medication with food.
      - ☐ Instruct the client not to discontinue dosage abruptly

- Furosemide (Lasix)
  - Loop diuretic used to reduce swelling caused by fluid retention
  - Nursing Considerations
    - Monitor for swelling.
    - Monitor the airway.
    - Provide humidity to reduce swelling.
    - Monitor blood pressure and serum electrolytes.
    - Monitor urine output.
  - Client Education
    - Instruct the client to take dose in the morning.
    - Advise the client to stand upright slowly to prevent postural hypotension.

Complications

- Hemorrhage
  - Bleeding at the incision site due to a loosened surgical tie, excessive coughing, or movement
  - Nursing Actions
    - The surgical dressing and incision need to be assessed for excessive drainage or bleeding during the postoperative period.
    - Inspect the surgical dressing for bleeding, especially at the back of the neck, and change the dressing as directed.
    - Expect about 50 mL of drainage in the first 24 hr.
    - If no drainage is found, check for drain kinking or the need to reestablish suction.
    - Expect only scant drainage after 24 hr.
    - Support the client's head and neck with pillows or sandbags. If the client needs to be transferred from a stretcher to the bed, support the client's head and neck in good body alignment.
  - Client Education
    - To avoid pressure on the suture line, encourage the client to avoid neck flexion or extension.
    - Instruct the client to cough and deep breath while supporting the client's neck.
    - Show the client how to change positions while supporting the back of the client's neck.

- Thyroid/Storm

  - Also known as thyrotoxic crisis, thyroid storm results from a sudden surge of large amounts of thyroid hormones into the bloodstream, causing an even greater increase in body metabolism. This is a medical emergency with a high mortality rate.

  - Precipitating factors include infection, trauma, and emotional stress, all of which increase demands on body metabolism. It can also occur following a subtotal thyroidectomy as a result of manipulation of the gland during surgery.

  - Findings are hyperthermia, hypertension, delirium, vomiting, abdominal pain, hyperglycemia, and tachydysrhythmias.

  - Nursing Actions

    - Maintain a patent airway.

    - Provide continuous cardiac monitoring for dysrhythmias.

    - Administer acetaminophen to decrease the client's temperature.

      □ Caution – Aspirin is contraindicated because it releases thyroxine from protein-binding sites and increases free thyroxine levels.

    - Provide cool sponge baths or apply ice packs to the client's axilla and groin areas to decrease fever. If fever continues, obtain a prescription for a cooling blanket for hyperthermia.

    - Administer propylthiouracil to prevent further synthesis and release of thyroid hormones.

    - Administer propranolol to block sympathetic nervous system effects.

    - Administer IV fluids to provide adequate hydration and prevent vascular collapse. Fluid volume deficit may occur because of increased fluid excretion by the kidneys or excessive diaphoresis. Carefully monitor intake and output hourly to prevent fluid overload or inadequate replacement.

    - Administer sodium iodide as prescribed, 1 hr after administering PTU.

      □ Caution – If given before PTU, sodium iodide can exacerbate symptoms in susceptible people.

    - Administer small doses of insulin as prescribed to control hyperglycemia. Hyperglycemia can occur because of the hypermetabolic state.

    - Administer supplemental O_2 to meet increased oxygen demands.

  - Client Education

    - Provide the client and family support and information about the client's condition and all procedures. Advise the client to notify the health care provider of fever, increased restlessness, palpitations, or chest pain.

- Airway Obstruction

  - Hemorrhage, tracheal collapse, tracheal mucus accumulation, laryngeal edema, and vocal cord paralysis can cause respiratory obstruction, with sudden stridor and restlessness.

- Nursing Actions
  - A tracheostomy tray should be kept near the client at all times during the immediate recovery period.
  - Maintain the bed in a high-Fowler's position to decrease edema and swelling of the neck.
  - If the client reports that the dressing feels tight, the health care provider should be alerted immediately.
  - Listen at the client's neck for respiratory stridor.
  - Provide humidified air.
  - Have suction equipment at the client's bedside.
  - Medicate as prescribed to reduce swelling.
- Client Education
  - Instruct the client to notify the nurse of tightness or difficulty breathing.

- Hypocalcemia and tetany
  - Damage to parathyroid gland causes hypocalcemia and tetany.
  - Nursing Actions
    - Monitor for signs of hypocalcemia (tingling of the fingers and toes, carpopedal spasms, convulsions).
    - Test for Chvostek's and Trousseau's signs, which are indicators of neuromuscular irritability from hypocalcemia.
    - Have IV calcium gluconate available for emergency administration.
    - Maintain seizure precautions.
  - Client Education
    - Advise the client to notify the nurse of any tingling sensation of the mouth, tingling of distal extremities, or muscle twitching.

- Nerve damage
  - Nerve damage can lead to vocal cord paralysis and vocal disturbances.
  - Incisional damage or swelling can cause nerve damage.
  - Nursing Actions
    - Teach the client that he will be hoarse, he will be able to speak only rarely, and he will need to rest his voice for several days.
    - After the procedure, monitor the client's ability to speak with each measurement of vital signs.
    - Assess the client's voice tone and quality and compare it to the preoperative voice.

- o Client Education
  - Remind the client that he will be asked to try to talk at intervals to check for nerve damage. Advise the client that a hoarse voice is not typically permanent.
- Client Outcomes
  - o The client will be able to get adequate sleep.
  - o The client will achieve and maintain appropriate weight and nutrition.
  - o The client will maintain a normal blood pressure and heart rate within the normal reference range.
  - o The client will be free of complications of hyperthyroidism.

CHAPTER 91: HYPERTHYROIDISM

 Application Exercises

Scenario: A nurse in an outpatient clinic is caring for a 46-year-old client who has symptoms of insomnia and anxiety, and feels as though his heart is racing. The client has lost 4.5 kg (10 lb) over the past 2 weeks without dieting.

1. The health care provider suspects Graves' disease. Which of the following laboratory test results should the nurse expect?

   A. Decreased thyrotropin receptor antibodies

   B. Decreased thyroid stimulating hormone

   C. Decreased free thyroxine index

   D. Decreased triiodothyronine

2. The client is diagnosed with hyperthyroidism. Which of the following findings should the nurse expect? (Select all that apply.)

   _____ Dry skin

   _____ Heat intolerance

   _____ Constipation

   _____ Exophthalmos

   _____ Palpitations

   _____ Weight loss

   _____ Low blood pressure

   _____ Bradycardia

3. Which of the following medications should the nurse expect to administer? (Select all that apply.)

   _____ Propylthiouracil (PTU)

   _____ Metoprolol (Lopressor)

   _____ Insulin

   _____ Amoxicillin (Amoxil)

   _____ Docusate sodium (Colace)

4. A nurse is assessing a client who is in hyperthyroid crisis. What assessment findings should the nurse expect and what interventions should be implemented?

5. A nurse in a surgical unit is preparing to receive a client from the postanesthesia care unit following a total thyroidectomy. The nurse prepares the client's room by supplying which of the following equipment to prevent or treat complications? (Select all that apply.)

_____ Laryngoscope

_____ Suction equipment

_____ Humidified air

_____ Flashlight

_____ Tracheostomy tray

_____ Oxygen set up

_____ Thoracotomy tray

6. Why is it important to support the client's head and neck with pillows or sandbags?

7. A nurse is caring for a client following a thyroidectomy. Which of the following client interventions should the nurse delegate to an assistive personnel (AP)?

A. Assess the client for signs of tetany.

B. Obtain the client's vital signs.

C. Replace the surgical dressing as needed.

D. Administer pain medication.

CHAPTER 91: HYPERTHYROIDISM

 Application Exercises Answer Key

Scenario: A nurse in an outpatient clinic is caring for a 46-year-old client who has symptoms of insomnia and anxiety, and feels as though his heart is racing. The client has lost 4.5 kg (10 lb) over the past 2 weeks without dieting.

1. The health care provider suspects Graves' disease. Which of the following laboratory test results should the nurse expect?

    A. Decreased thyrotropin receptor antibodies

    B. Decreased thyroid stimulating hormone

    C. Decreased free thyroxine index

    D. Decreased triiodothyronine

    A client with Graves' disease will have a decreased TSH due to elevated serum thyroid hormone. TSH-RAb, FTI, and T_3 will all be elevated.

 NCLEX® Connection: Reduction of Risk Potential, Laboratory Values

2. The client is diagnosed with hyperthyroidism. Which of the following findings should the nurse expect? (Select all that apply.)

    _____ Dry skin

    __X__ **Heat intolerance**

    _____ Constipation

    __X__ **Exophthalmos**

    __X__ **Palpitations**

    __X__ **Weight loss**

    _____ Low blood pressure

    _____ Bradycardia

    Heat intolerance, exophthalmos, palpitations, and weight loss are findings consistent with hyperthyroidism. Dry skin, constipation, low blood pressure, and bradycardia are expected findings of hypothyroidism.

 NCLEX® Connection: Reduction of Risk Potential, System Specific Assessment

3. Which of the following medications should the nurse expect to administer? (Select all that apply.)

    __X__   **Propylthiouracil (PTU)**

    __X__   **Metoprolol (Lopressor)**

    __X__   **Insulin**

    _____   Amoxicillin (Amoxil)

    _____   Docusate sodium (Colace)

Propylthiouracil blocks the synthesis of thyroid hormone. Metoprolol is a beta-adrenergic blocker that treats sympathetic nervous system effects, such as tachycardia and palpitations. Insulin is used to manage hyperglycemia. There is no indication that the client has an infection; therefore, the client does not need an antibiotic. A client who has hyperthyroidism most likely has diarrhea, so docusate sodium (a stool softener) is contraindicated.

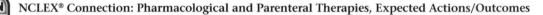 NCLEX® Connection: Pharmacological and Parenteral Therapies, Expected Actions/Outcomes

---

4. A nurse is assessing a client who is in hyperthyroid crisis. What assessment findings should the nurse expect and what interventions should be implemented?

Thyroid storm, also called thyroid crisis or thyrotoxicosis, usually occurs with Graves' disease. The condition develops rapidly and can be life-threatening. Thyroid storm is often precipitated by trauma or infection. The rapid increase in metabolic rate leads to hypertension, nausea, diaphoresis, fever, and tachycardia.

Priority nursing management includes maintaining a patent airway, offering a cooling blanket for hyperthermia, administering antipyretic as prescribed, administering supplementary oxygen therapy as prescribed, and administering pharmacological interventions as ordered (propylthiouracil, methimazole, sodium iodide solution, propranolol, glucocorticoids).

NCLEX® Connection: Physiological Adaptation, Pathophysiology

5. A nurse in a surgical unit is preparing to receive a client from the postanesthesia care unit following a total thyroidectomy. The nurse prepares the client's room by supplying which of the following equipment to prevent or treat complications? (Select all that apply.)

X	**Laryngoscope**
X	**Suction equipment**
X	**Humidified air**
_____	Flashlight
X	**Tracheostomy tray**
X	**Oxygen set up**
_____	Thoracotomy tray

The nurse should provide the client a laryngoscope, bedside suction to remove secretions or blood, air humidification to reduce swelling, tracheostomy tray, and oxygen in case of an obstructed airway. A flashlight and a thoracotomy tray are not necessary.

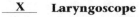 NCLEX® Connection: Reduction of Risk Potential: Potential for Complications of Diagnostic Tests/ Treatments/ Procedures

6. Why is it important to support the client's head and neck with pillows or sandbags?

Pillows or sandbags are used to immobilize the client's head and neck in order to prevent flexion and hyper-extension of the neck, which could strain the suture line and cause disruption of the sutures and hemorrhage.

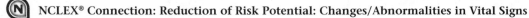 NCLEX® Connection: Reduction of Risk Potential: Potential for Complications of Diagnostic Tests/ Treatments/ Procedures

7. A nurse is caring for a client following a thyroidectomy. Which of the following client interventions could the nurse delegate to an assistive personnel (AP)?

A. Assess client for signs of tetany.

B. Obtain client's vital signs.

C. Replace surgical dressing as needed.

D. Administer pain medication.

Obtaining the client's vital signs is within the scope of practice of an assistive personnel. Assessment, dressing changes, and administration of medication is not within the scope of practice of an assistive personnel.

NCLEX® Connection: Reduction of Risk Potential: Changes/Abnormalities in Vital Signs

UNIT 12	NURSING CARE OF CLIENTS WITH ENDOCRINE DISORDERS
Section	Thyroid Disorders

Chapter 92   Hypothyroidism

Overview

- Hypothyroidism is a condition in which there is an inadequate amount of circulating thyroid hormones triiodothyronine (T_3) and thyroxine (T_4), causing a decrease in metabolic rate that affects all body systems.

- Classifications of hypothyroidism by etiology

  ○ Primary – Primary hypothyroidism stems from dysfunction of the thyroid gland. This is the most common type of hypothyroidism and is caused by disease (autoimmune thyroiditis – Hashimoto's disease) or loss of the thyroid gland (iodine deficiency, surgical removal of the gland).

  ○ Secondary – Secondary hypothyroidism is caused by failure of the anterior pituitary gland to stimulate the thyroid gland or failure of the target tissues to respond to the thyroid hormones (pituitary tumors).

  ○ Tertiary – Tertiary hypothyroidism is caused by failure of the hypothalamus to produce thyroid-releasing factor.

- Hypothyroidism is also classified by age of onset.

  ○ Cretinism – Cretinism is a state of severe hypothyroidism found in infants. When infants do not produce normal amounts of thyroid hormones, their central nervous system development and skeletal maturation are altered, resulting in retardation of mental growth, physical growth, or both.

  ○ Juvenile hypothyroidism – Juvenile hypothyroidism is most often caused by chronic autoimmune thyroiditis and affects the growth and sexual maturation of the child. Signs and symptoms are similar to adult hypothyroidism, and the treatment reverses most of the clinical manifestations of the disease.

  ○ Adult hypothyroidism

- Because older adult clients with hypothyroidism may have confusing signs and symptoms that mimic the aging process, hypothyroidism is often undiagnosed in older adult clients, which can lead to potentially serious side effects from medications (sedatives, opiates, anesthetics).

Assessment

- Risk Factors

  o The disorder is most prevalent in women, with the incidence rising significantly in people who are 40 to 50 years of age.

  o Many individuals with mild hypothyroidism are frequently undiagnosed, but the hormone disturbance may contribute to an acceleration of atherosclerosis or complications of medical treatment, (intraoperative hypotension, cardiac complications following surgery).

  o Use of medications (lithium [Eskalith], amiodarone)

  o Inadequate intake of iodine

- Subjective and Objective Data

  o Hypothyroidism is often characterized by vague and varied symptoms that develop slowly over time.

  o Early findings

    - Fatigue

    - Intolerance to cold

    - Decreased bowel motility

    - Weight gain

    - Pale skin

    - Thin, brittle fingernails

    - Depression

    - Thinning hair

    - Joint and/or muscle pain

  o Late findings

    - Slow thought process and speech

    - Thickening of the skin

    - Thinning of hair on the eyebrows

    - Dry, flaky skin

    - Swelling in face, hands, and feet (myxedema [non-pitting, mucinous edema])

    - Decreased acuity of taste and smell

    - Hoarse, raspy speech

    - Abnormal menstrual periods and decreased libido

○ Laboratory Tests

LABORATORY TEST	EXPECTED RESULTS WITH HYPOTHYROIDISM
T_3	• Decreased
Serum thyroid-stimulating hormone (TSH)	• Elevated with primary hypothyroidism • Decreased in secondary hypothyroidism
Free thyroxine index (FTI) and thyroxine (T_4) levels	• Decreased
Serum cholesterol	• Elevated
CBC	• Anemia

○ Diagnostic Procedures

■ Skull x-ray, computed tomography scan, and MRI

□ These procedures can help locate pituitary or hypothalamic lesions that may be the underlying cause of hypothyroidism.

■ Radioisotope (^{131} I) scan and uptake

□ Results will be less than 10% in a 24-hr period. In secondary hypothyroidism, intake increases with administration of exogenous TSH.

■ ECG

□ Sinus bradycardia and, flat or inverted T waves

Collaborative Care

• Nursing Care

○ Monitor for cardiovascular changes (low blood pressure, bradycardia, dysrhythmias).

○ If the client's mental status is compromised, orient periodically and provide safety measures.

○ Increase the client's activity level gradually, and provide frequent rest periods to avoid fatigue and decrease myocardial oxygen demands.

○ Apply antiembolism stockings and elevate the client's legs to assist venous return.

○ Encourage the client to cough and breathe deeply to prevent pulmonary complications.

○ Provide a low-calorie, high-bulk diet, and encourage activity to help prevent constipation and promote weight loss. Administer cathartics and stool softeners as needed. Avoid fiber laxatives, which interfere with absorption of levothyroxine.

○ Provide meticulous skin care. Turn and reposition the client every 2 hr if the client is on extended bed rest. Use alcohol-free skin care products and an emollient lotion after bathing.

(S)   o   Provide extra clothing and blankets for clients with decreased cold tolerance. Dress the client in layers, adjust room temperature, and encourage warm liquids if possible. Caution the client against using electric blankets or other electric heating devices because the combination of vasodilatation, decreased sensation, and decreased alertness may result in unrecognized burns.

   o   Encourage the client to verbalize feelings and fears about changes in body image. Return to the euthyroid (normal thyroid gland function) state takes some time. The client may need frequent reassurance that most of the physical manifestations are reversible.

(S)   o   Use caution due to alteration in metabolism.

- CNS depressants (barbiturates or sedatives) are contraindicated or given at a significantly decreased dose.

- External warming measures are contraindicated because they can produce vasodilatation and vascular collapse.

- Medications

   o   Thyroid hormone replacement therapy – levothyroxine (Synthroid)

- Thyroid hormone replacement therapy is a treatment of choice.

- It increases the effects of warfarin (Coumadin) and can increase the need for insulin and digoxin (Lanoxin).

(G)   ■   Use caution when starting thyroid hormone replacement with older adult clients and those who have coronary artery disease to avoid coronary ischemia because of increased oxygen demands of the heart. It is preferable to start with much lower doses and increase gradually, taking 1 to 2 months to reach full replacement doses.

- Nursing Considerations

  □ Administer thyroid hormone replacement therapy, as prescribed.

  □ Monitor for cardiovascular compromise (e.g., chest pain, palpitations, rapid heart rate, shortness of breath) during early thyroid therapy.

- Client Education

  □ Instruct the client that treatment begins slowly and the dosage is increased every 2 to 3 weeks until the desired response is obtained. Serum TSH will need to be drawn at scheduled times to ensure appropriate dosage.

  □ Instruct the client to monitor for and report signs and symptoms of hyperthyroidism, (irritability, tremors, tachycardia, palpitations, heat intolerance).

  □ Inform the client that the treatment is considered to be lifelong, requiring ongoing medical assessment of thyroid function.

- Interdisciplinary Care

   o   A home health nurse may need to visit the client and assess for side effects during the first few weeks of therapy.

- Client Outcomes
  - The client's TSH will return to the expected reference range.

Complications

- Myxedema coma
  - Myxedema coma is a life-threatening condition that occurs when hypothyroidism is untreated or when a stressor, such as infection, affects an individual who has hypothyroidism. Clients who have been taking levothyroxine sodium and suddenly stop the medication are also at risk.
  - Clients with myxedema coma experience:
    - Significantly depressed respirations (hypoxia, hypercapnia)
    - Decreased cardiac output
    - Worsening cerebral hypoxia
    - Stupor
    - Hypothermia
    - Bradycardia
    - Hypotension
    - Hypoglycemia
    - Hyponatremia
  - Nursing Actions
    - Maintain airway patency with ventilatory support if necessary.
    - Maintain circulation through IV fluid replacement.
    - Provide continuous ECG monitoring.
    - Monitor ABGs to detect hypoxia and metabolic acidosis.
    - Warm the client with blankets.
    - Monitor the client's body temperature until stable.
    - Replace thyroid hormone by administering large doses of levothyroxine (Synthroid) IV as prescribed. Monitor vital signs because rapid correction of hypothyroidism can cause adverse cardiac effects.
    - Monitor intake and output and daily weights. With treatment, urine output should increase and body weight should decrease; failure to do so should be reported to the health provider.
    - Replace fluids and other substances, such as glucose, as needed.
    - Administer corticosteroids as prescribed.
    - Check for possible sources of infection (blood, sputum, urine), which may have precipitated the coma. Treat any underlying illness.

CHAPTER 92: HYPOTHYROIDISM

 Application Exercises

Scenario: A nurse in an outpatient clinic is seeing a 46-year-old client for symptoms of fatigue, cold intolerance, dry skin, hoarseness, weight gain, and fluid retention. Based on her symptoms, thyroid studies are performed and reveal an elevated thyroid stimulating hormone (TSH) and decreased T_3 and T_4 levels. The client is prescribed levothyroxine sodium (Synthroid) 0.1 mg by mouth daily and instructed to return to the clinic in 1 month to have a TSH drawn.

1. What is the significance of the client's laboratory findings?

2. The nurse recognizes that the client's TSH is a reliable indicator of the efficacy of the levothyroxine sodium because

    A. the TSH will have a value of zero when an euthyroid state is re-established.

    B. the TSH will return to its normal reference range when an euthyroid state is re-established.

    C. the TSH will increase above its reference range when a therapeutic medication level is reached.

    D. the TSH will decrease below its reference range when a therapeutic medication level is reached.

3. Which of the following should the nurse teach the client about her condition and the prescribed medication? (Select all that apply.)

    _____ Expected medication side effects, such as nervousness, heat intolerance, and diarrhea.

    _____ Medication should not be discontinued without the advice of the provider.

    _____ Follow-up serum TSH levels should be obtained.

    _____ Alopecia should be reported.

    _____ Fiber laxatives should be used for constipation.

CHAPTER 92: HYPOTHYROIDISM

 Application Exercises Answer Key

Scenario: A nurse in an outpatient clinic is seeing a 46-year-old client for symptoms of fatigue, cold intolerance, dry skin, hoarseness, weight gain, and fluid retention. Based on her symptoms, thyroid studies are performed and reveal an elevated thyroid stimulating hormone (TSH) and decreased T_3 and T_4 levels. The client is prescribed levothyroxine sodium (Synthroid) 0.1 mg by mouth daily and instructed to return to the clinic in 1 month to have a TSH drawn.

---

1. What is the significance of the client's laboratory findings?

When the serum T_3 and T_4 levels fall below normal, the pituitary gland is stimulated to release TSH in an attempt to raise the T_3 and T_4 levels back to normal. If the thyroid cannot produce T_3 and T_4 because of disease, the TSH will continue to elevate, but production of T_3 and T_4 will not be able to increase. These laboratory findings indicate primary hypothyroidism.

 NCLEX® Connection: Reduction of Risk Potential, Laboratory Values

2. The nurse recognizes that the client's TSH is a reliable indicator of the efficacy of the levothyroxine sodium because

A. the TSH will have a value of zero when an euthyroid state is re-established.

B. the TSH will return to its normal reference range when an euthyroid state is re-established.

C. the TSH will increase above its reference range when a therapeutic medication level is reached.

D. the TSH will decrease below its reference range when a therapeutic medication level is reached.

The TSH will return to its normal reference range when the level of T_4 is re-established and an euthyroid state exists.

 NCLEX® Connection: Reduction of Risk Potential, Laboratory Values

3. Which of the following should the nurse teach the client about her condition and the prescribed medication? (Select all that apply.)

_____ Expected medication side effects, such as nervousness, heat intolerance, and diarrhea.

___X___ **Medication should not be discontinued without the advice of the provider.**

___X___ **Follow-up serum TSH levels should be obtained.**

_____ Alopecia should be reported.

_____ Fiber laxatives should be used for constipation.

The client should be taught how to take and monitor for expected effects of levothyroxine. However nervousness, heat intolerance, and diarrhea, are adverse effects and may indicate that a decrease in dosage is indicated. The dose of levothyroxine will also be monitored by the TSH level to avoid dosages that are too high or low. Alopecia is a physical change consistent with hypothyroidism and does not need to be reported. Fiber laxatives should not be recommended as they can interfere with the absorption of levothyroxine.

Ⓝ **NCLEX® Connection: Pharmacological and Parenteral Therapies, Adverse Effects/ Contraindications/Side Effects/Interactions**

Overview

- Cushing's disease and Cushing's syndrome are caused by an over secretion of the adrenal cortex.

- The adrenal cortex produces:

  - Mineralocorticoids – Aldosterone (increases sodium absorption, causes potassium excretion in the kidney)

  - Glucocorticoids – Cortisol (affects glucose, protein, and fat metabolism; the body's response to stress, and the body's immune function)

  - Sex hormones – Androgens and estrogens

- With Cushing's disease, there is an excess of glucocorticoids, resulting in increased cortisol and increased androgens.

Health Promotion and Disease Prevention

- Advise the client to take prescribed medications as instructed and monitor for adverse reactions. Advise the client that medication therapy may be lifelong.

- Advise the client to eat foods high in calcium and vitamin D. The client should not use alcohol or caffeine. Advise the client to monitor for signs of gastric bleeding, such as coffee-ground emesis or black, tarry stools.

- Advise the client to avoid infection by using good hygiene and avoiding crowds or individuals who are infected.

- Advise the client that residual muscle weakness may be present and home assistance may be needed.

- Instruct the client to monitor weight every day and report weight gain.

Assessment

- Risk Factors

    o Endogenous causes of increased cortisol (Cushing's disease)

    - Adrenal hyperplasia

    - Adrenocortical carcinoma

    - Carcinomas of the lung, gastrointestinal (GI) tract, or pancreas (These tumors can secrete ACTH.)

    - Pituitary carcinoma that secretes adrenocorticotropic hormone (ACTH)

    o Exogenous causes of increased cortisol (Cushing's syndrome) include the therapeutic use of glucocorticoids for:

    - Organ transplant

    - Chemotherapy

    - Autoimmune diseases

    - Asthma

    - Allergies

    - Chronic inflammatory diseases

- Subjective Data

    o Weakness

    o Fatigue

    o Back and joint pain

    o Altered emotional state (may include irritability or depression)

- Objective Data

    o Physical Assessment Findings

    - Evidence of decreased immune function and decreased inflammatory response (increased incidence of infections without the accompanying fever, swelling, drainage, and redness)

    - Thin, fragile skin

    - Bruising and petechiae (fragile blood vessels)

    - Hypertension (sodium and water retention)

    - Tachycardia

    - Weight gain

    - Dependent edema – Changes in fat distribution, including the characteristic fat distribution of moon face, truncal obesity, and fat collection on the back of the neck (buffalo hump)

- Fractures (osteoporosis)

- Muscle wasting (particularly in the extremities)

- Impaired glucose tolerance

- Hirsutism

- Acne

- Red cheeks

- Striae (reddened lines on abdomen and thighs)

- Emotional lability

o Laboratory Tests

- Elevated plasma cortisol levels in the absence of acute illness or stress are diagnostic for Cushing's disease/syndrome. Urine cortisol levels (24-hr urine collection) Contain elevated levels of free cortisol.

- Plasma adrenocorticotropic hormone (ACTH) levels:

  □ Hypersecretion of ACTH by the anterior pituitary results in elevated ACTH levels.

  □ Disorder of the adrenal cortex or medication therapy results in decreased ACTH levels.

- Serum potassium and calcium levels – Decreased

- Serum glucose level – Increased

- Serum sodium level – Increased

- Lymphocytes – Decreased

- Dexamethasone suppression tests – Tests vary in length and amount of dexamethasone administered. Twenty-four hr urine collections reveal suppression of cortisol excretion in clients without Cushing's disease. Nonsuppression of cortisol excretion is indicative of Cushing's disease. Medications are withheld and stress is reduced prior to and during testing. False positive results may occur in clients with acute illness and alcoholism.

o Diagnostic Procedures

- X-ray, magnetic resonance imaging, and CT scans may be performed to identify lesions of the pituitary gland, adrenal gland, lung, gastrointestinal tract, or pancreas.

- Radiological imaging may be performed to determine the source of adrenal insufficiency, (tumor, adrenal atrophy).

- Nursing Actions
  - Establish an IV line if needed.
  - Determine allergies.
  - Explain the procedure to the client.
  - Provide padding, pillows, and/or blankets to provide comfort.
- Client Education
  - Explain to the client that the tests are noninvasive and not painful.

Collaborative Care

- Nursing Care

  - Dietary alterations – Decrease sodium intake and increase intake of potassium, protein, and calcium.

  - Monitor intake and output.

  - Obtain daily weight.

  - Assess for signs of hypervolemia, (edema, distended neck veins, shortness of breath presence of adventitious breath sounds).

  - Maintain a safe environment to minimize the risk of pathological fractures and skin trauma.

  - Prevent infection by performing frequent hand hygiene.

  - Encourage physical activity within the client's limitations.

  - Provide meticulous skin care.

  - Monitor for and protect against skin breakdown and infection.

- Medications

  - Treatment is dependent upon the cause. For Cushing's syndrome, tapering off glucocorticoids or managing the symptoms may be necessary.

  - Aminoglutethimide (Cytadren)
    - Adrenal corticosteroid inhibitor
    - Aminoglutethimide decreases adrenal hormone synthesis to provide short-term symptom relief for clients with Cushing's syndrome.
    - Nursing Considerations
      - Use temporarily until surgery or other treatment is finished, usually no more than 3 months.
      - Monitor blood pressure for hypotension.
      - Monitor fluids and electrolytes for clients with gastric effects.

- ■ Client Education
    - □ Advise the client not to drive or operate machinery until medication effects are known.
    - □ Advise the client that the medication may cause nausea, drowsiness, dizziness, or rash.
    - □ Advise the client relief is temporary. Symptoms will return if medication is discontinued.
    - □ Inform the client that the medication may be taken with food to relieve gastric effects.
  - ○ Ketoconazole (Nizoral)
    - ■ Adrenal corticosteroid inhibitor
    - ■ Ketoconazole is an antifungal agent that when taken in high dosages inhibits adrenal corticosteroid synthesis.
    - ■ Nursing Considerations
      - □ Can be used in addition to radiation or surgery.
      - □ Monitor liver enzymes and monitor for signs of liver toxicity, (yellow sclera, dark-colored urine).
      - □ Monitor fluids and electrolytes for clients who have gastric effects.
    - ■ Client Education
      - □ Advise the client that the medication can cause nausea, vomiting, or dizziness.
      - □ Advise the client relief is temporary. Symptoms will return if the medication is discontinued.
      - □ Inform the client that the medication may be taken with food to relieve gastric effects.
- ● Interdisciplinary Care
  - ○ A nutritionist may be consulted to advise the client about restricting fluids and consuming a low-sodium, high-protein diet.
- ● Therapeutic Procedures
  - ○ Chemotherapy with cytotoxic agents for Cushing's disease caused by a tumor.
    - ■ Nursing Actions
      - □ Monitor for adverse effects, for example, thrombocytopenia or nausea and vomiting, depending on the chemotherapeutic agent.
      - □ Monitor WBC, absolute neutrophil count, platelet count, hemoglobin, and hematocrit.
      - □ Assess the client for bruising and bleeding gums.
      - □ Administer an antiemetic as prescribed.

- ■ Client Education

    - □ Instruct the client to avoid crowds and contact with individuals who are infected.

    - □ Advise the client to monitor for bleeding, such as tarry stools or coffee-ground emesis.

    - □ Advise the client that alopecia may occur.

- ○ Radiation therapy

    - ■ Nursing Actions

        - □ Provide skin care and assess for skin damage.

        - □ Intervene for skin and alopecia effects.

    - ■ Client Education

        - □ Advise the client to:

            - ‣ Avoid removing radiation markings.

            - ‣ Avoid applying lotions, other than those prescribed by the radiologist to affected areas.

            - ‣ Avoid exposing irradiated areas to sun.

            - ‣ Expect fatigue and altered taste due to radiation.

- ● Surgical Interventions

    - ○ Hypophysectomy

        - ■ Surgical removal of the pituitary gland (depending on the cause of Cushing's disease)

        - ■ Nursing Actions

            - □ Monitor and correct electrolytes, especially sodium, potassium, and chloride. Monitor and adjust serum glucose levels. Monitor ECG.

            - □ Protect the client from developing an infection using good hand hygiene and avoiding contact with individuals who have infections. Use caution to prevent a fracture by providing assistance getting out of bed and raising side rails.

            - □ Monitor for bleeding. Monitor nasal drainage for a possible cerebral spinal fluid (CSF) leak. Assess drainage for the presence of glucose or a halo sign (yellow on the edge and clear in the middle), which may indicate CSF.

            - □ Assess neurologic condition every hour for the first 24 hr and then every 4 hr.

            - □ Administer glucocorticoids as prescribed to prevent an abrupt drop in cortisol level.

            - □ Administer stool softeners as prescribed to prevent straining.

- ■ Client Education
  - □ Advise the client to use caution preoperatively to prevent infection or fractures.
  - □ Advise the client a transsphenoidal hypophysectomy is accessed through the sphenoid sinus via the nasal cavity or under the upper lip. The client may have nasal packing postoperatively. A drip pad will be placed under the nose for bloody drainage. The client will need to breathe through his mouth. Advise the client to avoid coughing, blowing his nose, or sneezing.
  - □ Instruct the client to avoid bending over and straining to prevent increased intracranial pressure.
  - □ Instruct the client to avoid brushing teeth for 2 weeks. Advise the client to floss and rinse his mouth.
  - □ Advise the client to notify the health care provider of sweet-tasting drainage, drainage that makes a halo (yellow on the edge and clear in the middle), or clear drainage from the nose, which may indicate CSF leak. Another indication may include a headache.
  - □ Advise the client to notify the provider of excessive bleeding, confusion, or headache.
- ○ Adrenalectomy
  - ■ Surgical removal of the adrenal gland, (may be unilateral [one gland] or bilateral [both glands]).
  - ■ Nursing Actions
    - □ Provide glucocorticoid and hormone replacement as needed.
    - □ Monitor for adrenal crisis due to an abrupt drop in cortisol level. Findings may include hypotension, tachycardia, tachypnea, nausea, and headache.
    - □ Monitor vital signs and hemodynamic levels frequently initially (every 15 min).
    - □ Monitor fluids and electrolytes.
    - □ Monitor the incision site for bleeding.
    - □ Monitor bowel sounds.
    - □ Provide pain medication as needed. Administer stool softeners as needed.
    - □ Slowly introduce foods.
    - □ Assess the abdomen for distention and tenderness. Monitor the incision site for redness, discharge, and swelling.
  - ■ Client Education
    - □ Teach the client about postoperative pain management, deep breathing, and anti-embolism care.
    - □ Advise the client of the need to take glucocorticoids, mineralocorticoids, and hormone replacements.

- Client Outcomes

  o The client will maintain adequate nutritional intake.

  o The client will maintain a constant weight with balanced fluid intake and output.

  o The client will be free of pain.

  o The client will be free of infection or fracture.

Complications

- Perforated viscera/ulceration

  o Decreases production of protective mucus in the lining of the stomach due to an increase in cortisol

  o Nursing Actions

    ▪ Monitor for evidence of GI bleeding (tarry, black stool, coffee-ground emesis).

    ▪ Administer anti-ulcer medications as prescribed.

  o Client Education

    ▪ Advise the client to monitor for GI bleeding and to avoid alcohol, caffeine, and smoking.

- Risk for bone fractures due to hypocalcemia

  o Nursing Actions

    ▪ Use caution when moving the client.

    ▪ Provide assistance when ambulating.

    ▪ Clear floors to prevent falls.

  o Client Education

    ▪ Encourage a diet high in calcium and vitamin D.

    ▪ Advise the client to avoid dangerous activities.

- Risk for infection due to immunosuppression

  o Immunosuppression and reduced inflammatory response occur due to elevated glucocorticoid levels.

  o Nursing Actions

    ▪ Monitor for subtle signs of infection, (fatigue, fever, localized swelling or redness).

  o Client Education

    ▪ Instruct the client about measures to minimize exposure to infectious organisms (avoid ill people and crowds, use good hand hygiene).

    ▪ Report signs of infection to the provider.

- Risk for adrenal crisis (also known as acute adrenal insufficiency)

  o Sudden drop in corticosteroids due to sudden withdrawal of medication or tumor removal

  o May develop with abrupt withdrawal of steroid medication

  o Nursing Actions

    ▪ Signs include hypotension, hyperkalemia, abdominal pain, weakness, and weight loss.

    ▪ Administration of glucocorticoids treats acute adrenal insufficiency.

  o Client Education

    ▪ Instruct the client to gradually taper the medication.

    ▪ During times of stress, additional glucocorticoids may be needed to prevent adrenal crisis.

CHAPTER 93: CUSHING'S DISEASE/SYNDROME

(A) Application Exercises

1. A nurse is caring for a client who has Cushing's disease. The nurse should know that this client is at risk for developing which of the following? (Select all that apply.)

_____ Infection

_____ Gastric ulcer

_____ Renal failure

_____ Bone fractures

_____ Dysphagia

2. A nurse is caring for a client who has Cushing's disease. Serum laboratory findings for this client may include which of the following? (Select all that apply.)

_____ Sodium 150 mEq/L

_____ Potassium 3.3 mEq/L

_____ Calcium 8.0 mg/dL

_____ BUN 30 mg/dL

_____ Creatinine 1.6 mg/dL

_____ Glucose 145 mg/dL

3. A nurse is caring for a client who has Cushing's disease and has excessive cortisol levels. Which of the following is the priority assessment?

A. Daily weights

B. Bowel sounds

C. Pupils

D. Pedal pulses

4. A nurse is caring for a client following a transsphenoidal hypophysectomy. The nurse tests the client's nasal drainage for a cerebral spinal fluid (CSF) leak. Which of the following positive laboratory results is an indication of a CSF leak?

A. RBCs

B. Ketones

C. Glucose

D. WBCs

CHAPTER 93: CUSHING'S DISEASE/SYNDROME

 Application Exercises Answer Key

1. A nurse is caring for a client who has Cushing's disease. The nurse should know that this client is at risk for developing which of the following? (Select all that apply.)

__X__	**Infection**
__X__	**Gastric ulcer**
_____	Renal failure
__X__	**Bone fractures**
_____	Dysphagia

A client who has Cushing's disease has excessive cortisol levels, which may increase the risk of infection, gastric ulcers, and pathological bone fractures. Immunosuppression and a reduced inflammatory response due to elevated glucocorticoid levels increase the risk for infection. High cortisol levels may decrease production of the protective mucus in the lining of the stomach, which may lead to gastric ulcers. Hypocalcemia due to excess cortisol may cause bone density loss and fractures. A client who has Cushing's disease is not at risk for renal failure or dysphagia.

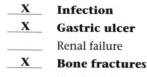 **NCLEX® Connection: Physiological Adaptation, Pathophysiology**

2. A nurse is caring for a client who has Cushing's disease. Serum laboratory findings for this client may include which of the following? (Select all that apply.)

__X__	**Sodium 150 mEq/L**
__X__	**Potassium 3.3 mEq/L**
__X__	**Calcium 8.0 mg/dL**
_____	BUN 30 mg/dL
_____	Creatinine 1.6 mg/dL
__X__	**Glucose 145 mg/dL**

Excessive glucocorticoids can cause sodium and water retention, which may lead to fluid overload, hypertension, and heart failure. Reduced glucose metabolism may cause hyperglycemia. Hypocalcemia and hypokalemia are also consistent in a client who has Cushing's disease. BUN and creatinine levels should not be elevated.

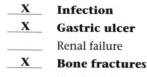 **NCLEX® Connection: Reduction of Risk Potential, Laboratory Values**

3. A nurse is caring for a client who has Cushing's disease and has excessive cortisol levels. Which of the following is the priority assessment?

    A. Daily weights

    B. Bowel sounds

    C. Pupils

    D. Pedal pulses

    The greatest risk to a client who has Cushing's disease is fluid retention, which can lead to hypertension and heart failure. The nurse should weigh the client daily, check extremities for peripheral edema, assess neck veins for distention, and monitor cardiac rhythm and breath sounds. The other assessments are important but are not the priority at this time.

    Ⓝ NCLEX® Connection: Reduction of Risk Potential, System Specific Assessment

4. A nurse is caring for a client following a transsphenoidal hypophysectomy. The nurse tests the client's nasal drainage for a cerebral spinal fluid (CSF) leak. Which of the following positive laboratory results is an indication of a CSF leak?

    A. RBCs

    B. Ketones

    C. Glucose

    D. WBCs

    Glucose found in the client's nasal drainage indicates a CSF leak. A halo sign (yellow around the edge and clear in the middle) is another indication CSF may be in the nasal drainage. Neurologic status and nasal drainage should be assessed to monitor for possible CSF leak. Presence of RBCs, ketones, or WBCs in nasal drainage is not an indicator of a CSF leak.

    Ⓝ NCLEX® Connection: Reduction of Risk Potential, Diagnostic Tests

UNIT 12	NURSING CARE OF CLIENTS WITH ENDOCRINE DISORDERS
Section	Adrenal Disorders
Chapter 94	Addison's Disease and Adrenal Crisis

Ⓞ Overview

- Addison's disease is an adrenocortical insufficiency. It is caused by damage or dysfunction of the adrenal cortex. The adrenal cortex produces:

  o Mineralocorticoids – Aldosterone (increases sodium absorption, causes potassium excretion in the kidney)

  o Glucocorticoids – Cortisol (affects glucose, protein, and fat metabolism; the body's response to stress; and the body's immune function)

  o Sex hormones – Androgens and estrogens

- With Addison's disease, the production of mineralocorticoids and glucocorticoids is diminished, resulting in decreased aldosterone and cortisol.

- Adrenal crisis, also known as acute adrenal insufficiency, has a rapid onset. It is a medical emergency. If it is not quickly diagnosed and properly treated, the prognosis is poor.

Ⓖ
- Older adult clients are less able to tolerate the complications of Addison's disease and adrenal crisis and will need more frequent monitoring.

Assessment

- Risk Factors

  o Causes of primary Addison's disease:

  - Idiopathic autoimmune dysfunction (majority of cases)

  - Tuberculosis

  - Histoplasmosis

  - Adrenalectomy

  - Cancer

  o Causes of secondary Addison's disease:

  - Steroid withdrawal

  - Hypophysectomy

  - Pituitary neoplasm

- An adrenal crisis is caused by an acute adrenocortical insufficiency that may be due to:
  - Sepsis
  - Trauma
  - Stress (myocardial infarction, surgery, anesthesia, hypothermia, volume loss, hypoglycemia)
  - Adrenal hemorrhage
  - Steroid withdrawal
- Subjective and Objective Data
  - Physical Assessment Findings
    - Signs and symptoms of chronic Addison's disease develop slowly.
    - Signs and symptoms of adrenal crisis develop rapidly.
    - Signs and symptoms:
      - Hyperpigmentation
      - Weakness and fatigue
      - Nausea and vomiting
      - Dizziness with orthostatic hypotension
      - Severe hypotension (adrenal crisis)
      - Dehydration
      - Hyponatremia
      - Hyperkalemia
      - Hypoglycemia
      - Hypercalcemia
  - Laboratory Tests
    - Serum electrolytes – Increased K+, decreased Na+, and increased calcium
    - BUN and creatinine – Increased
    - Serum glucose – Decreased
    - Serum cortisol – Decreased
    - Adrenocorticotropic hormone (ACTH) stimulation test – ACTH is infused, and the cortisol response is measured. With primary adrenal insufficiency, plasma cortisol levels do not rise.

- o Diagnostic Procedures
  - ECG
    - □ Used to assess for ECG changes or dysrhythmias associated with electrolyte imbalance.
    - □ Nursing Actions
      - ‣ Apply electrodes using conductive gel.
    - □ Client Education
      - ‣ Explain all procedures to the client.
  - X-ray, CT scan, and magnetic resonance imaging scan
    - □ Radiological imaging to determine source of adrenal insufficiency, such as a tumor or adrenal atrophy
    - □ Nursing Actions
      - ‣ Establish an IV line if needed.
      - ‣ Determine allergies.
      - ‣ Explain the procedure to the client.
      - ‣ Provide padding, pillows, and/or blankets to provide comfort.
    - □ Client Education
      - ‣ Explain to the client that tests are noninvasive and not painful.

Collaborative Care

- Nursing Care
  - o Monitor the client for fluid deficits and hyponatremia. Administer saline infusions to restore fluid volume. Observe for signs and symptoms of dehydration. Obtain orthostatic vital signs.
  - o Administer prescribed hydrocortisone boluses and a continuous infusion or periodic boluses.
  - o Monitor for and treat hyperkalemia:
    - Obtain a serum potassium and ECG.
    - Administer sodium polystyrene sulfonate (Kayexalate), insulin, calcium, glucose, and sodium bicarbonate as prescribed.
  - o Monitor for and treat hypoglycemia:
    - Perform frequent checks of the client's neurologic status, monitor for signs and symptoms of hypoglycemia, and check serum glucose.
    - Administer food and/or supplemental glucose.

- ○ Maintain a safe environment:
  - Provide assistance ambulating.
  - Raise side rails.
  - Prevent falls by keeping floors clear.
- Medications
  - ○ Hydrocortisone (Cortef), Prednisone (Deltasone), and Cortisone (Cortisone Acetate)
    - Glucocorticoid is used as an adrenocorticoid replacement for adrenal insufficiency and as an anti-inflammatory.
    - Nursing Considerations
      - □ Monitor weight, blood pressure, and electrolytes.
      - □ Increase dosage during periods of stress or illness if necessary.
      - □ Taper dose if discontinuing to avoid adrenal crisis.
      - □ Give with food to reduce gastric effects.
    - Client Education
      - □ Advise the client to:
        - ▸ Take medication as directed.
        - ▸ Avoid discontinuing the medication abruptly.
        - ▸ Report symptoms of Cushing's syndrome (round face, edema, weight gain).
        - ▸ Advise the client to take the medication with food.
        - ▸ Report symptoms of adrenal insufficiency (fever, fatigue, muscle weakness, anorexia).
  - ○ Fludrocortisone (Florinef)
    - Fludrocortisone is a mineralocorticoid used as a replacement in adrenal insufficiency.
    - Nursing Considerations
      - □ Monitor weight, blood pressure, and electrolytes.
      - □ Hypertension may be a side effect.
      - □ Dosage may need to be increased during periods of stress or illness.
    - Client Education
      - □ Advise the client to take the medication as directed.
      - □ Warn the client to expect mild peripheral edema.
- Interdisciplinary Care
  - ○ Home assistance for fluid, medication, and dietary management may be required.

- Care After Discharge

  ○ Client Education

    ■ Advise the client to

      □ Take prescribed medications as instructed and monitor for adverse reactions.

      □ Avoid using alcohol and caffeine.

      □ Monitor for signs of gastric bleeding (coffee-ground; emesis tarry, black stool).

      □ Monitor for hypoglycemia (diaphoresis, shaking, tachycardia, headache).

      □ Report symptoms of adrenal insufficiency, (fever, fatigue, muscle weakness, dizziness, anorexia).

      □ To prevent adrenal crises, instruct clients who have Addison's disease to increase corticosteroid doses as directed by a provider, during times of stress.

    ■ Inform the client that medication therapy may be lifelong.

- Client Outcomes

  ○ The client will maintain balanced electrolytes and glucose levels.

  ○ The client will maintain a normal blood pressure with balanced fluid intake and output.

Complications

- Addisonian Crisis

  ○ Addisonian crisis occurs when there is an acute drop in adrenocorticoids due to sudden discontinuation of glucocorticoid medications or when induced by severe trauma, infection, or stress.

  ○ Nursing Actions

    ■ Establish an IV line and replace saline and volume with a 0.9% sodium chloride infusion.

    ■ Monitor ECG and electrolytes.

    ■ Monitor vital signs.

    ■ Administer adrenocorticoids as prescribed.

  ○ Client Education

    ■ Advise the client to notify the provider of any infection, trauma, or stress that may increase the need for adrenocorticoids.

    ■ Advise the client to take the medication as directed.

    ■ Advise the client not to discontinue the medication abruptly.

- Hypoglycemia

  - Insufficient glucocorticoid causes increased insulin sensitivity and decreased glycogen, which leads to hypoglycemia.

  - Nursing Actions

    - Monitor glucose levels.

  - Client Education

    - Advise the client and family to monitor for hypoglycemia.

      - Symptoms may include diaphoresis, shaking, tachycardia, and headache.

    - Instruct the client to have a 15-gram carbohydrate snack readily available.

- Hyperkalemia/Hyponatremia

  - Decrease in aldosterone levels can cause an increased excretion of sodium and a decreased excretion of potassium.

  - Nursing Actions

    - Monitor electrolytes and ECG.

  - Client Education

    - Advise the client to take the medications as directed.

    - Instruct the client to report signs of hyperkalemia (nausea, cardiac palpitations/missed beat).

CHAPTER 94: ADDISON'S DISEASE AND ADRENAL CRISIS

 Application Exercises

1. A nurse is caring for a client who has Addison's disease and is taking hydrocortisone (Cortef). Which of the following medication instructions is appropriate for the nurse to include? (Select all that apply.)

_____ Take the medication on an empty stomach.

_____ Notify the provider of any illness or stress.

_____ Report any symptoms of weakness or dizziness.

_____ Do not discontinue the medication suddenly.

_____ Eat a low-sodium diet.

2. A nurse is reviewing serum laboratory results for a client who has Addison's disease. Which of the following findings should the nurse expect? (Select all that apply.)

_____ Sodium 130 mEq/L

_____ Potassium 5.1 mEq/L

_____ Calcium 10.6 mg/dL

_____ Magnesium 2.5 mg/dL

_____ Glucose 65mg/dL

_____ Phosphorus 2.4 mg/dL

3. A nurse is caring for a client who has an acute adrenal insufficiency (adrenal crisis). The nurse should understand that this is an emergency event that may be precipitated by a sudden decrease in circulating

A. cortisol.

B. thyrotropin.

C. prolactin.

D. vasopressin.

CHAPTER 94: ADDISON'S DISEASE AND ADRENAL CRISIS

 Application Exercises Answer Key

1. A nurse is caring for a client who has Addison's disease and is taking hydrocortisone (Cortef). Which of the following medication instructions is appropriate for the nurse to include? (Select all that apply.)

	Take the medication on an empty stomach.
X	**Notify the provider of any illness or stress.**
X	**Report any symptoms of weakness or dizziness.**
X	**Do not discontinue the medication suddenly.**
	Eat a low-sodium diet.

The client should be advised to take the medication as directed and not to discontinue it abruptly. The client should take the medication with food to prevent gastrointestinal irritation and symptoms of adrenal insufficiency (fever, fatigue, muscle weakness, dizziness, anorexia) should be reported. The client should notify her provider of any infection, trauma, or stress that may increase the need for adrenocorticoids. A client who has Addison's disease may have hyponatremia. Therefore, a low-sodium diet should not be advised.

Ⓝ NCLEX® Connection: Physiological Adaptation, Illness Management

2. A nurse is reviewing serum laboratory results for a client who has Addison's disease. Which of the following findings should the nurse expect? (Select all that apply.)

X	**Sodium 130 mEq/L**
X	**Potassium 5.1 mEq/L**
X	**Calcium 10.6 mg/dL**
	Magnesium 2.5 mg/dL
X	**Glucose 65 mg/dL**
	Phosphorus 2.4 mg/dL

Insufficient glucocorticoids may cause sodium and water excretion that can lead to hyponatremia. Reduction in cortisol can cause hypoglycemia. Hypercalcemia and hyperkalemia are also consistent findings in clients who have Addison's disease. Magnesium and phosphorus levels should not be affected in clients who have Addison's disease. However, BUN and creatinine may be elevated due to a decreased glomerular filtration rate.

Ⓝ NCLEX® Connection: Reduction of Risk Potential, Laboratory Values

3. A nurse is caring for a client who has an acute adrenal insufficiency (adrenal crisis). The nurse should understand that this is an emergency event that may be precipitated by a sudden decrease in circulating

    A. cortisol.

    B. thyrotropin.

    C. prolactin.

    D. vasopressin.

Adrenal crisis has a rapid onset and may be precipitated by a sudden decrease in circulating adrenal cortical steroids. It is a medical emergency and if it is not promptly diagnosed and properly treated, the prognosis is poor. An adrenal crisis is characterized by hyperkalemia, hypovolemia, hypoglycemia, and cortisol deficits. The nurse should advise the client to notify the provider of any infection, trauma, or stress that can increase the need for adrenocorticoids. Insulin can be used to promote the movement of potassium into cells, which can temporarily reduce life-threatening hyperkalemia. The client should be advised to take medication as directed and to not discontinue it abruptly. Thyrotropin is excreted by the anterior pituitary gland to stimulate the thyroid hormones. Prolactin is released by the anterior pituitary gland to stimulate breast milk production. Vasopressin is released by the posterior pituitary gland and promotes the reabsorption of water.

Ⓝ NCLEX® Connection: Physiological Adaptation, Medical Emergencies

Overview

- A pheochromocytoma is a tumor of the center of the adrenal gland, the adrenal medulla. It is a rare tumor, and only about 10% of pheochromocytomas are malignant.

- Pheochromocytomas produce and store catecholamines, such as epinephrine and norepinephrine. The excess epinephrine and norepinephrine produce sympathetic nervous system effects.

- If the catecholamine surge of a pheochromocytoma is recognized promptly and treated appropriately, it is potentially curable. If the diagnosis is missed, the client may suffer severe cardiac and neurologic damage.

- The cause of pheochromocytomas is not known.

Assessment

- Risk Factors

    ○ Occurs more often in clients with

        ■ Neurofibromatosis

        ■ Multiple endocrine neoplasia syndromes

        ■ Age between 40 and 60 years

    ○ Precipitating causes of a catecholamine surge by a pheochromocytoma

        ■ Anesthesia

        ■ Opiates and opiate antagonists (naloxone)

        ■ Dopamine antagonists (droperidol, phenothiazines)

        ■ Medications that inhibit catecholamine reuptake (tricyclic antidepressants)

        ■ Childbirth

- Radiographic contrast media

- Foods high in tyramine (wine, aged cheese)

- Increases in intra-abdominal pressure (abdominal palpation) – Can cause a hypertensive episode

- Older adult clients may be less able to tolerate elevations in blood pressure caused by pheochromocytomas.

- Subjective and Objective Data

  o Pain in chest/abdomen accompanied by nausea and vomiting

  o Hypertension

  o Headache

  o Palpitations

  o Diaphoresis

  o Heat intolerance

  o Tremors

  o Apprehension

  o Laboratory Tests

    - Vanillylmandelic acid (VMA) testing – 24-hr urine collection for VMA, a breakdown product of catecholamines

      □ A normal VMA level is 2 to 7 mg/24 hr. High levels at rest indicate a pheochromocytoma.

  o Diagnostic Procedures

    - Clonidine suppression test

      □ If a client does not have a pheochromocytoma, clonidine (Catapres) suppresses catecholamine release and decreases the serum level of catecholamines (decreased blood pressure). If the client does have a pheochromocytoma, the clonidine has no effect (no decreased blood pressure).

    - Administration of phentolamine (Regitine)

      □ Phentolamine is used to control hypertensive crisis. A rapid decrease in systolic blood pressure of 35 mm Hg or greater and a diastolic blood pressure of 25 mm Hg or greater with the administration of phentolamine (Regitine), an alpha blocker, is diagnostic.

Collaborative Care

- Nursing Care

  - Do not palpate the abdomen. This may cause catecholamine release, which may lead to a hypertensive crisis.

  - Monitor ECG changes and fluid and electrolyte laboratory values. Blood sugar levels should also be monitored closely.

  - Provide emotional support to the client and family. Encourage verbalization of feelings about the disease.

- Medications

  - Alpha adrenergic blockers – Prazosin (Minipress) and phenoxybenzamine (Dibenzyline)

    - Given before surgery to regulate hypertension

    - Nursing Considerations

      - Always obtain the client's blood pressure before administering the medication.

      - Start with a low dose of medication.

      - Watch for orthostatic hypotension.

      - Monitor blood pressure 2 hr after administering the initial dose.

    - Client Education

      - Instruct the client to change positions slowly and notify the nurse if feelings of lightheadedness occur.

      - Have the client take the medication with food.

  - Beta blockers – Metoprolol (Lopressor)

    - Given before surgery to regulate hypertension

    - Nursing Considerations

      - Always obtain the client's blood pressure and pulse before administering the medication.

      - Watch for bradycardia (heart rate less than 60/min); if bradycardia occurs, hold medication and notify the provider.

      - Watch for orthostatic hypotension.

      - Use cautiously with clients who have diabetes mellitus.

- ■ Client Education
    - □ Provide the client with knowledge about the disease, the reasons for the diagnostic tests, the need for yearly testing of metanephrine, the need to monitor blood pressure, and the symptoms of high blood pressure.
    - □ Instruct the client to change positions slowly and notify the nurse if feelings of lightheadedness occur.
    - □ Have the client take the medication with food.
  - ○ Glucocorticoids – Prednisone (Deltasone)
    - ■ Given after surgery for adrenal suppression, to replace a drop in cortisol levels
- • Interdisciplinary Care
  - ○ Endocrinology services may be consulted to manage adrenal disease.
- • Surgical Interventions
  - ○ Unilateral or bilateral adrenalectomy surgery is the preferred therapeutic procedure.
    - ■ The removal of one or both adrenal glands to excise the tumor
    - ■ Nursing Actions
      - □ Blood pressure must be carefully controlled preoperatively and postoperatively.
      - □ Monitor all vital signs and check I&O.
      - □ Monitor ECG and electrolytes.
      - □ Preoperatively, use alpha blockers initially and then beta blockers to control hypertension.
      - □ Postoperatively, monitor for hypotension and hypovolemia, due to the sudden decrease in catecholamines.
      - □ Administer postoperative medications. Monitor for effects and side effects.
      - □ Assess for signs of postoperative bleeding, such as tachycardia, hypotension, and a firm abdomen.
    - ■ Client Education
      - □ Teach the client that after a bilateral adrenalectomy, lifelong glucocorticoid and mineralocorticoid replacement is required.
      - □ Teach the client that after a unilateral adrenalectomy, glucocorticoid supplementation may be needed until the one gland is able to produce enough.

- Care After Discharge

  o Home health services may be indicated regarding incision care, medication regimen, and blood pressure follow-up.

  o Client Education

    ▪ Teach client how to properly take blood pressure and interpret readings.

    ▪ Promote good hand hygiene to prevent infection.

    ▪ Encourage the client to assess skin daily for skin breakdown and sensitivity.

    ▪ Teach the client to take daily weights and keep a daily record to monitor for fluid excess.

    ▪ Teach the client to notify the health care provider if there is a weight gain of 3 lbs or more in a week.

    ▪ Encourage the client to wear a medical identification bracelet.

    ▪ Promote a diet rich in vitamins, calories, and minerals.

    ▪ Encourage smoking cessation, if the client smokes.

    ▪ Encourage the client to avoid caffeinated beverages.

- Client Outcomes

  o The client will maintain baseline blood pressure.

  o The client will maintain a weight that is within 10% of his ideal body weight.

  o The client will maintain a diet regimen high in vitamins, calories, and minerals.

  o The client will take medications as prescribed.

Complications

- Hypertensive crisis

  o This is the most significant complication of a pheochromocytoma.

  o Nursing Actions

    ▪ Closely monitor the client's blood pressure and observe for any signs or symptoms that may indicate a hypertensive crisis.

    ▪ Administer alpha blockers as prescribed (phentolamine IV, phenoxybenzamine).

CHAPTER 95: PHEOCHROMOCYTOMA

(A) Application Exercises

Scenario: A nurse is caring for a client who has a pheochromocytoma and is scheduled to have surgery in several days.

1. The nurse knows that pheochromocytomas produce catecholamines that stimulate adrenergic receptors. Why has the provider prescribed phenoxybenzamine (Dibenzyline) only and not phenoxybenzamine and a beta-blocker?

2. Why is amitriptyline (Elavil), a tricyclic antidepressant, contraindicated for this client?

3. Why is this client at risk for developing hypertension?

4. Why are neurologic checks important in this situation?

5. Why might this client be tachycardic and diaphoretic?

6. A nurse is caring for a client who is having a catecholamine surge. Which of the following are possible precipitating causes of the surge? (Select all that apply.)

_____   General anesthesia

_____   Local anesthesia

_____   Morphine

_____   Naloxone (Narcan)

_____   Levodopa with carbidopa (Sinemet)

_____   Haloperidol (Haldol)

_____   Orange sherbet

_____   Red wine

_____   Coffee

7. A nurse is caring for a client who is suspected to have a pheochromocytoma. The nurse knows that the clonidine suppression test is used as a diagnostic test to detect pheochromocytoma for what reason?

CHAPTER 95: PHEOCHROMOCYTOMA

 Application Exercises Answer Key

Scenario: A nurse is caring for a client who has a pheochromocytoma and is scheduled to have surgery in several days.

1. The nurse knows that pheochromocytomas produce catecholamines that stimulate adrenergic receptors. Why has the provider prescribed phenoxybenzamine (Dibenzyline) only and not phenoxybenzamine and a beta-blocker?

   Phenoxybenzamine is an alpha-adrenergic blocker. If a beta-blocker is administered before alpha blockade is complete, there will be unopposed stimulation of the alpha receptors.

    NCLEX® Connection: Pharmacological and Parenteral Therapies, Expected Actions/ Outcomes

2. Why is amitriptyline (Elavil), a tricyclic antidepressant, contraindicated for this client?

   Amitriptyline inhibits the reuptake of catecholamines. This will result in sustained high levels of epinephrine and sympathetic stimulation.

    NCLEX® Connection: Pharmacological and Parenteral Therapies, Adverse Effects/ Contraindications/Side Effects/Interactions

3. Why is this client at risk for developing hypertension?

   Pheochromocytomas secrete catecholamines. These catecholamines directly stimulate the alpha receptors, which causes vasoconstriction.

    NCLEX® Connection: Physiological Adaptation, Pathophysiology

4. Why are neurologic checks important in this situation?

   An elevated blood pressure can cause neurologic effects.

    NCLEX® Connection: Physiological Adaptation, Pathophysiology

5. Why might this client be tachycardic and diaphoretic?

> **Catecholamines stimulate beta receptors in the heart, and they cause an increase in sweat gland secretion.**

 NCLEX® Connection: Physiological Adaptation, Pathophysiology

6. A nurse is caring for a client who is having a catecholamine surge. Which of the following are possible precipitating causes of the surge? (Select all that apply.)

__X__	**General anesthesia**
_____	Local anesthesia
__X__	**Morphine**
__X__	**Naloxone (Narcan)**
_____	Levodopa with carbidopa (Sinemet)
__X__	**Haloperidol (Haldol)**
_____	Orange sherbet
__X__	**Red wine**
__X__	**Coffee**

> **General anesthesia, opioids (morphine), opioid antagonists (naloxone), dopamine antagonists (haloperidol), foods/beverages high in tyramine (red wine), and catecholamine stimulants (vanilla, coffee) can precipitate a catecholamine surge. Local anesthesia, levodopa with carbidopa, and orange sherbet are not associated with catecholamine surge.**

 NCLEX® Connection: Physiological Adaptation, Pathophysiology

7. A nurse is caring for a client who is suspected to have a pheochromocytoma. The nurse knows that the clonidine suppression test is used as a diagnostic test to detect pheochromocytoma for what reason?

> **Clonidine normally decreases sympathetic outflow and lowers heart rate and blood pressure by decreasing catecholamine release. If the client has a pheochromocytoma, there will be higher than normal levels of catecholamines, and these vital sign changes will not occur with clonidine administration.**

 NCLEX® Connection: Reduction of Risk Potential, Diagnostic Tests

Overview

- Diabetes mellitus is characterized by chronic hyperglycemia due to inadequate insulin secretion and/or the effectiveness of endogenous insulin (insulin resistance).

- Diabetes mellitus is a contributing factor to development of cardiovascular disease, hypertension, renal failure, blindness, and stroke as individuals age.

Health Promotion and Disease Prevention

- Diabetic Screening

  o Test urine for glucose and ketones during routine examinations to evaluate the need for further testing.

- Client Education

  o Teach the client that exercise and good nutrition are necessary for controlling diabetes.

  o Teach the client how to monitor blood glucose levels as prescribed.

  o Teach the client with diabetes that foot care and skin care are priorities.

Assessment

- Risk Factors

  o Genetics may predispose an individual to the occurrence of type 1 or type 2 diabetes.

  o Toxins and viruses can predispose an individual to diabetes by destroying the beta cells leading to type 1 diabetes mellitus.

  o Obesity, physical inactivity, high triglycerides (greater than 250 mg/dL), and hypertension may lead to the development of insulin resistance and type 2 diabetes.

  o Secondary causes of diabetes include pancreatitis and Cushing's syndrome.

Ⓖ
- ○ Because of the deterioration of the function of all organs, the older adult clients are at risk for:
  - ■ Kidney and liver dysfunction leading to altered urinary output and altered metabolism of medications.
  - ■ Vision alterations (yellowing of lens, decreased ability of depth perception, cataracts) as well as eye changes that may be related to diabetic retinopathy.
  - ○ Vision and hearing deficits may interfere with the understanding of teaching, reading of materials, and preparation of medications.
  - ○ Tissue deterioration secondary to aging may impact the client's ability to prepare food, care for self, perform ADLs, perform foot/wound care, and perform glucose monitoring.
  - ○ A fixed income may mean that there are limited funds for buying diabetic supplies, wound care supplies, insulin, and medications; this may result in complications.
  - ○ Older adult clients may not be able to drive to the health care provider's office, grocery store, or pharmacy. Assess support systems available for older adult clients.

- • Subjective and Objective Data
  - ■ Blood glucose

AUTONOMIC NERVOUS SYSTEM RESPONSES – RAPID ONSET	IMPAIRED CEREBRAL FUNCTION – GRADUAL ONSET
• Hunger, lightheadedness, and shakiness	• Strange or unusual feelings
• Nausea	• Decreased level of consciousness
• Anxiety and irritability	• Difficulty in thinking and inability to concentrate
• Pale, cool skin	• Change in emotional behavior
• Diaphoresis	• Slurred speech
• Irritability	• Headache and blurred vision
• Normal or shallow respirations	• Seizures leading to coma
• Tachycardia and palpitations	

  - ■ Hyperglycemia – Blood glucose level usually greater than 250 mg/dL
  - ■ Thirst
  - ■ Frequent urination
  - ■ Hunger
  - ■ Skin that is warm, dry, and flushed with poor turgor
  - ■ Dry mucous membranes
  - ■ Soft eyeballs

- Weakness
- Malaise
- Rapid, weak pulse and hypotension
- Rapid, deep respirations (Kussmaul respirations, with acetone/fruity odor due to ketones)

  ○ Laboratory Tests

- Diagnostic criteria for diabetes include two findings (on separate days) of one of the following:
  □ Symptoms of diabetes plus casual plasma glucose concentration of greater than 200 mg/dL (without regard to time since last meal)
  □ Fasting blood glucose greater than 126 mg/dL
  □ Two-hour glucose greater than 200 mg/dL with an oral glucose tolerance test

- Fasting blood glucose
  □ Nursing Actions
    ▸ Postpone administration of antidiabetic medication until after the level is drawn.
  □ Client Education
    ▸ Ensure that the client has fasted (no food or drink other than water) for the 8 hr prior to the blood draw.

- Oral glucose tolerance test
  □ A fasting blood glucose level is drawn at the start of the test. The client is then instructed to consume a specified amount of glucose. Blood glucose levels are drawn every 30 min for 2 hr. The clients must be assessed for hypoglycemia throughout the procedure.
  □ Client Education
    ▸ Instruct the client to consume a balanced diet for 3 days prior to the test. Then instruct the client to fast for 10 to 12 hr prior to the test.

- Glycosylated hemoglobin (HbA1c)
  □ The normal reference range is 4% to 6%, but an acceptable target for clients who have diabetes may be 6.5% to 8%, with a target goal of less than 7%. HbA1c is the best indicator of the average blood glucose level for the past 120 days. Assists in evaluating treatment effectiveness and compliance.

- ○ Diagnostic Procedures
  - ■ Self-monitored blood glucose (SMBG)
    - □ Nursing Action
      - ▸ Follow or ensure that the client follows the proper procedure for blood sample collection and use of a glucose meter. Supplemental short-acting insulin may be prescribed for elevated pre-meal glucose levels.
    - □ Client Education
      - ▸ Instruct the client to check the accuracy of the strips with the control solution provided.
      - ▸ Advise the client to keep a record of the SMBG that includes time, date, serum glucose level, insulin dose, food intake, and other events that may alter glucose metabolism, such as activity level or illness.

Collaborative Care

- • Nursing Care
  - ○ Monitor
    - ■ Blood glucose levels and factors affecting levels (other medications)
    - ■ I & O and weight
    - ■ Skin integrity and healing status of any wounds, (Feet and folds of the skin should be monitored closely.)
    - ■ Sensory alterations (tingling, numbness)
    - ■ Visual alterations
    - ■ Presence of recurrent infections
    - ■ Dietary practices
    - ■ Exercise patterns
    - ■ The client's self-monitoring blood glucose skill proficiency
    - ■ The client's self-medication administration proficiency
  - ○ Teach the client proper foot care.
    - ■ Inspect feet daily. Wash feet daily with mild soap and warm water.
    - ■ Pat feet dry gently, especially between the toes.
    - ■ Use mild foot powder (powder with cornstarch) on sweaty feet.
    - ■ Do not use commercial remedies for the removal of calluses or corns.
    - ■ Consult a podiatrist.
    - ■ The best time to perform nail care is after a bath/shower.
    - ■ Separate overlapping toes with cotton or lamb's wool.

- Avoid open-toe, open-heel shoes. Leather shoes are preferred to plastic ones. Wear shoes that fit correctly. Wear slippers with soles. Do not go barefoot. Shake out shoes before putting them on.

- Wear clean, absorbent socks or stockings that are made of cotton or wool and have not been mended.

- Do not use hot water bottles or heating pads to warm feet. Wear socks for warmth.

- Avoid prolonged sitting, standing, and crossing of legs.

o Teach the client to follow agency policies for nail care. Some protocols allow for trimming toenails straight across with clippers and filing edges with an emery board or nail file. If clippers or scissors are contraindicated, the client should file the nails straight across.

o Teach the client to cleanse cuts with warm water and mild soap, gently dry, and apply a dry dressing. Instruct the clients to monitor healing and to seek intervention promptly.

o Provide nutritional guidelines.

- Plan meals to achieve appropriate timing of food intake, activity, onset, and peak of insulin. Calories and food composition should be similar each day.

- Eat at regular intervals and do not skip meals.

- Count grams of carbohydrates consumed.

- Recognize that 15 g of carbohydrates are equal to 1 carbohydrate exchange.

- Restrict calories and increase physical activity as appropriate to facilitate weight loss (for clients who are obese) or to prevent obesity.

- Include fiber in the diet to increase carbohydrate metabolism and to help control cholesterol levels.

- Use artificial sweeteners.

- Keep fat content below 30% of the total caloric intake.

o Teach the client appropriate techniques for SMBG, including obtaining blood samples, recording and responding to results, and correctly handling supplies and equipment.

o Teach the client guidelines to follow when sick.

- Monitor blood glucose every 3 to 4 hr.

- Continue to take insulin or oral antidiabetic agents.

- Consume 4 oz of sugar-free, non-caffeinated liquid every 0.5 hr to prevent dehydration.

- Meet carbohydrate needs through soft food if possible. If not, consume liquids equal to usual carbohydrate content.

- Test urine for ketones and report to provider if they are abnormal (the level should be negative to small).

- Rest.

- Call the health care provider if:

  □ Blood glucose is greater than 240 mg/dL.

  □ Fever is greater than 38.9° C (102° F), does not respond to acetaminophen, or lasts more than 12 hr.

  □ Feeling disoriented or confused.

  □ Experiencing rapid breathing.

  □ Vomiting occurs more than once.

  □ Diarrhea occurs more than five times or for longer than 24 hr.

  □ Unable to tolerate liquids.

  □ Illness lasts longer than 2 days.

○ Advise the client to eat at regular intervals, avoid alcohol intake, and adjust insulin to exercise and diet to avoid hypoglycemia.

○ Teach the client measures to take in response to signs and symptoms of hypoglycemia (shakiness, diaphoresis, anxiety, nervousness, chills, nausea, headache, weakness, confusion).

- Check blood glucose level.

- Follow guidelines outlined by the health care provider/diabetes educator. Guidelines may include:

  □ Treat with 15 to 20 g carbohydrates.

    ▸ Examples – 4 oz orange juice, 2 oz grape juice, 8 oz milk, glucose tablets per manufacturer's suggestion to equal 15 g

  □ Recheck blood glucose in 15 min.

  □ If still low (less than 70 mg/dL), give 15 to 20 g more of carbohydrates.

  □ Recheck blood glucose in 15 min.

  □ If blood glucose is within normal limits, take 7 g protein (if the next meal is more than an hour away).

    ▸ Example – 1 oz of cheese (1 string cheese), 2 tablespoons of peanut butter, or 8 oz of milk

- If the client is unconscious or unable to swallow, administer glucagon SC or IM (repeat in 10 min if still unconscious) and notify the health care provider.

- o Teach the client signs and symptoms of hyperglycemia (hot, dry skin and fruity breath) and measures to take in response to hyperglycemia.

    - Encourage oral fluid intake.

    - Administer insulin as prescribed.

    - Restrict exercise when blood glucose levels are greater than 250 mg/dL.

    - Test urine for ketones and report if abnormal.

    - Consult the provider if symptoms progress.

  - o Encourage the client to wear a medical identification wristband.

- Medications

  - o Clients who have type 1 diabetes are on an insulin regimen that frequently consists of more than one type of insulin (rapid, short, intermediate, and long acting). Insulin given in this manner is administered one or more times per day and based on a client's blood glucose level. Some clients who have type 2 diabetes or women who have gestational diabetes may require insulin if glycemic control is unable to be obtained with diet, exercise, and oral hypoglycemics.

  - o Some clients are placed on an insulin pump, which is a small pump that is worn externally, contains insulin, and delivers insulin as programmed via a needle inserted into the subcutaneous tissue. The needle should be changed at least every 3 days.

  - o Clients who have type 2 diabetes can usually regulate their blood glucose with diet and exercise with the addition of oral hypoglycemics as needed.

TYPE	TRADE NAME	ONSET	PEAK	DURATION
Rapid acting	Insulin lispro (Humalog)	Less than 15 min	0.5 to 1 hr	3 to 4 hr
Short acting	Regular insulin (Humulin R)	0.5 to 1 hr	2 to 3 hr	5 to 7 hr
Intermediate acting	NPH insulin (Humulin N)	1 to 2 hr	4 to 12 hr	18 to 24 hr
Long acting	insulin glargine (Lantus)	1 hr	none	10.4 to 24 hr

    - Nursing Considerations

      - □ Observe the client perform self-administration of insulin and offer additional instruction as indicated.

      - □ Do not mix insulin glargine (Lantus) with other insulins due to incompatibility.

      - □ Provide information regarding oral antidiabetic medications.

        - ▸ Administer as prescribed (for example, 30 min before first main meal for most oral blood glucose lowering agents or with the first bite of each main meal for alpha-glucosidase inhibitors).

        - ▸ Avoid alcohol with sulfonylurea agents (disulfiram-like reaction).

- ▸ Monitor renal function (biguanides).

- ▸ Monitor liver function (thiazolidinediones and alpha-glucosidase inhibitors).

- ▸ Advise women of childbearing age taking thiazolidinediones that additional contraception methods may be needed since these medications reduce the blood levels of some oral contraceptives.

- ■ Client Education

  - ▢ Provide information regarding self-administration of insulin.

    - ▸ Rotate injection sites (prevent lipohypertrophy) within one anatomic site (prevent day-to-day changes in absorption rates).

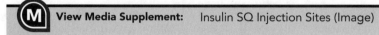

View Media Supplement: Insulin SQ Injection Sites (Image)

    - ▸ Inject at a 90° angle (45° angle if thin). Aspiration for blood is not necessary.

    - ▸ When mixing a rapid- or short-acting insulin with a longer-acting insulin, draw up the shorter-acting insulin into the syringe first and then the longer-acting insulin (this reduces the risk of introducing the longer-acting insulin into the shorter-acting insulin vial).

- ○ Oral hypoglycemics

  - ■ Biguanides – Metformin HCL (Glucophage)

    - ▢ Reduces the production of glucose through suppression of gluconeogenesis

    - ▢ Nursing Considerations

      - ▸ Monitor significance of gastrointestinal (GI) effects (anorexia, nausea, vomiting).

      - ▸ Monitor for lactic acidosis, especially in clients with renal insufficiency or liver dysfunction.

    - ▢ Client Education

      - ▸ Instruct the client to take vitamin B_{12} and folic acid supplements.

      - ▸ Instruct the client to contact the provider if signs of lactic acidosis (myalgia, sluggishness, somnolence, hyperventilation) are experienced.

      - ▸ Instruct the client that this medication may be taken during pregnancy for gestational diabetes.

  - ■ Sulfonylureas – Tolbutamide (Orinase), chlorpropamide (Diabinese), and glyburide (DiaBeta, Micronase)

    - ▢ Stimulates insulin release from the pancreas

- □ Nursing Considerations
  - ▸ Monitor for hypoglycemia. Beta blockers can mask tachycardia typically seen during hypoglycemia. Adjust teaching regarding symptoms of hypoglycemia accordingly.
- □ Client Education
  - ▸ Instruct the client to avoid use during pregnancy.
  - ▸ Instruct the client to avoid alcohol due to disulfiram effect.

- ■ Meglitinides – Repaglinide (Prandin) and nateglinide (Starlix)
  - □ Stimulates insulin release from pancreas
  - □ Nursing Considerations
    - ▸ Monitor for hypoglycemia.
    - ▸ Do not administer with gemfibrozil (Lopid).
  - □ Client Education
    - ▸ Wear a medical identification wristband due to the risk of hypoglycemia.

- ■ Thiazolidinediones – Rosiglitazone (Avandia) and pioglitazone (Actos)
  - □ Increases cellular response to insulin by decreasing insulin resistance
  - □ Nursing Considerations
    - ▸ Monitor for fluid retention, especially in clients with a history of heart failure.
    - ▸ Monitor the client's LDL and triglycerides for elevations.
  - □ Client Education
    - ▸ Instruct the client to have serum alanine aminotransferase (ALT) checked every 6 months after baseline.

- ■ Alpha-Glucosidase Inhibitors – Acarbose (Precose) and miglitol (Glyset)
  - □ Slows carbohydrate absorption and digestion
  - □ Nursing Considerations
    - ▸ Alert the client of GI discomfort common with these medications (abdominal distention, cramps, excessive gas, diarrhea).
    - ▸ Monitor for iron deficiency anemia (hemoglobin and iron levels).
  - □ Client Education
    - ▸ Instruct the client to have liver function tests performed every 3 months or as prescribed.
    - ▸ Report jaundice immediately.

- ▪ Gliptins – Sitagliptin (Januvia)
  - ▫ Augments naturally occurring incretin hormones, which promote release of insulin and decrease secretion of glucagon
  - ▫ Nursing Considerations
    - ▸ These medications have very few side effects but upper respiratory symptoms (nasal and throat inflammation) may be present.
  - ▫ Client Education
    - ▸ Instruct the client to report persistent upper respiratory symptoms.

- • Interdisciplinary Care
  - ○ Refer the client to a diabetes educator for comprehensive education in diabetes management.

- • Client Outcomes
  - ○ The client will have blood glucose levels within an acceptable range.
  - ○ The client will be able to self-administer insulin.
  - ○ The client will be able to monitor for complications and intervene as necessary.

Complications

- • Consistent maintenance of blood glucose levels within the normal reference range is the best protection against the complications of diabetes mellitus. Normal reference ranges may vary and will usually range from 70 to 120 mg/dL.
  - ○ Cardiovascular and cerebrovascular disease
    - ▪ Hypertension, myocardial infarction, and stroke
    - ▪ Nursing Actions
      - ▫ Monitor blood pressure.
    - ▪ Client Education
      - ▫ Encourage checks of cholesterol (HDL, LDL, and triglycerides) yearly and monitoring of blood pressure and HbA1c levels every 3 months.
      - ▫ Encourage participation in regular activity.
      - ▫ Encourage a diet of low-fat meals that is high in fruits, vegetables, and whole grain foods.
      - ▫ Teach the client to report shortness of breath, headaches (persistent and transient), numbness in distal extremities, swelling of feet, infrequent urination, and changes in vision.
      - ▫ Encourage a dietary consult.

- ○ Impaired vision and blindness
  - ▪ Caused by diabetic retinopathy
  - ▪ Client Education
    - □ Encourage yearly eye exams to ensure the health of the eyes and to protect vision.
    - □ Encourage management of blood glucose levels.
- ○ Foot injury
  - ▪ Caused by sensory neuropathy, ischemia, and infection
  - ▪ Nursing Actions
    - □ Monitor blood glucose levels.
    - □ Provide foot care.
  - ▪ Client Education
    - □ Encourage annual exams by a podiatrist.
    - □ Instruct the client to examine feet daily.
    - □ Provide foot care instructions.
- ○ Renal failure
  - ▪ Damage to the kidneys from prolonged elevated blood glucose levels and dehydration
  - ▪ Nursing Actions
    - □ Monitor hydration and renal function (I & O, creatinine levels).
    - □ Report an hourly output of less than 30 mL/hr.
    - □ Monitor blood pressure.
  - ▪ Client Education
    - □ Encourage yearly urine analysis, BUN, and creatinine clearance.
    - □ Encourage the client to avoid soda, alcohol, and toxic levels of acetaminophen.
    - □ Teach the client to consume 2 to 3 L of fluid per day from food and beverage sources and to drink an adequate amount of water
    - □ Tell the client to report decrease in output to the provider.

View Media Supplement:
- Diabetic Retinopathy (Image)
- Diabetic Foot Ulcers (Images)

CHAPTER 96: DIABETES MELLITUS MANAGEMENT

(A) Application Exercises

1. A nurse is caring for a client whose blood glucose is 49 mg/dL. The client is lethargic but arousable. Which of the following is the priority nursing action?

    A. Re-check blood glucose in 15 min.

    B. Give 7 g of protein.

    C. Give 15 to 20 g of carbohydrates.

    D. Report findings to the client's health care provider.

2. A client's medication record reads: Lispro insulin 10 units subcutaneously 0800. Which of the following actions should the nurse take when administering this medication?

    A. Check the client's blood glucose immediately after administration.

    B. Administer the medication when the breakfast tray arrives.

    C. Administer the medication within 30 min of the scheduled time.

    D. Clarify the prescription because the medication is usually given at bedtime.

3. A client's blood glucose level is 257 mg/dL at 0800, and the health care provider's prescription for sliding scale insulin for this blood glucose result is 6 units of Regular insulin (Humulin R) subcutaneously. This client also receives 12 units of insulin glargine (Lantus) subcutaneously every morning. Which of the following methods should the nurse use to draw up and administer the insulin?

    A. In one insulin syringe, draw up 6 units of Regular insulin. In a separate insulin syringe, draw up 12 units of insulin glargine and give two separate injections.

    B. Draw up the Regular insulin first, and then draw up the insulin glargine in the same syringe. Administer one injection that contains both insulins.

    C. Draw up the insulin glargine first, and then draw up the Regular insulin in the same syringe. Administer one injection that contains both insulins.

    D. Give only the 6 units of Regular insulin as indicated on the sliding scale prescription.

4. An adult client who has type 1 diabetes mellitus is admitted to the hospital for circulatory impairment to the lower extremity and an open draining wound on the right foot. The client manages her own blood glucose monitoring and insulin injections at home. Her instructions include blood glucose monitoring before meals and at bedtime. It is 0800. In what order should the nurse perform the following interventions?

    _____ Complete the morning assessment.

    _____ Teach the client about complications of diabetes and circulation.

    _____ Perform morning care and grooming.

    _____ Administer the morning insulin injection.

    _____ Take vital signs.

    _____ Perform a finger stick for blood glucose monitoring.

    _____ Assist with the breakfast tray.

CHAPTER 96: DIABETES MELLITUS MANAGEMENT

 Application Exercises Answer Key

1. A nurse is caring for a client whose blood glucose is 49 mg/dL. The client is lethargic but arousable. Which of the following is the priority nursing action?

    A. Re-check blood glucose in 15 min.

    B. Give 7 g of protein.

    C. Give 15 to 20 g of carbohydrates.

    D. Report findings to the client's health care provider.

    The greatest risk to the client is a lack of glucose for cell metabolism. Therefore, the priority action is to give 15 to 20 g of carbohydrates to raise the client's serum blood glucose level. Next, the client's blood glucose should be checked in 15 min. If the blood glucose remains below 70 mg/dL, give 15 g more of carbohydrates should be given. The client's blood glucose should be re-checked in 15 min. This would be repeated until the client's blood glucose is above 70 mg/dL, then 7 g of protein should be given. Findings should be reported to the client's health care provider and actions should be documented.

    NCLEX® Connection: Reduction of Risk Potential, System Specific Assessment

2. A client's medication record reads: Lispro insulin 10 units subcutaneously 0800. Which of the following actions should the nurse take when administering this medication?

    A. Check the client's blood glucose immediately after administration.

    B. Administer the medication when the breakfast tray arrives.

    C. Administer the medication within 30 min of the scheduled time.

    D. Clarify the prescription because the medication is usually given at bedtime.

    Insulin lispro (Humalog) is a rapid-acting insulin with an onset of less than 15 min. Administering the insulin at the time the breakfast tray arrives will ensure adequate blood glucose at the time of peak action. The client's blood glucose level should be checked prior to insulin administration to prevent an episode of hypoglycemia. This medication is given prior to meals, and may be given 2 to 3 times/day.

    NCLEX® Connection: Pharmacological and Parenteral Therapies, Expected Actions/ Outcomes

3. A client's blood glucose level is 257 mg/dL at 0800, and the health care provider's prescription for sliding scale insulin for this blood glucose result is 6 units of Regular insulin (Humulin R) subcutaneously. This client also receives 12 units of insulin glargine (Lantus) subcutaneously every morning. Which of the following methods should the nurse use to draw up and administer the insulin?

A. In one insulin syringe, draw up 6 units of Regular insulin. In a separate insulin syringe, draw up 12 units of insulin glargine and give two separate injections.

B. Draw up the Regular insulin first, and then draw up the insulin glargine in the same syringe. Administer one injection that contains both insulins.

C. Draw up the insulin glargine first, and then draw up the Regular insulin in the same syringe. Administer one injection that contains both insulins.

D. Give only the 6 units of Regular insulin as indicated on the sliding scale prescription.

The insulin should be drawn in two syringes and given as two separate SC injections. Insulin glargine and Regular insulin are not compatible and cannot be given in the same syringe.

 NCLEX® Connection: Pharmacological and Parenteral Therapies, Adverse Effects/ Contraindications/Side Effects/Interactions

4. An adult client who has type 1 diabetes mellitus is admitted to the hospital for circulatory impairment to the lower extremity and an open draining wound on the right foot. The client manages her own blood glucose monitoring and insulin injections at home. Her instructions include blood glucose monitoring before meals and at bedtime. It is 0800. In what order should the nurse perform the following interventions?

4	Complete the morning assessment.
7	Teach the client about complications of diabetes and circulation.
6	Perform morning care and grooming.
3	Administer the morning insulin injection.
1	Take vital signs.
2	Perform a finger stick for blood glucose monitoring.
5	Assist with the breakfast tray.

The nurse should obtain the client's vital signs and then check the client's blood glucose level. Insulin should be given approximately 30 min prior to a meal, so it should be given after the blood glucose level is drawn. The nurse should then complete the morning assessment, assist with the breakfast tray, and complete morning care and grooming. Education about the complications of diabetes mellitus should be performed when the nurse has adequate time and the client is not tired or distracted by other activities.

 NCLEX® Connection: Reduction of Risk Potential, Potential for Complications From Surgical Procedures and Health Alterations

Overview

- Diabetic ketoacidosis (DKA) is an acute, life-threatening condition characterized by hyperglycemia (greater than 300 mg/dL) resulting in the breakdown of body fat for energy and an accumulation of ketones in the blood and urine. The onset is rapid, and the mortality rate of DKA is 1% to 10%.

- Hyperglycemic-hyperosmolar state (HHS) is an acute, life-threatening condition characterized by profound hyperglycemia (greater than 600 mg/dL), dehydration, and an absence of ketosis. The onset generally occurs over several days, and the mortality rate of HHS is up to 15% or more.

Assessment

- Risk Factors

  - DKA is more common in clients with type 1 diabetes mellitus.

  - HHS is more common in older adult clients and in clients with untreated or undiagnosed type 2 diabetes mellitus.

  - Physiological changes in cardiac and pulmonary function may place older adult clients at greater risk for fluid overload (precipitate heart failure exacerbation) from fluid replacement therapy.

  - Any condition that increases carbohydrate metabolism, such as stress, illness, infection, surgery, or trauma that requires an increased need for insulin or that produces a lack of sufficient insulin (such as new onset of diabetes mellitus or nonadherence to a diabetic regimen)

- Subjective Data

  - Nausea, vomiting, and/or abdominal pain (DKA/metabolic acidosis)

  - Reports of frequent urination, thirst, and hunger

  - Reports of confusion

- Objective Data

  - Physical Assessment Findings

    - Polyuria, polydipsia, and polyphagia (early signs)

    - Change in mental status

    - Signs of dehydration (dry mucous membranes, weight loss, sunken eyeballs resulting from fluid loss such as polyuria)

    - Kussmaul respiration pattern, rapid and deep respirations, fruity breath (DKA/metabolic acidosis)

    - Generalized seizures and reversible paralysis (HHS)

  - Laboratory Tests

    - Therapeutic management is guided by serial laboratory analysis.

DIAGNOSTIC PROCEDURE	DKA	HHS
Serum glucose levels	Greater than 300 mg/dL	Greater than 600 mg/dL
Serum electrolytes • Sodium (Na) • Potassium (K)	• Na^+- Increased due to water loss • K^+- Initially low due to diuresis, which may increase due to acidosis	• Na^+- Increased due to water loss • K^+- Initially low due to diuresis
Serum renal studies • BUN • Creatinine	• Increased secondary to dehydration	• Increased secondary to dehydration
Ketone levels • Serum • Urine	• Present in serum and urine	• Absent in serum and urine
Serum osmolarity	• High	• Very high
Serum pH (ABG)	• Metabolic acidosis with respiratory compensation (Kussmaul respirations)	• Absence of acidosis

Collaborative Care

- Nursing Care

  - Always treat the underlying cause (infectious process).

  - Provide rapid isotonic fluid (0.9% sodium chloride) replacement to maintain perfusion to vital organs. Monitor the client for evidence of fluid volume excess due to the need for large quantities of fluid.

  - Follow with a hypotonic fluid (0.45% sodium chloride) to continue replacing losses to total body fluid.

- When serum glucose levels approach 250 mg/dL, add glucose to IV fluids to minimize the risk of cerebral edema associated with drastic changes in serum osmolality.

- Administer Regular insulin (Humulin R) 0.1 unit/kg as an IV bolus dose and then follow with a continuous IV infusion of Regular insulin at 0.1 unit/kg/hr.

- Monitor glucose levels hourly.

- Monitor serum potassium levels. Potassium levels will initially be elevated with insulin therapy, but potassium will shift into cells and the client will need to be monitored for hypokalemia. Provide potassium replacement therapy in all replacement IV fluids, as indicated by laboratory values. Make sure urinary output is adequate before administering potassium.

- Administer sodium bicarbonate by slow IV infusion for severe acidosis (pH of less than 7.0). Monitor potassium levels because a correcting acidosis too quickly may lead to hypokalemia.

- ⓖ Considerations for older adult clients

  - Encourage older adult clients to wear medical alert bracelets.

  - Teach older adult clients to monitor blood glucose every 1 to 4 hr when ill.

  - Emphasize the importance of not skipping an insulin dose when ill.

  - Maintain hydration because older adult clients may have a diminished thirst sensation.

  - Changes in mental status may keep older adult clients from seeking treatment.

- Client Education

  - Provide the client with education to prevent reoccurrence.

    - Take measures to decrease the risk of dehydration.

    - Monitor glucose every 4 hr when ill and continue to take insulin.

    - Consume liquids with carbohydrates and electrolytes (sports drinks) when unable to eat solid food.

    - Notify the health care provider if illness lasts more than 1 day.

- Therapeutic Outcomes

  - The client will maintain appropriate levels of blood glucose.

  - The client will monitor for signs of impeding complications and notify the health care provider immediately if any occur.

CHAPTER 97: COMPLICATIONS OF DIABETES MELLITUS

(A) Application Exercises

1. A nurse is administering insulin by continuous IV infusion to a client who has diabetic ketoacidosis (DKA). Explain why the nurse should monitor the client for hypokalemia.

2. A nurse is caring for a client who is in a hyperosmolar-hyperglycemic state (HHS). Which of the following findings is consistent with HHS? (Select all that apply.)

_____ Abdominal pain

_____ Confusion

_____ Polyuria

_____ Polydipsia

_____ pH 7.24

3. A nurse is caring for a client who has diabetic ketoacidosis (DKA). What type of IV fluids should the nurse expect to administer initially and subsequently as blood glucose decreases?

4. What type of acid-base imbalance is likely in a client with diabetic ketoacidosis (DKA)? How should the nurse recognize compensation for this acid-base disorder?

CHAPTER 97: COMPLICATIONS OF DIABETES MELLITUS

 Application Exercises Answer Key

1. A nurse is administering insulin by continuous IV infusion to a client who has diabetic ketoacidosis (DKA). Explain why the nurse should monitor the client for hypokalemia.

   With insulin therapy, potassium will shift from the intravascular space into cells rapidly. Therefore, the client should be monitored for hypokalemia. Potassium replacement should be administered while making sure urinary output is adequate prior to administration.

 NCLEX® Connection: Reduction of Risk Potential, Potential for Complications of Diagnostic Tests/Treatments/Procedures

2. A nurse is caring for a client who is in a hyperosmolar-hyperglycemic state (HHS). Which of the following findings is consistent with HHS? (Select all that apply.)

	Abdominal pain
X	**Confusion**
X	**Polyuria**
X	**Polydipsia**
	pH 7.24

   The client with HHS will not have abdominal pain, which is a symptom of acidosis. Confusion from dehydration may be present, as well as thirst and frequent urination. The client will also have a normal pH (7.35 to 7.45) instead of being acidotic (7.24).

 NCLEX® Connection: Reduction of Risk Potential, System Specific Assessment

3. A nurse is caring for a client who has diabetic ketoacidosis (DKA). What type of IV fluids should the nurse expect to administer initially and subsequently as blood glucose decreases?

   Initially, 0.9% sodium chloride (an isotonic solution) should be infused rapidly to expand blood volume and maintain perfusion to vital organs. Then, a hypotonic solution, such as 0.45% sodium chloride, should be infused to replace losses to total body fluid. As blood glucose decreases, a 5% dextrose in 0.45% sodium chloride solution should be administered to maintain adequate blood glucose levels and prevent cerebral edema.

 NCLEX® Connection: Physiological Adaptation, Medical Emergencies

4. What type of acid-base imbalance is likely in a client with diabetic ketoacidosis (DKA)? How should the nurse recognize compensation for this acid-base disorder?

   Metabolic acidosis secondary to breakdown of fats for energy manifested by ketosis is most likely. Rapid, deep respirations (Kussmaul's respirations) will show compensation for the acidosis as the body blows off carbon dioxide, a respiratory acid.

 NCLEX® Connection: Physiological Adaptation, Fluid and Electrolyte Imbalances

UNIT 13: NURSING CARE OF CLIENTS WITH IMMUNE SYSTEM DISORDERS AND INFECTIOUS DISORDERS

- Diagnostic and Therapeutic Procedures
- Immune Disorders
- Autoimmune Disorders
- Cancer-Related Disorders
- Infectious Disorders

NCLEX® CONNECTIONS

When reviewing the chapters in this unit, keep in mind the relevant sections of the NCLEX® outline, in particular:

CLIENT NEEDS: HEALTH PROMOTION AND MAINTENANCE	CLIENT NEEDS: PHARMACOLOGICAL AND PARENTERAL THERAPIES	CLIENT NEEDS: REDUCTION OF RISK POTENTIAL
Relevant topics/tasks include:	Relevant topics/tasks include:	Relevant topics/tasks include:
• Health Promotion/Disease Prevention	• Medication Administration	• Alterations in Body Systems
○ Educate the client on actions to promote/maintain health and prevent disease.	○ Administer and document medications given by parenteral routes.	○ Identify signs, symptoms, and incubation periods of infectious diseases.
• Health Screening	• Parenteral/Intravenous Therapy	○ Provide care for the client with an infectious disease.
○ Apply knowledge of pathophysiology to health screening.	○ Monitor the use of an infusion pump.	○ Evaluate the client's response to treatment for an infectious disease.
• High-Risk Behaviors	• Pharmacological Pain Management	
○ Provide information for the prevention of high-risk health behaviors.	○ Administer and document pharmacological pain management appropriate for client age and diagnoses.	

UNIT 13	NURSING CARE OF CLIENTS WITH IMMUNE SYSTEM DISORDERS AND INFECTIOUS DISORDERS
Section	Diagnostic and Therapeutic Procedures
Chapter 98	**Immune and Infectious Disorders Diagnostic Procedures**

Overview

- Diagnostic procedures for immune and infectious disorders involve identification of pathogenic microorganisms. The most accurate and definitive way to identify microorganisms and cell characteristics is by examining blood, body fluids, and tissue samples under a microscope.

- Immune and infectious disorders diagnostic procedures that nurses should be knowledgeable about

  ○ Serum WBC count with differential

  ○ Radioallergosorbent test

  ○ Skin testing for allergens

- Effective treatment of infectious disease begins with identification of the pathogenic microorganism.

White Blood Cells

- WBCs, or leukocytes, stimulate the inflammatory response and offer protection against various types of infection and foreign antigens.

- There are five types of WBCs. Laboratory analysis of these various types of circulating WBCs is called the differential. The differential on the laboratory report is listed so the percentages of cells equal 100%. This number is arrived at by counting the number of each type of cell in a representative sample of 100 WBCs and multiplying it by 100. If the percent of one type of cell increases, the percents of other types decrease accordingly.

- Interpretation of Findings

  ○ The normal reference range for WBCs is 5,000 to 10,000/mm^3. A healthy older adult can have a range of 3,000 to 9,000/mm^3.

  ○ A total WBC count less than 4,300/mm^3 is called leukopenia. It may indicate a compromised inflammatory response or viral infection.

  ○ A count greater than 10,000/mm^3 is called leukocytosis. It may indicate an inflammatory response to a pathogen or a disease process.

- ○ A neutrophil count less than 2,000/mm³ is called neutropenia. Neutropenia occurs in clients who are immunocompromised, are undergoing chemotherapy, or have a process that reduces the production of neutrophils. A client with neutropenia is at an increased risk for infection.

  - ■ Clients who have neutropenia may also have an absolute neutrophil count calculated by multiplying the total WBC count by the summed number of neutrophils and bands and then dividing by 100. Neutropenic precautions (a private room; designated equipment; restricted exposure to live plants, ingestion of fresh fruits, and vegetables) will be instituted if the client's ANC is 1.0 or less.

- ○ An increase in "banded," or immature neutrophils indicates an infectious process is present and is called a "left shift." This occurs in response to an increased production of neutrophils in response to the infection, allowing the release of some before full maturity is reached.

TYPE OF WBC	PERCENT OF CIRCULATING WBCS	INCREASED IN RELATION TO:	DECREASED IN RELATION TO:	ADDITIONAL INFORMATION
Neutrophils	55% to 75%	• Acute bacterial infections • Fungal infections	• Sepsis • Radiation therapy, aplastic anemia, chemotherapy, and influenza	• The majority of neutrophils are segmented (mature) with a lesser amount being banded (not fully mature). • Immature neutrophils should not be found in the blood.
Lymphocytes (T cells and B cells)	20% to 40%	• Chronic bacterial or viral infection • Viruses such as mononucleosis, mumps, and measles • Bacteria such as hepatitis • Lymphocytic leukemia, multiple myeloma	• Leukemia • Sepsis	• T-lymphocytes initiate cell-mediated immunity. • B-lymphocytes initiate humoral immunity.

TYPE OF WBC	PERCENT OF CIRCULATING WBCS	INCREASED IN RELATION TO:	DECREASED IN RELATION TO:	ADDITIONAL INFORMATION
Monocytes	2% to 8%	• Chronic inflammation • Protozoal infections • Tuberculosis • Viral infections such as mononucleosis, mumps, and measles	Corticosteroids	
Eosinophils	1% to 4%	• Allergic reactions • Parasitic infections • Chronic inflammation • Hodgkin's disease	• Stress • Corticosteroids	
Basophils	0.5% to 1%	Leukemia	• Acute allergic/ hypersensitivity reaction • Hyperthyroidism	

Radioallergosorbent Test

- A radioallergosorbent test (RAST) is done on a sample of a client's blood to determine sensitivity to various allergens. It may be done in conjunction with skin testing or as an alternative when the risk of a hypersensitivity reaction to an allergen exists.

- The advantage to RAST testing is that it will not precipitate a dangerous allergic reaction in the client and is quicker to administer.

- The disadvantage to RAST testing is that it is available for fewer antigens, may be less sensitive than skin testing, and is more expensive

- Indications

  ○ Potential Diagnoses

    ▪ Suspected environmental and food allergies

  ○ Client Presentation

    ▪ Report of hypersensitivity reactions

    ▪ Presence of hives, asthma, and/or gastrointestinal dysfunction

- Interpretation of Findings

    - During the test, various radiolabeled allergens are exposed to the client's blood and the amount of the client's immunoglobulin E (IgE) that is attracted to each specific allergen is measured according to standardized values. If an allergen is not attracted, this is considered a negative result. If a client's IgE is attracted to an allergen, the amount is measured on a scale of 1 to 5 with the higher number indicating a higher level from sensitivity.

- Intraprocedure

    - Nursing Actions

        - Draw a blood sample.

- Postprocedure

    - Nursing Actions

        - Inform the client of when to expect results (usually takes at least a week).

Skin Testing for Allergens

- Skin testing for allergens involves the use of intradermal injections or scratching the superficial layer (scratch or prick test) of the skin with small amounts of suspected allergens.

- Intradermal testing runs a higher risk of hypersensitivity reactions and is usually done if the scratch test is inconclusive.

- Indications

    - Potential Diagnoses

        - Suspected environmental and food allergies

    - Client Presentation

        - Presence of hives, asthma, and/or gastrointestinal dysfunction

- Interpretation of Findings

    - Allergens that provoke a localized reaction (wheal and flare) are considered a positive reaction to that allergen.

    - The larger the reaction the stronger the allergy.

- Preprocedure

    - Nursing Actions

        - Prepare the client's skin for application of various allergens using soap and water (client's back or forearm are usually used for testing).

        - Alcohol may be used to remove oil from the client's skin.

        - Have equipment available for a possible anaphylaxis reaction.

- ○ Client Education
  - Instruct the client to avoid taking corticosteroids and antihistamines 5 days prior to the testing.

- Intraprocedure
  - ○ Nursing Actions
    - The client's skin is scratched or pricked with a needle after application of a drop of an allergen.
    - Standard pattern of application should be used so identification of the allergen can be done according to the location of the reaction.
    - Application of saline (negative control reaction) and histamine (positive control for reaction) should be done as a baseline for expected reactions.
    - An assessment of reactions is done after 15 to 20 min.

- Postprocedure
  - ○ Nursing Actions
    - Assess the client's skin for areas of reaction and document the allergen that is responsible.
    - Remove all solutions from the client's skin.
    - Inform the client when results will be available.
    - Recommend an antihistamine or topical corticosteroid if the client experiences itching secondary to the testing.
  - ○ Client Education
    - Teach desensitizing options and avoidance therapies to the client related to identifying allergens.
    - Advise the client to follow a special diet that eliminates allergens (gluten-free).

CHAPTER 98: IMMUNE AND INFECTIOUS DISORDERS DIAGNOSTIC PROCEDURES

Ⓐ Application Exercises

Scenario: A client comes to clinic with reports of urinary frequency and urgency. The nurse suspects a urinary tract infection and sends a urine specimen for culture and sensitivity to the laboratory. While awaiting culture and sensitivity results, the client is started on amikacin (Amikin) 15 mg/kg/day. She is allergic to sulfa medications. The results of the urine culture and sensitivity are as follows:

Urine midstream clean catch

Final Report:

Colony count: Greater than 100,000 colonies

Bacteria type: *Escherichia coli* (heavy growth)

Sensitivity:

MEDICATION	SUSCEPTIBILITY {R = RESISTANT, S = SENSITIVE TO MEDICATION (LEVELS 1 TO 4)}
Trimethoprim-sulfamethoxazole	S 4+
Amikacin	S 3+
Gentamicin	R
Tobramycin	S 1+
Cephalosporin	S
Ciprofloxacin	R
Amoxicillin	S 2+

1. Which of the following findings indicates the client has a urinary tract infection?

    A. Colony count greater than 100,000 colonies

    B. Susceptibility of R to gentamicin

    C. Report of urinary urgency and frequency

    D. Prescription for amikacin

2. According to the above data, which of the following medications should the nurse be sure the client is taking?

    A. Tobramycin

    B. Amikacin

    C. Ciprofloxacin

    D. Trimethoprim-sulfamethoxazole

3. A nurse is preparing to administer a scratch test on a client who has suspected multiple food and environmental allergies. Which of the following actions should the nurse perform prior to beginning the procedure? (Select all that apply.)

_____ Cleanse the client's skin with povidone-iodine (Betadine).

_____ Ask the client about previous reactions to allergens.

_____ Ask the client about medications taken over the past several days.

_____ Tell the client to expect itching at one site.

_____ Obtain emergency resuscitation equipment.

CHAPTER 98: IMMUNE AND INFECTIOUS DISORDERS DIAGNOSTIC PROCEDURES

(A) Application Exercises Answer Key

Scenario: A client comes to clinic with reports of urinary frequency and urgency. The nurse suspects a urinary tract infection and sends a urine specimen for culture and sensitivity to the laboratory. While awaiting culture and sensitivity results, the client is started on amikacin (Amikin) 15 mg/kg/day. She is allergic to sulfa medications. The results of the urine culture and sensitivity are as follows:

Urine midstream clean catch

Final report:

Colony count: Greater than 100,000 colonies

Bacteria type: *Escherichia coli* (heavy growth)

Sensitivity:

MEDICATION	SUSCEPTIBILITY	
Trimethoprim-sulfamethoxazole	S 4+	
Amikacin	S 3+	
Gentamicin	R	
Tobramycin	S 1+	
Cephalosporin	S	
Ciprofloxacin	R	R = Resistant
Amoxicillin	S 2+	S = Sensitive to medication (levels 1 to 4)

1. Which of the following findings indicates that the client has a urinary tract infection?

   A. Colony count greater than 100,000 colonies
   B. Susceptibility of R to gentamicin
   C. Report of urinary urgency and frequency
   D. Prescription for amikacin

   Heavy growth of greater than 100,000 colonies definitively diagnoses an infection. Susceptibility of "R" means that the antigen is not sensitive to the medication. While the report of urinary urgency and frequency is indicative of a urinary tract infection (UTI), it is not definitive for the diagnosis. The prescription for the broad-spectrum antibiotic amikacin was given to begin treatment for the most common type of bacteria found in urinary tract infections, E. coli, prior to definitively diagnosing with a culture.

    NCLEX® Connection: Physiological Adaptation, Infectious Disease

2. According to the above data, which of the following medications should the nurse be sure the client is taking?

    A. Tobramycin

    B. Amikacin

    C. Ciprofloxacin

    D. Trimethoprim-sulfamethoxazole

The client is receiving the most appropriate medication. Appropriate medications are those with 3 to 4+ degrees of sensitivity. Based on these results, the most sensitive medication is trimethoprim-sulfamethoxazole; however, the client is allergic to sulfa. Subsequently, the correct answer is amikacin, because it demonstrates a 3+ sensitivity to *E. coli*.

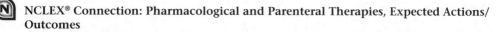 **NCLEX® Connection: Pharmacological and Parenteral Therapies, Expected Actions/ Outcomes**

3. A nurse is preparing to administer a scratch test on a client who has suspected multiple food and environmental allergies. Which of the following actions should the nurse perform prior to beginning the procedure? (Select all that apply.)

    _____ Cleanse the client's skin with povidone-iodine (Betadine).

    __**X**__ **Ask the client about previous reactions to allergens.**

    __**X**__ **Ask the client about medications taken over the past several days.**

    __**X**__ **Tell the client to expect itching at one site.**

    __**X**__ **Obtain emergency resuscitation equipment.**

The nurse should ask if the client has had any previous reactions to allergens that could indicate an increased risk of an anaphylactic reaction. Emergency equipment should be available even if the client denies such a reaction. The client should be asked if any antihistamines or corticosteroids were taken within 5 days of testing due to their ability to suppress reactions. Since histamine will be applied as a control site, the client will experience itching at this site. The nurse should use soap and water to cleanse the skin, not povidone-iodine, which could interfere with an allergen and elicit a response.

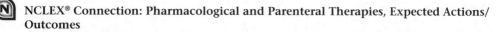 **NCLEX® Connection: Reduction of Risk Potential, Potential for Complications of Diagnostic Tests/Treatments/Procedures**

UNIT 13	NURSING CARE OF CLIENTS WITH IMMUNE SYSTEM DISORDERS AND INFECTIOUS DISORDERS
Section	Diagnostic and Therapeutic Procedures
Chapter 99	Immunizations

Overview

- Administration of a vaccine causes production of antibodies that prevent illness from a specific microbe.

- Adaptive immunity allows the body to make antibodies in response to a foreign organism. Adaptive immunity can be active or passive or natural or artificial.

- Active-natural immunity develops when the body produces antibodies in response to exposure to a live pathogen. Active-artificial immunity develops when a vaccine is given and the body produces antibodies in response to exposure to a killed or attenuated virus.

- Passive-natural occurs when antibodies are passed from the mother to the fetus/newborn through the placenta and then breastfeeding. Passive-artificial immunity occurs after antibodies in the form of immune globulins are administered to an individual who requires immediate protection against a disease where exposure has already occurred.

- Vaccines may be made from killed viruses or live, attenuated (or weakened) viruses.

Medication Classification: Vaccinations

- The 2010 Centers for Disease Control and Prevention (CDC) vaccination recommendations for adults (18 years and older) (Go to www.cdc.gov for updates.)

  o Tetanus diphtheria (Td) booster – Give booster every 10 years. For adults 19 to 64 years of age who did not receive a dose of tetanus diphtheria, pertussis (Tdap) previously, substitute one dose with Tdap.

  o Measles, mumps and rubella vaccine (MMR) – Give one to two doses at ages 19 to 49.

  o Varicella vaccine – Give two doses to adults who do not have evidence of a previous infection. A second dose should be given to adults who have had only one previous dose.

  o Pneumococcal polysaccharide vaccine (PPSV) – Vaccinate adults who are immunocompromised, who have a chronic disease, who smoke cigarettes, or who live in a long-term care facility. CDC guidelines should be followed for revaccination. Give one dose to adults older than 65 years of age who have not previously been vaccinated nor have history of disease.

o   Hepatitis A – Two doses for high-risk individuals

o   Hepatitis B – Three doses for high-risk individuals

o   Seasonal influenza vaccine – Give one dose annually. Recommended for all adults older than 50; health care providers, including those who care for young children; individuals who have chronic medical conditions such as cerebral palsy, asthma, and diabetes mellitus; individuals who are immunocompromised; and individuals living in long-term care settings. Note that the live attenuated vaccine (LAIV), given as a nasal spray is only indicated for adults under age 50 or for those who are not pregnant or immunocompromised.

o   Meningococcal conjugate vaccine (MCV4) – Given to students entering college and living in college dormitories, if not previously immunized. Meningococcal polysaccharide vaccine (MPSV) is recommended for adults older than 56 years of age. Revaccination may be recommended after 5 years for adults at high risk for infection, such as adults without a spleen, military recruits, or adults traveling to a country that is hyperendemic or epidemic.

o   Human papilloma virus (HPV2 or HPV4) – Given in three doses and recommended for females up to age 26 who were not vaccinated as children. The second dose should be administered 2 months after the first dose, and the third dose should be administered 6 months after the first dose.

   ■   HPV4 – This vaccine is given to males up to age 26

o   Herpes zoster vaccine – Recommended for all adults over age 60 years.

Purpose

- Expected Pharmacological Action

   o   Immunizations produce antibodies that provide active immunity. Immunizations may take months to have an effect, but provide long-lasting protection against infectious diseases.

- Therapeutic Uses

   o   Eradication of infectious diseases (polio, smallpox)

   o   Prevention of childhood and adult infectious diseases and their complications (measles, diphtheria, mumps, rubella, tetanus, H. influenza)

Contraindications/Precautions

- An anaphylactic reaction to a vaccine is a contraindication for further doses of that vaccine.

- An anaphylactic reaction to a vaccine is a contraindication to use of other vaccines containing the same substance.

- Moderate or severe illnesses with or without fever are contraindications for use of a vaccine. With acute febrile illness, vaccination is deferred until symptoms resolve. The common cold and other minor illnesses are not contraindications.

○ Contraindications to vaccinations require the primary care provider to analyze data and weigh the risks that come with or without vaccinating.

○ Individuals who are immunocompromised are defined by the CDC as those who have hematologic or solid tumors, who have congenital immunodeficiency, or are receiving long-term immunosuppressive therapy, including corticosteroids.

IMMUNIZATIONS	SIDE EFFECTS	CONTRAINDICATIONS
Td or DTaP	• Local reaction at injection site	• Severe febrile illness • A history of prior anaphylactic reaction to the DTaP vaccination • An occurrence of encephalopathy 7 days after the administration of the DTaP immunization • An occurrence of seizures within 3 days of the vaccination • A history of uncontrollable crying that could not be consoled by parents after receiving prior vaccination; may last more than 3 hr and occurs within 48 hr of the vaccination
MMR	• Local reactions such as rash; fever; and swollen glands in cheeks, neck, and under the jaw • Possibility of joint pain lasting for days to weeks. • Risk for anaphylaxis and thrombocytopenia	• Pregnancy • Allergy to gelatin and neomycin (Mycifradin) • Clients who are immunocompromised (with HIV infection or from medication administration) • Recent transfusion with blood products
Varicella vaccine (two doses)	• Varicella-like rash that may be local or generalized, such as vesicles on the body • Fever, malaise, and anorexia	• Pregnancy ○ Women who are pregnant should avoid close proximity to children who are recently vaccinated. • Cancers of blood and lymphatic system • Allergy to gelatin and neomycin • Clients who are immunocompromised (with HIV infection or from medication administration)

IMMUNIZATIONS	SIDE EFFECTS	CONTRAINDICATIONS
Pneumococcal vaccine (PCV) (one or two doses)	• Mild local reactions, fever, and no serious adverse effects	• Pregnancy
Hepatitis A (two doses) Hepatitis B (three doses)	• Local reaction at injection site	• Hep A ○ Pregnancy may be a contraindication • Hep B ○ A prior history of anaphylactic reaction ○ An allergy to baker's yeast
Seasonal influenza vaccine (one dose annually)	• Inactivated – Mild local reaction, and fever • Live attenuated – Headache, cough, and fever • Rare – Risk for Guillain-Barré syndrome, manifested by ascending paralysis beginning with weakness of lower extremities and progressing to difficulty breathing or respiratory arrest	• Live attenuated influenza vaccine administered as a nasal spray is contraindicated for adults who are older than 50, are immunocompromised, or have a chronic disease. • History of Guillain-Barré syndrome
Meningococcal Conjugate vaccine (MCV4) (one or more doses)	• Mild local reaction and rare risk of allergic response	• History of Guillain-Barré syndrome
Human papilloma virus (HPV2 or HPV4) vaccine (three doses) The second dose should be administered 2 months after the first dose; the third dose should be administered 6 months after the first dose.	• Mild local reaction and fever • Fainting has occurred shortly after receiving vaccination • Rare – Risk for Guillain-Barré syndrome	• Pregnancy
Herpes zoster		• Clients who are immunocompromised (with HIV infection or from medication administration)

Medication/Food Interactions

- None significant

Nursing Administration

- For adults

  - Give subcutaneous vaccinations in outer aspect of the upper arm or anterolateral thigh.

  - Give intramuscular vaccinations into the deltoid muscle for adults.

- For clients of all ages

  - Have emergency medications and equipment on standby in case the client experiences an allergic response such as anaphylaxis (rare).

  - Follow storage and reconstitution directions. If reconstituted, use within 30 min.

  - Provide written vaccine information sheets and review the content with clients.

  - Instruct clients to observe for complications and to notify the provider if side effects occur.

  - Document administration of vaccines including date, route, site, type, manufacturer, lot number, and expiration of vaccine. Also document the client's name, address, and signature.

Nursing Evaluation of Medication Effectiveness

- Depending on the therapeutic intent of the vaccine, effectiveness may be evidenced by:

  - Improvement of local reaction with absence of pain, fever, and swelling at the site of injection.

  - Development of immunity.

CHAPTER 99: IMMUNIZATIONS

Ⓐ Application Exercises

1. A client is asking a nurse about strategies to promote comfort after receiving an immunization. Which of the following strategies should the nurse recommend? (Select all that apply.)

_____ Massage the site.

_____ Apply a cool compress to the site.

_____ Take acetaminophen or ibuprofen.

_____ Encourage the use of the affected extremity.

_____ Apply an antimicrobial ointment.

2. A client has been exposed to Hepatitis A and has not received the vaccine for this disease. The nurse is preparing to give the client an IM injection of immunoglobulin to impart which of the following types of immunity?

A. Active-natural

B. Active-artificial

C. Passive-natural

D. Passive-artificial

3. Which of the following questions should a nurse ask a client who is preparing to receive a varicella vaccine?

A. "Are you allergic to aluminum?"

B. "Are you allergic to baker's yeast?"

C. "Are you pregnant?"

D. "Have you had a recent blood transfusion?"

CHAPTER 99: IMMUNIZATIONS

 Application Exercises Answer Key

1. A client is asking a nurse about strategies to promote comfort after receiving an immunization. Which of the following strategies should the nurse recommend? (Select all that apply.)

_____	Massage the site.
__X__	**Apply a cool compress to the site.**
__X__	**Take acetaminophen or ibuprofen.**
__X__	**Encourage the use of the affected extremity.**
_____	Apply an antimicrobial ointment.

Cool compresses, administration of acetaminophen or ibuprofen, and encouraging gentle use of the extremity are all comfort strategies useful for discomfort in an injection site. Massaging the site is not recommended for an extended period of time after the injection, and use of an antimicrobial ointment is not indicated.

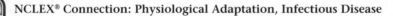

NCLEX® Connection: Reduction of Risk Potential, Potential for Complications of Diagnostic Tests/Treatments/Procedures

2. A client has been exposed to Hepatitis A and has not received the vaccine for this disease. The nurse is preparing to give the client an IM injection of immunoglobulin to impart which of the following types of immunity?

A. Active-natural

B. Active-artificial

C. Passive-natural

D. Passive-artificial

Passive artificial immunity will allow the client to receive some protection against Hepatitis A quicker than the body would be able to respond. This type of protection is temporary, so a Hepatitis A immunization should be administered when the client is not receiving immunoglobulins.

NCLEX® Connection: Physiological Adaptation, Infectious Disease

3. Which of the following questions should a nurse ask a client who is preparing to receive a varicella vaccine?

      A. "Are you allergic to aluminum?"

      B. "Are you allergic to baker's yeast?"

      C. "Are you pregnant?"

      D. "Have you had a recent blood transfusion?"

Prior to administering a varicella vaccination, the nurse should ask the client if she is pregnant. If so, the client should wait until after the pregnancy to be vaccinated. Immunization against Hepatitis A and B are contraindicated in individuals who are allergic to aluminum and baker's yeast. Clients who have recently received a blood transfusion should not receive an MMR vaccine.

(N) **NCLEX® Connection: Physiological Adaptation, Infectious Disease**

UNIT 13   NURSING CARE OF CLIENTS WITH IMMUNE SYSTEM DISORDERS
            AND INFECTIOUS DISORDERS

Section   Immune Disorders

Chapter 100 HIV/AIDS

Overview

- Human immunodeficiency virus (HIV) is a retrovirus that is transmitted through blood and body fluids (semen, vaginal secretions).

- HIV targets CD4+ lymphocytes, also known as T-cells or T-lymphocytes.

    o   T-cells work in concert with B-lymphocytes. Both are part of specific acquired (adaptive) immunity.

    o   HIV integrates its RNA into host cell DNA through reverse transcriptase, reshaping the host's immune system.

- HIV is found in feces, urine, tears, saliva, cerebrospinal fluid, cervical cells, lymph nodes, corneal tissue, and brain tissue, but epidemiologic studies indicate that these are unlikely sources of infection.

- All women who are pregnant should be screened for HIV.

- HIV infection is one continuous disease process with three stages.

    o   Primary HIV-1 infection

        ▪   Manifestations occur within 2 to 4 weeks of infection.

        ▪   Symptoms are similar to those of influenza.

        ▪   This stage is marked by a rapid rise in the HIV viral load, decreased CD4+ cells, and increased CD8 cells.

        ▪   The resolution of clinical manifestations coincides with the decline in viral HIV copies.

        ▪   Lymphadenopathy persists throughout the disease process.

    o   Chronic asymptomatic infection

        ▪   This stage may be prolonged and clinically silent (asymptomatic).

        ▪   The client may remain asymptomatic for 10 years or more.

        ▪   Anti-HIV antibodies are produced (HIV positive).

- Over time, the virus begins active replication using the host's genetic machinery.
  - CD4+ cells are destroyed.
  - The viral load increases.
  - Dramatic loss of immunity begins.
- AIDS
  - This stage is characterized by life-threatening opportunistic infections.
  - This is the end stage of HIV infection.
  - Without treatment, death occurs within 3 to 5 years.
  - All people with AIDS have HIV, but not all people with HIV have AIDS.

Health Promotion and Disease Prevention

- Teach the client how the virus is transmitted and ways to prevent infection.
- Encourage the client to maintain up-to-date immunizations, including yearly seasonal influenza and pneumococcal polysaccharide vaccine (PPSV).

Assessment

- Risk Factors
  - Unprotected sex (vaginal, anal, oral)
  - Multiple sex partners
  - Occupational exposure (healthcare workers)
  - Perinatal exposure
  - Blood transfusions (not a significant source of infection in the U.S.)
  - Intravenous drug use with a contaminated needle
  - HIV infection may go undiagnosed in older adult clients due to the similarity of its manifestations to other illnesses that are common in this age group.
  - Older adults are more susceptible to fluid and electrolyte imbalances, malnutrition, skin alterations, and wasting syndrome than younger adults.
  - Older women experience vaginal dryness and thinning of the vaginal wall, increasing their susceptibility to HIV infection.
- Subjective Data
  - Chills
  - Anorexia, nausea, and weight loss
  - Weakness and fatigue
  - Headache
  - Night sweats

- Objective Data
  - Physical Assessment Findings and Laboratory Data
    - A confirmed case classification meets the laboratory criteria for a diagnosis of HIV infection and one of the four HIV infection stages (stage 1, stage 2, stage 3, or unknown).

STAGE	DEFINING CONDITIONS	CD4+ T-LYMPHOCYTE COUNT	CD4+ T-LYMPHOCYTE PERCENTAGE OF TOTAL LYMPHOCYTES
Stage 1	• None	500 cells/mEq/L or more	29 or more
Stage 2	• One or more of the infections of Stage 3	200 to 499 cells/mEq/L	14 to 28
Stage 3 (AIDS)*	• Candidiasis of the esophagus, bronchi, trachea, or lungs • Herpes simplex – Chronic ulcers (of more than 1 month's duration) • HIV-related encephalopathy • Disseminated or extrapulmonary histoplasmosis • Kaposi's sarcoma • Burkitt's lymphoma • Mycobacterium tuberculosis of any site • *Pneumocystis jirovecii* pneumonia • Recurrent pneumonia • Progressive multifocal leukoencephalopathy • Recurrent *Salmonella septicemia* • Wasting syndrome attributed to HIV	less than 200 cells/mEq/L	less than 14
Stage unknown	• No information available	No information available	No information available

*Documentation of an AIDS-defining condition supersedes a CD4+ T-lymphocyte count of 200 cells/mEq/L or more and a CD4+ T-lymphocyte percentage of total lymphocytes of more than 14.

RN ADULT MEDICAL SURGICAL NURSING

Human Immunodeficiency Virus Infection (HIV) (retrieved 3/18/10 from http://www.cdc.gov). To read more about HIV, go to the Web site of the Centers for Disease Control and Prevention (http://www.cdc.gov).

- CBC and differential – Abnormal (anemia, thrombocytopenia, leukopenia)

- Platelet Count – Decreased less than 150,000/mm^3

  o Diagnostic Procedures

  - HIV determination

    □ Positive result from an HIV antibody screening test (reactive enzyme immunoassay [EIA]) confirmed by a positive result from a supplemental HIV antibody test (Western blot or indirect immunofluorescence assay test)

    □ Positive result or report of a detectable quantity from any of the following HIV virologic (non-antibody) tests:

      ▸ HIV nucleic acid (DNA or RNA) detection test (polymerase chain reaction [PCR])

      ▸ HIV p24 antigen test, including neutralization assay

      ▸ HIV isolation (viral culture)

  - Liver profile, biopsies, and testing of stool for parasites

    □ Nursing Actions

      ▸ Prepare the client for the test.

    □ Client Education

      ▸ Inform the client about the details of the test, such as length and what to expect.

  - Brain or lung MRI or CT scan

    □ Detailed image of the brain or lung to detect abnormalities

    □ Nursing Actions

      ▸ Prepare the client for the procedure.

    □ Client Education

      ▸ Inform the client about the length of time the test takes (sometimes up to 1 hr).

Collaborative Care

- Nursing Care

  - Assess risk factors (sexual practices, IV drug use).

  - Monitor fluid intake/urinary output.

- ■ Obtain daily weights to monitor weight loss.

- ■ Monitor nutritional intake.

- ■ Monitor electrolytes.

- ■ Assess skin integrity (rashes, open areas, bruising).

- ■ Assess the client's pain status.

- ■ Monitor vital signs (especially temperature).

- ■ Assess lung sounds/respiratory status (diminished lung sounds).

- ■ Assess neurological status (confusion, dementia, visual changes).

- o Encourage activity alternated with rest periods.

- o Administer supplemental oxygen as needed.

- o Provide analgesia as needed.

- o Provide skin care as needed.

- • Medications

  - o Highly active antiretroviral therapy (HAART) involves using 3 to 4 HIV medications in combination with other antiretroviral medications to reduce medication resistance, adverse effects, and dosages.

    - ■ Entry/infusion inhibitors – Enfuvirtide (Fuzeon)

      - □ Helps to decrease the amount of virus in the body and limit its spread

    - ■ Nucleoside reverse transcriptase inhibitors (NRTIs) – Zidovudine (Retrovir)

      - □ Interfere with the virus's ability to convert RNA into DNA

    - ■ Non-nucleoside reverse transcriptase inhibitors (NNRTIs) – Delavirdine (Rescriptor) and efavirenz (Sustiva)

      - □ Inhibit viral replication in cells

    - ■ Protease inhibitors – Amprenavir (Agenerase), nelfinavir (Viracept), saquinavir (Invirase), and indinavir (Crixivan)

      - □ Inhibit an enzyme needed for the virus to replicate

    - ■ Antineoplastic medication – Interleukin (Interferon)

      - □ Immunostimulant that enhances the immune response and reduces the production of cancer cells (used commonly with Kaposi's sarcoma)

  - o Nursing Considerations

    - ■ Monitor laboratory results (CBC, WBC, liver function tests). Antiretroviral medications may increase alanine aminotransferase (ALT), aspartate aminotransferase (AST), bilirubin, mean corpuscular volume (MCV), high-density lipoproteins (HDLs), total cholesterol, and triglycerides.

- o Client Education
  - ■ Educate the client about the side effects of the medications and ways to decrease the severity of the side effects.
  - ■ Educate the client about the need to take medications on a regular schedule and to not miss doses.

- Interdisciplinary Care
  - o Infectious disease services may be consulted to manage HIV.
  - o Respiratory services may be consulted to improve respiratory status.
  - o Nutritional services may be consulted for dietary supplementation.
  - o Rehabilitation services may be consulted for strengthening and improving the client's level of energy.

- Therapeutic Procedures
  - o Vitamins, herbal products, and shark cartilage may help alleviate the symptoms of HIV.
    - ■ Ask the client if she is taking herbal products. These can alter the effects of the prescribed medications.

- Care After Discharge
  - o Refer the client to local AIDS support groups as appropriate.
  - o Home health service may be indicated for clients who need help with strengthening and assistance regarding ADLs.
  - o Home health services may also provide assistance with IVs, dressing changes, and total parenteral nutrition (TPN).
  - o Respiratory services may be consulted for providing portable oxygen.
  - o Long-term care facilities may be indicated for clients with chronic HIV.
  - o Hospice services may be indicated for clients who have a late stage of HIV.
  - o Food services may be indicated for clients who are homebound and need meals prepared.
  - o Client Education
    - ■ Instruct the client to practice good hygiene and frequent hand hygiene to reduce the risk of infection.
    - ■ Instruct the client to avoid crowded areas or traveling to countries with poor sanitation.
    - ■ Encourage the client to avoid raw foods, such as vegetables and meats.
    - ■ Instruct the client to avoid cleaning pet litter boxes to reduce the risk of toxoplasmosis.

- Encourage the client to keep the home environment clean and to avoid being exposed to family and friends who have colds or flu viruses.

- Provide client teaching regarding:

  - Transmission, infection control measures, and safe sex practices

  - The importance of maintaining a well-balanced diet

  - Self-administration of prescribed medications and potential side effects

  - Signs/symptoms that need to be reported immediately (infection)

- Instruct the client to adhere to the antiretroviral dosing schedules.

- Instruct the client about the need for frequent follow-up monitoring of CD4+ and viral load counts.

- Encourage the use of constructive coping mechanisms.

- Assist the client with identifying primary support systems.

- Teach the client to report signs of infection immediately to the health care provider.

- Client Outcomes

  o The client will have adequate gas exchange.

  o The client will be free from pain.

  o The client will be able to maintain a weight within 10% of ideal body weight.

  o The client will adhere to the prescribed medication regimen.

Complications

- Opportunistic infections

  o Bacterial diseases, such as tuberculosis, bacterial pneumonia, and septicemia (blood poisoning)

  o HIV-associated malignancies, such as Kaposi's sarcoma, lymphoma, and squamous cell carcinoma

  o Viral diseases, such as those caused by cytomegalovirus, herpes simplex, and herpes zoster virus

  o Fungal diseases, such as PCP, candidiasis, cryptococcosis, and penicilliosis

  o Protozoal diseases, such as toxoplasmosis, microsporidiosis, cryptosporidiosis, isosporiasis, and leishmaniasis

  o Nursing Actions

    - Implement and maintain anti-retroviral medication therapy as prescribed.

    - Administer antineoplastics, antibiotics, analgesics, antifungals, and antidiarrheals as prescribed.

    - Administer appetite stimulants (to enhance nutrition).

- Monitor for skin breakdown.
- Maintain fluid intake.
- Maintain nutrition.
  - o Client Education
    - Teach the client to report signs of infection immediately to the health care provider.
- Wasting syndrome
  - o Nursing Actions
    - Maintain nutrition orally or by TPN if indicated.
    - Provide between-meal supplements/snacks.
    - Serve at least six small feedings with high protein value.
- Fluid/Electrolyte imbalance
  - o Nursing Actions
    - Monitor fluid/electrolyte status.
    - Report abnormal laboratory data promptly.
    - Maintain IV fluid replacement.
- Seizures (HIV encephalopathy)
  - o Nursing Actions
    - Maintain client safety.
    - Implement seizure precautions.

CHAPTER 100: HIV/AIDS

 Application Exercises

1. A client visits an outpatient clinic and reports night sweats and fatigue. He states that he has a cough, has been nauseated, and is having abdominal pain and frequent diarrhea. His temperature is 38.1° C (100.6° F) orally. He states that he is afraid he has HIV. Which of the following actions should be the nurse's priority? (Select all that apply.)

_____ Perform a physical assessment.

_____ Determine when current symptoms began.

_____ Teach the client about disease transmission.

_____ Draw blood for HIV testing.

_____ Offer emotional support.

_____ Initiate oxygen therapy.

_____ Initiate IV access for medications.

_____ Obtain a sexual history.

2. A nurse is caring for a client who is suspected of having HIV. Which of the following diagnostic tests and laboratory values are used to confirm HIV infection? (Select all that apply.)

_____ HIV p24 antigen test

_____ HIV isolation (viral culture)

_____ CD4+ T-lymphocyte count

_____ CD4+ T-lymphocyte percentage of total lymphocytes

_____ Cerebrospinal fluid (CSF) analysis

CHAPTER 100: HIV/AIDS

 Application Exercises Answer Key

1. A client visits an outpatient clinic and reports night sweats and fatigue. He states that he has a cough, has been nauseated, and is having abdominal pain and frequent diarrhea. His temperature is 38.1° C (100.6° F) orally. He states that he is afraid he has HIV. Which of the following actions should be the nurse's priority? (Select all that apply.)

X	**Perform a physical assessment.**
X	**Determine when current symptoms began.**
_____	Teach the client about disease transmission.
_____	Draw blood for HIV testing.
_____	Offer emotional support.
_____	Initiate oxygen therapy.
_____	Initiate IV access for medications.
X	**Obtain a sexual history.**

Using the nursing process, assessment is the highest priority. Therefore, the priority nursing interventions are to perform a physical assessment, determine when current symptoms began, and obtain a sexual history. The other options are interventions for the nurse to take, but none of them is a priority at this time.

 NCLEX® Connection: Physiological Adaptation, Infectious Disease

2. A nurse is caring for a client who is suspected of having HIV. Which of the following diagnostic tests and laboratory values are used to confirm HIV infection? (Select all that apply.)

X	**HIV p24 antigen test**
X	**HIV isolation (viral culture)**
_____	CD4+ T-lymphocyte count
_____	CD4+ T-lymphocyte percentage of total lymphocytes
_____	Cerebrospinal fluid (CSF) analysis

Positive results or reports of a detectable quantity from HIV p24 antigen test and HIV isolation (viral culture) confirm the presence of HIV infection. The CD4+ T-lymphocyte count and CD4+ T-lymphocyte percentage of total lymphocytes assist with classifying the stage of HIV infection. CSF analysis may be used to confirm meningitis.

NCLEX® Connection: Physiological Adaptation, Infectious Disease

UNIT 13   NURSING CARE OF CLIENTS WITH IMMUNE SYSTEM DISORDERS
            AND INFECTIOUS DISORDERS

Section   Autoimmune Disorders

Chapter 101 Systemic Lupus Erythematosus

Overview

- Systemic lupus erythematosus (SLE) is an autoimmune disorder in which an atypical immune response results in chronic inflammation and destruction of healthy tissue.

  - In autoimmune disorders, small antigens may bond with healthy tissue. The body then produces antibodies that attack the healthy tissue. This may be triggered by toxins, medications, bacteria, and/or viruses.

  - Control of symptoms and decrease in number of exacerbations is the goal of treatment, because there is no cure for autoimmune disorders.

  - Other autoimmune disorders are rheumatoid arthritis, vasculitis, multiple sclerosis, scleroderma (including Raynaud's phenomenon), and psoriasis.

  - Occurrence of autoimmune disorders increases with age.

- SLE varies in severity and progression. It is generally characterized by periods of exacerbations (flares) and remissions.

- SLE is classified as discoid or systemic. A temporary form of SLE may be medication-induced.

  - Discoid SLE primarily affects the skin. It is characterized by an erythematosus butterfly rash over the nose and cheeks and is generally self-limiting.

  - Systemic SLE affects the connective tissues of multiple organ systems and can lead to major organ failure.

  - Medication-induced SLE can be caused by medications (procainamide, hydralazine, isoniazid). Symptoms resolve when the medication is discontinued, and it does not cause renal or neurologic disease.

- SLE may be difficult to diagnose because of the vagueness of early symptoms.

Assessment

- Risk Factors

  - Females between the ages of 15 and 40 are at risk.

  - African American, Asian, or Native American descent poses a risk.

- o The incidence of lupus drops in women following menopause but remains steady in men.

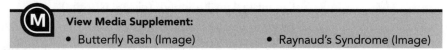

- o Diagnosis of SLE may be delayed in older adult clients because many of the clinical manifestations mimic other disorders or may be associated with reports common to the normal aging process.

  - Joint pain and swelling may significantly limit ADLs in older adult clients with comorbidities.

  - Older adult clients are at an increased risk for fractures if corticosteroid therapy is used.

- Subjective Data

  - o Fatigue/malaise

  - o Alopecia

  - o Anorexia/weight loss

  - o Depression

- Objective Data

  - o Physical Assessment Findings

    - Fever (also a major symptom of exacerbation)

    - Joint pain, swelling, and tenderness

    - Anemia

    - Lymphadenopathy

    - Raynaud's phenomenon (arteriolar vasospasm in response to cold/stress)

    - Findings consistent with organ involvement (kidney, heart, lungs and vasculature)

    - Butterfly rash on face

View Media Supplement:
- Butterfly Rash (Image)   • Raynaud's Syndrome (Image)

  - o Laboratory Tests

    - Autoantibodies

      - Antinuclear antibody (ANA) titer (antibody produced against one's own DNA) – Positive ANA titer in 90% of clients with lupus (normal is negative ANA titer at 1:20 dilution)

    - Anti-DNA – Positive (not specific for SLE but positive in the vast majority of clients with SLE)

- Extractible nuclear antibodies (ENAs) specific for selected parts of a cell's nucleus
  - Anti-Smith (anti-Sm) – Positive (highly specific for SLE)
  - Anti-RO (SSA) – Positive
  - Anti-LA (SSB) – Positive
  - Anti-RNP – Positive
  - Anti-phospholipids (AP) – Positive
- Serum complement (C3, C4) – Decreased
  - The complement system is made up of proteins (there are nine major complement proteins). These proteins work with the immune system and play a role in the development of inflammation. C3 and C4 are diagnostic for SLE because they decrease due to depletion secondary to an exaggerated inflammatory response.
- BUN and Serum Creatinine – Elevated (with renal involvement)
- Urinalysis – Positive for protein and RBCs (renal involvement)
- CBC – Pancytopenia

Collaborative Care

- Nursing Care
  - Assess/Monitor
    - Pain, mobility, and fatigue
    - Vital signs (especially blood pressure)
    - Systemic manifestations
      - Hypertension and edema (renal compromise)
      - Urine output (renal compromise)
      - Diminished breath sounds (pleural effusion)
      - Tachycardia and sharp inspiratory chest pain (pericarditis)
      - Rubor, pallor, and cyanosis of hands/feet (vasculitis/vasospasm, Raynaud's phenomenon)
      - Arthralgias, myalgias, and polyarthritis (joint and connective tissue involvement)
      - Changes in mental status that indicate neurologic involvement (psychoses, paresis, seizures)
      - BUN, serum creatinine, and urinary output for renal involvement
      - Nutritional status
  - Provide small, frequent meals if anorexia is a concern. Offer between-meal supplements.

- o Encourage the client to limit salt intake for fluid retention secondary to steroid therapy.

- o Provide emotional support to the client and family.

- Medications

  - o NSAIDs

    - Used to reduce inflammation

    - Nursing Considerations

      - □ NSAISs are contraindicated for clients with renal compromise.

      - □ Monitor for NSAID-induced hepatitis.

  - o Corticosteroids

    - Used for immunosuppression and to reduce inflammation

    - Nursing Considerations

      - □ Monitor for fluid retention, hypertension, and renal dysfunction.

    - Client Education

      - □ Do not stop taking steroids or decrease the dose abruptly.

  - o Immunosuppressant agents – Methotrexate and azathioprine (Imuran)

    - Used to suppress the immune response

    - Nursing Considerations

      - □ Monitor for toxic effects (bone marrow suppression, increased liver enzymes).

  - o Antimalarial – Hydroxychloroquine (Plaquenil)

    - Used for suppression of synovitis, fever, and fatigue

    - Nursing Considerations

      - □ Encourage frequent eye examinations.

- Interdisciplinary Care

  - o Physical and occupational may be used therapy for strengthening exercises and adaptive devices as needed.

  - o Refer clients to support groups as appropriate.

- Care After Discharge

  - o Client Education

    - Teach the client regarding the need to:

      - □ Avoid UV and sun exposure. The client should use sunscreen when outside and exposed to sunlight.

      - □ Use mild protein shampoo and avoid harsh hair treatments.

- □ Use steroid creams for skin rash.

- □ Report peripheral and periorbital edema promptly.

- □ Report signs/symptoms of infection related to immunosuppression.

- □ Avoid crowds and individuals who are sick, because illness can precipitate an exacerbation.

- Client Outcomes

  - ○ The client's laboratory values will indicate a decrease in immune and inflammatory response.

  - ○ The client will have extended periods of remission from the disease.

Complications

- Lupus nephritis (renal failure/glomerulonephritis)

  - ○ Clients whose SLE is unable to be managed with immunosuppressants and corticosteroids may experience renal failure secondary to glomerulonephritis. This is a major cause of death, and a renal transplant may be necessary.

  - ○ Nursing Actions

    - ▪ Monitor for periorbital and lower extremity swelling and hypertension. Monitor the client's renal status closely (creatinine, BUN).

  - ○ Client Education

    - ▪ Teach the client the importance of taking immunosuppressants and corticosteroids as prescribed.

    - ▪ Teach the client the significance of avoiding stress and illness.

- Pericarditis, and myocarditis (instruct the client to report chest pain)

  - ○ Inflammation of the heart, its vessels, and the surrounding sac can occur secondary to SLE.

  - ○ Nursing Actions

    - ▪ Monitor for chest pain, fatigue, arrhythmias, and fever.

  - ○ Client Education

    - ▪ Teach the client to:

      - □ Take immunosuppressants and corticosteroids as prescribed.

      - □ Avoid stress and illness.

      - □ Report chest pain to the provider.

CHAPTER 101: SYSTEMIC LUPUS ERYTHEMATOSUS

(A) Application Exercises

Scenario: A 32-year-old woman is experiencing an exacerbation of systemic lupus erythematosus (SLE). She reports fatigue, joint tenderness, and anorexia. Her knees are swollen, she has an oral temperature of 38.2° C (100.8° F), and her blood pressure is 152/90 mm Hg. Renal compromise is suspected.

1. Based on the client's data, which of the following abnormal laboratory findings should the nurse anticipate? (Select all that apply.)

   _____ Positive ANA

   _____ 2+ urine protein

   _____ Increased hemoglobin

   _____ Decreased white blood cell count

   _____ Elevated BUN

   _____ Increased hematocrit

   _____ Decreased serum complement

2. Which of the following instructions should the nurse include when teaching the client about self-care? (Select all that apply.)

   _____ Avoid sun exposure.

   _____ Report peripheral edema to the provider.

   _____ Avoid harsh hair treatments.

   _____ Avoid the use of steroid creams for skin rash.

   _____ Report a productive cough to the provider, even if a fever is not present.

   _____ Avoid crowds and individuals who are sick.

3. The client will be discharged with a prescription for prednisone (Deltasone) until symptoms improve. The nurse should teach the client about which of the following possible side effects from this medication? (Select all that apply.)

   _____ Orthostatic hypotension

   _____ Weight gain

   _____ Loss of appetite

   _____ Buffalo hump

   _____ Moon face

   _____ Abdominal striae

   _____ Hair loss

   _____ Elevated blood glucose

CHAPTER 101: SYSTEMIC LUPUS ERYTHEMATOSUS

 Application Exercises Answer Key

Scenario: A 32-year-old woman is experiencing an exacerbation of systemic lupus erythematosus (SLE). She reports fatigue, joint tenderness, and anorexia. Her knees are swollen, she has an oral temperature of 38.2° C (100.8° F), and her blood pressure is 152/90 mm Hg. Renal compromise is suspected.

1. Based on the client's data, which of the following abnormal laboratory findings should the nurse anticipate? (Select all that apply.)

  X   **Positive ANA**

  X   **2+ urine protein**

  _____ Increased hemoglobin

  _____ Decreased white blood cell count

  X   **Elevated BUN**

  _____ Increased hematocrit

  X   **Decreased serum complement**

Positive ANA titers and decreased serum complement are expected findings with SLE. Elevated BUN and urine protein provide information regarding renal involvement. Increases in hemoglobin and hematocrit are not expected findings and white blood cell count is usually elevated.

(N) **NCLEX® Connection: Reduction of Risk Potential, Laboratory Values**

2. Which of the following instructions should the nurse include when teaching the client about self-care? (Select all that apply.)

  X   **Avoid sun exposure.**

  X   **Report peripheral edema to the provider.**

  X   **Avoid harsh hair treatments.**

  _____ Avoid the use of steroid creams for skin rash.

  X   **Report a productive cough to the provider, even if a fever is not present.**

  X   **Avoid crowds and individuals who are sick.**

Clients with SLE should avoid sun exposure, report peripheral and periorbital edema to the provider; avoid harsh hair treatments, such as permanent waves; report a productive cough, even if fever is not present; and avoid crowds and individuals who are sick to decrease the risk of exposure. Steroid creams should be used for skin rashes.

(N) **NCLEX® Connection: Physiological Adaptation, Illness Management**

3. The client will be discharged with a prescription for prednisone (Deltasone) until symptoms improve. The nurse should teach the client about which of the following possible side effects from this medication? (Select all that apply.)

_____	Orthostatic hypotension
X	**Weight gain**
_____	Loss of appetite
X	**Buffalo hump**
X	**Moon face**
X	**Abdominal striae**
_____	Hair loss
X	**Elevated blood glucose**

Weight gain, buffalo hump (accumulation of fatty tissue between the scapula), moon face (rounding of the face due to accumulation of fatty tissue), abdominal striae, and elevated blood glucose are findings associated with long-term steroid use. Hypertension, rather than hypotension, is expected secondary to fluid retention and increased appetite and excessive hair growth (hirsutism) are additional possible side effects.

Ⓝ **NCLEX® Connection: Pharmacological and Parenteral Therapies, Adverse Effects/ Contraindications/Side Effects/Interactions**

UNIT 13	NURSING CARE OF CLIENTS WITH IMMUNE SYSTEM DISORDERS AND INFECTIOUS DISORDERS
Section	Autoimmune Disorders

Chapter 102 Rheumatoid Arthritis

Overview

- Rheumatoid arthritis (RA) is a chronic, progressive inflammatory disease that can affect tissues and organs but principally attacks the joints producing an inflammatory synovitis. It involves joints bilaterally and symmetrically, and it typically affects several joints at one time.

- RA is an autoimmune disease that is precipitated by WBCs attacking synovial tissue. The WBCs cause the synovial tissue to become inflamed and thickened. The inflammation can extend to the cartilage, bone, tendons, and ligaments that surround the joint. Joint deformity may result from these changes, decreasing the joint's range of motion and function.

- RA is also a systemic disease that can affect any connective tissue in the body. Common structures that are affected are the blood vessels, pleura surrounding the lungs, and pericardium. Iritis and scleritis can also develop in the eyes.

- The natural course of the disease is one of exacerbations and remissions.

Health Promotion and Disease Prevention

- Use adaptive devices that prevent development of deformity of inflamed joints during ADLs.

- Continue using affected joints and ambulating to maintain function and range of motion.

Assessment

- Risk Factors

  o Female gender

  o Age 20 to 50 years

  o Genetic predisposition

  o Epstein-Barr virus

  o Stress

- Early signs of RA (fatigue, joint discomfort) are vague and may be attributed to other disorders in older adult clients.

- Joint pain and dysfunction may have a greater effect on older adult clients than on younger adult clients, due to the presence of other chronic conditions.

- Older adult clients may be less able to overcome and/or cope with joint pain/ deformity.

- Subjective Data

  - Pain at rest and with movement

  - Morning stiffness

  - Pleuritic pain (pain upon inspiration)

  - Xerostomia (dry mouth)

  - Anorexia/weight loss

  - Fatigue

  - Paresthesias

  - Recent illness/stressor

- Objective Data

  - Clinical findings depend on the area affected by the disease process.

  - Joint swelling and deformity

    - Finger, hands, wrists, knees, and foot joints are generally affected.

    - Finger joints affected are the proximal interphalangeal and metacarpophalangeal joints.

    - Joints may become deformed merely by completing ADLs.

    - Ulnar deviation, swan neck, and boutonnière deformities are common in the fingers.

View Media Supplement: Rheumatoid Arthritis Changes (Image)

  - Subcutaneous nodules

  - Fever (generally low grade)

  - Muscle weakness/atrophy

  - Reddened sclera and/or abnormal shape of pupils

- o Laboratory Tests
  - Anti-CCP antibodies – Positive
    - □ This test detects antibodies to cyclic citrullinated peptide (anti-CCP). The result is positive in most people who have rheumatoid arthritis, even years before symptoms develop. The test is more sensitive for RA than rheumatoid factor (RF) antibodies.
  - RF antibody
    - □ Diagnostic level for rheumatoid arthritis is 1:40 to 1:60 (normal 1:20 or less).
    - □ High titers correlate with severe disease.
    - □ Other autoimmune diseases can also increase RF antibody.
  - Erythrocyte sedimentation rate (ESR) – Elevated
    - □ The increase is associated with the inflammation or infection in the body.
    - □ 20 to 40 mm/hr is mild inflammation.
    - □ 40 to 70 mm/hr is moderate inflammation.
    - □ 70 to 150 mm/hr is severe inflammation
    - □ Other autoimmune diseases can also increase ESR antibody.
  - C-reactive protein (may be done in place of ESR) – Positive
    - □ This test is useful for diagnosing disease or monitoring disease activity, and for monitoring the response to anti-inflammatory therapy.
  - Antinuclear antibody (ANA) titer (antibody produced against one's own DNA)
    - □ A positive ANA titer is associated with RA (it is normally negative at 1:20 dilution).
    - □ Other autoimmune diseases can also increase ANA.
  - Elevated WBCs
    - □ WBC count may be elevated during an exacerbation secondary to the inflammatory response.
- o Diagnostic Procedures
  - Arthrocentesis
    - □ Synovial fluid aspiration by needle
    - □ With RA, increased WBCs and RF are present in fluid.
    - □ Nursing Actions
      - ‣ Monitor for bleeding or a synovial fluid leak from the needle biopsy site.
    - □ Client Education
      - ‣ Take acetaminophen (Tylenol) for pain.

- X-ray

  □ X-rays are used to determine the degree of joint destruction and monitor its progression. They may provide adequate visualization and negate the need for more expensive radiologic tests, such a CTs and MRIs.

  □ Nursing Actions

    ▸ Assist the client into position.

  □ Client Education

    ▸ Instruct the client about the need to minimize movement during the procedure.

Collaborative Care

- Nursing Care

  ○ Apply heat or cold to the affected areas as indicated based on client response.

    - Morning stiffness (hot shower)

    - Pain in hands/fingers (heated paraffin)

    - Edema (cold therapy)

  ○ Assist with and encourage physical activity to maintain joint mobility (within the capabilities of the client).

  ○ Monitor the client for signs/symptoms of fatigue.

  ○ Teach the client measures to:

    - Maximize functional activity.

    - Minimize pain.

    - Conserve energy (space out activities, take rest periods).

  ○ Provide a safe environment.

    - Facilitate the use of assistive devices.

    - Remove unnecessary equipment/supplies.

  ○ Use progressive muscle relaxation.

  ○ Administer medications as prescribed.

  ○ Monitor for medication effectiveness (reduced pain, increased mobility).

  ○ Teach the client regarding signs/symptoms that need to be reported immediately (fever, infection, pain upon inspiration, pain in the substernal area of the chest).

- Medications

  ○ NSAIDs

    - NSAIDs provide analgesic, antipyretic, and anti-inflammatory effects. NSAIDs can cause considerable gastrointestinal (GI) distress.

- Nursing Considerations

  - Request a concurrent prescription for a GI-acid lowering agent (H2 receptor blocker, proton pump inhibitor) if GI distress reported.

  - Monitor for fluid retention, hypertension, and renal dysfunction.

- Client Education

  - Instruct the client to

    ▸ Take the medication with food or with a full glass of water or milk. If taking routinely, H_2 receptor blocker may also be prescribed.

    ▸ Observe for GI bleeding (coffee ground emesis; dark, tarry stools).

    ▸ Avoid alcohol, which can increase risk of GI complications.

  ○ Corticosteroids

    - Corticosteroids (prednisone) are strong anti-inflammatory medications that may be given for acute exacerbations or advanced forms of the disease. They are not given for long-term therapy due to significant side effects (osteoporosis, cataracts).

    - Nursing Considerations

      - Observe for cushingoid changes.

      - Monitor weight and blood pressure.

    - Client Education

      - Instruct the client to observe for changes in vision, blood glucose, and impaired healing.

      - Instruct the client to avoid crowds.

      - Instruct the client to follow the provider's prescription, such as alternate day dosing, tapering, and discontinuing medication.

  ○ Disease modifying anti-rheumatic drugs (DMARDs)

    - DMARDs work in a variety of ways to slow the progression of RA and suppress the immune system's reaction to RA that causes pain and inflammation. Relief of symptoms may not occur for several weeks.

    - Antimalarial agent – Hydroxychloroquine (Plaquenil)

    - Antibiotic – Minocycline (Minocin)

    - Sulfonamide – Sulfasalazine (Azulfidine)

    - Biologic response modifiers – Etanercept (Enbrel), infliximab (Remicade), adalimumab (Humira), and chelator penicillamine (Cuprimine)

    - Cytotoxic medications – Methotrexate (Rheumatrex), leflunomide (Arava), cyclophosphamide (Cytoxan), and azathioprine (Imuran)

- Interdisciplinary Care

  ○ Refer the client to support groups as appropriate.

- o Refer the client to occupational therapy for adaptive devices that can facilitate carrying out ADLs and prevent deformities.

- o A home health aide may be necessary for assistance with ADLs.

- Therapeutic Procedures

  - o Plasmapheresis

    - Removes circulating antibodies from plasma, decreasing attacks on the client's tissues

  - o May be done for a severe, life-threatening exacerbation.

- Surgical Interventions

  - o Total joint arthroplasty

    - May be done for a severely deformed joint that has not responded to medication therapy

- Client Outcomes

  - o The client will maintain full range of motion of joints.

  - o The client's pain will be managed so that ADLs can be comfortably carried out.

  - o The client will use adaptive devices so that ADLs can be independently carried out and deformities prevented.

Complications

- Sjögren's syndrome (triad of symptoms – dry eyes, dry mouth, and dry vagina)

  - o Caused by obstruction of secretory ducts and glands

  - o Nursing Actions

    - Provide the client with eye drops and artificial saliva, and recommend vaginal lubricants as needed.

    - Provide fluids with meals.

- Secondary osteoporosis

  - o Immobilization caused by arthritis can contribute to the development of osteoporosis.

  - o Nursing Actions

    - Encourage weight-bearing exercises as tolerated.

- Vasculitis (organ ischemia)

  - o Inflammation of arteries can disrupt blood flow, causing ischemia. Smaller arteries in the skin, eyes, and brain are most commonly affected in RA.

  - o Nursing Actions

    - Monitor for skin lesions, decrease in vision, and symptoms of cognitive dysfunction.

CHAPTER 102: RHEUMATOID ARTHRITIS

(A) Application Exercises

Scenario: A 47-year-old client visits an outpatient clinic due to an exacerbation of rheumatoid arthritis (RA). She is experiencing increased joint tenderness and swelling. She also has subcutaneous nodules in the metacarpophalangeal (MCP) and proximal interphalangeal (PIP) joints of her hands bilaterally.

1. Which of the following data is essential for the nurse to collect to plan care for this client? (Select all that apply.)

_____   Exacerbating factors

_____   History of recent illness

_____   Blood pressure

_____   Family members with disease

_____   Pain status

_____   Date of original diagnosis

_____   Temperature

_____   Range of motion

2. Which of the following laboratory tests are likely to be ordered for this client? (Select all that apply.)

_____   Urinalysis

_____   Erythrocyte sedimentation rate (ESR)

_____   Rheumatoid factor (RF)

_____   Arterial blood gases

_____   Antinuclear antibody (ANA) titer

_____   BUN

_____   Platelet count

_____   WBC count

3. The client wants to know if she should place ice on her swollen joints. Which of the following is an appropriate response from the nurse?

A. "Yes, ice will numb the painful joints."

B. "Yes, ice decreases swelling relieving pain."

C. "No, ice should never be used. Heat should be used."

D. "No, ice is hard and heavy. It can cause deformity."

CHAPTER 102: RHEUMATOID ARTHRITIS

(A) Application Exercises Answer Key

Scenario: A 47-year-old client visits an outpatient clinic due to an exacerbation of rheumatoid arthritis (RA). She is experiencing increased joint tenderness and swelling. She also has subcutaneous nodules in the metacarpophalangeal (MCP) and proximal interphalangeal (PIP) joints of her hands bilaterally.

1. Which of the following data is essential for the nurse to collect to plan care for this client? (Select all that apply.)

X	**Exacerbating factors**
X	**History of recent illness**
_____	Blood pressure
_____	Family members with disease
X	**Pain status**
_____	Date of original diagnosis
X	**Temperature**
X	**Range of motion**

Determination of whether or not the client's disease is manifesting with a low-grade fever and identification of exacerbating factors, such as a recent illness, are important for developing a comprehensive plan of care. Baselines regarding range of motion and pain status are needed for evaluation of intervention effectiveness. Blood pressure variations are not usually a component of RA and information about family members with RA and the date of original diagnosis will not provide data helpful for development of the client's plan of care.

(N) NCLEX® Connection: Reduction of Risk Potential, System Specific Assessment

2. Which of the following laboratory tests are likely to be ordered for this client? (Select all that apply.)

_____	Urinalysis
X	**Erythrocyte sedimentation rate (ESR)**
X	**Rheumatoid factor (RF)**
_____	Arterial blood gases
X	**Antinuclear antibody (ANA) titer**
_____	BUN
_____	Platelet count
X	**WBC count**

Elevations in ESR, RF, ANA titer, and WBC counts are consistent with diagnosis of RA.

(N) NCLEX® Connection: Reduction of Risk Potential, Laboratory Values

3. The client wants to know if she should place ice on her swollen joints. Which of the following is an appropriate response from the nurse?

    A. "Yes, ice will numb the painful joints."

    B. "Yes, ice decreases swelling relieving pain."

    C. "No, ice should never be used. Heat should be used."

    D. "No, ice is hard and heavy. It can cause deformity."

Ice can be used when swelling is present because it causes vasoconstriction, decreasing swelling and pain. It is not desirable to use ice to numb painful joints and can cause damaging vasoconstriction. Use of ice will not cause deformity and appropriate use of padding should enhance comfort. Heat is appropriate to use for stiffness.

NCLEX® Connection: Physiological Adaptation, Illness Management

UNIT 13	NURSING CARE OF CLIENTS WITH IMMUNE SYSTEM DISORDERS AND INFECTIOUS DISORDERS
Section	Cancer-Related Disorders

Chapter 103 General Principles of Cancer

Overview

- Cancer is a neoplastic disease process that involves abnormal cell growth and differentiation.

- The exact cause of cancer is unknown, but viruses, physical and chemical agents, hormones, genetics, and diet are thought to be factors that trigger abnormal cell growth.

- Cancer cells may invade surrounding tissues and/or spread to other areas of the body through lymph and blood vessels (metastasis).

- Cancers may arise from almost any tissue in the body.

  - Carcinomas arise from epithelial tissue.

  - Adenocarcinomas arise from glandular organs.

  - Sarcomas arise from mesenchymal tissue.

  - Leukemias are malignancies of the blood-forming cells.

  - Lymphomas arise from the lymph tissue.

  - Multiple myeloma arises from plasma cells and affects the bone.

- Screening and early diagnosis are the most important aspects of health education and care.

Risk Factors

- Age

  - The highest incidence of cancer occurs in older adults. Older adult women most commonly develop colorectal, breast, lung, pancreatic, and ovarian cancers.

    - Older adult men most commonly develop lung, colorectal, prostate, pancreatic, and gastric cancers.

- Race

  - Caucasian women over the age of 40 are more likely to develop breast cancer than are African-American, American-Indian, and Hispanic women. However, the death rate for each of these groups is higher than for Caucasian women.

  - Caucasian men are at an increased risk for testicular cancer, whereas African-American men are at an increased risk for prostate cancer.

- Genetic predisposition

- Exposure to chemicals, viruses, tobacco, and alcohol

- Exposure to certain viruses and bacteria

  - Liver cancer can develop after many years of infection with hepatitis B or hepatitis C.

  - Infection with human T-cell leukemia virus increases the risk of lymphoma and leukemia (indigenous to certain areas of the world, such as Africa and Melanesia).

  - Infection with Epstein-Barr virus has been linked to an increased risk of lymphoma.

  - Human papillomavirus (HPV) infection is the main cause of cervical cancer.

  - HIV increases the risk of lymphoma and Kaposi's sarcoma.

  - *Helicobacter pylori* may increase the risk of stomach cancer and lymphoma of the stomach lining.

- A diet high in fat and red meat and low in fiber

- Sun, ultraviolet light, or radiation exposure (radon)

- Sexual lifestyles (multiple sexual partners or STDs)

- Poverty, obesity, and chronic GERD

Assessment

- Signs and Symptoms (Clinical findings depend on the type and location of cancer.)

  - Seven warning signs *(CAUTION)* clients should watch for
    Change in bowel or bladder habits
    A sore that doesn't heal
    Unusual bleeding or discharge
    Thickening or lump in the breast or elsewhere
    Indigestion or difficulty swallowing
    Obvious change in warts or moles
    Nagging cough or hoarseness

○ Weight loss

○ Fatigue/Weakness

○ Pain (may not occur until late in the disease process)

○ Nausea/Anorexia

Diagnostic Procedures

- Genetic tests (BRCA1, BRCA2) – Mutations in these genes can predispose a woman to a high risk of breast cancer.

- Tissue biopsy – The definitive diagnosis of abnormal cancer cells

- CBC and differential – Screenings for leukemias

- Chest x-ray, computed tomography (CT) scan, magnetic resonance imaging (MRI), positron emission tomography (PET) scan, and single photon emission computed tomography (SPECT) scans are used to visualize tumors, metastasis, or progression of cancer.

- Tumor marker assays (carcinoembryonic antigen [CEA], cancer antigen 125 [CA-125], prostate-specific antigen [PSA], human chronic gonadotropin [beta-hCG], alpha fetoprotein [AFP]) – These are blood tests that screen for cancers of the colon, pancreas, liver, prostate, uterus, and ovaries. Elevated values are suggestive of cancer.

Staging

- The tumor-node-metastasis (TNM) system is used to stage cancer:

  ○ Tumor (T)

    ▪ TX – Unable to evaluate the primary tumor

    ▪ T0 – No evidence of primary tumor

    ▪ Tis – Tumor in situ

    ▪ T1, T2, T3, and T4 – Size and extent of tumor

  ○ Node (N)

    ▪ NX – Unable to evaluate regional lymph nodes

    ▪ N0 – No evidence of regional node involvement

    ▪ N1, N2, and N3 – Number of nodes that are involved and/or extent of spread

  ○ Metastasis (M)

    ▪ MX – Unable to evaluate distant metastasis

    ▪ M0 – No evidence of distant metastasis

    ▪ M1 – Presence of distant metastasis

Complications and Nursing Implications

- Oncologic Emergencies

  o Syndrome of inappropriate antidiuretic hormone (SIADH)

    - SIADH occurs when excessive levels of antidiuretic hormones are produced. Because antidiuretic hormones help the kidneys and body to conserve the correct amount of water, SIADH causes the body to retain water. This results in a dilution of electrolytes (such as sodium) in the blood. Most common in lung and brain cancers.

    - Nursing Actions

      □ Monitor the client for hyponatremia and low serum osmolality.

      □ Administer furosemide (Lasix), IV 0.9% sodium chloride (NaCl), and/or hypertonic saline as prescribed for severe hyponatremia.

      □ Closely monitor vital signs and serum sodium as Lasix will promote sodium excretion and hypertonic saline can cause fluid overload.

  o Hypercalcemia

    - A common complication of leukemia; breast, lung, head, and neck cancers; lymphomas; multiple myelomas; and bony metastases of any cancer.

    - Symptoms include anorexia, nausea, vomiting, shortened QT interval, kidney stones, bone pain, and changes in mental status.

    - Nursing Actions

      □ Administer 0.9% NaCl saline, furosemide (Lasix), pamidronate, and phosphates as prescribed.

  o Superior vena cava syndrome

    - Results from obstruction (metastases from breast or lung cancers) of venous return and engorgement of the vessels from the head and upper body. Symptoms include periorbital and facial edema, erythema of the upper body, dyspnea, and epistaxis.

    - Nursing Actions

      □ Position the client in a high-Fowler's position initially to facilitate lung expansion. Use high dose radiation therapy for emergency temporary relief.

  o Disseminated intravascular coagulation

    - A coagulation complication secondary to leukemia or adenocarcinomas.

    - Nursing Actions

      □ Observe the client for bleeding and apply pressure as needed.

      □ Be prepared to administer blood clotting factors that have been lost through bleeding and may need to be replaced with plasma transfusions. Heparin may also be used to slow the cascade of events that makes the body overuse its blood clotting factors.

CHAPTER 103: GENERAL PRINCIPLES OF CANCER

(A) Application Exercises

1. A nurse is teaching a client about the risk for cancer. Which of the following client statements indicates the need for further teaching?

   A. "I see a dermatologist regularly for the mole on my thigh."

   B. "I take Milk of Magnesia for occasional constipation."

   C. "I tan using an indoor tanning lotion instead of laying out in the sun."

   D. "I used to smoke but switched to chewing tobacco 3 years ago."

2. A nurse is teaching a client about maintaining a diet that may prevent certain cancers. The nurse should inform the client that the intake of which of the following may be beneficial? (Select all that apply.)

   _____ Low saturated fats

   _____ Fruits

   _____ Fiber

   _____ Red meats

   _____ Simple carbohydrates

   _____ Vegetables

   _____ Fish

3. A nurse is caring for a client who has lung cancer and is exhibiting signs of syndrome of inappropriate antidiuretic hormone. Which of the following findings are essential to report to the provider? (Select all that apply.)

   _____ Behavioral changes

   _____ Headache

   _____ Urine output 40 mL/hr

   _____ Nausea/Vomiting

   _____ Hyponatremia

   _____ High urine specific gravity

   _____ Lethargy

   _____ Seizures

CHAPTER 103: GENERAL PRINCIPLES OF CANCER

 Application Exercises Answer Key

1. A nurse is teaching a client about the risk for cancer. Which of the following client statements indicates the need for further teaching?

    A. "I see a dermatologist regularly for the mole on my thigh."

    B. "I take Milk of Magnesia for occasional constipation."

    C. "I tan using an indoor tanning lotion instead of laying out in the sun."

    D. "I used to smoke but switched to chewing tobacco 3 years ago."

Chewing tobacco can cause oral cancer and should be avoided, just as smoking tobacco should be avoided. The other statements indicate correct actions for the client to take regarding cancer risk.

NCLEX® Connection: Physiological Adaptation, Pathophysiology

2. A nurse is teaching a client about maintaining a diet that may prevent certain cancers. The nurse should inform the client that the intake of which of the following may be beneficial? (Select all that apply.)

     X   **Low saturated fats**

     X   **Fruits**

     X   **Fiber**

           Red meats

           Simple carbohydrates

     X   **Vegetables**

     X   **Fish**

Foods that are low in saturated fats and high in fiber, along with a diet high in fruits, vegetables, and fish provide protection against certain types of cancers. Red meat, and simple carbohydrates can increase a client's risk of cancer.

NCLEX® Connection: Basic Care and Comfort, Nutrition and Oral Hydration

3. A nurse is caring for a client who has lung cancer is and exhibiting signs of syndrome of inappropriate antidiuretic hormone. Which of the following findings are essential to report to the provider? (Select all that apply.)

__X__	**Behavioral changes**
__X__	**Headache**
_____	Urine output 40 mL/hr
__X__	**Nausea/Vomiting**
__X__	**Hyponatremia**
_____	High urine specific gravity
__X__	**Lethargy**
__X__	**Seizures**

SIADH occurs when excessive levels of antidiuretic hormones are secreted secondary to cancer or other disease processes. The syndrome causes the body to retain water and certain levels of electrolytes in the blood (sodium) to fall. As serum sodium falls, cellular swelling occurs. The brain is particularly susceptible to swelling and produces nausea, vomiting, behavioral changes, headache, and seizures, all of which should be reported to the health care provider immediately.

Ⓝ NCLEX® Connection: Physiological Adaptation, Alterations in Body Systems

UNIT 13	NURSING CARE OF CLIENTS WITH IMMUNE SYSTEM DISORDERS AND INFECTIOUS DISORDERS
Section	Cancer-Related Disorders

Chapter 104 Cancer Treatment Options

Overview

- Cancer treatment options focus on removing or destroying cancer cells and preventing the continued abnormal cell growth and differentiation.

- Cancer treatment options that nurses should be knowledgeable about

  o Chemotherapy

  o Radiation therapy

  o Hormonal therapy

  o Immunotherapy

- Many cancers are curable when diagnosed early.

Chemotherapy

- Chemotherapy involves the administration of systemic or local cytoxic medications that damage a cell's DNA or destroy rapidly dividing cells.

  o Chemotherapeutic agents are often selected in relation to their effect on various stages of cell division. Subsequently, combinations of anticancer medications are used to enhance destruction of cancer cells.

  o Many of the adverse effects of chemotherapeutic agents are related to the unintentional harm done to normal rapidly proliferating cells, such as those found in the gastrointestinal tract, hair follicles, and bone marrow.

  o Chemotherapy may be administered in a health care setting, provider's office, clinic, or home.

  o Depending on the agent, it can be given by the oral, parenteral, IV, intracavitary, or intrathecal route. Special training/certification is necessary for the administration of some agents.

    ▪ Implanted ports - May be implanted for therapy that is intended to be given on a long-term basis.

      □ The port is comprised of a small reservoir that is covered by a thick septum.

- □ The port is surgically implanted into a pocket in the client's chest wall. A catheter is then inserted into the subclavian vein with the tip in the vena cava.
  - ■ Access to the port should be done by:
    - □ Applying a local anesthetic to the skin if indicated.
    - □ Palpating the skin to locate the port body septum to ensure proper insertion of the needle.
    - □ Cleaning the skin with alcohol for at least 3 seconds and allowing it to dry prior to insertion of the needle.
    - □ Using a noncoring needle (may be straight or angled to prevent dislodgement).
    - □ Flushing after every use and at least once a month.
    - □ Following facility protocol to flush when deaccessing port (Flush with 10 mL of 0.9% NaCl followed by 5 mL of 10, 100 units/mL of heparin.).
  - ○ Extravasation of agents that are vesicants require special, immediate attention to minimize tissue damage. Selection of a neutralizing solution is dependent on vesicant.

- Indications
  - ○ Chemotherapy may be used to cure a disease, help control the progression of a disease, or as palliative treatment for individuals who have a terminal disease.
  - ○ Chemotherapy is most commonly used for treatment of cancer, but it may also be used for other disorders such as autoimmune diseases.

- Client Outcomes
  - ○ The client will identify strategies to minimize side effects.
  - ○ The client's diagnostic tests will reveal elimination or slowing of disease progression.
  - ○ The client will experience relief from cancer symptoms.

- Preprocedure
  - ○ Since administration of chemotherapeutic medications is limited to certified individuals, management of adverse effects is the primary focus of health care personnel.

- Complications
  - ○ Immunosuppression
    - ■ Immunosuppression due to bone marrow suppression by cytotoxic medications is the most significant adverse effect of chemotherapy.
    - ■ Nursing Actions
      - □ Monitor the client's temperature and white blood cell (WBC) count.
      - □ A fever greater than 37.8° C (100° F) should be immediately reported to the provider.

- ☐ Cultures should be done prior to initiating antimicrobial therapy.
- ☐ If the client's WBC drops below 1,000/mm³, place the client in a private room and initiate neutropenic precautions.
  - ▸ Have the client remain in his room unless he needs to leave for a diagnostic procedure or therapy. In this case place a mask on him during transport.
  - ▸ Protect the client from possible sources of infection (plants, change water in equipment daily, restrict client to room).
  - ▸ Have client, staff, and visitors perform frequent hand hygiene. Restrict visitors who are ill.
  - ▸ Avoid invasive procedures that could cause a break in tissue unless necessary (rectal temperatures, injections).
  - ▸ Keep designated equipment in the client's room (blood pressure machine, thermometer).
  - ▸ Administer colony-stimulating factors filgrastim (Neupogen, Neulasta) as prescribed to stimulate WBC production.
- ■ Client Education
  - ☐ Encourage the client to avoid crowds while undergoing chemotherapy.
  - ☐ Client instructions
    - ▸ Avoid eating fresh fruits and vegetables that could contain bacteria.
    - ▸ Avoid yard work, gardening, or changing a pet's litter box.
    - ▸ Avoid fluids that have been sitting at room temperature for greater than 1 hr.
    - ▸ Wash toothbrush daily in dishwasher or rinse in bleach solution.
    - ▸ Report fever > 37.8° C (100° F) or other symptoms of bacterial or viral infections immediately to the provider.
- ○ Nausea and vomiting/anorexia
  - ■ Many of the medications used for chemotherapy are emetogenic (induce vomiting) or cause anorexia as well as an altered taste in the mouth.
  - ■ Serotonin blockers, such as ondansetron (Zofran), have been found to be effective and are often given along with corticosteroids, phenothiazines, and antihistamines.
  - ■ Nursing Actions
    - ☐ Give the client antiemetic medications at times that are appropriate for a chemotherapeutic agent (prior to treatment, during treatment, after treatment).
    - ☐ Antiemetic medications may need to be given for several days after each treatment.

- □ Visual imagery and relaxation techniques may be useful adjuncts to antiemetics.

- □ Perform calorie counts to determine intake. Provide liquid supplements as needed. Add protein powders to food or tube feedings.

- □ Administer megestrol (Megace) to increase the client's appetite if prescribed.

- □ Perform mouth care prior to serving meals to enhance the client's appetite.

- ■ Client Education

  - □ Instruct the client about the administration of antiemetics and schedule them prior to meals.

  - □ Encourage the client to eat several small meals a day if better tolerated.

  - □ Suggest that the client select foods that are served cold and do not require cooking, which can emit odors that stimulate nausea.

  - □ Encourage consumption of high-protein, high-calorie, nutrient-dense foods and avoidance of low- or empty-calorie foods.

  - □ If the client has a metallic taste in the mouth, encourage the use of plastic eating utensils, sucking on hard candy, and avoiding red meats if the metallic taste worsens.

- ○ Alopecia

  - ■ Alopecia is a side effect of certain chemotherapeutic medications related to their interference with the life cycle of rapidly proliferating cells.

  - ■ Nursing Actions

    - □ Discuss with client the impact of alopecia on self image. Discuss options such as hats, turbans, and wigs to deal with hair loss.

    - □ Recommend soliciting information from the American Cancer Society regarding products for clients experiencing alopecia.

    - □ Reinforce with the client that alopecia is temporary and hair should return when chemotherapy is discontinued.

  - ■ Client Education

    - □ Instruct the client to avoid the use of damaging hair-care measures, such as electric rollers, hair dye, and permanent waves. Use of a soft hair brush or wide-tooth comb for grooming is preferred.

    - □ Suggest that the client cut her hair short before treatment to decrease weight on the hair follicle.

    - □ After hair loss, the client should protect the scalp from sun and can use a diaper rash ointment/cream for itching.

- ○ Mucositis

  - ■ Mucositis (also referred to as stomatitis) is inflammation of tissues in the mouth, such as the gums, tongue, roof and floor of the mouth, and inside the lips and cheeks.

- Nursing Actions

  □ Examine the client's mouth several times a day and inquire about the presence of oral lesions.

  □ Document the location and size of lesions that are present.

  □ Avoid using glycerin-based mouthwashes or mouth swabs.

  □ Administer a topical anesthetic prior to meals.

  □ Discourage selection of salty, acidic, or spicy foods on menu.

  □ Offer mouth care before and after each meal.

- Client Education

  □ Encourage the client to rinse her mouth with a solution of half 0.9% NaCl and half peroxide at least twice a day, and to brush her teeth using a soft-bristled toothbrush.

  □ Encourage the client to eat soft foods and supplements that are high in calories such as mashed potatoes, scrambled eggs, and cooked cereal. Other appropriate food sources are cold foods such as milk shakes, ice cream, frozen yogurt, bananas, and breakfast mixes.

○ Anemia and thrombocytopenia

- Anemia (decreased number of circulating red blood cells [RBCs]) and thrombocytopenia (decreased number of circulating platelets) occur secondary to bone marrow suppression.

- Nursing Actions for Anemia

  □ Monitor the client for fatigue, pallor, dizziness, and shortness of breath.

  □ Help the client manage anemia-related fatigue by scheduling activities with rest periods in between and using energy saving measures (sitting during showers and ADLs).

  □ Administer erythropoietic medications such as erythropoietin alfa (Epogen) and antianemic medications such as ferrous sulfate (Feosol) as prescribed.

  □ Monitor the client's Hgb to determine response to medications. Be prepared to administer blood if prescribed.

- Nursing Actions for Thrombocytopenia

  □ Monitor the client for petechiae, ecchymosis, bleeding of the gums, nosebleeds, occult or frank blood in stools, urine, and/or vomitus.

  □ Institute bleeding precautions (avoid IVs and injections, apply pressure for approximately 10 min after blood draws, handle client gently and avoid trauma).

  □ Administer thrombopoietic medications such as oprelvekin (Interleukin 11, Neumega), which may decrease the need for platelet transfusions and lessen the risk of bleeding. Monitor platelet count, and be prepared to administer platelets if the count falls below 30,000/mm^3.

- Client Education
  - Instruct the client to:
    - Use an electric razor instead of a razor blade when shaving.
    - Use a soft-bristled toothbrush.
    - Blow his nose only when necessary.
    - Wear shoes when ambulating.
    - Avoid the use of NSAIDs.

Radiation Therapy

- Radiation therapy involves the use of ionizing radiation to target tissues and destroy cells.
  - Side effects include skin changes, hair loss, and debilitating fatigue.
  - Radiation therapy can be administered internally with an implant (brachytherapy) or externally with a radiation beam.
  - Radiation therapy is used to cure some cancers, augment the treatment of other cancers, and hopefully increase a client's survival rate and time.
  - Radiation therapy can also be given preoperatively to decrease the size of a tumor or to treat metastatic tumors in clients who are in the terminal stage of their disease.
- Client Outcomes
  - The client will identify strategies to minimize side effects.
  - The client's diagnostic tests will reveal elimination or slowing of the disease process.
  - The client will experience relief from cancer symptoms.
- Internal Radiation Therapy
  - Brachytherapy is the term used to describe internal radiation that is placed close to the target tissue. This is done via placement in a body orifice (vagina) or body cavity (abdomen) or delivered via IV such as with radionuclide iodine, which is absorbed by the thyroid.
  - Nursing Actions
    - Ongoing Care
      - The client should be placed in a private room.
      - Appropriate signage should be placed on the door warning of the radiation source.
      - Health care personnel should wear a dosimeter film badge that records the amount of radiation exposure.
      - Visitors should be limited to 30-min visits and maintain a distance of 6 ft.
      - Visitors and health care personnel who are pregnant or under the age of 16 should not come into contact with the client.

- □ A lead container should be kept in the client's room if the delivery method could allow spontaneous loss of radioactive material. Tongs should also be available to use for placing radioactive material into a lead container.

- □ Precautions listed above should be carried out at home if the client is discharged during therapy.

- ○ Client Education

  - ▪ Inform client of the need to remain in a position necessary to prevent dislodgement the of radiation implant.

  - ▪ Instruct the client to call the nurse for assistance with elimination.

- • External Radiation Therapy

  - ○ External radiation or teletherapy is delivered over the course of several weeks and aimed at the body from an external source.

  - ○ Nursing Actions

    - ▪ Preparation of the Client

      - □ The client's skin over the targeted area is marked with "tattoos" that guide the positioning of the external radiation source.

    - ▪ Ongoing Care

      - □ Recommend that the client eat a diet that does not contain red meat. Radiation can cause dysgeusia, making foods such as red meat unpalatable.

      - □ Help the client manage fatigue by scheduling activities with rest periods in between and using energy-saving measures (sitting during showers and ADLs).

      - □ Treat symptoms related to the area of the body being irradiated.

        - ‣ Mouth – Mucositis, xerostomia

        - ‣ Neck – Difficulty swallowing

        - ‣ Abdomen – Gastroenteritis

  - ○ Client Education

    - ▪ Inform the client that fatigue is a common side effect of radiation therapy.

    - ▪ Gently wash the skin over the irradiated area with mild soap and water. Dry the area thoroughly using patting motions.

    - ▪ Do not remove radiation "tattoos" that are used to guide therapy.

    - ▪ Do not apply powders, ointments, lotions, or perfumes to the irradiated skin.

    - ▪ Wear soft clothing over the irradiated skin and avoid tight or constricting clothes.

    - ▪ Do not expose the irradiated skin to sun or a heat source.

Hormonal Therapy

- Hormone therapy is effective against tumors that are supported or suppressed by hormones.

- Indications

  - Hormone agonists, such as gonadotropin-releasing hormone agonists (GnRH) like leuprolide (Eligard, Lupron), are effective against tumors that require a particular hormone for support.

    - The use of androgenic hormones in a client who has estrogen-dependent cancer can suppress growth of this type of cancer.

    - Conversely, the use of estrogenic hormones for a testosterone-dependent cancer can suppress growth of this type of cancer.

  - Hormone antagonists are also effective against tumors that require a particular hormone for support.

    - The use of an anti-estrogen hormone in a client with estrogen-dependent cancer can suppress growth of this type of cancer.

    - The same is true for anti-testosterone hormones.

- Client Outcomes

  - The client will identify strategies to minimize side effects.

  - The client's diagnostic tests will reveal elimination or slowing of the disease process.

  - The client will experience relief from cancer symptoms.

- Nursing Actions

  - GnRH

    - Ongoing Care

      - Monitor the client's cardiac status, along with blood pressure and the occurrence of pulmonary edema.

    - Client Education

      - Inform male clients about the impact on sexual functioning (decreased libido, erectile dysfunction) and feminizing effects of hormone therapy (gynecomastia, hot flashes, bone loss).

      - Instruct the client to increase his intake of calcium and vitamin D.

  - Androgen antagonists – flutamide (Eulexin)

    - Ongoing Care

      - Monitor the client's liver enzymes and CBC.

- Client Education

  - Warn the client about the feminizing effects of hormone therapy (gynecomastia, erectile dysfunction).

  - Advise the client to notify the provider of sore throat or bruising.

- Estrogen antagonists – tamoxifen (Nolvadex), anastrozole (Arimidex), trastuzumab (Herceptin)

  - Ongoing Care

    - Monitor the client's CBC, clotting times, lipid profiles, calcium and cholesterol serum levels, and liver function for medication-related changes.

    - Neurologic and cardiovascular functioning should also be monitored for changes.

  - Client Education

    - Inform the client of side effects, which include nausea, vomiting, hot flashes, weight gain, vaginal bleeding, and increased risk of thrombosis.

    - Reinforce the need for yearly gynecologic exams and the need to take calcium and vitamin D supplements.

Immunotherapy

- Immunotherapy, or biologic response modifiers (BMRs), alter a client's biological response to cancerous tumor cells.

  - Interleukins and interferons are the two primary cytokines (immune response modulators) used in immunotherapy.

    - Interleukins help coordinate the inflammatory and immune responses of the body, in particular, the lymphocytes.

    - Interferons, when stimulated, can exert an antitumor effect by activating a variety of responses.

  - Cytokines are the primary BMRs currently used, and they work to enhance the immune system. They help the client's immune system recognize cancer cells and use the body's natural defenses to destroy them.

- Client Outcomes

  - The client will identify strategies to minimize side effects.

  - The client's diagnostic tests will reveal elimination or slowing of the disease process.

  - The client will experience relief from cancer symptoms.

- Nursing Actions

  - Interleukins

    - Ongoing Care

      - Monitor the client for influenza-like symptoms and edema.

- ○ Interferons
  - ■ Ongoing Care
    - □ Monitor the client for peripheral neuropathy that may affect vision, hearing, balance, and gait.
    - □ Take precautions for orthostatic hypotension.
  - ■ Client Education
    - □ Instruct the client to immediately report influenza-like symptoms or changes consistent with peripheral neuropathy.
    - □ Warn the client that skin rashes are common and use of a perfume-free moisturizer may be helpful.
    - □ Instruct the client to avoid the sun and swimming if skin symptoms arise

CHAPTER 104: CANCER TREATMENT OPTIONS

Ⓐ Application Exercises

1. A client who is undergoing chemotherapy is placed on neutropenic precautions. Which of the following actions is appropriate for the nurse to take? (Select all that apply.)

_____ Place the client on a high-fiber diet.

_____ Remove plants from the client's room.

_____ Have the client wear a mask during transport to radiology.

_____ Tell assistive personnel that the blood pressure machine cannot be removed from the room.

_____ Recommend a prescription for oprelvekin (Interleukin-11).

_____ Restrict the client from eating raw carrots.

2. A nurse is caring for a client who is undergoing a course of chemotherapy. The client is reporting severe nausea and has lost 7 lb since her last course of chemotherapy. Which of the following statements is appropriate for the nurse to make?

A. "Your nausea will lessen with each course of chemotherapy."

B. "Hot food is better tolerated because of the aroma it produces."

C. "Try eating several small meals throughout the day."

D. "Eat as much red meat as tolerated to keep your weight up."

3. A nurse is caring for a client who has a platelet count of 25,000/mm^3. Which of the following medications is appropriate for the nurse to recommend?

A. Oprelvekin (Interleukin-11)

B. Epoetin alfa (Epogen)

C. Filgrastim (Neupogen)

D. Megestrol (Megace)

4. A nurse is caring for a client who is being treated for cervical cancer with brachytherapy. When reviewing the client's restrictions, which of the following is appropriate to include? (Select all that apply.)

_____ Visitors can stay 30 min at a time.

_____ The client must stay on bed rest while the implant is in place.

_____ The client will have a catheter in place.

_____ The client will be placed on fiber laxatives.

_____ The client may not watch television with a radiation source in the room.

CHAPTER 104: CANCER TREATMENT OPTIONS

 Application Exercises Answer Key

1. A client who is undergoing chemotherapy is placed on neutropenic precautions. Which of the following actions is appropriate for the nurse to take? (Select all that apply.)

_____	Place the client on a high-fiber diet.
X	**Remove plants from the client's room.**
X	**Have the client wear a mask during transport to radiology.**
X	**Tell assistive personnel that the blood pressure machine cannot be removed from the room.**
_____	Recommend a prescription for oprelvekin (Interleukin-11).
X	**Restrict the client from eating raw carrots.**

Clients who are neutropenic should be protected from unnecessary contaminants. Removing plants from the room, restricting the ingestion of raw fruits and vegetables, using designated care equipment, and placing a mask on the client during transport are methods that can limit a client's exposure to infectious agents. There is no benefit from placing a client on a high-fiber diet and oprelvekin (Interleukin-11) is given to clients who are anemic.

 NCLEX® Connection: Safety and Infection Control, Standard/Transmission-Based/Other Precautions

2. A nurse is caring for a client who is undergoing a course of chemotherapy. The client is reporting severe nausea and has lost 7 lb since her last course of chemotherapy. Which of the following statements is appropriate for the nurse to make?

A. "Your nausea will lessen with each course of chemotherapy."

B. "Hot food is better tolerated because of the aroma it produces."

C. "Try eating several small meals throughout the day."

D. "Eat as much red meat as tolerated to keep your weight up."

Several small meals a day are usually better tolerated than larger meals for a client who has nausea. Nausea usually occurs to the same extent with each course of chemotherapy. Cold foods are tolerated better than warm foods because odors from warm foods can stimulate nausea. Red meat is not tolerated well in clients undergoing chemotherapy as the taste of meat is frequently altered and unpalatable.

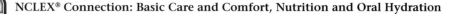 **NCLEX® Connection: Basic Care and Comfort, Nutrition and Oral Hydration**

3. A nurse is caring for a client who has a platelet count of 25,000/mm^3. Which of the following medications is appropriate for the nurse to recommend?

   A. Oprelvekin (Interleukin-11)

   B. Epoetin alfa (Epogen)

   C. Filgrastim (Neupogen)

   D. Megestrol (Megace)

   Oprelvekin is a thrombopoietic growth factor medication. It is appropriate to recommend this medication for a client who has a decreased platelet count. Epoetin alfa is used in the treatment of anemia; filgrastim stimulates WBC production; and megestrol is used to increase appetite.

 NCLEX® Connection: Pharmacological and Parenteral Therapies, Expected Actions/ Outcomes

4. A nurse is caring for a client is being treated for cervical cancer with brachytherapy. When reviewing the client's restrictions, which of the following is appropriate to include? (Select all that apply.)

X	**Visitors can stay 30 min at a time.**
X	**The client must stay on bed rest while the implant is in place.**
X	**The client will have a catheter in place.**
_____	The client will be placed on fiber laxatives.
_____	The client may not watch television with a radiation source in the room.

   Clients who are undergoing brachytherapy will have a radiation implant that must remain in place during the entire treatment. Since the client has cervical cancer, she will have a vaginal implant. Subsequently, the client will be on bed rest to avoid displacement of the implant during ambulation. A catheter will be necessary, and the client will be encouraged to not have a bowel movement unless necessary during the treatment. Fiber laxatives, which initiate bowel movements, would be contraindicated. Visitors may visit for 30 min at a time while maintaining a distance of 6 feet. Watching television during treatment is not contraindicated and can help the client manage boredom.

 NCLEX® Connection: Physiological Adaptation, Radiation Therapy

UNIT 13	NURSING CARE OF CLIENTS WITH IMMUNE SYSTEM DISORDERS AND INFECTIOUS DISORDERS
Section	Cancer-Related Disorders

Chapter 105 Pain Management for Clients with Cancer

Overview

- The management of cancer pain is necessary to optimize the quality of life of a person who has cancer.

- Not all clients who have cancer have pain.

- Cancer pain may be caused by the tumor or may be a result of the cancer treatment.

  ○ Direct cancer pain is caused by tumor pressure or cell invasion and may include tissue, bone, and nerve pain.

  ○ Pain due to cancer treatment may be caused by surgery, radiation, chemotherapy, or inactivity.

Definition of Pain

- Pain is subjective and may be indicative of tissue injury or impending tissue injury.

- Pain may have physical and emotional components.

- The reaction to pain varies from person to person and may be influenced by the age, gender, and culture.

- Pain may be acute or chronic.

  ○ Acute pain occurs suddenly and is short term. Acute cancer pain may be the result of surgery.

  ○ Chronic pain occurs gradually and lasts longer than 3 months. Chronic cancer pain is usually caused by the tumor and destruction or pressure of surrounding tissue.

- Type of pain

  ○ Neuropathic – Due to nerve damage; described as numb, tingling, shooting, or radiating pain

  ○ Visceral/Deep – Occurs in internal organs; may be difficult to identify. Characterized by deep, sharp pain.

  ○ Somatic – Occurs in bone or connective tissues; may be described as throbbing or dull

Assessment of Cancer Pain

- The most reliable indicator of pain is verbal expression of pain from the client.

- The nursing assessment should be performed using standard pain measures (location, quality, intensity, timing, setting, associated symptoms, aggravating/relieving factors).

- Pain assessment also involves observing and documenting nonverbal indicators and physiological changes.

  o Nonverbal indicators of acute pain

    ▪ Agitation and grimacing

    ▪ Elevated heart rate, respiratory rate, and/or blood pressure

    ▪ Diaphoresis and pupil dilation

    ▪ Splinting of a certain area

  o Nonverbal indicators of chronic pain

    ▪ Depression

    ▪ Lethargy

    ▪ Anger

    ▪ Weakness

- Barriers to effective pain management

  o Inadequate pain assessment

  o Knowledge of the health care professional regarding pharmacological pain management

    ▪ Reluctance by the clients to report pain

    ▪ Fear of addiction leading to noncompliance

    ▪ Inadequate dosing

Management of Cancer Pain

- Palliative cancer pain management is intended to provide comfort and reduce pain rather than to cure the cancer.

- The goal of palliative pain management is to reduce pain to improve quality of life while maintaining dignity and mental clarity.

- Methods of pain management

  ○ Removal or reduction in size of cancer

    ▪ Surgery, chemotherapy, and radiation therapy may reduce pain by removing cancer and pressure of tumor on tissues or organs.

      ☐ Surgical removal of tumor – Removal of cancer may include part of the body and result in change in organ function. The client may be fearful about survival and anxious about the loss of a body part.

      ☐ Radiation – Radiation may cause localized hair loss, skin changes, and severe fatigue.

      ☐ Chemotherapy – Killing of the cells may result in localized complications (stomatitis), or systemic complications, (nausea, vomiting, neutropenia).

- Nursing Actions

  ○ Nursing actions are specific to each surgery or procedure.

  ○ Client education

    ▪ Include information regarding the specific procedure or treatment.

    ▪ Include the family in care and management.

    ▪ Provide information about support groups, such as the American Cancer Society.

    ▪ Radiation – Instruct the client about specific skin care and to avoid sun exposure.

    ▪ Chemotherapy – Include information about avoiding infection and managing other adverse effects.

Medications

- Pharmacological management of pain includes NSAIDS, opioids, antidepressants, anticonvulsants, steroids, and local anesthetics. Some clients who have cancer pain may require regular use of analgesics for pain control.

CLASSIFICATION AND THERAPEUTIC INTENT	MEDICATION	NURSING CONSIDERATION	CLIENT EDUCATION
Nonopioid medications and nonsteroidal anti-inflammatory medications • Given for mild to moderate pain	• Acetaminophen (Tylenol) • Ketorolac (Toradol) • Aspirin (acetylsalicylic acid) • Ibuprofen (Motrin)	• Monitor for signs of gastrointestinal (GI) bleeding, such as bloody stools or emesis that looks like coffee grounds. • Monitor for bruising and bleeding. • Do not give acetaminophen to clients who have liver disease. • Monitor for tinnitus and hearing loss if NSAIDs are prescribed	• Take with food to prevent GI upset. • Be alert to GI or other bleeding and bruising. • Do not crush or chew enteric-coated products.
Opioids • Given for moderate to severe pain • May be given for breakthrough pain • Fentanyl (Sublimaze) is available for transdermal use.	• Morphine sulfate • Meperidine (Demerol) • Hydromorphone (Dilaudid) • Oxycodone (OxyContin) • Fentanyl (Sublimaze)	• Use with caution in older adult clients. • Monitor for respiratory depression. ○ Have naloxone (Narcan) available to reverse effects.	• Use medication as directed. • Prevent constipation with diet changes and stool softeners if needed. • Be aware that nausea may subside after a few days.
Antidepressants • Given to reduce associated depression, promote sleep, and increase serotonin levels that may improve feelings of well-being • May decrease neuropathic pain	• Amitriptyline (Elavil) • Desipramine (Norpramin) • Imipramine (Tofranil)	• Use with caution in older adult clients. • Do not give to clients who have seizure disorders or a history of cardiac problems. • Use with caution in young adult clients or clients who are at risk for suicide, because antidepressants may increase suicide risk.	• Notify the health care provider if depression increases or if thoughts of suicide occur. • Be aware that therapeutic effects may take 2 to 3 weeks to become established.

CLASSIFICATION AND THERAPEUTIC INTENT	MEDICATION	NURSING CONSIDERATION	CLIENT EDUCATION
Anticonvulsants • Given to treat neuralgia or neuropathic-type pain	• Gabapentin (Neurontin) • Valproic acid (Depakene) • Pregabalin (Lyrica)	• Monitor electrolytes. • Monitor medications levels. • Monitor for tremors.	• Avoid the use of alcohol. • Do not drive at the start of therapy. • Notify the health care provider if tremors occur.
Steroids • May reduce pain by reducing swelling	• Prednisolone (Prelone) • Dexamethasone (Decadron)	• Reduce dosage gradually. • Monitor for muscle weakness, joint pain, or fever. • Monitor serum glucose levels.	• Use only as directed. • Do not discontinue suddenly. • Take with food.
Adjunctive agents • Sympatholytic agents – Used to treat neuropathic pain ○ Used in conjunction with bupivacaine in epidural or other local infusions.	• Clonidine (Catapres)	• Monitor for hypotension.	• Change positions slowly, because these medications may cause postural hypotension.
• Skeletal muscle relaxants – May be used along with other pain medications for muscle spasms associated with cancer pain	• Baclofen (Lioresal)	• Monitor for seizure activity.	• Take with food. • Use caution when driving or operating machinery. • These medications may cause drowsiness and dizziness.

CLASSIFICATION AND THERAPEUTIC INTENT	MEDICATION	NURSING CONSIDERATION	CLIENT EDUCATION
Systemic local anesthetics • May be given via an infusion pump directly into the area of pain (intrathecal, intra-articular, intrapleural) to provide pain relief	• Lidocaine (Xylocaine) • Bupivacaine (Marcaine) • Ropivacaine (Naropin)	• Monitor for hypotension. • Monitor for signs of infection at the catheter insertion site. • Evaluate pain status. • Monitor for motor impairment and level of sedation. • May be used in combination with a narcotic or another medication, such as clonidine (Catapres).	• Monitor the infusion site for signs of infection, such as redness or swelling. • Monitor for fever. • Notify the health care provider of increased pain or decreased movement that may indicate a motor block. • Care for and protect the external catheter.
Topical anesthetics • Used to treat oral ulcers that may be caused by radiation or chemotherapy and neuropathic pain, such as in postmastectomy axillary pain	• Lidocaine HCL (Lidoderm patch) • Eutectic mixture of local anesthetic (EMLA) cream	• Monitor for pain relief and local skin reaction.	• Use as directed. • Use only on intact skin.

ADMINISTRATION METHOD	DESCRIPTION
Oral	• First choice for administration • Long-acting formulations are available.
Transdermal – Fentanyl (Sublimaze)	• Easy to administer • Slow onset • Long duration (48 to 72 hr)
Rectal	• Contraindicated for clients with a low WBC or low platelet count
Subcutaneous infusion – Morphine or hydromorphone	• Slow infusion rate (2 to 4 mL/hr) • Requires nursing support • Risk of infiltration • Rapid onset
Intravenous	• Requires nursing support • Risk of infiltration • Rapid onset

ADMINISTRATION METHOD	DESCRIPTION
Epidural or intrathecal	• Risk of infection, pruritus, and urinary retention • Requires nursing care to monitor, especially with increase in dosage

Anesthetic Interventions

- Regional nerve blocks

  ○ An anesthetic agent, such as bupivacaine, and/or a corticosteroid, is injected directly into a nerve root to provide pain relief.

    ▪ Used for an isolated area of pain

      □ For example, an intercostal nerve block may used to treat chest or abdominal wall pain

    ▪ The procedure may take from 15 min to 1 hr, depending upon the area receiving the block.

  ○ Nursing Actions

    ▪ Obtain baseline vital signs. Monitor blood pressure and vital signs during the procedure and for at least 1 hr following the procedure (follow established guidelines).

    ▪ Establish IV access before the procedure.

    ▪ Monitor for signs of systemic infusion, (metallic taste, ringing in ears, perioral numbness, seizures).

    ▪ Assess the insertion site for redness and swelling.

    ▪ Assess level of nerve block and pain.

    ▪ Protect area of numbness from injury.

  ○ Client Education

    ▪ Advise the client to monitor the injection site for swelling, redness, or drainage.

    ▪ Advise the client to protect the area of numbness from injury and to notify the health care provider of increased pain or signs of systemic infusion, (metallic taste, ringing in ears, perioral numbness, seizures).

- Epidural or intrathecal catheters

  ○ A local anesthetic or analgesic is injected into the epidural space (the space outside the dura mater of the spinal cord) or intrathecal space (the subarachnoid area within the spinal cord sheath that contains cerebrospinal fluid).

- An external catheter is surgically placed under the skin with an external port for long-term use.
    - ☐ Used for chronic pain management
    - ☐ May be attached to a continuous infusion or injected as needed
    - ☐ Used for upper abdominal pain, thoracic pain, and pain located below the umbilicus
  - ○ Nursing Actions
    - Monitor during insertion/injection and for at least 1 hr following insertion/injection (follow established guidelines) for hypotension, anaphylaxis, seizures, and dura puncture.
    - Monitor for respiratory depression and sedation.
    - Monitor the insertion site for hematoma and signs of an infection.
    - Assess the level of sensory block.
    - Evaluate leg strength prior to ambulating.
    - Local anesthetics block the sympathetic nervous system, causing peripheral vasodilation and hypotension. This may cause reduced stroke volume, cardiac output, and peripheral resistance. IV fluids may need to be increased to compensate for the sympathetic blocking effects of regional anesthetics.
  - ○ Client Education
    - Advise the client to notify the health care provider of signs of infection, (fever, swelling and redness, increase in pain or severe headache, sudden weakness to lower extremities, decrease in bowel or bladder control).
    - Notify the provider of signs of systemic infusion, (metallic taste, ringing in ears, perioral numbness, seizures).
    - Long-term reactions may include sexual dysfunction or amenorrhea.

Other Invasive Techniques

- Neurolytic ablation
  - ○ Involves interrupting the nerve pathway or destroying the nerve roots that are causing pain; usually involves a CT-guided probe and injection of chemicals, such as phenol or ethanol
    - For example, celiac plexus nerve ablation may be effective for pancreatic, stomach, abdominal, small bowel, and proximal colon pain.
    - The procedure is considered irreversible. However, nerve ablation may provide relief for several months until nerve fibers regenerate.
    - Nerve ablation may cause loss of sensory, motor, and autonomic function.
    - Use only when noninvasive methods are ineffective.

- Radiofrequency ablation

    o Electrical currency creates heat on a probe that is guided to the tumor or nerves and is used to destroy cancer cells or ablate nerve endings. This is often used for lung and bone tumors.

- Cryoanalgesia

    o Uses a needle-like probe to deliver extreme cold to interfere with pain conduction via nerve pathways

    o Nursing Actions

        ▪ Monitor vital signs, especially blood pressure, during and for at least 1 hr following the procedure (follow established guidelines).

        ▪ Monitor for signs of bleeding, such as tachycardia and hypotension.

        ▪ Monitor for skin irritation.

        ▪ Monitor for other effects such as diarrhea, loss of bladder or bowel control, or extremity weakness.

        ▪ Assess pain relief.

    o Client Education

        ▪ Instruct the client to apply ice if needed for pain at the insertion site.

        ▪ Continue to use pain medications as directed if needed.

        ▪ Notify the health care provider of an increase in pain or weakness of extremities.

Alternative Approaches

- Alternative approaches to pain management may be used in addition to pain medications or other techniques. Many of these provide some pain reduction with minimal side effects.

    o Transcutaneous electrical nerve stimulation (TENS)

        ▪ Low-voltage electrical impulses are transmitted through electrodes that are attached to the skin near or over the area of pain. This is usually used in conjunction with analgesics.

        ▪ Nursing Actions

            □ Use with conductive gel.

            □ Monitor electrode sites for burns or rash.

            □ Offer other pain medications if indicated.

            □ Do not use on clients who have pacemakers or infusion pumps.

- ■ Client Education

  - □ Advise the client to inspect the skin under the electrodes to monitor for burns or irritation.

  - □ Advise the client not to use if pregnant.

  - □ Advice the client not to use near the head or over the heart.

- ○ Relaxation techniques and imagery

  - ■ Useful during a procedure or a period of increased pain.

  - ■ Relaxation techniques include deep breathing, progressive relaxation, and meditation.

  - ■ Positive imagery involves visualizing a peaceful image and may be used with the aid of audiotapes.

  - ■ Relaxation and imagery may help reduce anxiety, stress, and related pain, and they may help the client to feel more in control of the pain.

- ○ Distraction

  - ■ Music, television, exercise, and family and friends may be effective distractions from pain and stress. Other distractions may include repetitive actions or movements or a visual focal point. A change of scenery may offer a distraction from pain.

- ○ Application of heat or cold, pressure, massage, or vibration

  - ■ Heat increases blood flow, relaxes muscles, and reduces joint stiffness. Cold decreases inflammation and causes local analgesia.

    - □ Do not use heat or cold directly on skin that is damaged by radiation.

  - ■ Massage and vibration may cause relaxation, distraction, and increased surface circulation.

- ○ Acupuncture

  - ■ Acupuncture is a technique that involves the use of small needles inserted into the skin at different depths to stimulate and alter nerve pathways.

- ○ Hypnosis

  - ■ Hypnosis involves using an altered state of awareness to redirect a person's perception of pain. It may be helpful to induce positive imagery, reduce anxiety, and improve coping.

- ○ Peer group support

  - ■ A support group helps provide emotional support for the client and the client's family. Other benefits to meeting with a support group include the presence of a social network, availability of information, and help in strengthening coping skills.

CHAPTER 105: PAIN MANAGEMENT FOR CLIENTS WITH CANCER

(A) Application Exercises

1. A nurse should know that which of the following is the most reliable indicator of pain?

   A. Vital signs

   B. Facial expression

   C. Verbal expression of pain

   D. Location of pain

2. A client who has chronic cancer pain has a permanent epidural catheter that is used for administration of a fentanyl/bupivacaine solution. For which of the following findings should the nurse monitor? (Select all that apply.)

   _____ Respiratory depression

   _____ Hypotension

   _____ Sedation

   _____ Muscle spasticity

   _____ Motor blockage

3. A nurse is caring for a client who is to undergo neurolytic ablation. The nurse should recognize that this treatment is used only when other measures have failed due to the risk of

   A. irreversible nerve damage.

   B. increased pain.

   C. myelosuppression.

   D. thrombocytopenia.

4. A nurse is caring for a client who has cancer. The goal of palliative pain management is to increase which of the following? (Select all that apply.)

   _____ Mental acuity

   _____ Physical mobility

   _____ Time spent at home

   _____ Quality of life

   _____ Pain relief

CHAPTER 105: PAIN MANAGEMENT FOR CLIENTS WITH CANCER

 Application Exercises Answer Key

1. A nurse should know that which of the following is the most reliable indicator of pain?

A. Vital signs

B. Facial expression

C. Verbal expression of pain

D. Location of pain

A client's verbal expression of pain is the most reliable indicator of pain. Nonverbal and physiologic indicators should be included in the pain assessment.

 NCLEX® Connection: Reduction of Risk Potential, System Specific Assessment

2. A client who has chronic cancer pain has a permanent epidural catheter that is used for administration of a fentanyl/bupivacaine solution. For which of the following findings should the nurse monitor? (Select all that apply.)

__X__	**Respiratory depression**
__X__	**Hypotension**
__X__	**Sedation**
_____	Muscle spasticity
__X__	**Motor blockage**

Side effects of epidural analgesia injected with an opioid and a local anesthetic may include respiratory depression, hypotension, sedation, and motor weakness. Vital signs should be assessed and fluids administered for hypotension, and muscle weakness should be evaluated prior to ambulation.

 NCLEX® Connection: Pharmacological and Parenteral Therapies, Pharmacological Pain Management

3. A nurse is caring for a client who is to undergo neurolytic ablation. The nurse should recognize that this treatment is used only when other measures have failed due to the risk of

A. irreversible nerve damage.

B. increased pain.

C. myelosuppression.

D. thrombocytopenia.

Neurolytic ablation causes permanent nerve destruction. It is usually used only after other methods have been unsuccessful. Increase in pain, myelosuppression, and thrombocytopenia are not related to neurolytic ablation.

NCLEX® Connection: Physiological Adaptation, Therapeutic Procedures

4. A nurse is caring for a client who has cancer. The goal of palliative pain management is to increase which of the following? (Select all that apply.)

	Mental acuity
X	**Physical mobility**
X	**Time spent at home**
X	**Quality of life**
X	**Pain relief**

The goal of palliative pain management is to reduce pain to improve quality of life while maintaining dignity and mental clarity. Maintaining mental clarity, rather than increasing it, is a goal of palliative therapy.

(N) NCLEX® Connection: Physiological Adaptation, Therapeutic Procedures

| UNIT 13 | NURSING CARE OF CLIENTS WITH IMMUNE SYSTEM DISORDERS AND INFECTIOUS DISORDERS |
| Section | Infectious Disorders |

Chapter 106 Bacterial, Viral, Fungal, and Parasitic Infections

Overview

- Pathogens are the microorganisms or microbes that cause infections.

  ○ Bacteria (*Staphylococcus aureus, Escherichia coli, Mycobacterium tuberculosis*)

  ○ Viruses – Organisms that use the host's genetic machinery to reproduce (HIV, hepatitis, herpes zoster, herpes simplex)

  ○ Fungi – Molds and yeasts (*Candida albicans*, Aspergillus)

  ○ Prions – Protein particles (new variant Creutzfeldt-Jakob disease)

  ○ Parasites – Protozoa (malaria, toxoplasmosis) and helminths (worms [flatworms, roundworms], flukes [Schistosoma])

- Virulence is the ability of a pathogen to invade and injure the host.

- Herpes zoster is a common viral infection that erupts years after exposure to chickenpox and invades a specific nerve tract.

Infection Process

- The infection process (chain of infection) includes:

  View Media Supplement: Chain of Infection (Image)

  ○ Causative agent (bacteria, virus, fungus, prion, parasite)

  ○ Reservoir (human, animal, water, soil, insects)

  ○ Portal of exit from (means for leaving) the host

    ■ Respiratory tract (droplet, airborne)

      □ *Myobacterium tuberculosis* and *Streptococcus pneumoniae*

    ■ Gastrointestinal tract

      □ Shigella, *Salmonella enteritidis, Salmonella typhi*, hepatitis A

- Genitourinary tract
  - *Escherichia coli*, hepatitis A, herpes simplex virus (type 1), HIV
- Skin/Mucous membranes
  - Herpes simplex virus and varicella
- Blood/Body fluids
  - HIV and hepatitis B and C

○ Mode of transmission

- Contact
  - Direct physical contact – Person to person
  - Indirect contact with an inanimate object – Object to person
  - Fecal-oral transmission – Handling food after using a restroom and failing to wash hands
- Droplet
  - Sneezing, coughing, and talking
- Airborne
  - Sneezing and coughing
- Vector borne
  - Animals or insects as intermediaries (ticks transmit Lyme disease; mosquitoes transmit West Nile and malaria)

○ Portal of entry to the host

- May be the same as the portal of exit

○ Susceptible host

- Compromised defense mechanisms (immunocompromised, breaks in skin) leave the host more susceptible to infections.

Immune Defenses

- Nonspecific innate-native immunity is that which allows the body to restrict entry or immediately respond to a foreign organism (antigen) through the activation of phagocytic cells, complement, and inflammation.

  ○ Nonspecific innate-native immunity provides temporary immunity but does not have memory of past exposures.

  ○ Intact skin is the body's first line of defense against microbial invasion.

  ○ The skin, mucous membranes, secretions, enzymes, phagocytic cells, and protective proteins work in concert to prevent infections.

- ○ Inflammatory response

  - Phagocytic cells (neutrophils, eosinophils, macrophages), the complement system, and interferons are involved.

  - An inflammatory response localizes the area of microbial invasion and prevents its spread.

- Specific adaptive immunity is that which allows the body to make antibodies in response to a foreign organism (antigen).

  - ○ Requires time to react to antigens

  - ○ Provides permanent immunity due to memory of past exposures

  - ○ Involves B and T lymphocytes

  - ○ Produces specific antibodies against specific antigens (immunoglobulins [IgA, IgD, IgE, IgG, IgM]).

Assessment

- Risk Factors

  - ○ Environmental factors

    - Excessive alcohol consumption

    - Smoking

    - Malnutrition

  - ○ Medication therapy (immunosuppressive agents)

    - Glucocorticosteroids

    - Antineoplastics

  - ○ Chronic diseases

    - Diabetes mellitus

    - Adrenal insufficiency

    - Renal failure

    - Hepatic failure

    - Chronic lung disease

  - ○ Older adults are at increased risk for infections due to:

    - Slowed response to antibiotic therapy

    - Slowed immune response

    - Loss of subcutaneous tissue and thinning of the skin

    - Decreased vascularity and slowed wound healing

    - Decreased cough and gag reflexes

- Chronic illnesses (diabetes mellitus, COPD, neurological or musculoskeletal impairments)

- Decreased gastric acid production

- Decreased mobility

- Bowel/Bladder incontinence

- Dementia

- Greater incidence of invasive devices (urinary catheters, feeding tubes, tracheostomies, intravenous lines)

- Subjective Data

  - Chills

  - Sore throat

  - Fatigue and malaise

  - Change in level of consciousness, nuchal rigidity, photophobia, headache

  - Nausea, vomiting, anorexia, abdominal cramping, and diarrhea

- Objective Data

  - Physical Assessment Findings

    - Fever

    - Enlarged lymph nodes

    - Dyspnea, cough, purulent sputum, and crackles in lung fields

    - Dysuria, urinary frequency, hematuria, and pyuria

    - Rash, skin lesions, purulent wound drainage, and erythema

    - Odynophagia, dysphagia, hyperemia, and enlarged tonsils

  - Laboratory Tests

    - White blood cell (WBC) count with differential

    - Culture and sensitivity

    - Erythrocyte sedimentation rate (ESR) – The rate at which red blood cells settle out of plasma

      - A normal value for adults is 15 to 20 mm/hr.

      - An increase indicates an active inflammatory process or infection.

    - Immunoglobulin electrophoresis

      - Determines the presence and quantity of specific immunoglobulins (IgG, IgA, IgM)

      - Used to detect hypersensitivity disorders, autoimmune disorders, chronic viral infections, immunodeficiency, multiple myeloma, and intrauterine infections

- Antibody screening tests
  - Detects the presence of antibodies against specific causative agents (bacteria, fungi, viruses, parasites)
  - A positive antibody test indicates that the client has been exposed to and developed antibodies to a specific pathogen, but it does not provide information about whether or not the client is currently infected (HIV antibodies).
- Auto-antibody screening tests
  - Detects the presence of antibodies against a person's own DNA (self-cells)
  - The presence of antibodies against self cells is associated with autoimmune conditions (systemic lupus erythematosus, rheumatoid arthritis).
- Antigen tests
  - Detects the presence of a specific pathogen (HIV)
  - Used to identify certain infections or disorders
- Stool for ova and parasites
  - Detects presence of hookworm ova in stool
  - Diagnostic Procedures
    - Gallium scan
      - A nuclear scan that uses a radioactive substance to identify hot spots of WBCs within the client's body
      - Radioactive gallium citrate is injected intravenously and accumulates in areas where inflammation is present.
    - X-rays, computed tomography (CT) scan, magnetic resonance imaging (MRI), and biopsies are used to determine the presence of infection, abscesses, and lesions.

Collaborative Care

- Nursing Care
  - Assess
    - Presence of risk factors for infection
    - Recent travel or exposure to an infectious disease
    - Behaviors that may put the client at increased risk
    - Signs and symptoms of fever (increased heart and respiratory rate, thirst, anorexia)
    - Presence of chills, which occur when temperature is rising, and diaphoresis, which occurs when temperature is decreasing
    - Presence of hyperpyrexia (greater than105.8), which can cause brain and organ damage

- ○ Implement infection control measures.

  - Perform frequent hand hygiene to prevent transmission of infection to other clients.

  - Maintain a clean environment.

  - Use personal protective equipment/barriers (gloves, masks, gowns, goggles).

  - Implement protective precautions as needed.

    - □ Standard (implemented for all clients)

    - □ Airborne (measles, varicella, tuberculosis)

    - □ Droplet (Haemophilus influenzae type B, pertussis, plague, *streptococcal pneumoniae*).

    - □ Contact (*Clostridium difficile*, herpes simplex virus, impetigo).

- ○ Provide diversional activities if needed.

- ○ Encourage increased fluid intake or maintain intravenous fluid replacement to prevent dehydration.

- Medications

  - ○ Antipyretics

    - Antipyretics (acetaminophen and aspirin) are used for fever and discomfort as prescribed.

    - Nursing Considerations

      - □ Monitor fever to determine effectiveness of medication.

      - □ Graph the client's temperature fluctuations on the medical record for trending.

  - ○ Antimicrobial therapy

    - Antimicrobial therapy kills or inhibits the growth of microorganisms (bacteria, fungi, viruses, protozoans). Antimicrobial medications either kill pathogens or prevent their growth. Anthelmintics are given for worm infestations. There are currently no treatments for prions.

    - Nursing Considerations

      - □ Administer antimicrobial therapy as prescribed.

      - □ Monitor for medication effectiveness (reduced fever, increased level of comfort, decreasing WBC count).

      - □ Maintain a medication schedule to assure consistent therapeutic blood levels of the antibiotic.

- Care After Discharge
  - Client Education
    - Teach the client regarding:
      - Any infection control measures needed at home
      - Self-administration of medication therapy
      - Complications that need to be reported immediately
- Client Outcomes
  - The client's fever will be reduced with the administration of an antipyretic.
  - The client's infectious process will resolve in relation to antimicrobial therapy.

Complications

- Multidrug-resistant infection
  - Antimicrobials are becoming less effective for some strains of pathogens, due to the pathogen's ability to adapt and become resistant to previously sensitive antibiotics. This significantly limits the number of antibiotics that are effective against the pathogen. Use of antibiotics, especially broad spectrum antibiotics, has significantly decreased to prevent new strains from evolving. Taking the measures below can ensure an antimicrobial is warranted and therapy has been effective.
  - Methicillin-resistant *Staphylococcus aureus* (MRSA) is a strain of *Staphylococcus aureus* that is resistant to all antibiotics, except vancomycin. Vancomycin-resistant *Staphylococcus aureus* (VRSA) is a strain of *Staphylococcus aureus* that is resistant to vancomycin but so far is sensitive to other antibiotics specific to the client's strain.
  - Nursing Actions
    - Obtain specimens for culture and sensitivity prior to initiation of antimicrobial therapy.
    - Monitor antimicrobial levels and ensure that therapeutic levels are maintained.
  - Client Education
    - Complete the full course of antimicrobial therapy.
    - Avoid overuse of antimicrobials.
- Sepsis
  - A systemic inflammatory response syndrome resulting from the body's response to a serious infection, usually bacterial (peritonitis, meningitis, pneumonia, wound infections, urinary tract infections)
  - Risk factors for sepsis include very young age, very old age, weakened immune system, and severe injuries (trauma). Sepsis can lead to widespread inflammation, blood clotting, organ failure, and shock.

- Blood cultures definitively diagnose sepsis. Systemic antimicrobials are prescribed accordingly. Vasopressors and anticoagulants may be prescribed for shock and blood clotting symptoms. Mechanical ventilation, dialysis, and other interventions may be needed for treatment of specific organ failure.

Herpes Zoster (Shingles)

- Herpes zoster is a viral infection. It initially produces chicken pox, after which the virus lies dormant in the dorsal root ganglia of the sensory cranial and spinal nerves. It is then reactivated as shingles later in life.

  - Shingles is usually preceded by a prodromal period of several days, during which pain, tingling, or burning may occur along the involved dermatome.

  - Shingles can be very painful and debilitating.

- Assessment

  - Risk Factors

    - Concurrent illness

    - Stress

    - Compromise to the immune system

    - Fatigue

    - Poor nutritional status

    - Older adult clients are more susceptible to herpes zoster infection. The immune function of older adults may also be compromised, so they should be assessed carefully for local or systemic signs of infection.

  - Subjective Data

    - Paresthesia

    - Pain that is unilateral and extends horizontally along a dermatome

  - Objective Data

    - Physical Assessment Findings

      - Vesicular, unilateral rash (the rash and lesions occur on the skin area innervated by the infected nerve)

      - Rash that is erythematous, vesicular, pustular, or crusting (depending on the stage)

      - Rash that usually resolves in 14 to 21 days

      - Low-grade fever

    - Laboratory Tests

      - Cultures provide a definitive diagnosis (but the virus grows so slowly that cultures are often of minimal diagnostic use).

      - Occasionally, an immunofluorescence assay can be done.

- Collaborative Care
  - Nursing Care
    - Assess/Monitor
      - Pain
      - Condition of the lesions
      - Presence of fever
      - Neurologic complications
      - Signs of infection
    - Use an air mattress or bed cradle for pain prevention/control of affected areas.
    - Isolate the client until the vesicles have crusted over.
    - Maintain strict wound care precautions.
    - Avoid exposing the client to infants, pregnant women who have not had chickenpox, and clients who are immunocompromised.
    - Moisten dressings with cool tap water or 5% aluminum acetate (Burow's solution) and apply to the affected skin for 30 to 60 min, four to six times per day as prescribed.
    - Use lotions to help relieve itching and discomfort.
    - Administer medications as prescribed.
  - Medications
    - Analgesics (NSAIDs, narcotics) enhance client comfort.
    - Anti-viral agents, such as acyclovir (Zovirax), may shorten the clinical course.
- Complications
  - Postherpetic neuralgia
    - Characterized by pain that persists for longer than 1 month following resolution of the vesicular rash
    - Tricyclic antidepressants may be prescribed
    - Postherpetic neuralgia is common in adults older than 60 years of age.

CHAPTER 106: BACTERIAL, VIRAL, FUNGAL, AND PARASITIC INFECTIONS

Ⓐ Application Exercises

1. For the scenarios listed below, select the corresponding mode of transmission. Some modes may be used more than once. Write A for airborne, CD for contact direct, CI for contact indirect, V for vector, and FO for fecal-oral.

_____ A client vomits on a nurse's uniform.

_____ A nurse receives an accidental needle stick.

_____ A mosquito bites a hiker in the woods.

_____ Someone with active TB coughs while riding a bus.

_____ A cook fails to wash his hands after using the bathroom.

_____ Someone sneezes into his hand and then shakes hands with another person.

2. Place the following nursing actions in the correct sequence for a client with an infectious disease of the respiratory system.

_____ Collect a specimen for culture and sensitivity.

_____ Implement droplet or airborne precautions.

_____ Assess lung sounds and respiratory rate.

_____ Teach the client about infection control at home.

_____ Maintain therapeutic antibiotic levels.

3. A nurse is caring for a client who has herpes zoster. Which of the following alterations in integument should the nurse expect to find?

A. Generalized pink body rash

B. Red circles with white centers

C. Red edematous rash on cheeks bilaterally

D. Linear clusters of fluid-containing vesicles with some crustings

4. Which of the following might a client experience immediately prior to an outbreak of shingles?

A. Fever and night sweats

B. Gastrointestinal distress, such as diarrhea

C. Petechial lesions on the trunk

D. Pain and tingling in a localized area of the body

CHAPTER 106: BACTERIAL, VIRAL, FUNGAL, AND PARASITIC INFECTIONS

 Application Exercises Answer Key

1. For the scenarios listed below, select the corresponding mode of transmission. Some modes may be used more than once. Write A for airborne, CD for contact direct, CI for contact indirect, V for vector, and FO for fecal-oral.

   CD   A client vomits on a nurse's uniform.

   CI   A nurse receives an accidental needle stick.

   V   A mosquito bites a hiker in the woods.

   A   Someone with active TB coughs while riding a bus.

   FO   A cook fails to wash his hands after using the bathroom.

   CD   Someone sneezes into his hand and then shakes hands with another person.

   Ⓝ NCLEX® Connection: Physiological Adaptation, Infectious Disease

2. Place the following nursing actions in the correct sequence for a client with an infectious disease of the respiratory system.

   3   **Collect a specimen for culture and sensitivity.**

   1   **Implement droplet or airborne precautions.**

   2   **Assess lung sounds and respiratory rate.**

   5   **Teach the client about infection control at home.**

   4   **Maintain therapeutic antibiotic levels.**

   Nurses must prioritize initiation of infection control precautions to protect others from acquiring the infection. Clients should be properly isolated immediately to prevent spread of infection. Assessment of the client should be done prior to implementing interventions. Specimens for culture and sensitivity should be drawn prior to initiating antibiotic therapy to accurately verify the presence of an infectious organism. Finally, maintaining antibiotic therapy levels and teaching the client about home care is necessary for successful eradication of the infection.

   Ⓝ NCLEX® Connection: Physiological Adaptation, Infectious Disease

3. A nurse is caring for a client who has herpes zoster. Which of the following alterations in integument should the nurse expect to find?

    A. Generalized pink body rash

    B. Red circles with white centers

    C. Red edematous rash on cheeks bilaterally

    D. Linear clusters of fluid-containing vesicles with some crustings

Herpes zoster is characterized by vesicles that follow along a dermatome and occur unilaterally. A pink body rash is indicative of an allergic reaction, red circles with white centers occur with ringworm, and a red edematous rash bilaterally on the cheeks is characteristic of systemic lupus erythematosus.

Ⓝ NCLEX® Connection: Reduction of Risk Potential, System Specific Assessment

4. Which of the following might a client experience immediately prior to an outbreak of shingles?

    A. Fever and night sweats

    B. Gastrointestinal distress, such as diarrhea

    C. Petechial lesions on the trunk

    D. Pain and tingling in a localized area of the body

Shingles is usually preceded by a prodromal period of several days. This involves pain, tingling, or burning along the involved dermatome. Fever, night sweats, gastrointestinal distress, and petechial lesions on the trunk are not expected findings for the client immediately prior to an outbreak of shingles.

Ⓝ NCLEX® Connection: Physiological Adaptation, Infectious Disease

UNIT 14: NURSING CARE OF PERIOPERATIVE CLIENTS

- Anesthesia and Moderate (Conscious) Sedation
- Preoperative Nursing Care
- Postoperative Nursing Care

NCLEX® CONNECTIONS

When reviewing the chapters in this unit, keep in mind the relevant sections of the NCLEX® outline, in particular:

CLIENT NEEDS: REDUCTION OF RISK POTENTIAL

Relevant topics/tasks include:
- Potential for Complications from Surgical Procedures and Health Alterations
  - Evaluate the client's response to postoperative interventions to prevent complications.
- Therapeutic Procedures
  - Provide pre and/or postoperative education.
  - Provide preoperative care.
  - Provide intraoperative care.
  - Manage the client during and following a procedure with moderate sedation.

CLIENT NEEDS: PHYSIOLOGICAL ADAPTATION

Relevant topics/tasks include:
- Alterations in Body Systems
  - Provide postoperative care.

UNIT 14	NURSING CARE OF PERIOPERATIVE CLIENTS

Chapter 107 Anesthesia and Moderate (Conscious) Sedation

Overview

- An anesthetic is a chemical agent that is administered prior to a surgical procedure to induce loss of consciousness, amnesia, and/or analgesia.

- Moderate (conscious) sedation is a type of anesthesia. A client does not lose consciousness, but induction of amnesia and analgesia is still achieved.

- There are different types of anesthesia used in the surgical setting, and the nurse should be familiar with their side effects.

ANESTHESIA

Overview

- Anesthesia is a state of depressed CNS activity, marked by depression of consciousness, loss of responsiveness to stimulation, and/or muscle relaxation.

- Anesthesia is classified as general or local.

  o General anesthesia – Causes loss of sensation, consciousness, and reflexes. It anesthesia is the method used when a client is undergoing major surgery, or one that will require complete muscle relaxation.

  o Local anesthesia – Causes loss of sensation without loss of consciousness. Local anesthetics block transmission along nerves. In turn, this provides for loss of autonomic function and muscle paralysis in a specific area of the body.

Risk Factors

- General anesthesia

  o Family history of malignant hyperthermia

  o Respiratory disease (hypoventilation)

  o Cardiac disease (dysrhythmias, altered cardiac output)

  o Gastric contents (aspiration)

  o Alcohol or drug abuse

- Local anesthesia complications

  o Allergy to ester-type anesthetics

  o Alterations in peripheral circulation

  (G) o Older adult clients are more susceptible to anesthetic agents than any other population.

  - Medications need to be titrated carefully to better control the incidence of unwanted effects.

  - Airway patency is the main priority in all situations, but cardiac problems can arise much more quickly in older adult clients.

  - The nurse should pay special attention when an older adult is undergoing a procedure, because the client's condition can deteriorate quickly.

General Anesthesia

- The phases of general anesthesia are

  o Induction – IV lines initiated, preoperative medications given, airway secured

  o Maintenance – Surgery performed, airway maintenance

  o Emergence – Surgery completed, removal of assistive airway devices

- Anesthetics used during general anesthesia are classified as either injectable or inhaled. Inhaled anesthetics are volatile gases or liquids that are dissolved in oxygen, and injectable anesthetics are given intravenously (IV).

  o Examples of inhalation anesthetic agents include halothane (Fluothane), isoflurane (Forane), and nitrous oxide.

  o Examples of IV anesthetic agents include benzodiazepines, etomidate (Amidate), propofol (Diprivan), ketamine (Ketalar), and droperidol plus fentanyl.

  o Inhalation anesthetics are eliminated predominantly through exhalation. The rate of elimination is dependent upon pulmonary ventilation and blood flow to the lungs. Postoperative administration of oxygen and encouraging the client to take deep breaths are important interventions.

- During administration of anesthetics, adjunct medications are also given. These substances are used to achieve further reactions as listed below:

ADJUNCT MEDICATION CLASS	MEDICATIONS	USE
Opioids	Fentanyl (Sublimaze) Sufentanil (Sufenta)	Sedation and analgesia
Benzodiazepines	Diazepam (Valium) Midazolam (Versed)	Amnesia and anxiety reduction

ADJUNCT MEDICATION CLASS	MEDICATIONS	USE
Anticholinergics	Atropine Glycopyrrolate (Robinul)	Dry up excessive secretions – Decrease the risk of aspiration
Antiemetics	Ondansetron (Zofran) Promethazine (Phenergan)	Nausea and vomiting reduction – Decrease the risk of aspiration
Sedatives	Pentobarbital (Nembutal) Secobarbital (Seconal)	Amnesia and sedation
Neuromuscular blocking agents	Succinylcholine (Anectine) Vecuronium (Norcuron)	Muscle relaxation for surgery and airway placement

- Nursing Interventions

  o Assure that consent has been signed by the client, because legal consent cannot be given by an adult who is medicated.

  o Have the client void before the medication is administered so he will not need to get out of bed.

  o Ensure that the bed is in the low position and that the side rails are raised for safety.

  o Monitor the client's airway and oxygen saturation.

  o Monitor and report laboratory values as appropriate (ABGs, CBC, and electrolytes).

  o Monitor the client's cardiac status (rhythm, heart rate, blood pressure).

  o Monitor the client's temperature.

  o Monitor drains, tubes, catheters, and IV access throughout anesthesia and surgery.

  o Assess the client's of level of sedation and anesthesia (level of consciousness, vital signs).

  o Notify the surgeon and anesthesiologist if abnormalities are noted.

Local Anesthesia

- There are three main methods of administration of local anesthesia

  o Topical – Applied directly to the skin or mucous membranes

  o Local infiltration – Injected directly into tissues through which a surgical incision is to be made.

  o Regional nerve block – Injected into or around specific nerves: four types of regional nerve blocks:

    ■ Spinal – Injected into the subarachnoid space cerebral spinal fluid (CSF), provides autonomic, sensory, and motor blockade to the body below the level in innervation that the area of the spine where the injection was made.

- ▪ Epidural – Injected into the epidural space in the thoracic or lumbar areas of the spine, and sensory pathways are blocked, but motor function remains.

- ▪ Bier – IV injection of anesthetic injected into an extremity following mechanical exsanguination with a tourniquet, and provides analgesia and a bloodless surgical site.

- ▪ Peripheral – injection of anesthetic into a specific nerve for analgesic and anesthetic use.

- Examples of local anesthetic agents include procaine (Novocain) and lidocaine (Xylocaine).

- Concurrent administration of a vasoconstrictor, usually epinephrine, is likely with local anesthetic administration to prolong the effects and to decrease the risk of systemic toxicity. This practice is avoided for distal injuries (finger) due to decreased circulation. Prolonged vasoconstriction could lead to tissue necrosis.

- Nursing Interventions

  - o Observe the client for systemic absorption (restlessness, excitement, seizures, tachycardia, tachypnea, hypertension).

  - o Monitor the client's airway and oxygen saturation.

  - o Monitor and report laboratory values as appropriate (ABGs, CBC, and electrolytes).

  - o Monitor the client's cardiac status (rhythm, heart rate, blood pressure).

  - o Monitor drains, tubes, catheters, and IV access throughout anesthesia and surgery

  - o Assess the client's level of sedation and anesthesia (level of consciousness, vital signs).

  - o Notify the surgeon and anesthesiologist if abnormalities are noted.

  - o Assess the client's motor function to ensure paralysis does not ensue (movement returns first, then sense of touch, pain, warmth, and finally, sensation of cold).

Complications

- Potential complications from use of anesthesia that the nurse should monitor for are:

COMPLICATION	SIGNS AND SYMPTOMS
Myocardial depression	Bradycardia, hypotension, cyanosis, edema
Anaphylaxis	Cardiac failure, allergic symptoms, abnormal vital signs
Malignant hyperthermia (with administration of succinylcholine)	Tachycardia, tachypnea, hypercarbia, dysrhythmias
Autonomic nervous system (ANS) system blockade (epidural and spinal)	Hypotension, bradycardia, nausea, vomiting
CSF leakage (spinal and epidural)	Headache

  - o Note: The nurse should notify the surgeon and anesthesiologist if any of the above signs and symptoms are noted.

MODERATE (CONSCIOUS) SEDATION

Overview

- Moderate sedation is the administration of sedatives and/or hypnotics to the point where the client is relaxed enough that minor procedures can be performed without discomfort, yet the client can respond to verbal stimuli, retains protective reflexes (gag reflex), is easily arousable, and, most importantly, independently maintains a patent airway.

- Only a qualified provider can administer moderate sedation. These include anesthesiologists, certified registered nurse anesthetists (CRNAs), attending provider, or RNs under the supervision of one of the previously mentioned providers.

- The nurse must continuously monitor a client who is undergoing moderate sedation. During the procedure, an RN must be present to monitor the client, with no other responsibilities during the procedure. This nurse is to remain with the client at all times before, during, and immediately after the procedure.

- Procedures that may require moderate sedation include, but are not limited to:

    ○ Minor surgical procedures (dental, podiatric, plastic, and ophthalmic procedures).

    ○ Diagnostic procedures (various types of endoscopy, bone marrow aspiration, lumbar puncture).

    ○ Cardioversion.

    ○ Wound care (suturing, dressing changes, incision and drainage of abscesses, burn debridement).

    ○ Reduction and immobilization of fractures.

    ○ Placement and removal of implanted devices, catheters, and tubes.

Risk Factors

    ○ Older adult clients are at a greater risk of adverse reactions to sedation medications.

    ○ Older adult clients have less physiologic reserve than younger clients, so care needs to be adjusted accordingly.

    ○ Nurses should be aware and maintain a safe environment for older adult clients, due to sensory limitations.

    ○ The nurse should pay careful attention to cardiac and respiratory status in the older adult clients, as problems may arise more quickly.

Medications

- Medications used during moderate sedation

  - Opioids – Morphine, fentanyl (Sublimaze), hydromorphone (Dilaudid), and meperidine (Demerol)

  - Anesthetics – Propofol (Diprivan)

  - Benzodiazepines – Midazolam (Versed), diazepam (Valium), lorazepam (Ativan)

- Dosages required for "light sedation" are highly individualized and require careful titration.

- Note: Naloxone hydrochloride (Narcan) or flumazenil (Romazicon) can be given to reverse moderate sedation when needed.

Nursing Interventions

- Preprocedure

  - Obtain a full history from the client, including allergies, medication usage, and pre-existing medical conditions (pulmonary disease). Any previous experiences with sedation or anesthesia should to be reported, especially any adverse reactions. Note the last dose of each medication, especially if it could alter the client's response (diuretic, antihypertensive, narcotic).

  - Provide the client with education about the procedure and the medications to be used.

  - Perform a full assessment on the client, including baseline vital signs, cardiac rhythm, and level of consciousness.

  - Determine the last time the client ate or drank (generally NPO for 4 hr before the procedure).

  - Establish IV access and administer fluids as prescribed.

  - Verify that the client signed the informed consent.

  - Attach monitoring equipment to the client.

  - Remove the client's dentures (in case intubation would become necessary).

- Intraprocedure

  - Remain with the client at all times. Allow other staff to assist the provider with the procedure, if indicated.

  - Continually assess and monitor the client's level of consciousness (Glasgow coma scale score), cardiac rhythm, respiratory status, and vital signs.

  - Ⓖ Maintain a safe environment for the older adult client due to sensory limitations.

  - Pay careful attention to cardiac and respiratory status for older adult clients, as problems can arise more quickly.

- ○ During the procedure, the following equipment must be present within immediate reach for routine monitoring and in case deep sedation with respiratory depression occurs:
    - Fully equipped crash cart that, includes emergency medications, airway and ventilatory equipment, and defibrillator.
    - A 100% oxygen source and administration supplies.
    - Airways and a positive-pressure breathing device.
    - A suction source and supplies.
    - IV supplies.
    - ECG monitor/display.
    - A noninvasive blood pressure monitor.
    - A pulse oximeter.
    - A means to monitor the client's body temperature.
    - A stethoscope.
- Postprocedure
    - ○ After completion of the procedure, the nurse who is monitoring should continue to record vital signs and level of consciousness until the client is fully awake and all assessment criteria return to pre-sedation levels. Only then can the nurse remove the monitor and all emergency equipment from the bedside.
    - ○ Typical discharge criteria
        - Level of consciousness as on admission
        - Vital signs stable for 30 to 90 min
        - Ability to cough and deep breathe
        - Ability to tolerate oral fluids
        - Ability to void
        - Absence of nausea, vomiting, shortness of breath, or dizziness

Complications

- Before, during, and after the procedure, emergency equipment is to remain at the client's bedside. Some complications that can arise from moderate sedation include:
    - ○ Airway obstruction
        - Insert airway and suction.
    - ○ Respiratory depression
        - Administer oxygen and reversal agents, such as naloxone (Narcan) and flumazenil (Romazicon).

- o Cardiac arrhythmias

  - ■ Set up a 12-lead ECG and provide antidysrhythmics and fluids.

- o Hypotension

  - ■ Provide fluids and vasopressors.

- o Anaphylaxis

  - ■ Administer epinephrine.

- Most hospitals and facilities require that for moderate sedation an RN needs certified in advanced cardiac life support (ACLS) or pediatric advanced life support (PALS) in case of an emergency. In all instances of complications, the sedation needs to be stopped and care given to the client to end the problem.

CHAPTER 107: ANESTHESIA AND MODERATE (CONSCIOUS) SEDATION

 Application Exercises

1. A young adult is having knee arthroscopy performed. After administration of midazolam (Versed), the nurse notices the client's blood pressure is 86/40 mm Hg, and his heart rate is 134/min. Which of the following should the nurse anticipate after informing the provider of the client's change in vital signs?

   A. Administer naloxone hydrochloride (Narcan).

   B. Administer morphine sulfate.

   C. Give 500 mL 0.9% sodium chloride via IV bolus.

   D. Stop the procedure.

2. After an anesthesiologist delivers nitrous oxide with a face mask to a client, which of the following is the priority assessment?

   A. Oxygen saturation

   B. Blood pressure

   C. Heart rate

   D. Temperature

3. Which of the following is an adverse side effect of inhalation anesthetics?

   A. Hypertension

   B. Increased intracranial pressure (ICP)

   C. Malignant hyperthermia

   D. Atrial tachycardia

Scenario: An adult female is brought into the emergency department for episodes of paroxysmal supraventricular tachycardia. After performing all other interventions, the provider decides to perform cardioversion and to administer midazolam (Versed) to relax the client for the procedure.

4. What steps need to be completed before the midazolam is given?

5. Which of the following equipment is needed at the client's bedside for the procedure? (Select all that apply.)

_____ Fully equipped crash cart, including emergency and resuscitative medications, airway and ventilatory equipment, and a defibrillator

_____ ECG monitor/display

_____ Noninvasive blood pressure monitor

_____ Pulse oximeter

_____ Means to monitor the client's body temperature

_____ Suture kit and removal tray

_____ Stethoscope

_____ 100% oxygen source and administration supplies

_____ Airways and positive-pressure breathing device

_____ Suction source and supplies

_____ IV supplies

_____ Indwelling urinary catheter

6. An older adult client is undergoing an endoscopy that will require moderate sedation. Which of the following findings in her history indicates the need for further assessment?

A. Allergy to bee stings

B. Gout

C. Gastrointestinal bleed

D. COPD

CHAPTER 107: ANESTHESIA AND MODERATE (CONSCIOUS) SEDATION

 Application Exercises Answer Key

1. A young adult is having knee arthroscopy performed. After administration of midazolam (Versed), the nurse notices the client's blood pressure is 86/40 mm Hg, and his heart rate is 134/min. Which of the following should the nurse anticipate after informing the primary care provider of the client's vital signs?

    A. Administer naloxone hydrochloride (Narcan).

    B. Administer morphine sulfate.

    C. Give 500 mL 0.9% sodium chloride via an IV bolus.

    D. Stop the procedure.

    A fluid bolus is appropriate for raising the client's blood pressure to maintain adequate cardiac output and tissue perfusion. None of the other options are indicated for this client.

 NCLEX® Connection: Reduction of Risk Potential, Potential for Complications from Surgical Procedures and Health Alterations

2. After an anesthesiologist delivers nitrous oxide with a face mask to a client, which of the following is the priority assessment?

    A. Oxygen saturation

    B. Blood pressure

    C. Heart rate

    D. Temperature

    According to the ABC priority-setting framework, assessment of oxygenation is the priority when administering a medication that has CNS and respiratory-depression effects. Blood pressure, heart rate and temperature are important assessments, but not the priority.

 NCLEX® Connection: Reduction of Risk Potential, Potential for Complications from Surgical Procedures and Health Alterations

3. Which of the following is an adverse side effect of inhalation anesthetics?

    A. Hypertension

    B. Increased intracranial pressure (ICP)

    C. Malignant hyperthermia

    D. Atrial tachycardia

    Malignant hyperthermia is a life-threatening risk of inhalation anesthesia. Prompt administration of 100% oxygen, dantrolene (skeletal muscle relaxant), and a cooling blanket is vital for survival. None of the other options is a side effect of inhalation anesthetics.

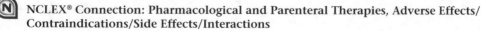 NCLEX® Connection: Pharmacological and Parenteral Therapies, Adverse Effects/ Contraindications/Side Effects/Interactions

Scenario: An adult female is brought into the emergency department for episodes of paroxysmal supraventricular tachycardia. After performing all other interventions, the provider decides to perform cardioversion and to administer midazolam (Versed) to relax the client for the procedure.

4. What steps need to be completed before the midazolam is given?

Obtain the client's full history, including allergies, medication usage, and pre-existing medical conditions (pulmonary disease). Any previous experiences with sedation or anesthesia need to be reported, especially any adverse reactions. Note the last dose of each medication, especially if it could alter the client's response (diuretic, antihypertensive, narcotic).

Provide education about the procedure to the client and the medications to be used. Perform a full assessment, including baseline vital signs, cardiac rhythm, and level of consciousness. Determine the last time the client ate or drank (generally NPO for 4 hr before the procedure). Establish IV access and administer fluids as prescribed. Verify that the client has signed the informed consent and attach monitoring equipment.

(N) NCLEX® Connection: Reduction of Risk Potential, Potential for Complications from Surgical Procedures and Health Alterations

5. Which of the following equipment is needed at the client's bedside for the procedure? (Select all that apply.)

   X   **Fully equipped crash cart, including emergency and resuscitative medications, airway and ventilatory equipment, and a defibrillator**

   X   **ECG monitor/display**

   X   **Noninvasive blood pressure monitor**

   X   **Pulse oximeter**

   X   **Means to monitor the client's body temperature**

         Suture kit and removal tray

   X   **Stethoscope**

   X   **100% oxygen source and administration supplies**

   X   **Airways and positive-pressure breathing device**

   X   **Suction source and supplies**

   X   **IV supplies**

         Indwelling urinary catheter

A suture kit and removal tray are not indicated for cardioversion. Laboratory vials and an indwelling urinary catheter are also not indicated for this procedure.

(N) NCLEX® Connection: Reduction of Risk Potential, Potential for Complications from Surgical Procedures and Health Alterations

6. A 68-year-old client is undergoing an endoscopy, which will require moderate sedation. Which of the following findings in her history indicates the need for further assessment?

    A. Allergic to bee stings

    B. Gout

    C. Gastrointestinal bleed

    D. Chronic obstructive pulmonary disease

    Chronic obstructive pulmonary disease poses a risk for possible airway compromise. Allergic to bee stings does not indicate a need for further assessment. Gout does not indicate a need for further assessment. Gastrointestinal bleed does not indicate a need for further assessment.

    NCLEX® Connection: Pharmacological and Parenteral Therapies, Adverse Effects/Contraindications/Side Effects/Interactions

Overview

- Surgery can take on many forms, including curative, palliative, cosmetic, and functional. Surgical procedures are performed on an inpatient, same-day, or outpatient-admission basis.

- Preoperative care takes place from the time a client is scheduled for surgery until care is transferred to the operating suite. Informed consent is obtained by the provider, and at that time all risks and benefits are explained to a client or surrogate.

- Assessment of risk factors is one of the major aspects of preoperative care. Preoperative care includes a thorough assessment of the client's physical, emotional, and psychosocial status prior to surgery.

Risk Factors

- Surgery

  - Infection (risk of sepsis)

  - Anemia (oxygenation, healing impact)

  - Hypovolemia from dehydration or blood loss (circulatory compromise)

  - Electrolyte imbalance through inadequate diet or disease process (dysrhythmias)

  - Age (older adults are at greater risk)

  - Pregnancy (fetal risk with anesthesia)

  - Respiratory disease (COPD, pneumonia, asthma)

  - Cardiovascular disease (cerebrovascular accident, heart failure, myocardial infarction, hypertension, dysrhythmias)

  - Diabetes mellitus (decreased intestinal motility, altered blood glucose levels, delayed healing)

  - Liver disease (altered medication metabolism)

  - Renal disease (altered elimination)

  - Endocrine disorders (hypo/hyperthyroidism, Addison's disease, Cushing's syndrome)

  - Immune system disorders (allergies, immunocompromise)

  - Coagulation defect (increased risk of bleeding)

- ○ Malnutrition (delayed healing)

- ○ Obesity (impact on anesthesia, elimination, and wound healing)

- ○ Use of some medications (antihypertensives, anticoagulants)

- ○ Substance use (tobacco, alcohol)

- ○ Family history (malignant hyperthermia)

- ○ Allergies (latex, anesthetic agents)

- ○ Older adult clients:

  - ■ Are at a greater risk of adverse reactions to preoperative medications.

  - ■ Have less physiologic reserve than younger clients, so care needs to be adjusted accordingly.

  - ■ May have sensory limitations, so the nurse must be alert to maintaining a safe environment.

  - ■ May have oral alterations (dentures, bridges, loose teeth) that may pose problems during intubation.

  - ■ Perspire less, which leads to dry, itchy skin that becomes fragile and easily abraded. Precautions need to be taken when moving and positioning these clients.

  - ■ Have decreased subcutaneous fat, which makes them more susceptible to temperature changes. They need to be covered with lightweight cotton blankets when they are moving to and from the operating room.

Diagnostic Procedures

- Urinalysis – Ruling out of infection

- Blood type and cross match – Transfusion readiness

- CBC – Infection/immune status

- Hgb and Hct – Fluid status, anemia

- Pregnancy test – Fetal risk of anesthesia

- Clotting studies (PT, INR, aPTT, platelet count)

- Electrolyte levels – Electrolyte imbalances

- Serum creatinine – Renal status

- ABGs – Oxygenation status

- Chest x-ray – Heart and lung status

- 12-lead ECG – Baseline heart rhythm, dysrhythmias

Preoperative Assessment

- Preoperative nursing assessments

    ○ Detailed history (including medical problems, allergies, medication use, substance abuse, psychosocial problems, and cultural considerations)

    ○ Anxiety level regarding the procedure

    ■ Older adult clients may be more fearful due to financial concerns and lack of social support.

    ○ Laboratory results

    ○ Head-to-toe assessment

    ○ Vital signs

Nursing Interventions

- Informed Consent

    ○ Once surgery has been discussed with the client or surrogate as treatment, it is the responsibility of the primary care provider to obtain consent after discussing the risks and benefits of the procedure. The nurse is not to obtain the consent for the provider in any circumstance.

    ○ The nurse can clarify any information that remains unclear after the provider's explanation of the procedure. The nurse may not, however provide any new or additional information not previously given by the provider.

    ○ The nurse's role is to witness the client's signing of the consent form after the client acknowledges understanding of the procedure.

    ○ Older adult clients may need to have surgical consent forms signed by a legal guardian.

RESPONSIBILITIES FOR INFORMED CONSENT		
THE PROVIDER	THE CLIENT	THE NURSE
Obtains informed consent To obtain informed consent, the provider must give the client: • A complete description of the treatment/procedure. • A description of the professionals who will be performing and participating in the treatment. • A description of the potential harm, pain, and/or discomfort that may occur. • Options for other treatments. • The right to refuse treatment.	**Gives informed consent** To give informed consent, the client must: • Give it voluntarily (there must be no coercion involved). • Be competent and of legal age or be an emancipated minor. When the client is unable to provide consent, another authorized person must give consent. • Receive enough information to make a decision based on an understanding of what is expected.	**Witnesses informed consent** To witness informed consent, the nurse must: • Ensure that the provider gave the client the necessary information. • Ensure that the client understood the information and is competent to give informed consent. • Have the client sign the informed consent document. • Notify the provider if the client has more questions or appears to not understand any of the information provided. (The provider is then responsible for giving clarification.) ○ The nurse documents questions the client has and notifies the provider. The nurse also documents any additional reinforcement of teaching. • Record the use of an interpreter in the client's medical record.

- Preoperative Teaching

  ○ Postoperative pain control techniques (medications, immobilization, patient-controlled analgesia pumps, splinting)

  ○ Demonstration and importance of coughing and deep breathing

  ○ Demonstration and importance of range-of-motion exercises and early ambulation for prevention of thrombi and respiratory complications

  ○ Invasive devices (drains, catheters, IV lines)

- ○ Postoperative diet
- ○ Use of the incentive spirometer

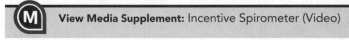

View Media Supplement: Incentive Spirometer (Video)

- ○ Preoperative instructions (avoid cigarette smoking for 24 hr preoperatively, medications to hold, bowel preparation)
  - ■ Clients who are taking acetylsalicylic acid (Aspirin) should be advised to stop taking it for 1 week before an elective surgery to decrease the risk of bleeding.
- ○ Care and restrictions relative to surgical procedure performed
- • Preoperative nursing actions
  - ○ Verify that the informed consent is accurately completed, signed, and witnessed.
  - ○ Administer enemas and/or laxatives either the night before and/or the morning of the surgery for clients undergoing bowel surgery.
  - ○ Regularly check the client's scheduled medication prescriptions. Some medications (antihypertensives, anticoagulants) may be held until after the procedure.
  - ○ Ensure that the client remains NPO for at least 6 to 8 hr before surgery with general anesthesia and 3 to 4 hr with local anesthesia to avoid aspiration. Note on the chart the last time the client ate or drank.
  - ○ Perform skin preparation, which may include cleansing with antimicrobial soap and clipping hair in areas that will be involved in the surgery.
  - ○ Ensure that jewelry, dentures, prosthetics, makeup, nail polish, and glasses are removed. These items can either be given to the family or locked away safely.
  - ○ Establish IV access.
  - ○ Administer preoperative medications (prophylactic antimicrobials, antiemetics, sedatives) as prescribed.
    - ■ Have the client void prior to administration.
    - ■ Monitor the client's response to the medications.
    - ■ Raise side rails following administration to prevent injury.
    - ■ The consent form must be signed before administration of preoperative medications.
  - ○ Ensure that the preoperative checklist is complete.

View Media Supplement: Preoperative Checklist (Image)

- ○ Transfer the client to the preanesthesia care unit.

Complications

- Complications during the postoperative period are usually related to the medications given preoperatively. These medications and their possible complications are as follows:

MEDICATION CLASS	POSSIBLE COMPLICATIONS
Sedatives (benzodiazepines, barbiturates)	Respiratory depression, drowsiness, dizziness
Opioids	Respiratory depression, drowsiness, dizziness, constipation
IV infusions (0.9% NaCl, Lactated Ringer's)	Heart failure, hypernatremia
Gastrointestinal medications (antiemetics, antacids, H_2 receptor blockers)	Alkalosis, cardiac abnormalities (certain H_2 receptor blockers), drowsiness

- For clients encountering severe anxiety and panic, reassurance will be necessary and sedation medications may be given.

- Be alert for any allergic reactions the client has to medications.

CHAPTER 108: PREOPERATIVE NURSING CARE

 Application Exercises

1. Which of the following preoperative client findings should be reported to a client's provider? (Select all that apply.)

_____ Potassium level of 3.9 mEq/L

_____ Sodium level of 145 mEq/L

_____ Creatinine level of 2.8 mg/dL

_____ Prothrombin time of 23 seconds

_____ Glucose level of 235 mg/dL

_____ WBC count of 17,850/mm^3

2. A nurse records a client's vital signs before transferring him to the preanesthesia unit for an exploratory laparotomy. The client's temperature is 39° C (102.2° F) orally. Which of the following actions should the nurse take?

   A. Contact and inform the provider about the temperature.

   B. Transfer the client to the preanesthesia unit and notify the receiving nurse about the temperature.

   C. Administer 650 mg of acetaminophen and recheck the temperature in 1 hr.

   D. Apply a cooling blanket and recheck the client's temperature in 30 min.

3. Which of the following are a nurse's responsibilities regarding informed consent for a procedure? (Select all that apply.)

_____ Ensure that the client signs the consent prior to administration of preoperative medications.

_____ Provide additional literature about the procedure if the client has questions.

_____ Clarify any points given by the provider about the procedure after the provider's explanation.

_____ Document the client signing the consent form in the chart.

_____ Delegate witnessing the client's signature on the consent form to an assigned assistive personnel.

CHAPTER 108: PREOPERATIVE NURSING CARE

 Application Exercises Answer Key

1. Which of the following preoperative client findings should be reported to a client's provider? (Select all that apply.)

_____	Potassium level of 3.9 mEq/L
_____	Sodium level of 145 mEq/L
X	**Creatinine level of 2.8 mg/dL**
X	**Prothrombin time of 23 seconds**
X	**Glucose level of 235 mg/dL**
X	**WBC count of 17,850/mm³**

Potassium and sodium levels are within normal ranges. Creatinine level is elevated, which indicates possible renal dysfunction. PT is prolonged, which poses concern for increased risk of bleeding due to delayed coagulation. The glucose level is high and intervention is needed (administration of insulin). WBC is elevated and possibly indicative of a preexisting infection that needs treatment prior to surgery.

 NCLEX® Connection: Reduction of Risk Potential, Potential for Complications of Diagnostic Tests/Treatments/Procedures

2. A nurse records a client's vital signs before transferring him to the preanesthesia unit for an exploratory laparotomy. The client's temperature is 39° C (102.2° F) orally. Which of the following actions should the nurse take?

A. Contact and inform the provider about the temperature.

B. Transfer the client to the preanesthesia unit and notify the receiving nurse about the temperature.

C. Administer 650 mg of acetaminophen and recheck the temperature in 1 hr.

D. Apply a cooling blanket and recheck the client's temperature in 30 min.

The client may have an infection, increasing the risk for complications following surgery; therefore, the provider should be notified. Additional assessments will likely be prescribed to investigate the possibility of an infectious process that needs to be treated prior to surgery.

 NCLEX® Connection: Reduction of Risk Potential, Potential for Complications of Diagnostic Tests/Treatments/Procedures

3. Which of the following are a nurse's responsibilities regarding informed consent for a procedure? (Select all that apply.)

X **Ensure that the client signs the consent prior to administration of preoperative medications.**

_____ Provide additional literature about the procedure if the client has questions.

X **Clarify any points given by the provider about the procedure after the provider's explanation.**

X **Document the client signing the consent form in the chart.**

_____ Delegate witnessing the client's signature on the consent form to an assigned assistive personnel.

The nurse should ensure that the client signed the consent form without being given any prior sedation. She should also clarify any points that remain unclear about the procedure after the provider's explanation and document the signing of the consent form in the chart. The nurse may not provide additional information regarding the procedure, and the nurse must witness the signing of the consent form. This cannot be delegated.

(N) NCLEX® Connection: Reduction of Risk Potential, Potential for Complications of Diagnostic Tests/Treatments/Procedures

Overview

- Transferring a client who is postoperative from the operating suite to the postanesthesia care unit (PACU) is the responsibility of the anesthesia provider who is either an anesthesiologist or a certified registered nurse anesthetist (CRNA). The circulating nurse will give the report to the PACU nurse.

- Postoperative care is usually provided initially in the PACU, where skilled nurses can closely monitor a client's recovery from anesthesia.

- In some instances a client is transferred from the operating suite directly to the intensive care unit. Initial postoperative care involves making assessments, providing medications, managing the client's pain, preventing complications, and determining when a client is ready to be discharged from the PACU.

- During the immediate postoperative stage, maintaining airway patency and ventilation and monitoring circulatory status are the main priorities for care.

- Postoperative clients who received general anesthesia require frequent assessment of their respiratory status. Postoperative clients who received epidural or spinal anesthesia require ongoing assessment of motor and sensory function.

- When a client is stable and is able to breathe on her own, she is either discharged to a postsurgical unit or to home if it was a same-day surgical procedure. Clients discharged home must also demonstrate that they can take fluids orally and safely ambulate to the bathroom and wheelchair with assistance. All clients who had same-day surgery should be accompanied by a significant other, family member, or other caregiver who can receive the discharge instructions and accompany the client home.

Risk Factors for Postoperative Complications

- Immobility (respiratory compromise, thrombophlebitis, pressure ulcer)

- Anemia (blood loss, oxygenation, and healing factors)

- Hypovolemia (tissue perfusion)

- Respiratory disease (respiratory compromise)

- Immune disorder (risk for infection, delayed healing)

- Diabetes mellitus (gastroparesis, delayed wound healing)

- Coagulation defect (increased risk of bleeding)

- Malnutrition (delayed healing)

- Obesity (wound healing, dehiscence, evisceration)

Ⓖ - Age-related respiratory, cardiovascular, and renal changes necessitate special attention to the postoperative recovery of older adults.

   ○ Older adult clients are more susceptible to cold temperatures, so additional warm blankets in the PACU may be required.

   ○ Responses to medications and anesthetics may delay an older adult client's return of orientation postoperatively.

   ○ Age-related physiologic changes may affect an older adult client's response to and elimination of postoperative medications. Monitor the client closely for appropriate response and possible adverse effects.

       ▪ Older adults perspire less, which leads to dry, itchy skin that becomes fragile and easily abraded. The use of paper tape for wound dressings may be appropriate, as well as lifting precautions.

       ▪ Take care to meet the nutritional needs of older adults to promote effective wound healing.

Diagnostic Procedures

- CBC (infection/immune status)

- Hgb and Hct (fluid status, anemia)

- Electrolyte levels (electrolyte balance)

- Serum creatinine (renal status)

- ABGs (oxygenation status)

- Laboratory tests (glucose) based on procedure and other health problems

PACU Assessments and Nursing Interventions

- Upon receiving a client from the operating suite, the unit nurse should immediately perform a full body assessment with priority given to airway, breathing, and circulation.

- Nursing monitoring and management

   ○ Airway

       ▪ An artificial airway is left in place until a client can maintain his airway on his own.

       ▪ Check the client's blood oxygen saturation levels (keep pulse oximetry on the client).

       ▪ Auscultate the client's lung sounds.

- Administer humidified oxygen to the client.
- Suction accumulated secretions if the client is unable to cough.
○ Circulation
  - Observe the client for bleeding (internally and externally).
  - Assess the client for signs of hypervolemia and hypovolemia.
  - Assess the client's skin color and condition.
  - Check the client's mucous membranes, lips, and nail beds.
  - Check the client's peripheral pulses.
  - Monitor ECG readings.
  - Monitor fluid and electrolyte balance.
○ Vital signs
  - Per agency protocol, obtain the client's until they are stable (every 15 min).
  - Provide heated blankets if the client is hypothermic.
○ Positioning
  - Position the client supine with head flat (prevent hypotension).
  - Put the client on his side if unresponsive or unconscious (risk of aspiration).
  - When the client is fully reactive, raise the head of the bed to facilitate respiratory expansion.
  - Do not elevate the client's legs higher than placement on a pillow if the client has received spinal anesthesia.
○ Response to anesthesia (sedation, nausea and/or vomiting)
  - Monitor the client's level of consciousness.
  - Assess the client for movement of and sensation in extremities.
  - Administer an antiemetic to the client for nausea and vomiting.
○ I&O
  - Check the client's bladder for distention.
  - Check urinary catheters for patency.
  - Observe the color, consistency, odor, and amount the client's of urine.
○ Take note of surgical wound, incision site, and/or dressing.
  - Observe drainage tubes for patency and proper function.
  - Check the client's dressings for excessive drainage.
○ Pain
  - Administer pain medication to the client as appropriate, secondary to recovery status.
  - Observe the client for respiratory depression and decreased oxygen saturation.

- Monitor the client's recovery from anesthesia by using the Aldrete scoring system. Each of the following five factors is given a score based upon the nurse's observations of the client. The five scores are totaled to determine the client's Aldrete Score.

MODIFIED ALDRETE SCORING SYSTEM		
FACTOR	ASSESSMENT/OBSERVATION	SCORE
Activity	Able to move 4 extremities	2
	Able to move 2 extremities	1
	Able to move 0 extremities	0
Consciousness	Fully awake	2
	Arousable	1
	Unarousable	0
Respiration	Breathe deeply and cough	2
	Dyspnea, hypoventilation	1
	Apneic	0
O_2 saturation	O_2 saturation maintained at 92% (at least) on room air	2
	Inhaled oxygen is necessary to maintain 0_2 saturation level at 92% (at least)	1
	O_2 saturation level is below 90% even though inhaled oxygen is being given	0
Circulation	Blood pressure is within 20% of preanesthesia level	2
	Blood pressure is within 20-49% of preanesthesia level	1
	Blood pressure is within 50% of preanesthesia level	0

- Criteria indicating readiness for discharge from the PACU

  o Aldrete Score of 8 to 10

  o Stable vital signs

  o No evidence of bleeding

  o Return of reflexes (gag, cough, swallow)

  o Wound drainage that is minimal to moderate

  o Urine output of at least 30 mL/hr

Unit Assessments and Nursing Interventions

- Upon receiving the client from the PACU, the unit nurse should immediately perform a full body assessment with priority given to airway, breathing, and circulation.

- Nursing monitoring and management

- o Airway
  - Monitor the oxygen saturation of the client's blood using a pulse oximeter.
  - Assist the client with coughing and deep breathing at least every 2 hr, and provide a pillow or folded blanket so that the client can splint as necessary for abdominal incision.
  - Assist the client with the use of an incentive spirometer at least every 2 hr.
  - Reposition the client every 2 hr and ambulate early and regularly.
- o Positioning
  - Do not put pillows under knees or elevate the knee gatch on the bed (decreases venous return).
  - Elevate the client's legs if shock develops.
- o Fluid status and oral comfort
  - Administer IV isotonic infusions (lactated Ringer's solution, 5% dextrose in lactated Ringer's solution) and maintain a patent IV line.
  - Encourage ice chips and fluids as prescribed/tolerated.
  - Provide frequent oral hygiene.
- o Pain
  - If prescribed, provide continuous pain relief through the use of a patient-controlled analgesia (PCA) pump. Epidural and intrathecal infusions are also available.
  - Assess the client's pain level frequently, using a standardized pain scale.
  - Encourage the client to ask for pain medication before the pain gets severe.
  - Assess the client for signs of pain, such as an increased pulse, respirations, or blood pressure; restlessness; and wincing or moaning during movement.
  - Monitor the client for side effects of opioids, such as nausea (encourage the client to change positions slowly), urinary retention, and constipation.
  - Provide analgesia 30 min before ambulation or other painful procedures.
- o Renal function (output should equal intake)
  - Monitor and report urinary outputs of less than 30 mL/hr.
  - Palpate the client's bladder following voiding to assess for bladder distention.
  - Consider using a bladder scan to assess suspected retention in regard to amount.
- o Bowel function
  - Maintain the client on NPO until return of the gag reflex (risk of aspiration) and peristalsis (risk of paralytic ileus).
  - Irrigate nasogastric (NG) suction tubes with saline as needed to maintain patency. Do not move the NG tubes in clients who are postoperative gastric surgery as ordered by the surgeon (risk to incision).

- Monitor the client's bowel sounds in all four quadrants as well as his ability to pass flatus.

- Advance the client's diet as prescribed and tolerated (clear liquids to regular).

● Prevent and monitor for thromboembolism (especially following abdominal and pelvic surgeries).

  ○ Apply pneumatic compression stockings and/or elastic stockings.

  ○ Reposition the client every 2 hr and ambulate early and regularly.

  ○ Administer low-level anticoagulants as prescribed.

  ○ Monitor the client's extremities for calf pain, warmth, erythema, and edema.

● Monitor the client's incisions and drain sites for bleeding and/or infection.

  ○ Monitor drainage from incisions/drain sites (should progress from sanguineous to serosanguineous to serous).

  ○ Monitor the incision site (expected findings include pink wound edges, slight swelling under sutures/staples, slight crusting of drainage). Report any signs of infection, including redness, excessive tenderness, and purulent drainage.

  ○ Monitor the client's wound drains (with each vital sign assessment). Empty as often as needed to maintain compression. Report increases in drainage (possible hemorrhage).

  View Media Supplement:
  - Penrose Drain (Image)
  - Hemovac Drain (Image)
  - Jackson-Pratt Drain (Image)

  ○ In most instances, the surgeon will change the dressing the first time. Subsequent dressing changes may be performed by the nurse using surgical aseptic technique.

  ○ Use an abdominal binder for clients who are obese or debilitated.

  ○ Encourage splinting with position changes.

  ○ Administer prophylactic antibiotics as prescribed.

  ○ Remove sutures or staples in 6 to 8 days as prescribed.

● Promote wound healing.

  ○ Encourage the client to consume a diet that is high in calories, protein, and vitamin C.

  ○ If the client has diabetes mellitus, maintain good glycemic control.

● Provide discharge teaching.

  ○ Medications (purpose, administration guidelines, adverse effects)

  ○ Activity restrictions (driving, stairs, limits on weight lifting, sexual activity)

  ○ Dietary guidelines, if applicable

  ○ Special treatment instructions (wound care, catheter care, use of assistive devices)

  ○ Emergency contact information and signs to report

Complications

- Airway obstruction

  - Nursing Actions

    - Monitor the client for choking, noisy, irregular respirations, decreased oxygen saturation values, and cyanosis, and intervene accordingly.

    - Keep emergency equipment at the bedside in the PACU.

- Hypoxia

  - Hypoxia is evidenced by a decrease in oxygen saturation.

  - Nursing Actions

    - Monitor the client's oxygenation status and administer oxygen as prescribed.

    - Encourage the client to cough and deep breathe.

    - Position the client to facilitate respiratory expansion.

- Hypovolemic shock

  - Postoperative shock can result from a massive loss of circulating blood volume.

  - Nursing Actions

    - Monitor the client for decreased blood pressure and urinary output, increased heart rate, and slow capillary refill.

    - Administer fluids and vasopressors as indicated.

- Paralytic ileus

  - A paralytic ileus can occur due to the absence of gastrointestinal peristaltic activity.

  - Nursing Actions

    - Monitor bowel sounds, encourage ambulation, advance the diet as tolerated, and administer prokinetic agents, such as metoclopramide (Reglan), as prescribed.

- Wound dehiscence or evisceration

  - Nursing Actions

    - Monitor risk factors (obesity, coughing, moving without splinting, diabetes mellitus).

    - If wound dehiscence or evisceration occurs, call for help, stay with the client, cover the wound with a sterile towel or dressing that is moistened with sterile saline, do not attempt to reinsert organs, monitor the client for shock, and notify the provider immediately.

View Media Supplement: Wound Evisceration (Video)

CHAPTER 109: POSTOPERATIVE NURSING CARE

Ⓐ Application Exercises

1. A nurse is determining if a client is ready to be discharged from the postanesthesia care unit to the postsurgical unit. Using the modified Aldrete scoring system, what is the score for a client who

> Is able to move her arms.
>
> Can cough and deep breathe.
>
> Has a blood pressure that is 35% of preanesthesia level.
>
> Responds when her name is called.
>
> Has an O_2 saturation of 92% without supplemental oxygen.

2. A nurse is caring for a client who had a hysterectomy and resumed a regular diet earlier in the day. The client is now reporting nausea and has vomited once. Which of the following actions should the nurse take first?

> A. Assess for bowel sounds.
>
> B. Administer an antiemetic.
>
> C. Check the client's pain level.
>
> D. Place the client on NPO status.

3. Identify the possible cause for each of the following postoperative client findings and list interventions for each.

POSTOPERATIVE CLIENT FINDING	CAUSE	INTERVENTION
Stridor and snoring (PACU)		
Jackson-Pratt drainage: two times output in previous hour		
Blood pressure 25% below preoperative blood pressure		
Ten minutes after use of patient controlled analgesia, client has pain rating of 8 on a scale from 0-10		
Erythematous swollen warm area on left calf; calf pain on dorsiflexion		
Urinary output for past 4 hr is 100 mL		
Sleeping, responds to command (PACU)		
pH 7.30, PaCO$_2$ 50 mm Hg		
Bowel sounds faint 24 hr after abdominal surgery		
Serosanguineous drainage beyond postoperative day 5		
WBC count of 9,800 mm^3 on postoperative day 1		
Wound edges: pink with slight swelling under sutures, scant amount of crusted serosanguineous drainage on postoperative day 2		
Hgb level of 8.2 g/dL on postoperative day 2 following hip arthroplasty surgery		
Scant amounts of blood in nasogastric contents in the first 24 hr postoperative gastric or bowel surgery		

CHAPTER 109: POSTOPERATIVE NURSING CARE

 Application Exercises Answer Key

1. A nurse is determining if a client is ready to be discharged from the postanesthesia care unit to the postsurgical unit. Using the modified Aldrete scoring system, what is the score for a client who

> Is able to move her arms. (**1**)
>
> Can cough and deep breathe. (**2**)
>
> Has a blood pressure that is 35% of preanesthesia level. (**1**)
>
> Responds when her name is called. (**2**)
>
> Has an O$_2$ saturation of 92% without supplemental oxygen. (**2**)
>
> **Total score equals 8**

 NCLEX® Connection: Reduction of Risk Potential, Therapeutic Procedures

2. A nurse is caring for a client who had a hysterectomy and resumed a regular diet earlier in the day. The client is now reporting nausea and has vomited once. Which of the following actions should the nurse take first?

> **A. Assess for bowel sounds.**
>
> B. Administer an antiemetic.
>
> C. Check the client's pain level.
>
> D. Place the client on NPO status.
>
> **Using the priority framework "assessment first," the first action the nurse should take is to assess the client's gastrointestinal system by listening for bowel sounds. Administering an antiemetic, checking the client's pain level, and placing the client on NPO status are all important, but not the first action the nurse should take.**

 NCLEX® Connection: Reduction of Risk Potential, Potential for Complications of Diagnostic Tests/Treatments/Procedures

3. Identify the possible cause for each of the following postoperative client findings and list interventions for each.

POSTOPERATIVE CLIENT FINDING	CAUSE	INTERVENTION
Stridor and snoring (PACU)	Possible tracheal/laryngeal spasm or blockage (mucus, edema, tongue)	Have emergency equipment on standby and restore airway (reposition, intubation).
Jackson-Pratt drainage: two times output in previous hour	Possible hemorrhage	Assess surgical site and vital signs, stat CBC, and notify the surgeon.
Blood pressure 25% below preoperative blood pressure	Cardiac depression, fluid-volume deficit, shock, hemorrhage, or medication effects	Monitor the client's blood pressure closely, provide fluids and/or vasopressors.
Ten minutes after use of patient controlled analgesia, client has pain rating of 8 on a scale from 0-10	Inadequate pain management protocol	Advocate for additional pain interventions and employ nonpharmacological comfort measures.
Erythematous swollen warm area on left calf; calf pain on dorsiflexion	Thrombophlebitis/deep vein thrombosis	Report findings to the provider promptly and maintain bed rest until thrombosis is ruled out or client is anticoagulated.
Urinary output for past 4 hr is 100 mL	Renal insufficiency	Promptly report hourly outputs of less than 30 mL/hr.
Sleeping, responds to command (PACU)	Expected finding following general anesthesia	Continue to routinely assess/monitor the client.
pH 7.30, $PaCO_2$ 50 mm Hg	Hypoventilation/respiratory acidosis	Encourage deep breathing to help mobilize secretions (suction).
Bowel sounds faint 24 hr after abdominal surgery	Expected findings due to effects of general anesthesia	Encourage ambulation and administer prokinetic agents as prescribed.
Serosanguineous drainage beyond postoperative day 5	Possible indication of ineffective healing and risk for wound dehiscence/evisceration	Report findings, encourage the client to avoid forceful coughing and straining, and to splint the incision with movement.
WBC count of 9,800 mm³ on postoperative day 1	No evidence of infection	Continue infection risk reduction interventions.

POSTOPERATIVE CLIENT FINDING	CAUSE	INTERVENTION
Wound edges: pink with slight swelling under sutures, scant amount of crusted serosanguineous drainage on postoperative day 2	**Expected findings of effective wound healing**	**Continue to monitor wound healing and to change dressings using proper technique.**
Hgb level of 8.2 g/dL on postoperative day 2 following hip arthroplasty surgery	**Surgical blood loss**	**Administer blood replacement products as prescribed, encourage energy conservation measures, administer erythropoietin and/or iron supplements as prescribed, administer oxygen as prescribed.**
Scant amounts of blood in nasogastric contents in the first 24 hr postoperative gastric or bowel surgery	**Expected finding**	**Report increases or bright red blood and do not reposition nasogastric tube due to risk of disrupting sutures.**

(N) NCLEX® Connection: Reduction of Risk Potential, Potential for Complications of Diagnostic Tests/Treatments/Procedures

References

Berman, A., Snyder, S. J., Kozier, B., & Erb, G. (2008). *Fundamentals of nursing: Concepts, process, and practice* (8th ed.). Upper Saddle River, NJ: Pearson Prentice Hall.

Dudek, S. G. (2010). *Nutrition essentials for nursing practice* (6th ed.). Philadelphia, PA: Lippincott Williams & Wilkins.

Ebersole, P., Hess, P., Touhy, T. A., Schmidt Logan, A., & Jett, K. (2008) *Toward healthy aging: Human needs and nursing response* (7th ed.). St. Louis, MO: Mosby.

Eliopoulos, C. (2009). *Gerontological nursing.* (7th ed.). Philadelphia, PA: Lippincott Williams & Wilkins.

Grodner, M., Long, S., & Walkingshaw, B. C. (2007). *Foundations and clinical applications of nutrition: A nursing approach* (4th ed.). St. Louis, MO: Mosby.

Ignatavicius, D. D., & Workman, M. L. (2010). *Medical-surgical nursing* (6th ed.). St. Louis, MO: Saunders.

Lowdermilk, D. L., & Perry, S. E. (2007). *Maternity & women's health care* (9th ed.). St. Louis, MO: Mosby.

Lehne, R. A. (2010). *Pharmacology for nursing care* (7th ed.). St. Louis, MO: Saunders.

LeMone, P., Burke, K., & Mohn-Brown, L. (2007). *Medical-surgical nursing care.* Upper Saddle River, NJ: Prentice-Hall.

Lilley, L. L., Harrington, S., & Snyder, J. S. (2007). *Pharmacology and the nursing process* (5th Ed.). St. Louis, MO: Mosby.

Potter, P. A., & Perry, A. G. (2009). *Fundamentals of nursing* (7th ed.). St. Louis, MO: Mosby.

Roach, S. S., & Ford, S. M. (2008). *Introductory clinical pharmacology.* Philadelphia, PA: Lippincott Williams & Wilkins.

Smeltzer, S. C., Bare, B. G., Hinkle, J. L., & Cheever, K. H. (2008). *Brunner and Suddarth's textbook of medical-surgical nursing* (11th ed.). Philadelphia, PA: Lippincott Williams & Wilkins.

Wilson, B. A., Shannon, M. T., & Shields, K. M. (2010). *Pearson nurse's drug guide 2010.* Upper Saddle River, NJ: Prentice-Hall.

Varcarolis, E. M., Carson, V. B., & Shoemaker, N. C. (2006). *Foundations of psychiatric mental health nursing: A clinical approach* (5th ed.). St. Louis, MO: Saunders.